INTEGRATIVE MEDICINE

THE PATIENT'S ESSENTIAL GUIDE TO CONVENTIONAL AND COMPLEMENTARY TREATMENTS FOR MORE THAN 300 COMMON DISORDERS

Co-Editors

Alan H. Pressman,
D.C., Ph.D., D.A.C.B.N., C.C.N.

Dr. Pressman's expertise on a wide range of topical health issues is heard by millions on his nationally syndicated radio show, "Healthline." He is currently the director of Gramercy Health Associates in New York City. A chiropractor and a board-certified dietitian/nutritionist, Dr. Pressman is the former chairman of the Department of Clinical Nutrition at New York Chiropractic College and served numerous terms as president for the Council on Nutrition of the American Chiropractic Association. He is also a diplomate and past president of the American Chiropractic Board of Nutrition and a fellow of the International & American Association of Clinical Nutritionists.

Donna Shelley, M.D., M.P.H.

Dr. Shelley is a board-certified physician in internal medicine. She was a founding member of the American College of Women's Health Physicians and of Mount Sinai Hospital's Women's Health Program in New York City. She also served as senior medical editor at Lifetime Medical Television. Currently, she is a director with the Division of Health Promotion and Disease Prevention, New York City Department of Health. Dr. Shelley is an active member of the American Women's Medical Association.

Contributing Writers

Carol G. Carlson

Carol Munson

Lauren David Peden

Stephanie Pedersen

Rebecca Valentine

Complementary Medicine Advisors

Dwight C. Byers
President, The International Institute of Reflexology
St. Petersburg, FL

Kara M. Dinda, M.S.
Education Director, American Botanical Council
Austin, TX

Mark Groven, ND
Bastyr University National Health Clinic
Seattle, WA

Cheryl Hoard
President, National Association for Holistic
    Aromatherapy
St. Louis, MO

Jeff Jenssen, D.C.
Advanced Chiropractic Center of Woodbridge, NJ
Clinton Chiropractic Center of Manhattan

Dr. Vasant D. Lad, B.A.M.S., M.A.Sc.
The Ayurvedic Institute
Albuquerque, NM

Kirin Mishra
Center Yoga, Lambertville, NJ
River Yoga, New Hope, PA

Barbara Mitchell, J.D., L.Ac.
Executive Director, National Acupuncture and Oriental
    Medicine Alliance
Olalla, WA

David Molony, Lisc. Ac., Dipl Ac. and C.H. (NCCAOM)
Executive Director, American Association of Oriental
    Medicine
Catasauqua, PA

Dinnie Pearson, BFA, CST, CIMI, CPMT
Integrational Bodywork
Philadelphia, PA

Patricia Rockwood
American Yoga Association
Sarasota, FL

Gretchen L. Schaff, PT
American Commission for Accreditation of Reflexology
    Education and Training (ACARET)
Private Practice, Elkins Park, PA

Patricia Warne
Desert Institute of the Healing Arts, Tucson, AZ
Connecting Point School of Massage and Spa
    Therapies, Telluride, CO

Julian Winston
Director Emeritus, National Center for Homeopathy
Editor, *Homeopathy Today* and *Homeopathy*
    New Zealand
Co-Director, Wellington College of Homeopathy
    (New Zealand)

INTEGRATIVE MEDICINE

THE PATIENT'S ESSENTIAL GUIDE TO CONVENTIONAL AND COMPLEMENTARY TREATMENTS FOR MORE THAN 300 COMMON DISORDERS

Co-Editors

Alan H. Pressman, D.C., Ph.D., D.A.C.B.N., C.C.N.

Donna Shelley, M.D., M.P.H.

Produced by The Philip Lief Group, Inc.

St. Martin's Press

New York

A NOTE TO READERS

This book is for informational purposes only. Readers are advised to consult a trained medical professional before acting on any of the information in this book. The fact that a particular therapy, treatment, herb, or supplement is discussed in the book in connection with an illness or condition does not mean that the author or publisher recommend its use for that particular condition. Similarly, the fact that an organization, telephone number, or Web site is listed in the book as a potential source of information does not mean that the author or publisher endorses any of the information they may provide or recommendations they may make.

Produced by The Philip Lief Group, Inc.

Book designed and illustrated by Max Crandall

Manufactured in the United States of America

Library of Congress Cataloging-in-Publication

ISBN 0-312-25379-6

First Edition: September 2000

10 9 8 7 6 5 4 3 2 1

CONTENTS

Contents

Contents

Contents

Contents

Contents

ACKNOWLEDGMENTS

To my son, Corey, and my daughter, Meghan, because they are my life.

—ALAN H. PRESSMAN

*Special thanks to my husband for his unwavering patience and support.
I gratefully acknowledge the encouragement, assistance, and steadfast support
of American Medical Women's Association staff Kelli Mills and Beth Feldpush
and Executive Director Eileen McGrath.*

—DONNA SHELLEY

FOREWORD

How many times have you left your doctor's office feeling confused, frustrated, or angry? While driving home, have you ever thought, "I should have asked more questions," or "I forgot to mention those symptoms," or "I don't feel comfortable with this treatment"? The unfortunate truth is that these days, conventional medicine can leave you feeling more like a number than a person.

As a result of the sweeping organizational changes that have transformed health care in recent years, many patients feel as though they have fewer choices and less power. Some feel frustrated that their insurance plans limit their treatment options; others are disillusioned by limited access to physicians and by cookie-cutter treatments that don't meet their individual needs. Yet, many of us—conditioned from childhood to see our doctors as authority figures—are hesitant to question our doctors' instructions, even if we aren't entirely comfortable with what we've been told.

These frustrations have helped fuel a renewed interest in complementary and alternative medicine (often abbreviated as CAM). Complementary therapies are those used *in addition to* conventional approaches, while alternative therapies are those used *in place of* conventional approaches. Many of the so-called "nontraditional" therapies

are actually centuries old but are now viewed as "new again." In an effort to learn more about these practices, information-hungry Americans are buying books, surfing the Net, watching the evening news, and subscribing to "natural" health newsletters and magazines. As a group, we are now spending a staggering $27 billion a year on treatments and books that fall under the CAM heading, and visits to nontraditional healers have jumped 50 percent in the last decade alone.

What's feeding this frenzy? To explain the snowballing appeal of complementary and alternative medicine, consider the following:

- CAM therapies are often as effective or more effective and less costly than conventional medical treatments.

- CAM practitioners generally begin with the gentlest treatments and monitor the results, moving to more aggressive therapies only if needed.

- CAM interventions are grounded in a total patient "mind-body-spirit" approach that focuses on the body's innate ability to heal itself and defend itself against disease.

- CAM practitioners recommend boosting the body's self-healing potential by making a commitment to a healthier lifestyle—often incorporating better nutrition, exercise, and stress reduction techniques—"natural" interventions that are associated with a host of health benefits and few, if any, adverse side effects.

Yet, despite the growing fervor for prevention and wellness strategies in our quest for optimal health, few of us are comfortable with the idea of abandoning conventional medicine, with its sophisticated technology and superb knowledge of human physiology. Most Americans grew up within the Western medicine model and recognize that conventional medicine is unequalled when it comes to acute care and emergency treatment. But wouldn't it be ideal if there were some way to combine the two—to take all that conventional medicine can offer and marry it with CAM's "best practice" therapies that emphasize prevention and are especially effective in treating long-term, chronic disorders?

That approach—increasingly referred to as *integrative medicine*—is what this book is about. Integrative medicine seeks to rationally and judiciously combine the best of what each approach can offer to arrive at a new kind of medicine: one that treats the whole individual rather than the disorder, one that is tailored to meet the particular needs of each patient, and one that encourages patients to become informed, active members of their health care team.

How to Use This Book

This book is organized in an easy-to-use A-to-Z format. Entries for medical disorders (such as arthritis) and common symptoms (such as fever) are listed alphabetically. Use the alphabet tabs, printed along the edge of each page, to help you locate the information you need.

Each entry includes the following data:

- **Signs and Symptoms.** A bulleted reference list outlines the most common signs and symptoms of the disorder.

- **Description.** This section provides a detailed overview of the condition, its most common known causes, who is most likely to be affected, and factors that place individuals at increased risk.

- **Conventional Medical Treatment.** The most common conventional approaches are described here, including an explanation of how the condition is diagnosed, prescription medications and procedures used in treatment, possible dangers of delayed treatment, and organizations you can contact for additional information and support.

- **Health Notes.** These lists feature bite-sized facts to help you understand the condition, along with prevention and wellness strategies.

- **Management Notes.** Sprinkled throughout the text are shaded boxes containing useful information about how to manage a particular disorder. For example, in the "Diabetes" entry, you will read about innovative computer programs designed to monitor important aspects of the disease, including blood sugar levels, weight, and blood pressure.

- **Complementary and Alternative Treatments.** This section covers a selection of CAM treatments that may be helpful in treating or managing the disorder. For easy reference, each modality is identified by its own icon (for example, Ayurvedic medicine is represented by a lotus blossom). If you are especially interested in a particular therapy, you can scan the entry to locate its icon. Each of the modalities covered in this section is discussed in more detail in the "Introduction to Complementary Therapies," beginning on page 1. The modalities include:

▲ *Nutrition and Supplementation* (the therapeutic use of proper diet, boosted with vitamin, mineral, and other supplements—often considered a natural "bridge" between conventional medicine and CAM treatments)

▲ *Aromatherapy* (the use of aromatic oils to facilitate and support the body's innate healing process)

▲ *Ayurvedic Medicine* (an ancient Indian healing system incorporating many aspects of an individual's life in the diagnosis and treatment of disease)

▲ *Bodywork and Somatic Practice* (a multitude of techniques ranging from massage to posture correction to energy rebalancing)

▲ *Chiropractic* (adjustment of the spinal column to facilitate proper functioning of the musculoskeletal system)

▲ *Herbal Therapy* (the use of plant-based remedies in many forms, including teas, capsules, tinctures, and ointments)

▲ *Homeopathy* (the treatment of a condition with a substance that produces the condition's symptoms, thereby stimulating the body's immune response)

▲ *Hydrotherapy* (the use of water—including whirlpool baths, ice packs, saunas, compresses, and mineral drinking waters—to treat various disorders)

▲ *Traditional Chinese Medicine* (an ancient medical system focusing on energy balancing and disease prevention and including the modalities of acupuncture, acupressure, and Chinese herbal therapy)

▲ *Yoga and Meditation* (disciplines that use stretching sequences, breathing techniques, and mental exercises to reduce stress and promote wellness).

• **For More Information.** At the end of each entry, you'll find a list of nationally recognized resources that specialize in the condition. These organizations can provide in-depth information about the disorder and frequently can offer much-needed support to patients and those who care for them. Addresses, telephone numbers, and Web addresses are included.

Symptom Boxes, inserted alphabetically throughout the book, describe a host of symptoms (such as "Coughing," "Fever," and "Shortness of Breath") common to a number of disorders. You will find information about causes, diseases that are associated with these symptoms, and conventional and complementary strategies for symptom management.

At the back of the book, a **Resources** section lists a number of Web sites you may want to consult for updated health and medical information. You will also find reference lists of the essential oils used in aromatherapy, common medicinal herbs and their Latin names, and herbal remedies used in traditional Chinese medicine. Illustrations show the body's acupoints and energy meridians and several common yoga poses. You will also find reflexology diagrams of the feet and hands.

Good health and the pursuit of wellness is a lifelong endeavor. We hope that this book will become an important tool in your quest for optimal health. Whether you use it to gain a better understanding of your condition, to learn more about conventional medicine's diagnostic and treatment methods, or to begin exploring the many complementary and alternative approaches available, you have taken a vital first step in becoming an active participant in your health care decisions.

A Brief Introduction to Complementary Therapies

Complementary therapies are derived from the theory that the body has an innate ability to heal itself, that each person has a powerful internal life-force that strives for health, balance, and vitality.

What Are Complementary Therapies?

Complementary therapies are referred to by many names—including alternative therapies, natural medicine, natural healing sciences, nature-oriented therapies, healing arts, and healing traditions. Sometimes these therapies are referred to collectively as *holistic medicine*. The word *holistic* refers to the concept of thinking of a person's body, mind, and spirit as integrated parts of one whole system dedicated to achieving and maintaining health and wellness.

The terminology of complementary medicine can sometimes be confusing. The public, the medical community, and complementary practitioners themselves use a number of terms interchangeably. As complementary medicine becomes more mainstream, the distinctions are becoming clearer. The word *alternative* refers to an approach used in place of traditional medicine. The term *complementary* implies that a therapy can be used in conjunction with conventional medicine. When complementary and/or alternative therapies are used together with conventional medicine in a fully coordinated approach to patient care, we speak of *integrative medicine*. This enlightened approach to diagnosis and treatment brings together the best of both traditions and has the further advantage of putting increased emphasis on disease prevention and general wellness. Each individual type of therapy within complementary/alternative medicine (often abbreviated as CAM) is called a *modality*. Modalities include, for example, chiropractic, herbal therapy, Ayurvedic medicine, and aromatherapy.

As a group, the complementary therapies are based on the notion that the body has an innate ability to heal itself, that each person has a powerful internal life-force that strives for health, balance, and vitality. On the other hand, conventional medicine—also called traditional or *allopathic* medicine—is based on the idea that the body requires outside intervention, such as pharmaceutical drugs or surgery, to heal.

All of the healing arts sciences share similar principles and common ground in their approach to health and well-being. The tools of these therapies are the gifts of nature and take the form of wholesome foods, nourishing herbs, botanical medicines, water, the healing power of touch, and the gentle, manipulative skill of the hands. The job of CAM practitioners is to facilitate and enhance the body's ability to heal, essentially activating the "flow" of the patient's own vital life-force. They believe that their role as health educators is an essential component of their work, and they strive to share information and explain core ideas, concepts, and techniques to patients to help them take an active role in maintaining their own health. (In fact, the Greek root of the word *physician* means "teacher.")

Complementary therapies focus on preventing illness, while traditional medicine concentrates on curing it.

Complementary therapies focus strongly on preventing illness, while traditional medicine mainly concentrates on curing it. Complementary practitioners counsel patients on how to modify their lifestyles in order to achieve, maintain, and enhance well-being over the course of a lifetime. Therapies may focus, for example, on healthy diet and the use of nutritional supplements; regular, moderate exercise; and the elimination of harmful habits or behaviors.

Complementary therapies are considered less intrusive than conventional medicine. The complementary approach is person-centered, while conventional medicine tends to be technology-based. In establishing the practitioner-patient relationship, the CAM practitioner begins by developing a supportive, caring relationship with the patient, which in itself has great healing power. This relates directly to the idea of holistic healing.

When diagnosing a condition, the practitioner takes into account every aspect of the person's life. Dietary and exercise habits, emotions, temperament, stress level, work life, recent life changes, interpersonal relationships, physical living environment, relationship with nature, and seasonal rhythms are just some of the areas considered.

Often several treatment options are recommended in a treatment plan that is highly individualized to the needs of the person. Practitioners take a "wait and watch" approach with each therapy, expecting that patients will heal at their own, individual rate. If a patient's condition does not improve within a reasonable time frame, the practitioner may advise moving on to another type of treatment or another modality.

How Do Complementary Therapies Work?

One of the principal goals of complementary therapies is to rid the body of accumulated wastes and toxins. Detoxification and cleansing are central to these healing programs. CAM practitioners believe that toxins block the flow of vital energy (known as *prana* in Ayurvedic medicine and *chi* in Traditional Chinese Medicine). Free flow of this energy throughout the body is integral to maintaining good health.

Another goal of many therapies is to correct imbalances within the body that lead to or aggravate pain, discomfort, illness, and disease. Imbalances leave our finely-tuned system unable to function efficiently. Complementary practitioners believe that imbalances trigger many dysfunctions—including poor nutrient absorption and blockage of neurological and circulatory pathways. This eventually reduces the flow of vital energy and leaves people vulnerable to illness and disease. Good health is viewed, then, as more than just the lack of illness. It represents the maintenance of proper balance and flow.

Ancient Healing Traditions

What is now known as complementary medicine actually has its roots in ancient civilizations. Through a process of trial and error, early people came to realize that certain plants had the power to cure. Our ancient ancestors also discovered that pressure on particular points on the body could stimulate healing in other parts of the body. From these notions, across the world and throughout the early eras of civilization, different traditions developed into highly-refined medical sciences. For example, Ayurveda—also known as "the science of life"—has been practiced for more than 5000 years. Traditional Chinese Medicine dates back 3000 years to the time when *The Yellow Emperor's Classic of Internal Medicine* was written.

Early settlers to the United States brought with them European herbal healing traditions, then blended them with the healing knowledge of the Native Americans. These traditions are still alive today throughout the American Southwest, where the custom of visiting *curanderas* (traditional healers) is common practice. In more modern times, new therapies have evolved and have taken their place alongside the traditional healing practices. These include chiropractic, reflexology, aromatherapy, and new forms of bodywork involving the physical manipulation of the body to relieve pain and stimulate healing.

As many of these modalities are becoming better known and more widely available, millions of Americans are seeking the advice of alternative and complementary health care practitioners. In 1993 Harvard University researcher Dr. David Eisenberg reported in the *New England Journal of Medicine* the results of a 1990 survey that showed one in three Americans was using at least one form of unconventional therapy. Dr. Eisenberg continued to track this trend, and in 1998 reported in the *Journal of the American Medical Association* that the figure had risen to 42 percent—a 25 percent increase. People in the United States are spending a whopping $27 billion a year on CAM treatments and advice—including vitamins, herbs, and books—largely out of their own pockets.

The surest sign that complementary and alternative therapies are becoming more mainstream is the growing trend for hospitals and medical centers to establish entire departments focusing on complementary care and for health insurers to reimburse for various complementary treatments. Acupuncture treatment is widely covered by health insurers, as is chiropractic, especially for treating back pain.

Given these trends, the medical and scientific community have started to take notice. In 1992 the U.S. Congress established the Office of Alternative Medicine (OAM) within the National Institutes of Health (NIH) and funded

Complementary practitioners believe that imbalances trigger many dysfunctions that eventually reduce the flow of vital energy and leave people vulnerable to illness and disease.

with a $2 million annual budget. In 1998 the office was renamed the National Center for Complementary and Alternative Medicine (NCCAM) and given $50 million in annual funding to sponsor research in complementary and alternative therapies through ten specialty centers. Early research focused on the efficacy of acupuncture treatments for various disorders. A joint study by the Agency for Health Care Policy and Research and the U.S. Department of Health and Human Services determined that chiropractic spinal manipulations can successfully address acute lower back pain in adults and should be tried prior to ordering CAT scans, magnetic resonance imaging (MRI), or surgery.

In the meantime, medical schools and mainstream healthcare organizations have started to incorporate CAM into their programs and services. Today more than half of the medical schools in the United States offer electives in nontraditional therapies. What's more, the American Medical Association (AMA) and its affiliate state and local medical societies are encouraging their members to familiarize themselves with conventional and alternative modalities in order to discuss these options with their patients.

Today more than half of the medical schools in the United States offer electives in nontraditional therapies.

Complementary Therapies Are "New" Again

There are several reasons why more and more Americans are gravitating toward complementary therapies. While most people readily admit that conventional medicine has no peer when it comes to emergency intervention and acute care, many patients are less satisfied with conventional medical approaches to the treatment of long-term or chronic illness. Conventional medicine attacks disease with costly synthetic treatments that may or may not relieve the symptom, but often come with unpleasant and unwanted side effects.

Today, more and more people are putting increased emphasis on disease prevention and wellness and are searching for treatments that are gentle on the body, support the mind and sensibilities, and nurture the spirit. Natural therapies are designed to promote optimal health, to strengthen the body so it can defend itself from disease. Patients who use natural remedies like the fact that such therapies are virtually free of side effects. A complementary practitioner always chooses the least intrusive therapy first, moving to stronger therapies only as needed. In addition, studies have found many natural therapies to be as or more effective, less dangerous, and more economical than conventional medical treatments.

Then, too, growing numbers of people have become alienated from the services that conventional medicine can offer in the managed healthcare environment. Many would characterize the current system as impersonal, intrusive, and unsettling. Generally, patients take between one and three minutes to give the doctor a complete explanation of their symptoms. Yet a recent report reveals that, on average, patients are interrupted by their physician 18 seconds into this description. The once-supportive family doctor has been replaced by a complex, high-tech, high-pressure medical system composed of many players. Some people never see the same doctor twice if their "primary care physician" is part of a group practice or health maintenance organization (HMO).

The media has jumped into the picture as well, as the public is fed daily stories about deaths from prescription drug interactions, malpractice lawsuits from surgeries, or hospital care gone awry. People are confused, frightened, and frustrated—and they're looking elsewhere for treatment.

Finding a Good Practitioner

You expect your conventional physician to have a license, such as an M.D., but how can you know that a CAM practitioner is qualified? With more and more complementary practitioners (such as acupuncturists, chiropractors, and massage therapists) seeking certification or licensure in the United States, the public has increased assurance that practitioners of complementary modalities have an appropriate level of education and skill. You can contact the state licensing board for the specialty or appropriate professional organizations for the names and qualifications of licensed practitioners in your area. (Turn to the individual modalities discussed later in this introduction, each of which lists organization addresses, toll-free numbers, and Web sites.) You can also use these organizational contacts to learn whether any complaints have been filed against a practitioner.

Once you've located a practitioner, what are the next steps? First of all, always ask to meet with a practitioner before agreeing to any treatment. (You also might be able to save yourself some time if you can make a phone appointment with the practitioner.) Prepare a list of questions to ask at your appointment, including:

- What are your credentials?

- What can you tell me about your experience in your area of specialty? (You also might ask why the practitioner chose that area of specialty— the answer might reveal something about the practitioner's personality, which may make you feel more comfortable.) How long have you been practicing?

- Please give me a complete explanation of the therapies you offer and the typical conditions those therapies are used for. (Or you may wish to ask about the therapies the practitioner uses for a particular condition you are suffering from or want to know more about.) Can you tell me about the results you've seen with this particular condition? (Make sure the practitioner has significant experience treating your particular condition.)

- How long does the therapy typically take (minutes, days, weeks? one appointment, several appointments?) and when can I realistically expect to see results? Agree with the practitioner, should you choose to undergo therapy, to set a time frame and a specific date on which to assess your progress and decide whether to continue or to consider a different therapy or practitioner. If the practitioner is unwilling to do this, consider that a "red flag."

*A **complementary practitioner** always chooses the least intrusive therapy first, moving to stronger therapies only as needed.*

- Would you be willing to ask one or more of your patients who have had this same therapy to speak with me about it?

- What is the cost of therapy? Are there any additional or "hidden" costs that I should know about, perhaps something that might occur down the line if not initially?

Following are some additional "watchdog" practices to keep an eye out for:

- Watch out for practitioners who bad-mouth conventional medicine. If you plan to work with the CAM practitioner in concert with your conventional physician, be sure that the practitioner knows about this and is agreeable and willing to communicate directly with your physician, if necessary or appropriate.

- Watch out for practitioners who are unable or unwilling to tell you the conditions or patient situations they do not feel comfortable treating, for example, conditions they do not treat (find out why) or for which they refer patients to others.

- Watch out for practitioners who do not have liability insurance. This is a must for *any* healthcare practitioner.

Safety Guidelines for Natural Therapies

Although complementary and alternative therapies are widely considered safe, common sense should always guide the use of herbs and supplements. The following are some general guidelines. Descriptions of the modalities and the individual diseases and disorders spell out more specific recommendations and cautions.

- Before beginning a natural therapy regimen of any kind, consult your physician for a diagnosis and to rule out a more serious disorder that could require conventional treatment and standard pharmaceuticals. The use of natural remedies could possibly mask the symptoms of a serious underlying condition.

- Inform all your healthcare practitioners before adding natural therapies to your treatment plan. Some herbs can cause allergic reactions, and some herbs and supplements don't mix well with conventional drugs.

Before beginning any natural therapy regimen, consult your physician for a diagnosis.

- Always use herbs under the care of a healthcare practitioner familiar with herbal medicine. This could be a naturopath, a specialist in botanical medicine, an Ayurvedic healer, an acupuncturist trained in Chinese herbal medicine, or a trained clinical herbalist. Your practitioner will devise a treatment strategy that takes into account your symptoms, your medical history, your age, the strength of the herb, and the results sought.

- Learn as much as you can about an herb before you take it. How much and how often should you take it? Does it work best as a capsule, tablet, tincture or tea? Are there any side effects? Are there any warnings?

- Buy from reputable manufacturers. The Food and Drug Administration (FDA) now requires that herbal preparations be labeled with the herb's scientific name, the amount of active ingredient, and the plant parts used. Product labels also should include the company's address, batch and lot numbers, expiration date, and dosage guidelines.

- Start with the lowest possible dose, and do not exceed maximum dosage unless your practitioner prescribes it. High doses of certain herbs and supplements (such as vitamin A) can cause toxicity if recommended levels are exceeded.

- If you are pregnant or nursing, consult a physician before undertaking an alternative therapy or using any herbs or supplements.

- Always keep essential oils, herbs, and supplements out of reach of children.

- Consult a physician before giving herbs to children under 12 or to adults over 65.

- Don't pick herbs yourself from chemically treated lawns or gardens.

- If you experience any side effects, such as headaches or diarrhea, immediately stop taking the herb and call your doctor. You can also call the FDA hotline at 800-332-1088.

> *Inform all your healthcare practitioners before adding natural therapies to your treatment plan.*

Guide to Complementary Medicine

Acupressure

See "Traditional Chinese Medicine" section.

Acupuncture

See "Traditional Chinese Medicine" section.

Aromatherapy

 Aromatherapy is the use of essential oils to assist the body's natural ability to heal itself. Essential oils are aromatic substances extracted from the flowers, fruits, seeds, leaves, wood, or roots of plants—those parts that give a plant its distinctive scent. They are not "oily" at all, but are highly volatile, meaning they readily evaporate. Essential oils are extracted by various methods, particularly steam distillation, resulting in an intensely concentrated fragrant oil rich in chemical compounds.

Throughout history, aromatic oils have been used for medicinal, cosmetic, and religious purposes. Ancient Hindus anointed themselves with aromatic oils when worshiping to chase away spiritual impurities. According to biblical history, Mary Magdalene anointed the feet of Jesus with spikenard oil. In more modern times, French medical doctor Jean Valnet used essential oils to treat serious medical conditions.

Today, aromatherapy is used to promote relaxation and to help ease various symptoms, such as the nausea that accompanies motion sickness. When used in conjunction with a relaxing massage, certain oils may rejuvenate, improve circulation, and have a balancing effect on the internal organs, say practitioners. Studies have also shown that particular oils can also have a calming or stimulating affect on the limbic system, the part of the brain that plays a central role in the production of emotions: joy, anger, contentment, and fear.

To prepare essential oils for massage purposes, add no more than 15 drops of the essential oil to one ounce of carrier oil (practitioners recommend almond or grapeseed oil, but vegetable oil will also work). Never use essential oils undiluted, unless specified. For baths, add 5 to 15 drops to water. To scent a room with a diffusor, add several drops. For use in a facial or respiratory steam, see "Hydrotherapy."

Use essential oils with caution, and never use them as a substitute for necessary medical care. Due to their intense concentration, they should never be taken internally. Keep all essential oils out of the reach of children and away from the eyes and mucous membranes. Some oils are lethal if ingested in high doses; others—such as pennyroyal, mugwort, wormwood, and tansy—should never be ingested. Certain essential oils can irritate the skin. When in doubt, test the skin for sensitivity, and if any sort of rash develops, discontinue use. Some oils, such as bergamot, can cause photosensitivity, so minimize your sun exposure when using these.

➤ *For a complete list of the essential oils mentioned in this book, along with their Latin names and usage information, see the resource listings at the back of this book.*

Throughout history, aromatic oils have been used for medicinal, cosmetic, and religious purposes.

For More Information
National Association for Holistic Aromatherapy
P.O. Box 17622
Boulder, CO 80308-7622
888-ASK-NAHA
www.naha.org

Ayurvedic Medicine

 Ayurveda, which has its roots in India, is one of the oldest healing therapies. Ancient Ayurvedic texts show that the practice has been in use for over 5000 years. *Ayurveda,* a Sanskrit word meaning "the science of life and longevity," includes the modalities of meditation, yoga, and Ayurvedic medicine, a healing system that integrates mind and body.

Ayurvedic philosophy is based on the principles of the five elements—space, air, fire, water, and earth—which make up the ethereal and physical matter of the earth. Each element is associated with certain attributes and behavioral patterns that exist in all aspects of nature. In the human body, the five elements create a specific individualized pattern, which is manifest in each person's *dosha,* or constitution.

The three basic types of doshas are *vata, pitta,* and *kapha.* Each person is a blend of the three, with one dosha usually dominating. This blend, or *prakruti,* results in unique personality traits and physical characteristics. To diagnose a condition, an Ayurvedic practitioner must first discover and understand an individual's prakruti:

- People with dominant vata dosha have a small bone structure, low body fat, underdeveloped muscles, quick movements, a changeable and excitable nature, the ability to learn quickly, a short memory span, irregular hunger patterns, and dry skin. Vatas also worry often and tire quickly. Vata types are prone to insomnia, nervous disorders, joint problems, and constipation.

- Pitta types have a medium build, moderate muscle tone, fair or ruddy skin, light eyes, a strong appetite, and sharp intelligence. They also tend to become irritable under stress and are competitive by nature. Pittas are prone to digestive troubles, skin conditions, and liver disorders.

- Kaphas have a heavy build, well-developed muscles, thick hair, large eyes, pale and moist skin, and a good memory. They tend to be kind and compassionate, though they are also sluggish and require excessive sleep. Kaphas are susceptible to disorders that involve excess mucus congestion, such as colds and sinusitis. An out-of-balance kapha is prone to obesity.

To determine a person's prakruti, an Ayurvedic practitioner will take the patient's pulse, which is the primary window to the innate prakruti, and examine the tongue, nails, face, hair, and skin. The practitioner will also take a detailed account of all aspects of the patient's lifestyle, environment, activity level, personal and family history, spiritual health, and sleeping and eating habits. Some practitioners use laboratory analysis of blood, urine, and stools as well. To stay healthy, Ayurveda teaches, one must keep *all* aspects of life in harmony.

Ayurvedic practitioners believe that diseases and medical conditions are the result of an excess or a deficiency of a particular dosha. In other words, a proper balance of all three doshas is the key to good physical and mental health. Treatment takes the form of a personalized dosha-balancing program and includes the following components:

> *To diagnose a condition, an Ayurvedic practitioner must first understand your unique personality traits, environment, lifestyle, and spiritual health.*

Diet to rebalance the constitution, prescribed according to season and dosha.

Exercise to improve circulation, boost metabolism, and energize the mind.

Meditation to enhance awareness of self and surroundings.

Herbs to rebuild the body.

Massage with medicated oils to remove toxins from the body.

Breathing exercises to relieve stress.

For More Information

The Ayurvedic Institute
11311 Menaul NE
Albuquerque, NM 87112
505-291-9698
FAX 505-294-7572
www.Ayurveda.com

Bodywork and Somatic Practices

 Bodywork and *somatic practices* are terms used to describe a number of ancient and modern complementary healthcare practices that support the healing process and promote well-being. There are myriad manual, energetic, and movement education methods and therapies that involve using the hands on and off the body. Techniques on the body use varying levels of pressure to release pain and tensions or to free energy in body systems and tissues for better health and comfort. Off-body hand techniques work in the auric field and address energy systems in and around the body, providing a gentle, integrated approach for body vitality and balance.

Bodywork is often used as an overall term to indicate a treatment, session, or lesson. More specifically, the term can refer to methods and therapies that focus mostly on pain and tension reduction, relaxation, better postural and structural function, and movement education.

Somatic practices refers to a body-mind approach that recognizes that stressed or unexpressed psychological states and emotions can result in physical and emotional tensions and imbalances in body function, well-being, or energy.

Body, mind, and spirit refers to the context of an entire, unique individual where these elements function in an integrated way. Somatic practice modalities, therefore, have a holistic focus and cover a wide range of styles and possibilities to address and resolve specific problems.

Alexander Technique F. M. Alexander, a turn-of-the-century Shakespearean actor, was able to cure his own voice loss by making changes in his posture. Based on this discovery, Alexander developed a way to re-educate the body to prevent or alleviate poor posture, muscular tension, and physical pain.

Techniques on the body use varying levels of pressure to release pain and tensions or to free energy in body systems for better health and comfort.

The Alexander Technique is a learning process, not a bodywork therapy. Students learn to identify tension-habit patterns and then establish new patterns of movement with the head gently balanced above a relaxed and elongated spine. The student wears comfortable clothes and receives both verbal and hand guidance cues in active movement activities or while lying on the massage table.

For More Information
American Society for the Alexander Technique
3010 Hennepin Avenue South
Minneapolis, MN 55408
800-473-0602
www.alexandertech.com

Aston-Patterning Judith Aston, a dancer who collaborated with Dr. Ida Rolf (see "Rolfing," below), developed in 1977 an educational approach she called Aston-Patterning, a process that combined movement education, bodywork, ergonomics, and fitness training. Aston-Patterning can help individuals achieve relief from acute or chronic pain, improve postural and movement patterns (either in everyday activities or in specialized contexts, such as sports or the performing arts), or pursue personal growth.

For More Information
Aston Training Center
P.O. Box 3568
Incline Village, NV 89450
775-831-8228
http://members.aol.com/SVUmassage/Aston.html

CranioSacral Therapy Research that osteopath John E. Upledger conducted in the 1970s led him to develop CranioSacral therapy (CST), an adaptable whole-body approach that enhances the craniosacral system, the membranes and cerebrospinal fluid that surrounds and protects the brain and spinal cord. The area extends from the bones of the skull, face, and mouth (which make up the cranium) down to the sacrum or tailbone. Imbalance or dysfunction in this system can result in sensory, motor, or neurological disabilities.

CST is a gentle, noninvasive therapy that uses a very light touch to identify and unblock areas of restriction within the craniosacral system. The goal is to help eliminate the negative effects of stress, strengthen resistance to disease, and enhance overall health. As a therapy, CST has been found to be effective in a broad spectrum of healthcare needs, for every age group from newborns to octogenarians. Clients typically lie on a massage table, although CST meets special needs off-table, such as work with toddlers or in hospital-type settings.

> *Off-body hand techniques address energy systems in and around the body, for vitality and balance.*

For More Information
Upledger Institute
11211 Prosperity Farms Road, D-325
Palm Beach Gardens, FL 33410-3449
800-233-5880
www.upledger@upledger.com

The Feldenkrais Method Dr. Moshe Feldenkrais was a nuclear physicist, an avid soccer player, and a judo expert who earned the first black belt in judo awarded in the Western hemisphere. He also developed a system of somatic education that raises student awareness of unconscious, ingrained movement habits.

The system is taught in two parts. *Awareness Through Movement* involves group lessons that involve light, effortless movements that focus primarily on how the student moves. *Functional Integration* involves one-on-one lessons that usually include gentle, directive touch to suggest a greater repertoire of movement possibilities that translate to the student's central nervous system.

Feldenkrais created thousands of ingenious lessons aimed at improving the quality of movement, thought, and behavior for people with certain chronic and acute injuries, cerebral palsy, stroke, and restrictions due to age. The system has also found support among athletes interested in enhanced body efficiency.

A Brief Introduction to Complementary Therapies

For More Information
The Feldenkrais Guild of North America
3611 SW Hood Avenue, #100
Portland, OR 97201
800-775-2118
www.feldenkrais.com

Hellerwork Joseph P. Heller learned to manipulate fascial tissue (the tissue that connects and supports body organs and other body structures) while studying with Dr. Ida Rolf.

Heller observed that people started talking about certain subjects when he worked on particular parts of their bodies. To the disciplines of soft tissue release and movement, Heller added a third element: the mind. He came to believe that bodies store emotions and attitudes. According to Heller, to change attitude is to change posture.

> *The touch mechanism creates a cascade of beneficial responses in the nervous system and endocrine system.*

Each Hellerwork session focuses on a certain part of the body or body process, along with a corresponding stage of development. For example, beginning sessions deal with breathing and standing as well as aspects of early childhood. Although relief from pain and tension may be benefits, the purpose of Hellerwork is to recondition the body and improve general well-being.

For More Information
Hellerwork International
406 Berry Street
Mount Shasta, CA 96067
800-392-3900
www.hellerwork.com

Massage Therapies Touch is an integral part of human well-being. It is so important, in fact, that studies of premature infants show that those who are stroked and touched gain weight faster and are more alert and active than those who are not touched. Therapeutic massage seeks to tap this power of touch to enhance overall health and to treat specific conditions.

The touch mechanism in humans creates a cascade of beneficial responses in the nervous and endocrine systems. These include relaxation, relief from pain, reduction of certain types of edema, increased range of motion, and a more positive attitude. Therefore, massage can deliver both psychological and physical benefits.

The primary aim of massage therapy is to manipulate the muscle and soft tissue to relieve tension in the body. A reduction in tension leads to increased circulation, which in turn helps eliminate metabolic wastes (such as lactic acid) by bringing fresh blood flow and oxygen to the tissues. This influx of oxygenated blood helps relieve tight, stiff muscles.

Massage therapy is available in many different styles that vary according to technique, degree of pressure, and areas of manipulation. Some therapies are gentle and nurturing; others work deep into the lower levels of muscle and tissue. Sports massage, for example, utilizes a deep, vigorous massage and is geared to therapeutic or corrective treatment, as in cases of injury or sports trauma.

Swedish massage is the most widely used technique and implements five basic strokes (all moving toward the heart) to stimulate the body's metabolic processes, increase the circulation of blood through the soft tissues of the body, and generally promote vitality. Swedish massage is firm, but quite relaxing.

In the past several years new types of massage have proliferated. Offshoots of Swedish massage include *infant massage*, a loving, nonverbal communication technique used by parents to enhance the infant-parent bond as well as enhance the baby's physical functions, relaxation response, and general well-being; *Kripalu massage*, a blend of Swedish massage, energy work, and yogic breathing exercises; *Lomilomi*, a system of massage that uses very large, broad movements and has a history of being passed on within Hawaiian families by *kahunas* or shamans; *prenatal/pregnancy massage*, a set of techniques designed to facilitate labor, help mothers cope with the physical and emotional strains of pregnancy and delivery, and help support mother and baby in the pregnancy and postpartum period.

Massage is administered with the client lying on a firm, padded table, undressed but draped in a sheet or towels. Oils or lotions are usually part of the experience. A practitioner's style, experience, and training, as well as your preference for varying degrees of pressure all come into play when choosing an approach that's right for you. Standards of practice now provide for many more licensed and/or certified massage therapists. Through referrals, professional and personal resources, and just asking questions, you will find modalities and practitioners to meet your needs.

For More Information
Associated Bodywork and Massage Professionals
28677 Buffalo Park Road
Evergreen, CO 80439-7347
800-458-2267
www.abmp.com

Premature infants who are stroked and touched gain weight faster and are more alert and active than those who are not touched.

Oriental Bodywork Therapy Oriental bodywork therapy is based on traditional Oriental medical principles for assessing and balancing the body's energy system to promote, maintain, and restore good health. It makes use of pressure and/or manipulation to treat the human body, mind, and spirit—including a person's electromagnetic energy field.

With the traditional Oriental medical principles come centuries of wisdom and myriad disciplines, including acupressure, shiatsu (in many styles), *Tui Na, Jin Shin Do,* and traditional Thai massage. The client is dressed in loose clothing and lies either on the floor or on a massage table. The therapist uses a combination of hands, elbows, knees, and feet to apply pressure to meridians and/or acupoints. Treatment also may include stretching and other techniques to influence total body balance.

A Brief Introduction to Complementary Therapies

For More Information
American Oriental Bodywork Therapy Association
Laurel Oak Corporate Center, Suite 408
1010 Haddenfield-Berlin Road
Voorhees, NJ 08043
609-782-1616
www.healthy.net/aobta

> *Polarity therapy looks at the body as a field of energy and seeks to release blocked energy currents that accompany symptoms of illness.*

Polarity Therapy Founded in the mid-1920s by Austrian-born naturopath Dr. Randolph Stone, polarity therapy was his vision of "energy medicine," a science of health (rather than disease) that addresses the person rather than the symptom. This therapy looks at the body as a field of energy and seeks to restore a client's balance and health by using the natural life-force currents that flow through a practitioner's hands to release blocked energy currents that accompany symptoms of illness.

In addition to the gentle balancing of the positive and negative energies of the body, polarity therapy also incorporates a dynamic system of movement therapy, a dietary regimen for cleansing and health building, body/mind/spirit psychology, and a deep understanding of energy, nature, and the healing process.

For More Information
American Polarity Therapy Association
P.O. Box 19858
Boulder, CO 80308
303-545-2080
www.polaritytherapy.org

Reflexology Reflexology is a manual technique used on specific reflex points and zones located along the energy meridians on the feet, hands, and ears to bring about psychological and physiological normalization and total body vitality. The therapist, by stimulating the feet with thumb and finger compression techniques, encourages positive changes throughout the body by releasing the body's own healing potential.

Several theories seek to explain the reflex action. Some reflexologists, working from the belief that energy pathways connect different parts of the body, theorize that mineral deposits, or waste products, form crystals in the feet. These deposits, they believe, prevent nerve and energy flow, and pressure on the feet breaks up the deposits and releases the flow. Others lean toward the theory that manipulating the feet releases endorphins, which block pain signals from reaching the higher nervous system.

Reflexology does not cure disease. Practitioners recommend it for relaxation, relieving pain, and revitalizing and balancing the body's systems. The reflexologist seeks to address the whole person, not just his or her symptoms or problems. Lotion or oil may be used as clients recline comfortably in a chair or on a massage table, minus socks and shoes.

➤ *See the resource listings at the back of this book for reflexology charts of the human foot and hand.*

For More Information
American Reflexology Certification Board
P.O. Box 620607
Littleton, CO 80162
303-933-6921

The International Institute of Reflexology
P.O. Box 12642
St. Petersburg, FL 33733
727-343-4811
www.reflexology-usa.net

Reiki Founded by Japanese Christian educator Dr. Mikao Usui and introduced in the United States in 1937 by his pupil Saichi Takata, Reiki is a profoundly simple energy healing system akin to the "laying on of hands." Based on the principle of *chi*, or universal life energy, Reiki is used for almost everything—from stress reduction to both physical and emotional healing. The practitioner places his or her hands very gently on the fully-clothed body, in a variety of established places on the head, chest, abdomen, and back. Treatments vary with each individual, but Reiki's greatest benefits occur when used in self-healing.

For More Information
The International Center for Reiki Training
21421 Hilltop Street, Unit 28
Southfield, MI 48034
800-322-8112
www.reiki.org

The Reiki Alliance
East 33135 Canyon Road
P.O. Box 41
Cataldo, ID 83810
208-682-3535
www.furumoto.org

> *The reflexologist encourages positive changes throughout the body by releasing the body's own healing potential.*

Rolfing Rolfing is a bodywork technique developed by American biochemist Ida P. Rolf in the 1940s after her own experience with a respiratory illness. When an osteopath manipulated one of her ribs back into place, Rolf experienced a recovery of health and realized the profound effect of body structure on psychological and physical well-being. Rolfing is used as an antidote to physical injury, poor posture, and emotional trauma.

The central idea behind Rolfing is that, over time, the fascia (the fibrous membrane that covers, supports, and separates muscle and connects skin with underlying tissue) becomes rigid and restricts movement. Lengthening and stretching techniques are used to loosen fascia adhesions and help the body realign itself with gravity. Practitioners use their fingers, knuckles, and elbows in often painful manipulation to release fascia, one area at a time. Clients complete a series of 10 sessions, each focusing on restoring flexibility and alignment to a different area of the body. Besides increasing mobility and optimizing health, energy, circulation, and resilience, Rolfing can provide a sense of lightness, relaxation, mental clarity, and enhanced well-being. It also may help those recuperating from injury or suffering from chronic pain.

For More Information
Rolf Institute for Structural Integration
205 Canyon Boulevard
Boulder, CO 80302
303-449-5903
www.rolf.org

Trager work can relieve chronic pain and can promote joint mobility, relaxation, heightened energy and vitality, and effortless posture and carriage.

Therapeutic Touch Therapeutic Touch (TT) was developed jointly by a professor of nursing, Dolores Krieger, Ph.D., R.N., and a spiritual healer, Dora Kunz, in the 1970s. TT is a contemporary interpretation of ancient healing practices, and as in Reiki, is built on the concept of a universal energy or life-force that can be tapped and directed toward the healing process. The goal is to clear and balance the recipient's energy field in order to activate his or her innate capacity for healing. The recipient is fully clothed and sits, stands, or lies while the practitioner rhythmically sweeps the energy field a few inches off the body to detect, then clear, areas of congestion or imbalance. Some clients report seeing colors or experiencing warmth and feelings of relaxation and integration. TT is used extensively in hospitals, healthcare settings, and in the home to help treat a variety of conditions.

For More Information
Nurse Healers Professional Associates
11250 Roger Bacon Drive, Suite 8
Reston, VA 20190
703-234-4149
www.therapeutic-touch.org

Therapeutic Touch Instruction
6609 S. Spencer Road
Newtown, KS 67114
316-283-9146
http://bdenison.sbcusa.com

The Trager Approach Trager work is a bodywork system developed by American medical practitioner Dr. Milton Trager in the 1920s. Its goals are to improve physical mobility and mental clarity and promote deep relaxation. It makes extensive use of touch and encourages the client, dressed in loose-fitting clothes or a bathing suit, to "free" different parts of the body. The approach consists of simple exercises called *Mentastics;* and deep, nonintrusive, hands-on tablework consisting of fluid, gentle, rocking movements. The idea is to use motion in the muscles and joints to produce positive sensory feelings, which are then fed back to the central nervous system, resulting in an experience of light, free flexibility. Trager work can be effective in relieving chronic pain and in promoting greater joint mobility, deeper states of relaxation, heightened levels of energy and vitality, and more effortless posture and carriage.

For More Information
Trager Institute
21 Locust Avenue
Mill Valley, CA 94941-2806
415-388-2688
www.trager.com

Trigger Point Myotherapy Trigger points are tender areas in muscles, tendons, and fascia that radiate pain to other regions of the body. Trigger point myotherapy is a therapeutic modality for the relief and control of myofascial pain and dysfunction in these pain areas. The goal of treatment is to reduce or eliminate myofascial pain and restore function. Treatment consists of trigger point compression, myomassage, passive stretching, and a regimen of corrective exercises, stress reduction techniques, and nutrition.

Trigger point therapy is frequently used by medical doctors, chiropractors, and physical therapists as well as by massage and bodywork practitioners to address a score of pain syndromes, including chronic neck and back pain.

For More Information
National Association for Trigger Point Myotherapy
P.O. Box 68
Warmouth Port, MA 02675-0068
508-896-4484

Chiropractic

Chiropractic is an alternative therapy based on the belief that illness originates in the spine. This hands-on therapy (the word *chiropractic* comes from the Greek and means "done by hand") enhances the body's innate self-healing capabilities. Today's system and theory was founded in 1895 by Daniel David Palmer, who recognized a relationship between the spine and health when he adjusted a deaf man's vertebrae and the man's hearing improved.

Chiropractic care focuses on the relationship among the spinal column and the nervous, muscular, and circulatory systems—and their combined effects on a patient's overall health. The brain, organs, and cellular systems are in constant intercommunication, sending and receiving messages that are vital to optimum body functioning. These messages travel in the form of nerve impulses along the spinal cord and through the rest of the nervous system. Pressure caused by *subluxation,* or misaligned vertebrae, impedes the transfer of

> *Chiropractic can be particularly beneficial in treating back pain, neck pain, and headache.*

nerve signals and may result in health problems. Chiropractic treatment aims to restore proper neuromusculoskeletal function—and thus improve health—by physically adjusting the misaligned vertebrae. This is a natural, drug-free, surgery-free treatment that allows the body to heal itself.

Scientific studies as well as anecdotal evidence suggest that chiropractic care can be particularly beneficial in treating back pain, neck pain, and headache. Other disorders it may help include peripheral joint injuries (such as tennis elbow, abnormal jaw function, and carpal tunnel syndrome), arthritis, and bursitis.

Chiropractic doctors receive academic and clinical training in accredited chiropractic colleges.

For More Information
American Chiropractic Association
1701 Clarendon Boulevard
Arlington, VA 22209
800-986-4636
www.americhiro.org

International Chiropractors Association
1110 North Glebe Road, Suite 1000
Arlington, VA 22201
800-423-4690
www.chiropractic.org

Approximately 25 percent of all prescription drugs are isolated from plant sources or synthesized from plant compounds.

Herbal Therapy

 The use of plants—their roots, stems, bark, leaves, flowers, fruits, and seeds—to achieve wellness is thought to be one of the oldest modes of healthcare. In fact, evidence of herbal remedies has been found at the burial site of a Neanderthal man who lived 60,000 years ago. Recorded evidence of early herbal use can be found in the *Ebers Paprus,* an ancient Egyptian medical text believed to have been written in the sixteenth century B.C. This work describes hundreds of treatments, including the use of mint to aid digestion and aloe vera to heal cuts.

Today, plants remain an integral part of medicine. About 80 percent of the world's population in developing countries uses plant-based medicine, according to the World Health Organization (WHO). Herbal therapies are popular and frequently prescribed in European countries, especially Germany.

In fact, approximately 25 percent of all prescription drugs are still isolated from plant sources or synthesized from plant compounds. For example, a commonly prescribed heart medication, digoxin, is derived from foxglove *(Digitalis lanata),* and the cancer drug taxol is isolated from the bark of the Pacific yew *(T. brevifolia).*

Until the 1930s, doctors in the United States relied heavily on herbal remedies. Then use declined with advancements in medical technology and the production of synthetic drugs. Now the scene is shifting once again. Recent trends show renewed interest in herbal treatments, which cost less than pharmaceutical preparations and often have fewer side effects. Americans are now spending approximately $5 billion a year on herbal products.

Herbal remedies are available in a variety of forms: as fresh leaves, dried leaves, powders, capsules, tinctures (glycerine or alcohol), and ointments. Commercially packaged products are regulated by the FDA under the Dietary Supplement Health and Education Act (DSHEA). This law requires the use of labels similar to the ones found on food and nutritional supplements.

When buying herbal remedies, seek out companies that voluntarily regulate themselves in order to control quality and meet a high standard of safety. Look for these clues on the label:

Discuss your herbal therapy with your primary care physician, because some herbs interact dangerously with prescription medications.

- recommended daily dose
- percentage of active ingredient
- milligrams of each ingredient per dose
- side effects/precautions
- lot/batch number
- expiration date
- address and phone number of the manufacturer
- FDA registration of manufacturing facilities
- compliance to standards of Good Manufacturing Practice
- independent laboratory verification of the amount of active ingredients and the absence of contaminants and adulterants

Always follow package directions for recommended dosage and duration of use. Herbal remedies are generally slow-acting, but overdosing or extending treatment beyond the recommended course is not better, and could be harmful. Some herbs—lobelia, for example—are safe in low doses but toxic in high amounts. (Fortunately, lobelia isn't widely distributed in commercial products.) Other herbs—aloe and bromelain are good examples—are safe for short-term use, but should not be used on a long-term basis.

For the most part, herbal remedies are gentler to the body than prescription drugs. But adverse side effects are still possible, so before starting a regimen, consult with a healthcare professional who is knowledgeable about herbal remedies. The American Herbalists Guild (AHG) can help you locate a qualified herbalist in your area.

Take special precautions if you are pregnant or have a serious health condition. Also, if you are taking prescription medications, be sure to discuss your herbal therapy with your primary care physician, because some herbs interact dangerously with pharmaceuticals. Ma huang, for example, interacts negatively with theophylline, caffeine, monoamine oxidase inhibitors, reserpine, dexamethasone, and amitriptyline.

Also, you will need to stop taking herbs at least two to three weeks before having surgery, as certain herbal remedies may have dangerous interactions with some anesthetics, deepening their effect or causing problems with blood pressure and bleeding.

A Brief Introduction to Complementary Therapies

For More Information
American Botanical Council
P.O. Box 144345
Austin, TX 78714-4345
512-926-4900
www.herbalgram.org

The American Herbalists Guild (AHG)
P.O. Box 70
Roosevelt, UT 84066
435-722-8434
www.healthy.net/herbalists

Americans are now spending approximately $5 billion a year on herbal products.

12 Popular Herbal Remedies The following are some of the most popular herbs and their common uses:

Aloe vera *(A. barbadensis)*—the gel is used externally to treat burns, abrasions, and other minor skin injuries; the dried leaf sap is used internally as a laxative

Cranberry *(Vaccinium macrocarpon)*—the juice of the berry is used internally to help prevent urinary tract infections

Dandelion *(Taraxacum officinale)*—the herb and root are used internally for dyspepsia, loss of appetite, flatulence, and as a diuretic

Echinacea *(Echinacea purpurea)*—the herb is used internally to reduce the duration and symptoms of upper respiratory infections

Evening primrose *(Oenothera biennis)*—the seed oil is used internally to treat premenstrual syndrome (PMS) symptoms

Feverfew *(Tanacetum parthenium)*—the leaf is used internally to lessen the severity of migraine headaches and has been used for arthritic conditions

Garlic *(Allium sativum)*—the powdered clove is used internally to treat high cholesterol and triglyceride levels; exhibits anti-bacterial, anti-fungal, antiviral, and anti-hypertensive properties

German chamomile *(Matricaria recutita)*—the flower is used internally as a popular remedy for indigestion and flatulence; also often used as a mild sedative at bedtime

Ginger *(Zingiber officinale)*—the root is used internally to treat nausea, motion sickness, and vomiting

Hawthorn *(Cratagus oxyacantha)*—the leaves and flowers or berries are used internally as a heart tonic and to treat mild forms of angina

Peppermint *(Mentha piperita)*—the leaves are used internally to calm the stomach and intestinal tract; the oil is helpful for irritable bowel syndrome and inflammation of the gums

Psyllium *(Plantago ovata and P. major)*—the seed or seed husk is used internally as a bulk laxative

Source: American Botanical Council

Preparing Basic Herbal Remedies

Infusion. Steep the dried herb (usually flowers or leaves) in 1 cup of boiling water for 10 to 15 minutes. The amount of herb varies, depending on the remedy, but it's often 1 to 2 teaspoons. Many dried herbs are available in convenient tea bags. If the herb is available only in bulk, use a mesh tea bag or strain the tea before drinking.

Decoction. Simmer the herb (usually in root or bark form) in 1 cup of water for 10 to 20 minutes. Strain. The amount of herb varies, depending on the remedy, but it's often 1 ounce of whole root or bark, 1 tablespoon minced, or 1 teaspoon powdered.

Tincture. Combine the herb and vodka or 95 percent proof grain alcohol in a glass jar, making sure the alcohol completely covers the herb. The proportion of herb to alcohol varies, depending on the remedy, but the typical tincture is 1 part herb to 2 parts alcohol. Store in a dark room or closet for 2 to 6 weeks, depending on the remedy. Strain the resulting liquid (tincture) into brown bottles to protect it from light.

➤ *For a complete list of common herbs and their Latin names, see the resource listings at the back of this book.*

Homeopathy

In 1790 Samuel Hahnemann, a highly respected German physician, rediscovered Hippocrates's theory that substances producing symptoms similar to those of a natural disease may be used to treat the disease itself. The result forms the basis for the natural therapy that Hahnemann called *homeopathy*.

The term—which comes from the Greek words *homoios*, meaning "similar," and *pathos*, meaning "to suffer"—reflects Hahnemann's fundamental concept "the law of similars." This principle states that a remedy can cure a specific disease if it is capable of producing the symptoms of the disease in the absence of the disorder itself.

Homeopathic practitioners, who may also be medical doctors, recommend a remedy only after carefully matching the drug profile with the patient's symptom pattern. In order to establish this pattern, the practitioner conducts a detailed personal interview. The patient's physical, psychological, and emotional symptoms are taken into account.

Homeopathic remedies are available commercially in tablet, liquid, wafer, ointment, and granular form and are marked with dilution ratios that show the proportion of active substance to inactive base. Ratios expressed as *c* consist of 1 part active tincture (concentrated extract) and 99 parts alcohol base; those expressed as *x* consist of 1 part active tincture and 9 parts alcohol base. The number preceding the *c* or *x* indicates the number of times the remedy

> *Homeopathy holds that a remedy can effect a cure if it is capable of producing the symptoms of the disease in the absence of the disorder itself.*

Paradoxically, the more diluted a homeopathic remedy is, the more potent or effective it is.

Popular Homeopathic Remedies

Following are some of the more popular homeopathic remedies and their common uses:

Aconitum napellus (**monkshood**)—used to treat fever and inflammation where there has been sudden onset after exposure to cold or fright

Allium cepa (**red onion**)—used to treat hay fever that is accompanied by fever and burning nasal discharge

Antimonium tartaricum (**tartar emetic**)—used to treat bronchitis cough and mucus in the lungs of a patient who is pale and cold

Apis mellifica (**honeybee**)—used to treat insect bites and bee stings that are red, sting, and feel better after cold applications

Arnica (**leopards bane**)—used to treat bruises and other minor injuries

Bryonia (**white bryonia**)—used for acute headaches that are made worse by motion, such as moving the head or eyes

Calcarea phosphorica (**phosphate of lime**)—used to speed healing of broken bones or to help during teething

Chamomilla (**German chamomile**)—used to treat pain and sensitivity, especially toothaches

Euphrasia (**eye bright**)—used to treat hay fever accompanied by burning eyes

Ferrum phos (**iron phosphate**)—used to treat ear infections, colds, fever, and nosebleeds

Gelsemium (**yellow jasmine**)—used to treat flu accompanied by chills and weakness

Kali bichromicum (**bichromate of potash**)—used to treat a headache that comes with sinus problems

Lycopodium (**club moss**)—used to treat indigestion, heartburn, and anxiety

Magnesia phosphorica (**phosphate of magnesia**)—used to treat general pain as well as leg and menstrual cramps that feel better after warm applications

Pulsatilla (**wind flower**)—used to ease the symptoms of premenstrual syndrome (PMS), especially when accompanied by depression

Spongia tosta (**roasted sponge**)—used to treat coughs and croup

Veratrum album (**white hellebore**)—used to treat a patient who is very weak and who is vomiting and defecating at the same time

has been diluted. For example, a remedy labeled "6c" has first been diluted 1 part to 99 parts. Then the resulting compound is mixed 1 part to 99 parts base, and the process is repeated 6 times.

Paradoxically, the more diluted a homeopathic remedy is, the more potent or effective it is. Practitioners usually suggest starting with the 30th potency. If no improvement is seen within three doses, consider a different remedy. If you use a lower potency (a 6c or 6x, for example), you might need to repeat the medication more often.

Homeopathic therapies have been used for more than 200 years to treat a wide range of common illnesses, such as colds, the flu, and sore throats. Because of their low toxicity, the treatments are ideal for infants and children. The healing rate depends on the individual. In all cases, homeopathic remedies should be discontinued as soon as the patient feels better.

Medical emergencies involving acute illness or injury—for example, a severe infection or a broken leg—are best handled with conventional medical treatment.

For More Information
National Center for Homeopathy
801 North Fairfax, #306
Alexandria, VA 22314
703-548-7790
www.homeopathic.org

Hydrotherapy

 Hydrotherapy—the use of water to relieve symptoms of health problems—has its roots in the beginning of civilization. The ancient Romans, Egyptians, Hebrews, Native Americans, and many other peoples used water to treat a variety of health conditions. Native Americans, for example, used sweat lodges for cleansing and ceremonial purposes. Ancient Scandinavians used saunas to detoxify the blood after long hard winters without fresh food.

Johann S. Hahn (1696–1773), widely considered the father of modern-day hydrotherapy, successfully treated the deadly smallpox virus with his hydrotherapy methods. John Harvey Kellogg (1852–1943), brother of the famous breakfast cereal tycoon, used a variety of hydrotherapy treatments in his famous Battle Creek Sanitorium. Today, as in the past, resorts built around natural hot springs offer relief from health problems to those who drink and bathe in the mineral-filled waters.

For treatment purposes, water can be used internally and externally in a great number of applications, including whirlpool baths, ice packs, saunas, douches, colonic irrigation, sitz baths, compresses, wraps, and mineral drinking waters. Hot water treatments are used to relax muscles and increase joint mobility. Cold water treatments, on the other hand, can relieve pain and reduce inflammation. Alternating the hot and cold treatments (contrast therapy) increases blood circulation through the elimination organs (kidneys, liver, and skin), thereby detoxifying the system and improving the quality of the blood.

Resorts built around natural hot springs offer relief from health problems to those who drink and bathe in the mineral-filled waters.

Hyperthermia treatments elevate the body's temperature to mimic fever, thereby stimulating the natural immune response.

Common Hydrotherapy Treatments

Cold compresses. These are useful for preventing congestion, lowering fever, relieving headaches, and reducing inflammation. To make a cold compress, fill a bowl with ice water, dip in a clean cloth, wring out excess water, and apply the cloth to the affected area. Repeat as necessary. For added therapeutic effect, add 3 to 4 drops of an essential oil to the water. (See "Aromatherapy" in this section for suggestions.)

Cold-water friction rub. Dip a washcloth in 50- to 60-degree water and wrap the cloth around your hand. Vigorously rub your arms, legs, feet, chest, and abdomen, dipping the cloth into the cool water as necessary to freshen. Dry yourself briskly.

Cold-water treading. To increase general vitality and stimulate the immune and lymphatic systems, walk in very cool water that reaches midcalf height. You can do this in a stream or lake, in a wading pool, or even in your own bathtub.

Colonic irrigation. This is a process designed to treat those with problems related to digestion, assimilation of nutrients, and elimination. The irrigation must be performed by an experienced colonic therapist who cleanses the colon by flushing it with water of various temperatures.

Constitutional therapy. To enhance the immune response, improve overall cellular function, promote detoxification, and help balance the nervous system. This therapy should be administered only by an experienced hydrotherapist who would apply alternating hot and cold towels to the front and back of the body, focusing on the chest, abdomen, and lower back.

Contrast therapy. This is the application of alternating hot and cold cloths to help improve circulation to an affected area.

Home baths. To relieve poison ivy irritation, re-acidify skin, and reduce fatigue, add 1 cup apple cider vinegar to a warm bath. To calm the nerves, reduce pain, or heal wounds and bruises, add 6 to 12 drops of lavender essential oil to a warm bath. For aches, pains, and swollen joints, add 1 pound of Epsom salts to a warm bath. To treat sunburn or itching, soothe and soften skin, or treat skin irritation, add 1 cup of finely-ground uncooked oatmeal (use a food processor or blender) to a warm bath.

Hot baths for hands and feet. These are helpful for congestive headaches, nosebleeds, leg cramps, menstrual cramps, and insomnia. The hot water pulls congestion away from areas of inflammation. Soak hands or feet in hot water for 10 to 15 minutes.

Hot compresses. A hot compress, or *fomentation,* is helpful for treating lung infections, delayed menstruation, and sciatica. To prepare a hot compress, follow the directions for a cold compress, except use hot water. Cover the compress with a towel and plastic wrap or a plastic bag. Change the compress every 3 to 10 minutes. Repeat as necessary.

Hyperthermia treatments. This therapy is designed to purposefully elevate body temperature to mimic fever, thereby elevating the white blood cell count and stimulating the body's natural immune response. Treatment may include hot compresses, steam therapy, sauna, sunbathing, or exercise.

Ice packs. To treat for sprains, other injuries, and acute inflammation, wrap ice in a plastic bag and towel and apply to the affected area in a 20-minutes-on, 20-minutes-off pattern for the first 24 to 36 hours. Applications should not exceed 20 minutes, as extended exposure to extreme cold can damage the skin.

Mustard plaster. This is a poultice (see "Poultice" below) that uses mustard (or ginger or cayenne) as a counter-irritant. The spice creates a superficial irritation to the skin, thereby drawing blood to the surface which promotes healing and relieves deeply congested or irritated tissue.

Poultice. This is a soft, moist cloth treated with herbs or clay, applied hot to a given area to create a moist, local heat. A poultice can be effective in drawing toxins from an inflamed area or from an insect bite.

Sitz baths. Use a hot sitz bath to treat infections of the bladder, vagina, or prostate as well as bowel problems and hemorrhoids. Cold sitz baths are useful for treating uterine prolapse and incontinence. Sit in water that's navel-high for 10 to 15 minutes.

Steam and saunas. Steam rooms, or saunas, are used to detoxify the system and to create artificial fevers (to fight infection). Do not stay in a steam room for more than 15 to 20 minutes.

Steam inhalation. Steam helps relieve congestion. It also helps open and cleanse the pores, thereby detoxifying the system. To prepare, simply fill a large basin or bowl with plenty of just-boiled water. Place a large towel over your head to trap the steam and stand or sit with your head about a foot above the steaming water. Close your eyes and inhale deeply. Add boiling water, as necessary, to keep the basin steaming. Avoid inhalation therapy if you have asthma.

For More Information

To view abstracts of over 900 studies on the medical benefits of this treatment modality, use the National Center for Complementary and Alternative Medicine's search engine at:
http://nccam.nih.gov/nccam/resources/cam-ci/search.cgi
Enter *Hydrotherapy* for "Term" and *All* for "Search Categories."

Nutrition and Supplementation

The Recommended Daily Allowances (RDAs), a useful starting point, are today considered largely inadequate.

 Nutrition A vital part of physiology, medicine, and other biological sciences, nutrition is the study of food and the way it nourishes the body. Its association with wellness dates back to Hippocrates, who considered food a single nutrient. In 1747 a British physician named

Lind conducted the first controlled nutrition experiment in which he tried to cure scurvy by treating sailors with lemon juice, lime juice, nutmeg, cider, vinegar, or seawater. Lemon juice and lime juice passed the tests, but vitamin C itself wasn't isolated for another two centuries. By 1912 scientists had isolated three macronutrients (major nutrients): carbohydrates, fats, and proteins. The discovery of the micronutrients (vitamins and minerals) as well as the various components of carbohydrates, fats, and proteins would come later.

Until fairly recently, the focus of nutritional science was on fighting deficiency diseases—including scurvy, pellagra, beriberi, and rickets. The Recommended Dietary Allowances (RDAs) were published in 1941 by the National Academy of Sciences (NAS) to guide meal planning for institutions, such as schools and hospitals. Today, thanks to years of research on the relationship between various nutrients and disease and disease prevention, we know that sound nutrition is a key pathway to optimal health. The RDAs, a useful starting point, are considered largely inadequate. In the mid 1990s the NAS issued new guidelines, the Dietary Reference Intakes (DRIs), that look toward optimal health and recommend much higher ranges for each nutrient.

By way of explanation, let's look at vitamin C. Sixty milligrams of C was long considered the amount needed to ward off scurvy. However, most Americans are not falling victim to scurvy. They're looking for a dosage that provides top-notch immunity, one that helps them maintain good health under conditions of physical or emotional stress. They're asking how much vitamin C they should take for a maximum health benefit. They're also asking how much can they take before it causes harm.

Yet optimizing health is more than just making up for shortfalls in vitamins or minerals. It's looking at dietary excesses as well, and that's no small matter. Recent studies show that 55 percent of Americans are overweight. The reasons are complex, of course, but eating too much food—especially items high in fat and sugar—plays a big part. All those excesses increase the risk of developing a serious illness—chiefly cancer, heart disease, and diabetes. Another concern of nutrition experts is whether or not you are digesting and absorbing your foods adequately. You may be on the best possible diet, but it won't do you any good if the nutrients aren't getting into your cells.

Most nutritionists and healthcare providers favor a whole-foods diet that emphasizes fruits, vegetables, legumes, and whole grains.

For basic nutrition information, check well-researched magazines and books (including this one) for guidelines. You'll discover that most nutritionists, certified or registered dietitians, and other healthcare providers favor a whole-foods diet that emphasizes plant-based foods—fruits, vegetables, legumes, and whole grains. Other foods included in a whole-foods plan are reasonable amounts of fish, poultry, and low-fat dairy products. What this diet limits is the intake of red meats, high-fat foods, sugar, sodium, and processed foods.

The case for a diet high in plant foods is easy to make. Research shows that a vegetarian lifestyle (one in which vegetable protein from legumes, nuts, and whole grains replaces protein from meat, poultry, and fish) may reduce your risk for heart disease, diabetes, colon cancer, hypertension, obesity, osteoporosis, and diverticular disease.

For custom and therapeutic diets—such as those designed to promote weight loss, lower cholesterol, address lactose intolerance or food allergies, prevent osteoporosis, or prepare an athlete for competition—seek the advice of nutritionists, certified and registered dietitians who work closely with healthcare providers. When consulting a certified or registered nutrition specialist, expect detailed questions about lifestyle, exercise habits, food likes and dislikes, and eating patterns. A comprehensive dietary plan takes into account many aspects of your life.

Supplementation Most nutritionists recommend getting the vitamins and minerals you need from whole foods, but they also recognize that it's nearly impossible to achieve the optimal intake of some nutrients without supplementing. Vitamin E is a good example. Several studies have shown that 100

> *A plant-based diet may reduce your risk for heart disease, diabetes, colon cancer, hypertension, obesity, and osteoporosis.*

Basic Dietary Guidelines

These are the food recommendations established jointly by the U.S. Departments of Agriculture and Health and Human Services.

Breads, Cereals, Rice, and Pasta. Try to get 6 to 11 servings from this group daily. It supplies complex carbohydrates, fiber, and minerals. One serving equals 1 slice of bread; 1/2 cup cooked cereal, rice, or pasta; 1/2 bagel or muffin; or 1 ounce dry cereal. For maximum fiber, use whole-grain products.

Fruits. Reach for 2 to 4 servings daily. Fruits provide vitamins A and C, potassium, and fiber. One serving equals 1 medium apple, banana, orange, peach; 1/2 cup chopped, cooked, or canned fruit; or 3/4 cup juice.

Vegetables. Go for 3 to 5 servings daily. Vegetables, especially the deep-yellow and deep-green varieties, are packed with vitamins, minerals, and fiber. One serving equals 1 cup raw leafy greens, 1/2 cup cooked vegetables, or 3/4 cup juice.

Meat, Poultry, Fish, Dried Beans, Eggs, and Nuts. Get 2 to 3 servings from this group daily. These foods are sources of protein, B vitamins, iron, and zinc. One serving equals 2 to 3 ounces of cooked lean meat, poultry, or fish (about the size of a deck of cards); 1 egg; or 1/2 cup cooked beans. To keep fat intake low, choose legumes, lean meats and fish, and skinless poultry breast meat.

Milk, Yogurt, and Cheese. Aim for 2 to 3 servings from this group. Dairy products are a source of protein, vitamins, and minerals—especially calcium and some B vitamins. One serving equals 1 cup (8 ounces) of milk or yogurt; 1 1/2 ounces of a natural cheese, such as cheddar or Swiss; or 2 ounces of processed cheese, such as American. Use fat-free or reduced-fat products to keep your fat intake low.

Fats, Oils, and Sweets. Limit intake. This group includes butter, margarine, oils, candy, soda, cakes, cookies, and similar foods. One serving equals 1 teaspoon butter, margarine, or oil.

IU (International Unit) to 400 IU of vitamin E is the daily dose recommended for preventing heart disease. Good food sources are nuts, nut butters, and vegetable oils. Unfortunately, it's very difficult to get more than 25 IU of E from diet alone.

Calcium is another example. Nutrition experts recommend that women over 50 take 1200 milligrams of calcium daily to reduce their risk of developing osteoporosis. Yet most women fall far short of that goal unless they take a supplement.

> *It's nearly impossible to achieve the optimal intake of some nutrients without supplementing.*

If you have a specific health concern and decide to take nutritional supplements, do so in combination with a well-balanced diet. There is absolutely no substitute for the long-term health benefits of a whole-foods diet rich in plant nutrients (phytonutrients), protein, and fiber. Supplements can fill in the gaps, but by themselves they can't make up for a diet that's packed with junk foods, processed foods, and empty calories—soda, candy, cookies, doughnuts, and the like.

Before purchasing supplements, consult a nutritionist or a healthcare provider who is knowledgeable in nutrition. This is especially important if you are pregnant or breastfeeding, chronically ill, under 18 years old, or taking prescription or over-the-counter medications. Follow recommended dosage guidelines, since some nutrients (such as the fat-soluble vitamins A, D, E, and K) are toxic in excessive amounts.

For More Information

American Dietetic Association
216 West Jackson Boulevard
Chicago, IL 60606-6995
312-899-0040
www.eatright.org

The Council on Nutrition of the
American Chiropractic Association
6855 Browntown Road
Front Royal, VA 22630
540-635-8844

International Food Information Council
1100 Connecticut Avenue, NW
Suite 430
Washington, DC 20036
202-296-6540
http://ificinfo.health.org

Traditional Chinese Medicine

 Traditional Chinese Medicine (TCM) has been practiced in China and Eastern Asia for nearly 5000 years. Since its inception, this medical system has focused primarily on disease prevention rather than treatment. Specifically, it seeks to protect the health of the body, mind,

21 Vitamins and Minerals at a Glance
Vitamins

Vitamin A. Known as the vitamin needed for good night vision, vitamin A is also essential for growth and development as well as for healthy skin, hair, and mucous membranes. Good food sources of this nutrient include dark-yellow, orange, and green fruits and vegetables and fortified fat-free milk. Vitamin A is fat-soluble, stored in the body, and can be toxic if taken in excessive amounts.

Beta-carotene. This important nutrient is converted into vitamin A in the body, and is a carotenoid. As a potent antioxidant it may reduce the risk of cancer and may protect against other health disorders. Excess amounts of beta-carotene are unhealthy; take it as part of a multivitamin and through a balanced diet. Excellent food sources include sweet potatoes, carrots, squash, mangoes, spinach, cantaloupe, apricots, pumpkin, kale, and collards.

Vitamin B_1. Also known as thiamine, this vitamin is necessary for the metabolism of carbohydrates, fats, and proteins. Mild deficiencies may take the form of fatigue, moodiness, and loss of appetite. Excellent food sources include lean pork, milk, peas, legumes, soybeans, and peanuts. If you take a multivitamin supplement, always be sure it includes vitamin B_1. Thiamine is water soluble and is not stored in the body.

Vitamin B_2. Also called riboflavin, this B vitamin aids in the metabolism of carbohydrates, fats, and proteins. It's also important for healthy skin and mucous membranes, good eye function, and a healthy nervous system. The signs of mild deficiency are wide ranging and include cracks in the corners of the mouth, sensitivity to light, and skin rashes. The best food sources of riboflavin are enriched grain products, some dairy products, eggs, almonds, and dark-green vegetables, such as broccoli. If you take a multivitamin supplement, always be sure it includes vitamin B_2. Riboflavin is water-soluble and is not stored in the body.

Vitamin B_3. Commonly known as niacin—and the cure for pellagra—this nutrient helps release energy from food, build red blood cells, synthesize hormones, and promote proper nervous system functioning. When used in megadoses, niacin becomes a drug and has gotten lots of press for its cholesterol-lowering abilities. Mild deficiencies may include indigestion, appetite loss, headaches, and anxiety. Good food sources include lean meats, poultry, fish, nuts and nut butters, and enriched flour. If you take a multivitamin supplement, be sure it includes vitamin B_3. Niacin is water-soluble.

Folate. Also commonly called folic acid or folacin, this B vitamin is critical for the growth and repair of cells. It helps protect against cervical cancer and heart disease and reduces the risk of developing neural tube birth defects (spina bifida, to be specific). Excellent food sources include avocados, asparagus, broccoli, brussel sprouts, beans, beets, celery, corn, eggs, fish, green leafy vegetables, nuts, seeds, oatmeal, peas, orange juice, fortified cereals, and wheat germ. Excess intake of this nutrient can mask a vitamin B_{12} deficiency. If you

Supplements can fill in the gaps, but they can't make up for a diet that's packed with junk foods, processed foods, and empty calories.

take a multivitamin supplement, always be sure it includes folate. Folate is water-soluble.

Vitamin B$_5$. Also known as pantothenic acid, this nutrient is an integral part of the vitamin B complex, and is needed for food metabolism. It also aids in synthesizing hormones and encouraging normal growth and development. Deficiencies of this nutrient are extremely rare because it's readily available in so many foods, including eggs, brown rice, salmon, beans, nuts, lentils, peas, and sweet potatoes.

Vitamin B$_6$. Also known as pyrodoxine, this nutrient supports the metabolism of protein and aids in the transmission of nerve impulses. Vitamin B$_6$ is necessary for a healthy immune system and prevents heart disease and hardening of the arteries. When prescribed in megadoses as a drug, it may alleviate carpal tunnel syndrome and PMS. Signs of mild deficiency may include acne, insomnia, and fatigue. Rich sources of B$_6$ are abundant and include whole grains, lean meats, poultry, fish, corn, nuts, potatoes, prune juice, bananas, and avocados. If you take a multivitamin supplement, always be sure it includes vitamin B$_6$. Though pyrodoxine is water soluble, excess amounts may be toxic and cause neurological damage with tingling and numbness in the hands and feet.

Vitamin B$_{12}$. This is yet another vitamin in the B complex group, and its primary role is to metabolize food and synthesize red blood cells. It also plays a critical role in producing RNA, DNA, and myelin, the protective layer over nerve endings. Symptoms of mild deficiency include weakness, weight loss, and tingling in the arms and legs; severe deficiencies result in pernicious anemia. Food sources include fish, eggs, and dairy products. B$_{12}$ is water-soluble and is usually given as an injection when large doses are needed.

Biotin. This nutrient works in conjunction with the other B vitamins to metabolize carbohydrates, fats, and proteins. It's also key to maintaining healthy skin and hair. Signs of deficiency are diverse and include hair loss, nausea, and fatigue. Good food sources of biotin include cheese, salmon, sunflower seeds, nuts, broccoli, and sweet potatoes. If you take a multivitamin supplement, be sure it includes biotin. Biotin is water-soluble.

Vitamin C. A powerful antioxidant and infection fighter, vitamin C has the ability to ward off and, if necessary, cure scurvy. It's also vital to healing wounds and bruises, and it may help protect against some cancers, cataracts, and heart disease. Minor deficiencies may appear as bleeding gums or the slow healing of cuts and scrapes. Outstanding sources of this nutrient include citrus fruits, bell peppers, strawberries, broccoli, tomatoes, cantaloupe, kiwi fruit, leafy green vegetables, papayas, brussel sprouts, and apple and cranberry juices. Vitamin C is water-soluble; however, excess amounts may cause diarrhea.

Vitamin D. This much-needed nutrient works closely with calcium to keep bones healthy and strong and to prevent rickets, a deficiency disorder. It also encourages proper nerve function and muscle contraction. Unlike most vitamins, which must be provided by food, vitamin D can be manufactured by the body with the help of sunshine. Requirements for producing 200 mg of this

Vitamin C is a powerful antioxidant and infection fighter and may help protect against some cancers, cataracts, and heart disease.

nutrient are as little as 10 minutes exposure to midday sun daily. Food sources are few: fortified milk, cereal, and fatty fish, such tuna and salmon. Vitamin D is fat-soluble and toxic in large amounts.

Vitamin E. A powerful antioxidant that helps regulate the immune and endocrine systems, vitamin E has received favorable reports on its possible role in guarding against certain cancers, cataracts, and heart disease. Deficiencies are rare. Vitamin E is fat-soluble, and food sources include vegetable oils, nuts, and avocados. Choose natural vitamin E (d-alpha tocopherol or RRR-alpha tocopherol) whenever possible.

Minerals

Calcium. This hard-working mineral is essential for developing and maintaining healthy bones and teeth. It's also critical for proper muscle contraction, blood clotting, and nerve-impulse transmission. With vitamin D, it fends off rickets and may lessen the risk of colorectal cancer. Good sources include dark-green leafy vegetables, dairy products, almonds, sardines (with bones), and salmon (with bones).

Chromium. This micronutrient helps regulate blood sugar and aids in sugar metabolism. Food sources of chromium include lean meats, poultry, molasses, whole grains, eggs, and cheese. Because the mineral is toxic in large amounts, it's best obtained from food or a multinutrient supplement.

Copper. Small amounts of this mineral are vital to health. It helps form hemoglobin, facilitates absorption of iron, assists in the regulation of blood pressure, and strengthens blood vessels. Deficiencies are rare except in people with malabsorption disorders. Foods sources include seafood, nuts, seeds, and blackstrap molasses.

Iron. A key nutrient for red blood cell formation and function, iron plays a significant role in the transport of oxygen from the lungs to body tissues. Most people get enough iron from food, but women before menstruation may require a slight boost. Good sources include red meat, chicken, whole grains, nuts, and dried fruits (especially raisins). Foods rich in Vitamin C enhance iron absorption. Coffee, tea, antacids, and excess calcium, magnesium, and zinc inhibit iron absorption. Iron supplements should be taken on a doctor's advice only.

Magnesium. This mineral can reduce the risk of heart disease and increase energy. When combined with calcium, magnesium aids in building strong teeth and bones. It also eases muscle pain. Nutritionists recommend consuming calcium and magnesium in a 2:1 ratio for a healthy balance. Too much magnesium without the proper amount of calcium may cause diarrhea in some people. Food sources include almonds, spinach, Swiss chard, sunflower seeds, halibut or mackerel, tofu, wheat bran, brown rice, avocados, and beans.

Calcium is essential for healthy bones and teeth, for muscle contraction, blood clotting, and the transmission of nerve impulses.

Potassium. When consumed daily, this mineral is effective in lowering high blood pressure and reducing the risk of stroke. Good food sources include beet greens, avocados, apricots, beans, potatoes, clams, yogurt, fish, orange juice, and bananas.

Selenium. Essential for normal growth and development, selenium's antioxidant effects complement those of vitamin E. Recent studies have found that selenium can prevent colon, lung, and prostate cancers. Generally speaking, selenium deficiencies are rare; most people can get enough through diet because so little of the nutrient is needed. Sources include whole grains, fish, oysters, poultry, brazil nuts, asparagus, garlic, mushrooms, and eggs.

Zinc. This mineral plays a critical role in immune system functioning, the repair of body tissue, and ability to taste and smell. Symptoms of minor deficiencies include loss of hair, appetite, and taste; slow healing of wounds; and fatigue. Too much zinc, however, can lead to impaired immune function and can cause nausea, headaches, poor muscle coordination, and other symptoms. Look to food to boost zinc levels, using a supplement only on a doctor's advice. Good food sources include eggs, cashews, almonds, soybeans, peanuts, cheese, oysters, poultry, crab, lean meats, and whole wheat breads.

Key to Abbreviations
IU—International Unit (a standardized measure for fat-soluble vitamins A, D, E)
mcg—microgram
mg—milligram

---

and spirit. In the early days of TCM, a family would retain the services of a physician, who was in charge of maintaining the health of the entire family for a monthly fee. If a family member became ill, it was considered a failure on the part of the physician, so he would treat the sick person free of charge.

The principles of Traditional Chinese Medicine have evolved over the millennia to explain the nature of the human organism. Two concepts are central to this healing system: balance and flow.

Two concepts are central to Traditional Chinese Medicine: balance and flow.

The practitioner helps the individual achieve internal balance as well as balance with the external environment. *Yin* and *yang* describe patterns and phenomena found in nature. They are opposing, yet complementary, forces (like the positive and negative forces of an electric current). They are not static, but rather, nurture and flow into one another. Each always contains an element of the other. Yin has the quality of the feminine and the water element. Its attributes are coldness, moistness, dimness, downward and inward movement, stillness, yielding, inhibition, slowness, and heaviness. Yang, on the other hand, has the quality of the masculine and the fire element. Its attributes are heat, dryness, brightness, upward and outward movement, lightness, activity, excitation, brightness, and rapidity.

Chi (also called *qi*) is the vital life-force that flows through all things, the energy that supports human growth and development. In the body, *chi* is channeled along a number of pathways called *meridians.* The meridians connect the different organ systems to each other and to the skin. When *chi* is flowing freely and in harmony, you remain healthy; when it is blocked or out of balance, illness results.

To restore health and prevent illness, the practitioner works to correct imbalances and reestablish the normal, healthy flow of energy throughout the body. Two of the chief practice methods of TCM, acupressure and acupuncture, seek to affect the flow of *chi* by stimulating specific points along the meridians.

A Traditional Chinese Medical practitioner relies on many symptom indicators and patterns to determine the landscape of a disease and to detect a state of excess or deficiency in the body. Diagnosis always involves close physical observation, which includes a reading of the pulse and an examination of the tongue.

To maintain well-being or treat imbalances, a TCM practitioner recommends ongoing modifications of lifestyle habits. As symptoms change, herbal formulas, dietary advice, acupressure and acupuncture treatments, fasting, massage *(tui na),* and exercise *(qi qong),* are adjusted accordingly.

To experience maximum benefit, it is important to seek out a qualified TCM practitioner. If you live in a large city with a substantial Asian population, you should be able to locate a TCM practitioner trained in China or Taiwan, or a board-certified practitioner trained at one of the programs accredited by the National Certification Commission for Acupuncture and Oriental Medicine (NCCAOM). If not, look for a medical doctor, osteopath, chiropractor, or licensed acupuncturist/herbalist who has at least 500 hours of training and who routinely applies this knowledge in clinical practice.

➤ *See the resource listings at the back of this book for drawings showing the body's energy meridians and acupoints.*

> *To restore health and prevent illness, the practitioner works to correct imbalances and reestablish the normal, healthy flow of energy throughout the body.*

Acupuncture One of the most powerful tools of Traditional Chinese Medicine, acupuncture treats certain disorders by inserting extremely fine stainless steel disposable needles into the skin at acupuncture points (often called *acupoints*). This is done to stimulate *chi,* the vital energy force that flows throughout the body. According to Traditional Chinese Medicine, when *chi* is out of balance, disease may set in.

Acupuncturists have identified more than 1000 acupuncture points in the human body. Some acupuncturists refer to *meridian points* of which there are more than 350 along 14 major meridians. During any given session, an acupuncturist may stimulate between 10 and 20 points. Generally, the needles are inserted just a fraction of an inch, but there are exceptions. The patient may feel a numbness or a slight tingling sensation at the insertion site, but no pain.

Acupuncturists have other ways to stimulate *chi* as well. Some use *moxibustion,* a Chinese herbal treatment in which cones of tightly bound smoldering mugwort *(Artemisia vulgaris)* leaves are attached to inserted needles. Others use the moxa cones without the needles. When used without needles,

Acupuncture influences the production of neurotransmitters —chemicals that transmit nerve impulses to the brain, changing our perception of pain.

the cones are placed directly on the skin at the acupuncture points and are allowed to burn down almost, but not quite, to the skin. Acupuncturists sometimes apply mild electrical current to the needles. Or they may use cupping to stimulate circulation or expel external cold, as when treating congestive lung conditions. To perform cupping, an acupuncturist heats the inside of a heavy glass cup with a candle to create a vacuum, then places the cup over the acupuncture point.

Acupuncture is known the world over as an effective treatment for many conditions. The World Health Organization (WHO) recognizes it for treating 43 common disorders, including asthma, food allergies, chronic diarrhea, constipation, premenstrual syndrome, sinusitis, bronchitis, hypertension, depression, anxiety, urinary stress incontinence, and nicotine addiction. In the United States, acupuncture has been so helpful in treating alcohol addiction that some state judiciary systems encourage its use in their detoxification programs.

Medical research has shown that acupuncture influences the production of neurotransmitters—chemicals that transmit nerve impulses to the brain, changing the brain's perception of pain. Because of its ability to relieve or block pain, acupuncture is used as a secondary anesthetic in 90 percent of head and neck surgeries performed in Bejing, China. Its primary use in the United States is pain reduction.

Throughout this country, acupuncture is an accredited masters degree level program recognized by the U.S. Department of Education. To locate a certified practitioner, call the American Association of Oriental Medicine, 888-500-7999.

For More Information
American Academy of Medical Acupuncture
5820 Wilshire Boulevard, Suite 500
Los Angeles, CA 90036
323-937-5514
www.medicalacupuncture.org

National Acupuncture and Oriental Medicine Alliance
14637 Starr Road, SE
Olalla, WA 98359
253-851-6896
www.acuall.org

Acupressure An easy, safe, noninvasive technique, acupressure falls within Traditional Chinese Medicine, along with acupuncture and Chinese herbal therapy. Acupressure is becoming increasingly popular in the West, even if the theory behind it isn't completely accepted by conventional practitioners of Western medicine.

According to Traditional Chinese Medicine, a network of energy pathways (called meridians) runs throughout the body, connecting the various organs. These pathways move *chi* (a vital life force that nourishes the body) and blood, regulate yin and yang (opposing yet complementary forces in the body), and moisten the joints and bones. When *chi* is out of balance, stagnant, or even overstimulated, disease can occur. An acupressure specialist seeks to interrupt and redirect out-of-kilter *chi*.

In actual practice, acupressure is simply applying finger, thumb, or hand pressure to acupressure points on the skin. These are also known as meridian points. There are 12 primary meridians—six that are associated with "yin" organs and six that are associated with "yang" organs. A network of fine capillaries extends from the primary meridians to connect every part of the body. The key to success is choosing the correct point or points to manipulate.

Acupressure can relieve a range of ailments, including everyday aches and soreness, such as backache, headache, neck pain, and sinus pain. It can also be effective in treating eyestrain, insomnia, constipation, motion sickness, and indigestion. Sports injuries often respond well to acupressure treatment.

With a little patience and a qualified instructor, many patients can learn to perform acupressure on themselves.

For More Information
American Association of Oriental Medicine
433 Front Street
Catasauqua, PA 18032
888-500-7999
www.aaom.org

Sports injuries often respond well to acupressure treatment.

Chinese Herbal Therapy Chinese herbal therapists make use of thousands of healing substances characterized by flavor (pungent, sour, sweet, bitter, and salty) and by four basic properties (hot, cold, warm, and cool) to help restore balance to the body's systems. Chinese herbs are usually prescribed in combinations of five to ten at a time and are generally prepared in soups or strong teas that are drunk at room temperature. Many herbs are also available in combination formulas, in pill form, as powders or tinctures, or as pastes that are applied to the skin. Like Western herbal remedies, Chinese herbal treatments call for patience as they take some time to work.

Caution: Chinese herbal medicine is not a "one-size-fits-all" therapy. The same cautions mentioned for Western herbal therapy (see page 18) apply to Chinese herbal therapy. Consult a trained herbalist or Chinese medical practitioner before taking any herbs. To avoid potentially serious interactions, it's important to tell all your healthcare providers about any prescription medicines and herbs you are taking.

➤ *For a list of common herbs and herbal formulas used in Traditional Chinese Medicine, see the resource listings at the back of this book.*

For More Information
American Association of Oriental Medicine
433 Front Street
Catasauqua, PA 18032
888-500-7999
www.aaom.org

National Certification Commission for
Acupuncture and Oriental Medicine
11 Canal Center Plaza, Suite 300
Alexandria, VA 22314
703-548-9004
www.nccaom.com

Yoga and Meditation

 Yoga Like Ayurveda, yoga has its roots in ancient India. Yet, while Ayurveda is considered the science of life, yoga is considered a science of self-discovery and for many people, a pathway to spiritual evolution. Although yoga is not a religion, practitioners generally strive to increase consciousness and practice mindful living.

Meditation is widely used to ease stress-related symptoms such as chronic pain, high blood pressure, panic, and headaches.

Patjanjali, one of the earliest scholars of yoga, identified eight "limbs" of classical yoga practice, beginning with two categories that describe essential ethical practices: restraints, or *yama* (nonviolence, truthfulness, not stealing, celibacy, and nonhoarding); and observances, or *niyama* (purity, contentment, tolerance, study, and remembrance). These are followed by physical exercises *(asana)*, breathing exercises *(pranayama)*, and withdrawal of the mind from the senses *(pratyahara)*. The classical practice of yoga involves all these techniques, although Westerners are most familiar with the physical exercises, or postures.

A well-rounded yoga routine involves body, breath, and mind in a balanced sequence of exercises, breathing techniques, and meditation. With regular practice you will see improvements in strength, flexibility, and emotional well-being, along with enhanced skills in concentration, relaxation, and stress management. Best results are obtained with daily practice, but yoga should never be forced or practiced to the point of pain.

Yoga has been shown to have a positive impact on many health problems. For example, regular yogic practice is a well-documented method for treating stress-related disorders. In addition, yoga exercises help maintain flexibility and strength, and are recommended for treating back, neck, and joint pain and stiffness. Some results pertaining to reducing elevated blood pressure and reversing heart disease have also been noted.

➤ *See the resource listings at the back of this book for drawings of some of the most common yoga poses, or asanas.*

For More Information
American Yoga Association
P.O. Box 19986
Sarasota, FL 34276-2986
941-927-4977
http://members.aol.com/amyogaassn

The Yoga Journal
2054 University Avenue
Berkeley, CA 94704
510-841-9200
www.yogajournal.com

Meditation Meditation, when practiced regularly, can bring a sense of peace and mindful living into daily life. It is a discipline that enhances mental control and relaxes the mind. Although the practice is used in Eastern cultures as a pathway to spiritual enlightenment, it has become widely accepted in many health systems for its ability to ease stress-related symptoms such as chronic pain, high blood pressure, panic, headaches, respiratory problems, insomnia, and premenstrual syndrome.

To do a simple meditation, first cleanse the breath with *pranayama* (see "Yoga," above). Then sit quietly and focus on a single thought, or a single sound, or on your breathing. Ignore all distractions and let your thoughts slip in and out of consciousness without judgment.

You can learn to meditate by using audiotapes and self-help books, but working with a trained instructor can help you develop your skills more quickly. Look for classes and workshops offered through hospitals, wellness centers, and continuing education programs.

For More Information
Insight Meditation Society
1030 Pleasant Street
Barre, MA 01005
978-355-4378
www.dharma.org

ABSCESS

Signs and Symptoms

- A localized pus-filled sore
- Possible swelling in the lymph glands closest to site of abscess
- Slight fever
- A general feeling of unwellness

Description

Though abscesses are most often thought of as occurring on the skin and gums, they can also develop in the tonsils, rectum, liver, lungs, brain, and between the outermost brain membrane and the bone of the spine or skull.

An abscess looks like a mound or a cyst. When a bacterial infection assaults a particular spot, tissue can be destroyed, causing a crater-like cavity.

Buying a Toothbrush

Using the right kind of toothbrush can help to prevent tooth decay that leads to abscesses. You should look for a soft or medium soft toothbrush with a small head that lets you get at every tooth. Stiff brushes often fail to clean crevices, and can even make gums bleed. Remember to change your toothbrush often—old brushes harbor bacteria and are ineffective when bent or frayed.

If you have a tendency toward gum disease or dental problems, ask your dentist if an electric toothbrush is right for you. These can often remove more plaque than regular toothbrushes, and may clean teeth more effectively below the gum line.

Health Notes

➤ *To prevent abscesses from developing, immediately clean and bandage all wounds.*

➤ *A daily diet high in the infection-fighter zinc and the antioxidant vitamins A, C, and E can help the body fight bacteria before the invaders have the chance to cause an abscess. See "Nutrition and Supplementation" in this entry for dosages.*

The body tries to ward off the infection with white blood cells, which congregate in the fresh crater—and continue congregating until there are so many of these white blood cells that the area becomes swollen.

Many abscesses occur at the site of an improperly treated minor wound—the perfect locale for invading bacteria to hunker down and set up operations. Other abscesses can occur after exposure to harmful bacteria that may lodge internally, causing an infection and abscess somewhere within the body.

Conventional Medical Treatment

If the abscess is accessible, your physician may lance it, drain the pus, irrigate the wound with saline, and pack it with gauze for 24 to 48 hours to absorb the discharge.

If the abscess has a diameter larger than 2 inches, is internal, or doesn't begin healing with the above measures, antibiotics are typically administered.

Complementary and Alternative Treatments

Nutrition and Supplementation

 Supplement your diet with nutrients that improve the immune system and fight infection. Zinc and vitamins A and C are preferred. Follow this daily supplementation guideline:

- zinc (30 mg in divided doses)
- vitamin A (100,000 IU for 5 days; decrease to 50,000 IU daily for 5 days, then to 25,000 IU daily; do not exceed 8000 IU daily if you are pregnant)
- vitamin C with bioflavonoids (5000 to 20,000 mg in divided doses)
- vitamin B complex (50 mg with food)
- vitamin E (400 to 600 IU) (Capsules can be opened and applied directly to the affected area.)
- garlic (as directed on label)

If you must take antibiotics, supplement with a prodophilus formula, following directions on label.

(For an *acute* condition, take supplements until your symptoms subside. If symptoms persist, seek the advice of your healthcare provider. For a *chronic* condition, consult your healthcare provider regarding the duration of treatment.)

Aromatherapy

 Tea tree oil makes a helpful antiseptic. To use it, place 4 drops in 1 cup water. Apply to the affected area 2 or 3 times daily. Other helpful essential oils, which can be used singularly or in combination, are lavender, bergamot, and German chamomile.

Herbal Therapy

 A number of herbs can be used for cleaning and healing an abscess. Try a strained and cooled decoction of burdock root. To make the decoction, boil 1 teaspoon of the root in 3 cups of water for 30 minutes; strain. Dip a clean cloth into the solution and place it on the affected area. Other helpful decoctions and infusions include dandelion root, red clover, and yellow dock root. Red clover and yellow dock can also be combined with the burdock.

Herbal products are available in health food stores and in some pharmacies and supermarkets. Follow package for specific directions.

If the abscess doesn't heal within a reasonable amount of time, or if it becomes larger or seriously inflamed, consult your doctor.

Homeopathy

 For an abscess caused by an imbedded foreign object, such as a splinter, a homeopathic practitioner may recommend *Silicea*, which helps bring an abscess to a head. Silicea also helps an open abscess drain. *Hepar sulph* can help the body re-absorb an abscess that's cold and very sensitive to touch. If an abscess doesn't heal in a reasonable amount of time, enlarges or deepens, or if the area around it reddens, consult your doctor.

Hydrotherapy

 To bring an abscess to a head, apply a poultice to the affected area. To speed healing and lessen pain, apply contrast therapy, alternating hot and cold cloths.

Traditional Chinese Medicine

 Chinese Herbal Therapy There are several Chinese herbs that can be used to cleanse an abscess and promote rapid healing.

Fresh garlic has long been heralded for its antiseptic and healing properties. Simply puree 3 to 5 fresh cloves and apply the poultice directly to the abscess for a few minutes, several times a day. Do not leave on too long, as it may burn the skin.

To temporarily relieve the pain of an infected tooth abscess, try *Liu Shen Wan* (Six Spirit Pills) or Bezoar Antidotal Tablets, which can be found at health food stores. Follow package directions.

ACNE

Signs and Symptoms

- Oily skin
- Enlarged pores
- Pus-filled or large, cyst-like pimples
- Whiteheads
- Blackheads

Description

Acne can range from mild—perhaps a few small pimples around the nose and chin—to severe—angry, red cyst-like nodules on the cheeks, jaw, and neck. While most people think of the condition as targeting just the face, acne is also common on the neck, back, shoulders, and buttocks.

Three out of four teens suffer from some grade of acne, from mild to severe. However, acne appears on people in all age groups. In fact, adult women make up a large portion of acne sufferers.

Contrary to popular belief, acne is not caused by eating fried food, drinking cola, or nibbling on chocolate. It occurs when sebum (a fatty secretion of the skin's sebaceous glands) and dead skin cells are manufactured faster than they can easily exit through the skin's pores. The trapped material solidifies into a plug of material that become stuck in the pore (also called the follicle). Blackheads, whiteheads, pimples, and acne cysts are all varying degrees of plugged pores.

So what causes the manufacture of sebum and dead skin cells to speed up? Hormones. Hormones are in abundance during adolescence: hence, the high incidence of teen acne. However, hormones are also present in birth control pills and increase during pregnancy and menstruation, explaining the acne many adult women suffer. While oily cosmetics and a pollution-filled environment don't cause acne per se, they do aggravate even the mildest condition, causing angrier-than-usual breakouts.

Conventional Medical Treatment

There are two directions conventional medicine takes to treat acne: topical and oral. Topical (on the skin) treatments are usually tried first. Frequently used treatments include tretinoin (Retin A®), azelaic acid (Azelex®), benzoyl peroxide preparations (such as Benzac® and Desquam-X®), glycolic or salicylic acid preparations (Stridex®), clindamycin, and erythromycin. Applied once or twice a day, they work to dry the skin, help the pores shed the trapped material through exfoliation, and kill the bacteria that can turn whiteheads or blackheads into cyst-like bumps or oozing pustules.

If the acne is especially severe, oral medication may be prescribed to shrink the lesions and make the skin less habitable to infection-causing bacteria. These medications include isoretinoin (Accutane®) and antibiotics such as tetracycline. Side effects, unfortunately, are common. Accutane® dries the body's mucous membranes (causing, for example, dry mouth) and causes severe birth defects when taken during pregnancy. Tetracycline

Keeping a Hygiene Journal

The teenage years are often emotionally turbulent, and acne, which occurs most often in teens, can have a detrimental impact on already shaky self-esteem. Hygiene is integral in treating and preventing acne pimples, and some teens may find it easier to evaluate their skin and regulate an appropriate cleaning schedule by keeping a journal. Over a period of one week, encourage your teenager to keep a record of how often he or she bathes and washes his or her face, making a note of any special products used.

Health Notes

➤ *To avoid exacerbating acne, keep your skin's contact with surfaces that may contain oil or traces of oil to a minimum. Wash makeup brushes and sponges twice a week in mild soap (such as dish soap or shampoo), change pillow cases twice a week, wipe the phone daily with facial toner on a cotton ball, and pull your hair off your face (especially if you use hair conditioners or styling products with conditioning ingredients).*

➤ *Use tepid water and a mild soap to wash away dirt and makeup upon waking, before and after physical exertion, and before going to bed.*

➤ *Refrain from touching skin and picking pimples and blackheads—both habits spread acne-aggravating bacteria. Picking at acne can literally create a mountain out of a molehill.*

➤ *Drink 8 to 12 8-ounce glasses of water per day to flush toxins from the body.*

➤ *A nutritious daily menu of whole grains, five servings of fruit/vegetables, and adequate levels of infection-fighting nutrients, such as anti-oxidants and zinc, can help fight bacterial invaders.*

➤ *Because caffeine is a stimulant, it increases oil production in some individuals. If you suffer from acne, it's best to limit yourself to one cup of coffee or tea a day.*

should not be used during pregnancy because it can cause permanent discoloration of the child's teeth. Some newer contraceptive pills, such as Ortho Tri-Cyclen®, can also improve acne.

Regardless of which medical course is prescribed, most physicians recommend washing skin with a mild soap twice a day, wearing an oil-free sunscreen, and avoiding scrubbing, touching, or picking pimples, and using hot water on your skin. To keep the pores plug-free, some dermatologists will perform *extractions* (a procedure to squeeze the blocked material out of the skin) in their offices; others recommend a trip to the *esthetician*—a medically-trained skin care specialist—once or twice a month.

For More Information
The American Academy of Dermatology
930 North Meacham Road
Schaumberg, IL 60173
888-462-DERM
www.aad.org

Complementary and Alternative Treatments

Nutrition and Supplementation

 If a body contains more toxins than the kidneys and liver can eliminate, the skin's job is to "sweat" them out. When this happens, the integrity of the skin is compromised and skin disorders occur. A high-fiber diet helps keep the colon clean so it can assist in ridding the body of toxins before the skin has to take over. Avoid all forms of sugar as well as processed foods and iodized salt. Make sure your acne is not a result of an allergy by eliminating all dairy products from your diet for one month and monitoring any improvements in your skin. Eat foods rich in zinc, such as soybeans, whole grains, and sunflower seeds. Zinc is a necessary component in the oil-producing glands of the skin. It heals the infected tissue and prevents scarring.

In addition, the following daily supplements are helpful:

Most Important

• vitamin B complex (100 mg 3 times daily)—helps maintains healthy skin tone

• zinc (30 mg; do not exceed 100 mg total)—aids in healing tissue, helps prevent scarring

- essential fatty acids, such as flaxseed oil and primrose oil (as directed on label)—helps to repair damaged skin cells and dissolve fatty deposits that block pores

- chromium picolinate (as directed on label)—helps reduce skin infections

Also Recommended

- selenium (100 to 200 mcg)—fights infection

- vitamin C (1000 mg)—essential for the formation of collagen

- a prodophilus formula (as directed on label)—replaces "friendly" bacteria

- potassium (99 mg)—a deficiency has been associated with acne

- vitamin A (25,000 IU until healed, then reduce to 5000 IU daily; do not exceed 8000 IU daily if you are pregnant)—strengthens the skin tissue

- N-acetyl cysteine (600 mg)

(For an *acute* condition, take supplements until your symptoms subside. If symptoms persist, seek the advice of your healthcare provider. For a *chronic* condition, consult your healthcare provider regarding the duration of treatment.)

Aromatherapy

To fight infection and dry blemishes, apply 1 drop of tea tree oil directly to acne spots, as needed.

Ayurvedic

Ayurveda considers acne a pitta condition, so practitioners recommend following a pitta-pacifying diet, which favors bland foods, such as applesauce, oatmeal, and rice, to help combat breakouts. Some Ayurvedic practitioners may also suggest applying one of the following mixtures to reduce oiliness and speed drying: a turmeric-sandalwood paste, a turmeric-sandalwood cream, a chickpea flour paste, or a ground almond paste. Still others may advise drinking a cumin-coriander tea or aloe vera juice.

Bodywork and Somatic Practices

To provide good lymph and blood circulation, massage may help. (Avoid massage if there are rashes, open cuts, or sores.) CranioSacral Therapy rids the body of stress, strengthens the immune system, and balances fluid and energy flow throughout the body. However, best results come from addressing the body holistically, as in a variety of Oriental bodywork therapies, reflexology, or Reiki. Therapeutic Touch lowers inflammation and irritability and allows the body to heal more swiftly.

Herbal Therapy

Acne often responds favorably to a tincture of equal parts sarsaparilla, burdock, and cleavers. Take ½ teaspoon of the mixture several times daily. You can also try washing the affected area with a calendula-witch hazel solution. To make the solution, steep 1 ounce dried calendula in 2 cups boiling water for 10 minutes; strain and cool to room temperature. Mix with an equal amount of distilled witch hazel.

Some people find that taking capsules of currant seed oil or evening primrose oil (500 mg several times daily) can help clear the condition. Other useful herbs include alfalfa, echinacea, and yellow dock root. Herbal products are available in health food stores and in some pharmacies and supermarkets. Follow package for specific directions.

Homeopathy

Acne may respond to homeopathic treatment. However, the selection of a remedy—more than one is available—depends on *your* symptoms and the stage of the condition. Don't try treating this disorder yourself. See a homeopathic professional.

Hydrotherapy

Contrast applications (alternating hot and cold cloths) can help improve circulation and heal blemishes; apply daily. Remember to drink lots of water to flush toxins from your system.

In addition, try steam treatment. Steam helps open and cleanse pores, and thereby, often lessens blemishes. Simply fill a basin or large bowl with plenty of boiling water. Place a large towel over your head to trap the steam, and stand or sit with your head about a foot above the steaming water. Afterward, wash gently with a mild soap. *Note:* In some cases, steam may worsen the condition.

Traditional Chinese Medicine

Acupuncture There are more than 120 acupuncture points located in each ear. An acupuncturist may treat breakouts by manipulating the lung, internal secretion, testicle, and cheek points in and around the ear.

Additionally, since Chinese medical practitioners believe that there is a direct correlation between lung function and healthy skin, an acupuncturist may treat acne via the lung or large intestine meridians and via the liver/gallbladder to address any imbalance that is causing hormonal problems.

Acupressure Because acne is sometimes associated with an unhealthy diet or gastrointestinal problems, it can be treated by pressing the massage points located in the abdominal region, which will stimulate digestion and regulate bowel functions.

Some acupressurists may also treat skin disorders by massaging the stomach meridian located on the upper cheeks (just below the eye sockets), along with the gastrointestinal points found on the outer thighs and on the soles of the feet.

Chinese Herbal Therapy To bring blemishes to a head, apply a hot poultice made from a burdock infusion to the affected area twice a day. The undiluted juice from a fresh aloe vera leaf can be applied directly to the blemish to soothe and speed healing.

A decoction of 2 to 8 grams of powdered licorice can be used as a healing astringent wash. Simply apply to the affected area and leave it on for 5 minutes before rinsing with water *(do not use soap);* repeat up to 3 times a day, as needed.

Acne sufferers can also try these pre-made remedies: *Shi Wei Bai Du Tang* (Bupleurum and Schizonepeta Formula), Plum Flower's Margarite Acne Pills, or *Qing Zang Fan Gen Tang Jai Yi Yi Jen* (Ledebouriella and Coix Combination). All are available in health food stores; follow package directions.

Yoga and Meditation

Yoga can help fight acne in a variety of ways: by improving circulation, bringing nutrients to the skin, flushing away toxins, and releasing stress. Try these poses in a daily routine: Standing Sun, Knee Squeeze, Child, Cobra, Lion, and Moon Salutation.

ADENOID CONDITIONS

Signs and Symptoms

The following symptoms are present individually and in combination in some cases.

- Cough
- Restlessness
- Headache
- Impaired sense of smell

- Impaired sense of taste
- Mouth breathing
- Sleep apnea
- Snoring
- Nasal voice
- Earache
- Slight temporary hearing loss
- A feeling of fullness in the ear

Description

Like their better-known cousins, the tonsils, adenoids are lymph nodes of the throat. Unlike the tonsils, which are found in the back of the mouth, the adenoids are located at the top of the throat. Their job (like that of the tonsils) is to filter infectious organisms from the body. An interesting fact about adenoids is that they are present at birth and grow until a few years before puberty, when they reverse their course and start to shrink. By the onset of puberty, the adenoids have diminished to the point where they are just barely visible. They stay this size for life. What does all this mean? That adenoid problems generally affect young children.

In some children, the adenoids become infected—not just once, but chronically in an on-and-off fashion. In fewer children—usually older children—the adenoids don't shrink as they should, but instead continue to grow until they've entered the eustachian (auditory) tube, interfering with hearing. It's not known why some children have problems with their adenoids, though heredity

Health Note

➤ *A nutrient-dense diet, moderate exercise, and regular sleep can keep the immune system strong enough to fight off infectious organisms.*

and weak immune systems are believed to play a role.

Conventional Medical Treatment

To diagnose an adenoid condition, a physician notes the symptoms and physically examines the area. If a mild infection is present, antibiotics may be prescribed. If the adenoids are chronically infected or have grown into the eustachian tube, an *adenoidectomy* (an operation in which the adenoids are removed) may be necessary. Be aware that even after being removed, adenoids can grow back, although the "re-grown" glands rarely present a problem.

Complementary and Alternative Treatments

Nutrition and Supplementation

To treat adenoid problems, nutritionists recommend a diet to decongest the lymph nodes; this will reduce adenoid swelling and strengthen immunity. Hot green or black tea with lemon is beneficial, since teas contain anti-viral tannins. Raw chopped garlic in chicken broth is also good for treating adenoid problems.

The following supplements can be taken to treat adenoid conditions:

- vitamin C (1000 mg)
- zinc, 1 15-mg. lozenge, twice daily
- vitamin B_6 (50 mg)
- vitamin A (25,000 IU for one week, then decrease dosage to 10,000 IU; do not exceed 8000 IU if you are pregnant)
- vitamin E (400 IU)

(For an *acute* condition, take supplements until your symptoms subside. If symptoms persist, seek the advice of your healthcare provider. For a *chronic* condition, consult your healthcare provider regarding the duration of treatment.)

Chiropractic

The chiropractor typically finds subluxations in the cervical section of the spine (upper neck) and performs specific chiropractic adjustments (SCAs) to correct the problem. Chiropractic work on people who suffer from adenoid conditions can help eliminate nerve interference and allow the natural healing process to occur.

Homeopathy

Adenoid disorders may respond to homeopathic treatment. However, the selection of a remedy—more than one is available—depends on *your* symptoms and the stage of the condition. Don't try treating this disorder yourself. See a homeopathic professional.

Traditional Chinese Medicine

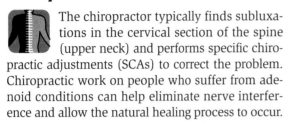

Acupuncture Acupuncture can be used to strengthen the immune system, which can, in turn, help prevent adenoid problems from developing. It can also be used to help alleviate the inflammation of infected adenoid glands.

Acupressure If swollen adenoids cause a sore throat, a practitioner may use acupressure to relieve the pain by manipulating the Stomach point 9 (located on the throat), Lung point 11 (on the thumb), and Large Intestine point 4 (which lies beneath the thumb and index finger).

Chinese Herbal Therapy *Liu Shen Wan* (Six Spirit Pills) may be taken to help alleviate the pain and swelling associated with inflamed adenoids. Follow the directions on the package, especially when administering the medication to children. To boost general immunity, garlic capsules can be purchased in health food stores and offer many of the same preventative and curative benefits of raw garlic, without the overpowering aroma. Follow package instructions. Propolis tincture also works well.

AGE SPOTS

Signs and Symptoms

- Flat, sharply demarcated patches of increased pigmentation that are usually brown in color
- Found most often on forearms, hands, and face, though they can be anywhere on the body that has been exposed to sunlight

Description

Age spots—also known as liver spots, *chloasma*, moth patches, or hyperpigmentation—are deposits of excess melanin that range from the size of a freckle to a few inches across. Usually seen in clusters, age spots can become large enough to arch over the length of the upper lip or can appear as large tracts of pigmented areas on the arms.

Although some people call them liver spots, these pigmented patches have nothing to do with the liver. Ultraviolet light and the body's melanin-producing melanocytes are actually responsible for age spots. Think of the melanocytes as factories that churn out melanin—the pigment that gives color to the hair and skin. Ultraviolet light is the energy that fuels the factories. Exposure to sunlight causes the melanocytes to produce increased amounts of pigmentation, resulting in darkened areas of skin (suntan, for example). Age

Trouble Spots

Generally, you should keep an eye out for patches that are scaly and gray, rather than brown. These patches, caused by overexposure to the sun, are called *keratoses,* and unlike the benign age spots, these *can* occasionally develop into cancer. If you think you've noticed any such marks, it is best to have them checked by your physician.

spots are a result of a lifetime of exposure to ultraviolet rays, though they normally do not appear until the third or fourth decade of life.

While both sexes get age spots, women are more prone to developing pigmented spots on their faces because female hormones heighten the effects of ultraviolet rays on the melanocytes. This is why pregnant women or those on birth control pills sometimes develop an overall mask or large facial patches of hyperpigmented skin, known as either chloasma or the mask of pregnancy.

While age spots may bother people aesthetically, they are medically insignificant. They never become cancerous.

Conventional Medical Treatment

Dermatologists are the conventional medical expert of choice to treat hyperpigmentation. Dermatologists often recommend two daily applications of a solution containing hydroquinone, a bleaching agent derived from the quinine plant, which is the standard treatment to break up melanin deposits in the skin. Retinoic acid, glycolic acid, and/or azelaic acid are often used in conjunction with hydroquinone to boost hydroquinone's penetration, resulting in a stronger lightening effect.

Bleaching hyperpigmented areas can be very difficult. The more chronic the sun damage, the longer it takes to see results. While some see improvement within a month of treatment, others don't see improvement for close to a year. Some people never see a total disappearance of pigmented areas after using the above formulas. If the pigmentation doesn't respond to any of these treatments, your dermatologist may remove age spots by freezing them with liquid nitrogen *(cryotherapy).*

Whatever therapy you choose, use sunblock and avoid the sun religiously if you don't want the spots to re-darken. While dermatological treatments lighten hyperpigmentation, they don't shut down the factory that causes the condition. In other words, supply the melanocytes with fuel (sun's rays) and they will once again crank up their output of melanin—and the pigment will return.

For More Information
The American Academy of Dermatology
930 North Meacham Road
Schaumberg, IL 60173
888-462-DERM
www.aad.org

Health Notes

➤ *Ultraviolet light is in the air when it snows, when the fog rolls in, when it rains—some even gets through glass windows. That means every morning—regardless of the weather, regardless of whether you'll be going outside—apply a sunblock with an effective UVA/UVB blocker. Look for a product with a Sun Protection Factor (SPF) of 15 or higher and check the ingredient label for zinc oxide or Parsol 1789, also known as avobenzone. These two sunblocking ingredients are the strongest currently available. Don't forget to reapply the sunblock after doing dishes, washing hands, or sweating.*

➤ *To lighten already existing age spots, try a dab of lemon juice or a commercial skin-bleaching cream.*

Complementary and Alternative Treatments

Nutrition and Supplementation

 Age spots are the result of a buildup of wastes caused by free radical damage in skin cells. Follow a fasting program to rid the body of toxins and cleanse the liver. Your diet should consist of 50 percent organically grown raw fruits and vegetables as well as grains, cereals, seeds, and nuts. Try to get most of your protein from vegetables, and totally eliminate animal protein from your diet for one month. Because age spots indicate that cells are full of accumulated wastes, it's a good idea to avoid sugar, saturated fats, red meat, processed foods, caffeine, and tobacco.

The following daily supplements may improve your condition:

Most Important

- vitamin B complex (100 mg 3 times daily)— helps older people assimilate of all nutrients

- vitamin C with bioflavonoids (3000 to 6000 mg, in divided doses)—an antioxidant and free radical scavenger

- *Lactobacillus bulgaricus* (as directed on label)—aids in liver regeneration and digestion

- pantothenic acid (50 mg 3 times daily)— boosts proper functioning of adrenal glands

- zinc (30 mg)

Also Recommended

- selenium (200 mcg)

- glutathione or N-acetyl cysteine (200 mg of either)

- vitamin B_5 (pantothenic acid) (50 mg 3 times daily)—supports adrenal gland function

- lecithin (1200 mg 3 times daily)—essential for healthy cell membranes

- L-carnitine (as directed on label)—assists in removing fat from the body

- superoxide dismutase (SOD) (as directed on label)—strong antioxidants

- vitamin A (5,000 IU; do not exceed 8,000 IU if you are pregnant)

(Consult your healthcare provider regarding the duration of treatment.)

Traditional Chinese Medicine

 Chinese Herbal Therapy Ginseng tablets are thought to have many restorative benefits and can be used to combat age spots; take one 3-gram tablet twice daily on an empty stomach. Another useful herb is *Ho Shou Wu,* which is available in pill form.

AIDS

Signs and Symptoms

A combination of any of the following:

- Constant unexplained fatigue
- Unexplained rashes
- Swollen lymph nodes
- Body aches
- Unexplained weight loss
- Easy bruising
- Shortness of breath
- Night sweats
- Ongoing, low-grade fever

- Persistent diarrhea
- Persistent cough
- Sore throat
- Oral yeast infection
- Purplish or grayish Kaposi's sarcoma lesions on the skin or inside the mouth
- Susceptibility to common illnesses, such as colds and pneumonia
- Susceptibility to sexually transmitted disease, such as syphilis
- Cancers, such as cervical cancer, non-Hodgkin's lymphoma, or primary brain lymphoma
- Susceptibility to skin conditions, such as seborrhea dermatitis, alopecia, herpes simplex, or herpes zoster
- Confusion

Description

Acquired Immune Deficiency Syndrome (AIDS) is caused by the human immunodeficiency virus (HIV) which can live in human blood, plasma, breast milk, semen, and vaginal secretions. The virus can be transmitted in a number of ways:

- via a blood transfusion of AIDS-tainted blood
- by direct contact between AIDS-infected blood and an opening in the skin (either an existing cut, torn cuticle, or other wound)
- by a prick from a needle that is tainted with AIDS-infected blood
- being born to a mother who has AIDS
- being breastfed by a mother who has AIDS
- by the exchange of fluids during oral, vaginal, or anal intercourse
- by artificial insemination from an infected donor

The virus has also been found in sweat, saliva and tears, though in such low concentrations that scientists believe these don't represent a transmission risk.

AIDS attacks the immune system, lowering the body's ability to prevent and fight opportunistic illnesses, such as pneumonia, yeast infections, tuberculosis, toxoplasmosis, cancers, and the common cold. In the end, it isn't AIDS that kills a person, it's one of these opportunistic illnesses that the body is unable to fight.

Approximately one to two months after being infected with HIV, a person may come down with what appears to be a cold, the flu, or mononucleosis, often accompanied by a rash. Lasting from one to three weeks, this "cold" occurs when the body attempts to fight the virus by creating antibodies. After this, the individual may immediately develop full-blown AIDS. However, the more common scenario is that two to 13 years pass after this strange "cold" occurs before full-blown AIDS appears. On average, an individual with full-blown AIDS lives only two to three years.

Conventional Medical Treatment

At this time, there is neither a cure for AIDS, nor a vaccine to prevent one from getting the disease. A blood test can confirm the presence of HIV within the body. The accepted medical course of treatment includes treating individual symptoms and infections as they arise, and administering medications that boost the immune system's ability to function. One of the most well-known of these drugs is azidothymidine (AZT).

There are strains of HIV, however, that are resistant to AZT. In these cases, saquinavir, ritonair, indinavir, or nelfinavir—or a combination of the four—are prescribed. Called protease inhibitors, these viral enzymes are thought to lessen HIV's potency. Because the virus can build a resistance to protease inhibitors, they are often used in combination (called "drug cocktails") or are alternated. In advanced stages of AIDS, protease inhibitors are also used in combination with AZT to improve immune system function.

Of course, we know much more about preventing AIDS than we do about curing it. See the tips throughout this entry for proven strategies.

For More Information
AIDS Action Committee
131 Clarendon Street
Boston, MA 02116
800-235-2331
TTY: 617-450-1427
www.aac.org

AIDS Clinical Trials Information Services
800-874-2572

American Foundation for AIDS Research (AMFAR)
120 Wall Street, 13th Floor
New York, NY 10005
212-806-1600
www.amfar.org

Bastyr University AIDS Research Center
14500 Juanita Drive, NE
Kenmore, WA 98028
425-602-3172
www.bastyr.edu/research

Gay Men's Health Crisis (GMHC)
119 W 24th Street
New York, NY 10011-3629
212-807-6664
www.gmhc.org

National Association of People With AIDS (NAPWA)
1413 K Street, NW, 7th Floor
Washington, DC 20005
202-898-0414
www.napwa.org

Complementary and Alternative Treatments

Nutrition and Supplementation

 One of the greatest threats to the AIDS patient is malnutrition and muscle wasting. Nutritional requirements increase, but many patients have lower appetites and increased difficulty in digesting food. Your healthcare provider can determine whether you are malabsorbing nutrients by conducting a comprehensive digestive stool analysis. In people with severely compromised immune systems, high-quality nutrition is key. Focus on the quality, rather than the quantity, of food consumed; but do note that in this case it is better to choose non-organic foods, as they will contain less bacteria, which is important considering the poor immune function of people with AIDS.

To minimize muscle wasting, eat a high-calorie diet and aim to obtain 40 percent of your calorie intake from high-quality protein sources, concentrating on lamb, fish, chicken, and eggs (ensure they are non-organic and cook them well to avoid bacterial contamination). Milkshakes provide a protein-rich drink, and skim milk powder can be stirred into foods such as casseroles, desserts, and sauces to add extra protein. Ask your healthcare provider about high-protein supplement drinks to boost your protein and calorie intake.

Increase your intake of fresh fruits and vegetables. Eat unripened papaya and fresh pineapple often; these supply enzymes that provide the body with energy. Oriental mushrooms (shiitake and maitake) boost the immune system, and shiitake mushrooms contain lentinan, which helps fight viruses. Garlic contains protein, vitamins A and C, thiamine, calcium, potassium, copper, and selenium. It also provides allicin, an anti-bacterial and anti-viral agent. Garlic works best when taken raw. Sea vegetables, such as kombu, nori, and dulse, contain minerals not found in foods grown on land. Dulse removes radiation from the body.

Freshly-made juice can be an important source of concentrated nutrients, antioxidants, and raw enzymes, which help the body digest foods. One AIDS researcher suggests this juice recipe for strengthening the immune system, increasing energy, and flushing the liver and lymphatic system: Wash a whole organic lemon, cut into quarters, and puree in a blender. Add 1 cup water and 1 tablespoon cold-pressed, extra virgin olive, oil. Sweeten, if desired, with a few tablespoons of fresh organic orange juice. Blend, strain, and drink. A daily intake of this juice can raise T-cell counts and decrease viral load.

Foods to avoid include junk foods, peanuts, sugar and sugar products, and anything containing caffeine. Limit your consumption of soy products, which contain enzyme inhibitors, but do not eliminate them completely, as they are a good source of protein. Increase calorie consumption by eating avocados, nut butters, almonds, and sunflower seeds.

The list of nutritional deficiencies is endless. Only a specialist can tell you what nutritional supplementation is ideal for you. The following daily list is not all-inclusive, but it will give you a good start.

- vitamin C with bioflavonoids (10,000 to 20,000 mg in divided doses)—builds immunity and protects against secondary infections. Take in buffered form to protect the stomach

- vitamin B_6 (100 mg) builds red blood cells and activates natural killer cells

- mixed carotenoid formula (as directed by healthcare provider)—increases T-cell numbers, which protects against infections (The body converts carotenoids into vitamin A, but it's safer in large doses than vitamin A.)

- a prodophilus formula (as directed on label 3 times daily)—supplies friendly bacteria for liver and intestinal tract function; also fights candida infection, often associated with HIV

- bovine colostrum (as directed on label)—controls AIDS-related diarrhea

- coenzyme Q10 (100 mg) circulation and energy; stimulates the immune system

- zinc (30 mg)—crucial for tissue repair

- lipoic acid (200 mg)—strong antioxidant

- colloidal silver (as directed on label)—promotes healing of skin lesions

- shark cartilage (as directed on label)—inhibits tumor growth (Use 100 percent pure dried shark cartilage.)

- egg lecithin (20 g in divided doses on empty stomach)—protects cells

- glutathione (as directed on label, on empty stomach)—inhibits the formation of free radicals; protects immune cells

- grape seed extract (as directed on label)—a powerful antioxidant that protects the cells

- raw thymus glandular (as directed on label)—enhances T-cell production

- selenium (200 mcg)—free radical scavenger that enhances the immune system

(Consult your healthcare provider regarding the duration of treatment.)

Aromatherapy

Aromatherapy may be used to help support the immune system and combined with massage to relax and soothe sore muscles. Essential oils to try include tea tree, lavender, oregano, and thyme (linalol).

Bodywork and Somatic Practices

Depending on the level of health and stamina, choose modalities that are very gentle for those who are frail (Therapeutic Touch, Reiki, CranioSacral Therapy, and polarity therapy). If the person is well enough to go to an office setting to receive work, then most other complementary therapies will comfort, and possibly help in supporting immune system function.

Herbal Therapy

Numerous herbs currently being studied for their strong anti-bacterial and anti-viral properties have possible benefits in treating AIDS. Those most commonly used now include astragalus, echinacea, licorice, goldenseal, garlic, reishi, and St. John's wort.

Herbal products are available in health food stores and in some pharmacies and supermarkets. Follow package for specific directions.

Remember to consult your doctor before embarking on any new regimen; proper care is extremely important.

Traditional Chinese Medicine

Acupuncture Numerous scientific studies have demonstrated that acupuncture is highly beneficial in the treatment of AIDS and HIV, largely by reducing stress and strengthening the body's immune system. In addition, acupuncture has been shown to dramatically reduce AIDS-related night sweats, fatigue, diarrhea, and skin problems in as few as four to six treatments.

Acupuncture has also been shown to improve AIDS sufferers' T-cell counts. A new treatment in which homeopathic remedies are injected into acupuncture points is now under investigation. Acupuncture sessions aimed at treating AIDS and HIV generally last about 45 minutes. Disposable, pre-sterilized needles are used to protect both the acupuncturist and the client.

Acupressure Acupressure can be used to treat AIDS-related symptoms, such as fatigue (the practitioner will work specific kidney, lung, large intestine, stomach, and conception vessel points) and diarrhea (in which stomach, spleen, and large intestine points are massaged). It can also be used to relieve stress, which may exacerbate the disease. Care must be taken not to use too much pressure during the massage, so as not to over-stimulate the immune-suppressing adrenal gland.

Chinese Herbal Therapy AIDS can be treated with a variety of Chinese herbal therapies, including The Duke of Chou's Centenarian Liquor, which boosts overall immunity, and Vermilion Elixir Wine, which nourishes the blood, brings the internal organs into harmony, and improves vitality. Both of these preparations contain more than 15 different ingredients and should be prepared and administered by a qualified herbalist following diagnosis by a TCM practitioner.

Perhaps the best known Chinese herbal immune deficiency remedy is astragalus, which works by reducing perspiration and fatigue and increasing overall energy. Astragalus is also thought to inhibit the spread of HIV, and studies have shown that it reduces the number of T-suppressor cells in AIDS patients. Take a decoction of 4 to 6 grams twice a day on an empty stomach. You can also make a liquor by steeping 80 to 100 grams of the sliced astragalus root in 1 liter of spirits for 2 to 3 months. Take 1 ounce of this preparation twice a day on an empty stomach (dilute each dose with 1 to 2 ounces of water if it's too strong). Astragalus's immune-boosting properties are heightened when it's combined with ginseng, angelica, licorice, and schisandra. To improve the flow of *chi* and restore energy balance, try Astragalus Combination, which is available at health food stores.

Recent studies have also indicated that extracts or decoctions of bitter melon may be useful in helping to raise HIV-impaired T-cell counts (although it can take up to six months of treatment to see results).

Yoga and Meditation

There are several yoga poses that help boost the immune system. These include the Shoulder Stand, Cobra, Locust, Bow, and various twisting poses. Meditation is an excellent way to cope with stress and counteract negative emotions. The breathing exercise Breath of Fire is also helpful.

ALCOHOL ABUSE

Signs and Symptoms

- Tendency to drink too much alcohol in one sitting

- Drinking daily, particularly during the day

- Desire to continue drinking even after others have said you've had too much

- Preoccupation with recreational drinking

- Denial that you drink too much

- Irritation and/or arguing with friends and family who express concern about the amount you drink

- Underestimating or lying to friends and family about the amount you drink

- Drinking—even one or two beers or glasses of wine—when alone

- Drinking to help induce relaxation, relieve pains, or put oneself to sleep

- Regret over words said or actions performed while drinking

- Repeated unsuccessful attempts to reduce the amount you drink or stop altogether

- Feelings of guilt about the amount you drink

- Increased susceptibility to anxiety, depression, and/or insomnia

- Severe mood swings

- Loss of memory and/or concentration

- Blackouts (in some cases) or inability to remember what happened the night before

- The inability to remember what happened the night before, even though you didn't black out (in some cases)

- Unpredictable and inappropriate behavior, such as anger, hostility, or irritability

- Driving accidents or arrests while under the influence of alcohol (in some cases)

- Employment problems, including tardiness, absenteeism, low productivity and/or interpersonal problems (in some cases)

- Hand tremors upon waking (in some cases)

Description

Alcohol abuse, alcoholism, alcohol dependency, alcohol addiction—all describe a condition in which a person drinks too much. "Too much" may seem like a subjective term, but according to experts the precise number of drinks means very little, since different people become tipsy after drinking different amounts. What matters is that

Are You Addicted to Alcohol?

Even if you don't think you drink too much, answer the following questions (called the CAGE questionnaire) to assess whether you may have a drinking problem:

1. Have you ever felt that you should **C**ut down on your drinking?

2. Have you ever been **A**nnoyed by people telling you that you should cut down or quit drinking?

3. Do you ever feel **G**uilty about your drinking?

4. Have you ever had a drink as an "**E**ye opener" first thing in the morning to relieve the shakes?

If you answered "yes" to any of these questions, this could indicate an alcohol problem.

Source: Mayfiled, D., McLeod, G., Hall, P., "The CAGE Questionnaire: Validation of a New Screening Instrument," *American Journal of Psychiatry* 131:1121-1123, 1974.

Health Notes

➤ *If you have a parent or other family members who are or were dependent on alcohol, there's an increased chance that you will have the same tendency. Be careful about the amount you drink or avoid alcohol altogether.*

➤ *If you are unable to get through a week without drinking more nights than not, or if you can't (or don't) stop at just one drink, immediately seek help from your local chapter of Alcoholics Anonymous or a trained psychotherapist before your dependency grows stronger.*

a person has difficulty letting a day go by without consuming alcohol.

While the precise cause of alcoholism is not known, researchers have determined that there is a genetic disposition toward alcohol dependency and that the condition affects more men than women. A common scenario involves someone whose mother or father was "a heavy drinker." When that person becomes an adult, he or she discovers that having a couple glasses of wine or beer with dinner reduce the day's stress. Even though such drinking doesn't change life circumstances or results in a hangover, this person continues drinking. Over time, two beers becomes a six pack, which becomes a night filled with drinking, and so on. This drinking can affect relationships and short-term as well as long-term health. If the person drives, there may be accidents or brushes with the law. It's a vicious cycle, and to cope with the new stresses being caused by alcohol consumption, the person may begin drinking during the day as well.

Conventional Medical Treatment

If you suspect that you or someone you care about is abusing alcohol, a visit with a physician is a smart idea. While medical treatment isn't normally used to treat alcoholism per se, it is necessary to discover whether one's health has in some way been damaged—for instance, if drinking has caused a vitamin deficiency or cirrhosis of the liver. To treat the alcoholism itself, your physician may recommend psychotherapy and/or group therapy, and in severe cases, an inpatient detox rehabilitation facility. The most well-known therapy group for alcoholics is Alcoholics Anonymous, or AA. In AA, you are asked to attend weekly, twice-weekly, or even nightly meetings, depending on how much help you need. During the meetings, you report your progress, talk about what problems and emotions you are facing, and listen to others do the same. In turn, group members offer advice, wisdom, and support. In addition to group help, the organization asks that you eradicate all forms of alcohol from your life, since most alcoholics are unable to stop at just one or two glasses of wine. (Support groups, such as Al-Anon, are available for friends and family members of alcoholics as well.)

In severe cases, some physicians may treat an alcoholic with the drug disulfram, which in some people lessens the desire to drink. The side effects of this drug, however, can be as unpleasant as a hangover: nausea, vomiting, headache, loss of mental acuity, and gastric distress.

For More Information

Al-Anon Family Group Headquarters, Inc.
1600 Corporate Landing Parkway
Virginia Beach, VA 23454-5617
800-4AL-ANON
www.al-anon.org

Alcoholic Anonymous Headquarters
P.O. Box 459, Grand Central Station
New York, NY 10163
212-870-3400
www.aa.org

National Council on Alcoholism and Drug Dependence
12 West 21st Street
New York, NY 10010
800-622-2255
www.ncadd.org

National Institute on Alcohol Abuse and
Alcoholism
6000 Executive Boulevard, Willco Building
Bethesda, MD 20892-7003
301-443-3860
www.niaaa.nih.gov

Individuals who wish to help address the
dangers of drunk driving can contact:
MADD (Mothers Against Drunk Driving)
PO Box 541688
Dallas, TX 75354
800-438-MADD
www.madd.org

Complementary and Alternative Treatments

Nutrition and Supplementation

 The best starting point is to consult a
nutritionally-oriented doctor who can
assess your specific nutritional needs,
for example, by conducting a functional liver
detoxification profile. However, there are general
problems that arise from alcohol abuse that you
can begin treating on your own. Eat a whole-foods
diet containing plenty of raw fruits and vegetables, whole grains, and legumes. As muscle wasting is often a problem, aim to obtain about 40
percent of calories from protein. Eliminate fried
foods and saturated fat from your diet. These foods
place undue stress on your liver, the organ that
has already suffered the most. Above all else,
avoid *all* alcohol.

Because alcohol abuse damages every cell in
the body and compromises the immune system,
alcoholics need to supplement *all* the known vitamins and minerals. The following daily guideline
is a good place to start; consult a healthcare provider to tailor a supplementation program to your
particular needs.

Most Important

- free-form amino acid complex (500 mg 3
  times daily on empty stomach)—for brain and
  liver function

- N-acetyl cysteine (500 mg, working up to 1000
  mg daily)—for regeneration of liver cells

- glutathione (650 mg)

- vitamin B complex injections (as prescribed
  by healthcare provider)—corrects deficiencies,
  supplemented with vitamin B_5 (pantothenic
  acid) (100 mg 3 times daily)—counteracts
  stress and aids in alcohol detoxification, and
  vitamin B_1 (thiamine) (200 mg 3 times
  daily)—especially lacking in alcoholics

- methionine (1000 mg daily, taken with water
  or juice but not with milk or food). To assist
  with absorption, take with 25 mg vitamin B_6
  and 100 mg vitamin C—boosts glutathione's
  availability to the liver

Also Recommended

- vitamin E (400 IU daily)

- evening primrose oil (1000 mg 3 times daily
  with food)—a good source of essential fatty
  acids

- vitamin C with bioflavonoids (3000 to10,000
  mg in divided doses)—a powerful antioxidant
  with healing potential; helps the body resist
  infection

- a prodophilus formula (as directed on label)

- lecithin capsules (1200 mg 3 times daily before meals)—may protect against cirrhosis and
  helps correct liver degeneration

- calcium (2000 mg at bedtime)—has a sedative
  effect

- phosphatidyl serine and phosphatidyl choline
  (take as directed on label)

- magnesium (1000 mg at bedtime)—works
  with calcium

- multivitamin and mineral complex (as directed on label)

- zinc (30 mg, not to exceed a total of 100 mg
  daily from all supplements)—helps improve a
  depressed metabolism

- L-glutamine (2 g)

- live cell therapy/glandular therapy (as directed on label)

- lipoic acid (200 to 250mg)

Aromatherapy

The essential oils of fennel, juniper, and rosemary may help clear the body of toxins that accumulate from excessive drinking.

Herbal Therapy

A variety of herbal preparations are good for treating the various side effects of alcohol abuse. Milk thistle helps repair damage to the liver. Valerian has a calming effect. Burdock root helps cleanse the blood. Other beneficial herbal remedies include dandelion root and red clover.

Herbal products are available in health food stores and in some pharmacies and supermarkets. Follow package for specific directions.

Homeopathy

Alcohol abuse may respond to homeopathic treatment. However, the selection of a remedy—more than one is available—depends on *your* symptoms and the stage of the condition. Don't try treating this disorder yourself. See a homeopathic professional.

Traditional Chinese Medicine

Acupuncture Auriculotherapy, also known as ear acupuncture, has been well-documented in the treatment and prevention of alcohol addiction. In fact, acupuncture is so successful that many substance abuse treatment programs now include it as a mandatory part of their rehabilitation process.

According to conventional medicine theory, acupuncture works by redirecting the endorphins in the body, which lessens cravings, relieves anxiety, and minimizes the symptoms of alcohol withdrawal. Typically, the liver, kidney, spleen, stomach, and brain points in the ear are manipulated.

When using whole-body acupuncture, the practitioner targets the heart, kidney, and liver points, since these are the organs most affected by excessive alcohol consumption. Additional points may be used to relieve withdrawal-related symptoms, such as insomnia, agitation, loss of appetite, and headache. Once the needles are inserted, electrical currents may be applied to enhance the treatment. In general, 10 to 12 treatments are required to see a noticeable improvement, and improvement is always most complete when the practitioner makes a complete Traditional Chinese Medicine diagnosis.

Chinese Herbal Therapy To improve alcohol-induced liver toxicity (including cirrhosis), some herbalists recommend *San Huang Xie Xin Tan,* a combination of coptis *(huang lien)* and rhubarb root *(da huang),* or *Fang Feng Tong Sheng,* a combination of ledebouriella *(fang feng)* and platycodon *(jie geng).*

Depending on what causes are behind an individual's alcohol abuse, an herbalist may recommend several other combination preparations, including Bupleurum and Dragon Bone Formula *(chai hu jia long gu mu li tang),* which has a therapeutic effect on the heart and liver; Ginseng and Longan Formula, which strengthens the heart and spleen; or Concha Marguerita and Ligustrum Formula, which regulates Yin imbalances.

Li Gan Pian (Liver Strengthening Tablets) is available at health food stores; follow package directions. Burdock can be taken to detoxify the blood; take 3 to 10 grams daily.

ALLERGIES

Signs and Symptoms

- Skin rashes
- Hives or itching
- Itchy nose and eyes
- Watery and/or swollen eyes
- Swelling around lips or tongue
- Runny nose/sneezing
- Persistent cough unrelated to a cold or the flu
- Wheezing or trouble breathing
- Nasal congestion
- Nausea/vomiting
- Diarrhea
- Abdominal cramps
- Anaphylactic shock

Description

An allergy manifests itself in many ways. Some people get hives after eating strawberries, some feel sick to their stomach after smelling chemical fumes, others become congested and teary after exposure to pollen in the air, still others suffer from eye swelling after a bite of lobster. These signals are the immune system's response to the presence of substances it sees as harmful.

The catch is, often the substance isn't harmful at all; it may even be helpful. Yet for some reason the strawberry or lobster or pollen or other offending substance (allergen) sets off the body's production of histamine. Histamine is a chemical that occurs naturally in the body and acts as an irritating stimulant. Histamine causes the symptoms of allergy, such as a runny nose or sneezing—actions specifically designed to expel the intruder from the body.

Different allergens prompt the release of histamine into different parts of the body. For instance, when someone who is allergic to molds in the air is exposed to them, they trigger the body to dump histamine into the respiratory system. The result? The lining of the airways swell and mucus is secreted. This leads to coughing, wheezing, and shortness of breath. Certain food allergens can lead to histamine being dumped into the digestive tract, causing a churning and/or cramping stomach, nausea, and diarrhea.

The severity of an allergy also varies from person to person. Between two people who are allergic to ragweed, one may suffer from mild sniffles while the other may be forced indoors by stinging, teary eyes, violent sneezing, and a constricted throat.

Anaphylactic shock is a type of allergic reaction that can occur suddenly and is life-threatening. It usually occurs as a reaction to an insect sting or medication, such as penicillin.

It's not known why some people have allergies and some don't. The majority of people who suffer from allergies, however, have a close relative who suffers from allergies as well—even if that relation doesn't have the same allergy. Other people become allergic to a substance through overexposure. In other words, they become allergic to a substance they've been around for years.

Conventional Medical Treatment

Before prescribing medical treatment for your allergy, your physician or allergist must determine what you are allergic to. You may think you already know. However, for safety's sake, your doctor will thoroughly examine your lungs, skin, eyes, nose, ears, lungs, and abdomen. You will be asked to give a complete food history, family history, and detailed information about your workplace, household, pets, and plants. You may be asked to keep a diary of when your symptoms occur and what you eat.

Allergies

ⓐ

When the cause of your allergy is still unclear and symptoms are severe, a skin test can provide the basis for most diagnoses. During a skin test, small pricks are made in the skin and a minute amount of a common allergen is inserted in each wound. If a welt develops, you are allergic to that substance.

Since skin testing is not very accurate in diagnosing food allergies, your doctor may have you take a double-blind food allergy test. During the test—used to uncover food allergies—a physician administers a series of foods and placebos. The substances are administered in a disguised form to overcome the emotional attachments and prejudices that people have toward certain foods.

Another diagnostic option is the radioallergosorbent test (RAST). RAST is a blood test that pinpoints inhalant allergies by measuring the amounts of antibodies in a person's blood. These antibodies are what trigger the body to produce histamine. RAST is less reliable than skin tests.

Once the allergy has been determined, you will be advised to avoid the substance. Antihistamines, which block the action of the histamines, are the basic drug treatment of allergies. Some doctors calm severe allergy symptoms with anti-inflammatory drugs called corticosteroids. And for certain allergies, such as those to molds, pollens, and insect venom, immunotherapy (allergy shots) is often used.

For More Information
American Academy of Allergy, Asthma, and Immunology
611 Wells Street
Milwaukee, WI 53202
414-272-6071
www.aaaai.org

Seasonal Allergy Management for Children

According to the Asthma and Allergy Foundation of America, nearly four million children suffer from seasonal allergies (such as hay fever), which are at their worst during warm-weather months. The foundation has these tips for making life more pleasant during allergy season:

- Limit outdoor activities to the late afternoon, when pollen counts are at their lowest.

- Throughout the year, dust, dander, and mold can collect in air conditioning vents, between window blinds, under the stove and refrigerator, on top of books, and elsewhere. When spring arrives, do a thorough "spring cleaning" to do away with these.

- Keep your child from playing outdoors on recently mowed lawns or sports fields.

- Be aware that mold spore counts are high after heavy rain.

- Keep windows closed during warm weather to keep airborne allergens out of your home. If possible, use a fan or air conditioner to keep rooms cool.

Health Notes

➤ *To help prevent allergies in children, don't feed them egg whites, shellfish, or wheat before age 1.*

➤ *Never feed an infant under age 1 raw honey. It contains a bacteria that can be fatal to an infant's unsophisticated immune system.*

➤ *If you or your child is severely allergic to insect stings, ask your doctor about a prescription for an emergency kit that contains epinephrine in a syringe ready for injection.*

Food Allergies

As many as two out of five Americans believe they have food allergies. Yet despite all the talk we hear these days about "having trouble" with certain foods, less than 1 percent of the nation's population actually has a food allergy. The foodstuffs that most often provoke a true allergic reaction are the proteins in egg whites, peanuts, wheat, and soybeans. Other foods that can cause allergies are berries, shellfish, and yellow food dye no. 5.

What many food-sensitive people actually have are food intolerances, also known as food sensitivities. These involve the digestive tract, rather than the immune system. An example of a food sensitivity is lactose intolerance, which is the inability of the digestive system to digest the enzyme lactose found in dairy products.

Food Allergy Network
10400 Eaton Place, Suite 107
Fairfax, VA 22030-2208
703-691-3179
www.foodallergy.org

National Institute of Allergies and Infectious Diseases
Building 31, Room 7A50
31 Center Drive MSC 2520
Bethesda, MD 20892-2520
301-496-5717
www.niaid.nih.gov

Complementary and Alternative Treatments

Nutrition and Supplementation

 Regardless of the cause, allergic reactions begin with the immune system. Nutrients that strengthen the immune system include bee pollen, quercetin, coenzyme Q10, vitamins A and E, selenium, glutathione, and zinc. Juices from red, yellow, and green fruits and vegetables, consumed two to three times a day, will supply you with high amounts of phytochemicals. Food allergies can be determined by rotating your foods, eating a different group for four days each, and monitoring your body's reaction. Avoid bananas, beef, caffeine, chocolate, citrus, corn, dairy, oats, oysters, peanuts, processed and refined foods, salmon, strawberries, tomatoes, wheat, and white rice until you are certain you are not allergic to them. Avoid taking aspirin within three hours of eating, as it has been reported that taking aspirin before ingesting an allergen allows more of that food to be eaten before reaction sets in. Try a diet consisting only of lamb, rice, and pears for one week to cleanse the body of toxins. These foods are very hypoallergenic. After that week, add food back into the diet, one day at a time. If you experience a reaction, eliminate that food for another 60 days, then introduce it again. If the same reaction occurs, permanently eliminate that food.

Nutritionists recommend the following daily supplements:

Most Important

- bee pollen (start with a few granules and work up to 2 tsp)—strengthens the immune system (*Warning:* Discontinue if you experience a rash, wheezing, or discomfort.)

- calcium (use calcium chelate form, 1500 to 2000 mg)—helps reduce stress

- magnesium (750 mg)—balances calcium

- vitamin B complex (100 mg)—aids digestion and nerve function, supplemented with vitamin B_5 (pantothenic acid) (100 mg 3 times daily)—reduces stress, and vitamin B_{12} (300 mcg 3 times daily)—for proper assimilation of nutrients

- vitamin C with bioflavonoids (5000 to 20,000 mg in divided doses)—protects the body from allergens and moderates the inflammatory response

- quercetin (500 mg twice daily)—increases immunity and decreases reactions to certain allergens

Also Recommended

- bromelain (100 mg twice daily)—enhances absorption of quercetin and acts as an anti-inflammatory

- germanium (60 mg)—stimulates immune response

- vitamin A (10,000 IU; do not exceed 8000 if you are pregnant)—for proper immune function

- vitamin E (600 IU)

- zinc (50 mg, not to exceed a total of 100 mg from all supplements)

- vitamin D (600 IU)—aids in calcium metabolism

- flaxseed oil (taken as directed on label)—contains essential omega-3 fatty acids

(For an *acute* condition, take supplements until your symptoms subside. If symptoms persist, seek the advice of your healthcare provider. For a *chronic* condition, consult your healthcare provider regarding the duration of treatment.)

Aromatherapy

To relieve congestion caused by allergies, try massaging the following blend into your skin around the sinuses: 1 drop of lavender oil, 1 drop niaouli, and 1 teaspoon sunflower oil. You might also try placing a drop of the essential oil of eucalyptus or peppermint on a handkerchief or tissue and inhaling.

Ayurvedic

Kapha doshas are often bothered by seasonal allergies and experience sneezing, watery eyes, and congestion. For relief, try placing a small amount of ghee (clarified butter) in each nostril several times a day. Before starting any new regimen to treat allergies, consult your doctor.

Bodywork and Somatic Practices

For an all-systems approach, Cranio-Sacral Therapy will ease or clear up physical symptoms, particularly in the cranium, while SomatoEmotional Release addresses the underlying emotional and/or spiritual components. The same physical/emotional/mental/spiritual focus is true of polarity therapy, all the Oriental bodywork therapies, and reflexology. Both Therapeutic Touch and Reiki can calm the central nervous system, ease symptoms, and boost vitality for the healing process. Alexander, Trager, Aston, and Feldenkrais address the habitual stress patterns that may regularly irritate the condition. Trigger point myotherapy, Rolfing, and Hellerwork address musculoskeletal tensions in the soft tissue and postural misalignments, which lower vitality and well-being. Massage provides relaxation, improves the internal balance of bodily systems, and helps flush lymph and blood in head, neck and shoulders.

Herbal Therapy

The herbalist's approach to allergy treatment is to reduce the production of mucus, and with it, the body's inflammatory response to pollens and other irritants. Helpful teas include chamomile, elder flower, goldenrod, nettle, yarrow, and red sage. To make these teas, steep 1 teaspoon dried or fresh herb in 1 cup boiling water for 5 minutes; strain.

You also might use echinacea, astragalus, or goldenseal to strengthen the immune system in general. Prepare a standard infusion. Herbal products are available in health food stores and in some pharmacies and supermarkets. Follow package for specific directions.

Homeopathy

Allergies are a chronic condition and are best treated by an experienced healthcare provider. However, your homeopathic practitioner may suggest one of the following remedies to reduce symptoms:

- *Allium cepa*—if the discharge from your nose burns, and the discharge from your eyes is bland

- *Euphrasia*—if the discharge from your nose is bland, and the discharge from your eyes burns

- *Whethia*—for hay fever accompanied by itching of the palate and back of the throat

- *Sabadilla*—if your condition is marked by sneezing, runny nose, and red, irritated eyes

Hydrotherapy

 To treat the symptoms of allergy and to prevent recurrences, therapists often advise drinking at least 2 quarts of water daily. They also suggest steam inhalation. For instructions on how to prepare an inhalation, see "Hydrotherapy" in the "Introduction to Complementary Therapies" section. Avoid inhalation therapy if you have asthma.

Traditional Chinese Medicine

 Acupuncture Whether allergies are food-related or seasonal (such as hay fever), Chinese medicine considers allergies to be caused by a weakened or malfunctioning immune system, and practitioners treat them accordingly.

Many studies have proven acupuncture's efficacy in controlling, and even curing, allergy symptoms, including diarrhea caused by lactose intolerance and chronic migraines brought about by environmental toxins. Usually, acupuncturists utilize techniques designed to strengthen the immune system so it can operate at peak efficiency, thereby improving the body's ability to defend itself against allergens and other bacterial intruders. They may do this by stimulating various acupoints within the ear or by manipulating specific organ-related points found throughout the entire body.

Acupressure Hay fever and allergy symptoms, such as sneezing and itchiness, can be relieved by pressing on acupoint LI4, which corresponds with the large intestine and lies in the webbing between the thumb and index finger, near the bone at the base of the index finger. Firmly press on this point for 1 to 2 minutes when you feel an allergy attack coming on, then repeat on the opposite hand. (Pregnant women should not use this technique, as it may induce uterine contractions.)

An acupressurist may also manipulate Liver 3 (in the *v* between the big and middle toes), Stomach 36 (just below the knee), and certain ear points in order to reduce hay fever symptoms, along with Bladder 2 (on the thickest part of the inner eyebrow) and Stomach 3 (located on the laugh lines, directly beneath the pupils).

Chinese Herbal Therapy Chinese herbalists believe that many allergies are caused by energy, or *chi*, imbalances. Several Chinese herb formulas can be quite useful in lessening allergy symptoms and reducing the frequency of allergic reactions.

Licorice is sometimes prescribed to relieve allergy-related congestion and soothe allergic skin reactions. For congestion and internal symptoms, take a decoction of 1 to 4 grams twice a day, mixed with 1 to 3 grams of ginger root, which will help lessen bronchial spasms. For skin rashes, use the decoction on the affected area 3 times a day for 1 week. Apply the licorice broth to the area and let it sit for 5 minutes before rinsing with water *(don't use soap)*. People with high blood pressure should consult their healthcare provider before using licorice preparations, as long-term use may cause hypertension.

If the herbalist has diagnosed a yang deficiency, he or she may recommend Rehmannia Eight, or *Pe Min Kan Wan*, pills to combat the patient's runny nose, itchy eyes, fatigue, shortness of breath, and postnasal-drip-induced cough. *Bi Yan Pian*, meanwhile, is used to treat allergy-related congestion and sinus pain, while Lopanthus Anti-Febrile pills are used to control food allergies. All of these preparations are available at health food stores; follow package directions. As always, you will find more effective results when working a practitioner.

Yoga and Meditation

Many allergies worsen when you feel stressed and uptight. To relax and restore mind-body balance, try the Sun Salutation, Moon Salutation, Cobra, Boat, and Half Boat along with meditation. Also practice deep-breathing exercises to aid breathing and improve sleep. Two other breathing exercises—Alternate Nostril Breathing and Breath of Fire—can also bring some relief.

ALTITUDE SICKNESS

Signs and Symptoms

- Headache
- Lack of energy
- Lack of appetite
- Dizziness
- Weakness
- Fatigue
- Shortness of breath
- Nausea and vomiting
- Increased heart and respiratory rate
- Coughing and/or wheezing

Description

Altitude sickness is the general name for three specific altitude-induced illnesses:

- acute mountain sickness (which affects most people within 4 to 6 hours after reaching 8,000+ feet)
- high altitude pulmonary edema (begins 24 to 96 hours after 8,000+ feet and features abnormal fluid in the lungs)
- high altitude cerebral edema (occurs 48 to 72 hours after reaching 12,000+ feet and is marked by swelling of the brain)

Factors that contribute to altitude sickness include how long a person takes to reach a certain altitude, what the altitude is, and how long he or she remains at that height. Why do individuals become sick when at high altitudes? Experts don't completely understand why, but they believe it has something to do with the fact that at higher altitudes, there is less oxygen in the air, resulting in less oxygen being absorbed by the body. Those who are out of shape, fatigued, or unwell are especially affected by diminished oxygen levels, and thus, have a higher risk of getting altitude sickness—or getting a more severe case of it.

Warning!

Your first action should always be to move an altitude-sick person to a lower altitude. If that is not possible, place the individual in a Gamow bag. Only after one of these measures has been completed should alternative therapies be administered.

Health Notes

- *Avoid altitude sickness by giving your body time to acclimate to lowered oxygen levels before climbing higher. When you reach 8,000 feet above sea level, spend two to four days getting used to this altitude before climbing higher. And never climb more than 1,500 feet per day.*
- *If you are part of a mountain expedition, rest one day for every two days of climbing after reaching the 8,000-foot mark. Slow things down even further when you get to 14,000 feet by ascending no more than 500 feet per day and by resting one day between every climbing day.*
- *Deep breathing can help you keep your blood supplied with precious oxygen. For every four minutes spent in high altitudes, breathe deeply 12 times in a row.*
- *If you have some time to prepare for your climb, up your daily intake of coenzyme Q10 (30-50 milligrams) and vitamins C (2 grams) and E (400 IU) a week before. These nutrients are believed to help the body adjust to higher altitudes and improve physical endurance. Many experts tout coenzyme Q10 as being able to help the body's cells use oxygen.*

Conventional Medical Treatments

The most important step in caring for any of the altitude sicknesses is to descend to a lower altitude—even an altitude of 500 to 1,000 feet lower is helpful in allaying symptoms. Administered oxygen and bed rest also offer relief. Using a portable hyperbaric chamber—also called a Gamow bag—is another effective way to treat people with this condition.

Complementary and Alternative Treatments

Traditional Chinese Medicine

Acupuncture Acupuncture may be used on Pericardium 6 to open the chest and Ren Conception Vessel 12 to get the lung *chi* moving.

Chinese Herbal Therapy To combat altitude sickness, Chinese herbalists recommend sucking on a few slices of honey-cured ginseng until symptoms subside.

Siberian pseudo-ginseng is also useful in treating altitude sickness. It can be purchased at health food stores; take as directed.

Alzheimer's Disease

Signs and Symptoms

- Confusion
- Forgetfulness
- Tendency to get lost
- Tendency to misplace objects
- Tendency to repeat oneself
- Anxiety

- Delusions
- Decline in intellectual ability, including the ability to think abstractly and the ability to learn or understand new information
- Decline in social skills and social graces
- Inability to concentrate
- Impaired ability to think abstractly
- Inability to learn or understand new information
- Loss of interest in life and other people
- Personality change
- Increased irritability
- Restlessness
- Sleep disturbance

Description

You've probably heard some people mistakenly pronounce Alzheimer's disease as "old-timer's disease." This is an honest error when you consider that the elderly and near-elderly are the ones who are most often struck with Alzheimer's. Of the 4 million people in America who have Alzheimer's, the majority are in the 50-to-90-year age bracket. In fact, it most often strikes people aged 65 or older and afflicts 40 percent of all Americans aged 85 years and older.

Another common misconception is that Alzheimer's disease is the same as dementia. *Dementia* is a general term that means "decline in mental function." Alzheimer's is a specific form of worsening dementia (in fact, the most common) that gradually causes brain cells to degenerate until they cannot communicate with one another.

It is not known exactly what causes Alzheimer's. Obviously, a major risk factor for developing Alzheimer's is age. So are genetics and head trauma. Although it's not known exactly why, low education level is also a risk factor. Experts believe that "unexercised" brain cells are weaker and more susceptible to damage over the lifespan.

Conventional Medical Treatment

If you suspect that you or someone you care about has Alzheimer's disease, it's important to see a physician as soon as possible. Many treatable medical conditions can be mistaken for Alzheimer's, including reactions to medication, depression, hypothyroidism, brain tumor, and vitamin deficiency. Alzheimer's is diagnosed by eliminating other possible illnesses. If a physical and neurological exam, urine analysis, blood work, electrocardiography, MRI or CAT scan, lumbar puncture tests, and X-rays reveal that no other medical conditions are present, a physician may diagnose Alzheimer's. If the condition is diagnosed, the patient will need to get the patient's finances, personal affairs, and care-taking arrangements in order before the disease progresses.

Aluminum and Alzheimer's Disease

Because it is not known with certainty what causes Alzheimer's disease, there are no guaranteed prevention tips. One popular prevention theory casts aluminum as contributing to Alzheimer's. This is due to the larger-than-normal amount of aluminum found in the brains of many Alzheimer's victims during autopsies. It's not known, however, whether a neural malfunction causes the brain to hoard aluminum, or if the person was exposed to larger than average amounts of the mineral during life. Either way, some experts suggest avoiding aluminum cookware, aluminum food and beverage containers, antacids and anti-diarrheal drugs (which contain aluminum salt), antiperspirants that contain aluminum chlorhydrate, and any commercially prepared food that lists the preservatives sodium aluminum phosphate, aluminum ammonium sulfate, or aluminum potassium sulfate on its label.

Health Note

➤ *Free radicals have been linked in a lengthy list of age-related disorders, including Alzheimer's disease. It is believed that free radicals can be neutralized by substances called antioxidants. Vitamins E and C have been shown to decrease the levels of free radicals in the blood.*

Herbal Help for Alzheimer's

Researchers at the New York Institute for Medical Research reported positive results from a study in which they assigned 309 Alzheimer's patients either Ginkgo biloba extract or a placebo. After a year of study, they found that 26 percent of the subjects given the extract showed slight improvement in cognitive skills, compared to 14 percent of those given a placebo.

Because Alzheimer's patients often react unexpectedly to drugs, medications are typically not given—not even to counteract symptoms such as insomnia or irritability. There are several drugs— tacrine (Cognex®), donepezil (Aricept®), and estrogen—that may offer mild improvements in cognitive function. Unfortunately, there is no cure for the condition, and most people grow more and more ill, dying two to ten years after symptoms appear.

For More Information

The Alzheimer's Association National Office
919 North Michigan Avenue, Suite 1000
Chicago, IL 60611-1676
800-272-3900
www.alz.org

National Council on Aging
409 Third Street, SW, 2nd Floor
Washington, DC 20024
202-479-1200
www.ncoa.org

National Institute on Aging
Alzheimer Education Referral Center
P.O. Box 8250
Silver Spring, MD 20907-8250
800-438-4380
www.alzheimers.org

Complementary and Alternative Treatments

Nutrition and Supplementation

 Eat a diet rich in whole grains and fresh vegetables, avoiding processed and refined foods. Many processed foods contain harmful additives, including aluminum. Alzheimer victims have up to four times the normal amount of aluminum in the brain's nerve cells. It isn't just food we need to consider: aluminum is found in cookware, shampoos, deodorants, buffered aspirin, and antacid. Severe exposure to aluminum, coupled with a deficiency in several nutrients, may lead to a predisposition for Alzheimer's.

In addition, Alzheimer's sufferers have been found to have deficiencies in zinc, vitamins A and E, beta-carotene, iron, B_6, B_{12}, boron, potassium, and selenium. A deficiency in even one of these nutrients is detrimental to health, but multiple deficiencies in a body that is aging presents serious problems. To help rebalance the body, consult a specialist who can custom-tailor your diet and supplementation program. In the meantime, the following daily guidelines will prove helpful:

Most Important

- acetylcholine (500 mg 3 times daily on empty stomach)—a deficiency has been linked to dementia

- boron (3 mg)—improves brain function

- coenzyme Q10 (100 to 200 mg)—boosts the supply of oxygen to the brain

- lecithin capsules (1200 mg 3 times daily before meals)—improves memory

- multivitamin and mineral complex with potassium (99 mg)—balances electrolytes

- grape seed extract (as directed on label)—a powerful antioxidant that protects brain cells from free radical damage

- selenium (200 mcg daily)—an antioxidant for brain cell protection

- vitamin B complex (2 cc 3 times weekly or as prescribed by doctor)—important for proper brain function; aids food digestion (injections work best), supplemented with vitamin B_6 ($^1/_2$ cc once weekly or as prescribed by doctor)—a deficiency can cause depression and mental difficulties, and vitamin B_{12} (1 cc 3 times weekly or as prescribed by doctor)—important for brain function; Alzheimer's patients often are deficient in this vitamin

- zinc (50 to100 mg)—helps stop amyloid plaque formation

Also Recommended

- docosahexaenoic acid (DHA) (100 mg 3 times with meals)

- phosphatidyl serine (1000 mg)

- lipoic acid (300 mg)

- acetyl-l-carnitine (500 mg twice daily)—slows memory deterioration; take on empty stomach

- apple pectin (as directed on label)—aids in removing toxic metals such as mercury, which can lead to dementia

- vitamin C with bioflavonoids (6000 to10,000 mg in divided doses)—enhances immunity and increases energy level; take in buffered form

- vitamin E (start at 400 IU daily and increase slowly to 800 IU daily)—transports oxygen to brain cells and protects them from free radicals

- melatonin (3 mg at bedtime)—can improve sleep habits

- flaxseed oil (1 tblsp)—provides omega-3 fatty acids, which ultimately nourish brain cells

- N-acetyl cysteine (1000 mg)

(Consult your healthcare provider regarding the duration of treatment.)

Ayurvedic

For improving memory that's not quite what it used to be, some Ayurvedic practitioners suggest *triphala*, a combination of three herbs, and *Ginkgo biloba*. Be sure to consult with your doctor before starting a regimen with herbs.

Bodywork and Somatic Practices

There have been some anecdotal reports that CranioSacral Therapy can help slow the disease and provide some clarity; it definitely promotes relaxation and well-being. Oriental bodywork, massage, polarity therapy and reflexology also may bring good results in some individuals.

Herbal Therapy

Ginkgo biloba (60 mg 2 times daily) may increase cerebral circulation, and therefore, may be helpful in treating this progressive disease. Other herbs with possible memory and circulatory benefits are gotu kola, sage, fenugreek, and dandelion.

Herbal products are available in health food stores and in some pharmacies and supermarkets. Follow package for specific directions.

Hydrotherapy

Constitutional therapy applied several times weekly may help temper some of the symptoms associated with this disorder. Simply apply alternating hot and cold towels to the front and back of the body, focusing on the abdomen and lower back.

Traditional Chinese Medicine

 Acupuncture Acupuncturists have had success treating Alzheimer's disease by using scalp acupuncture to stimulate the meridians in the head, which opens blocked energy pathways and increases blood flow to nutrient-starved sections of the brain.

When treating Alzheimer's, acupuncture is often used in conjunction with Chinese herbs and with a Chinese exercise called *qigong*, a gentle therapeutic routine that improves the patient's cardiovascular condition and general circulation.

Chinese Herbal Therapy Gingko biloba has been so successful at improving brain functioning in Alzheimer's patients that it recently passed stringent FDA testing as an Alzheimer's remedy. In fact, after being treated with gingko, the FDA's research subjects—all of whom suffered from Alzheimer's—underwent an MRI (magnetic reso-

nance imaging), which demonstrated a marked improvement in their cerebral capabilities. Gingko is thought to work by improving circulation to the brain and increasing the synthesis of dopamine, norepinephrine, and other neurotransmitters; thereby repairing memory loss and enhancing intellectual functioning (such as the ability to process information). The recommended dose is 5 to 15 grams daily, taken in decoction or capsule form.

In addition, Spleen Restoration Decoction is often used to treat Alzheimer's-related senile dementia. It contains more than 12 different herbs and should be prepared by a qualified herbal specialist. A pre-made formula, called Spleen Restoration Pills, is available at health food stores.

Yoga and Meditation

 Improved blood flow and relaxation can help boost memory. Look to the following yoga poses for benefits: Shoulder Stand, Headstand, Plow, Camel, Bow, Cobra, Corpse, and Sun Salutation. For additional benefits, incorporate meditation into your daily routine.

ANAL FISSURES

Signs and Symptoms

- Streaks of blood coating your stool, and/or visible on toilet paper
- Anal itching
- Mild to moderate pain during defecation

Description

An anal fissure is a minor tear, or crack-like sore, that extends from the external anal sphincter muscle up into the anal canal. Anal fissures are more common in women than men.

Straining to pass hard stools is the primary cause of anal fissures. The anal tissue is only so pliant. When over-exerted, the tissue may tear instead of yield.

Conventional Medical Treatment

While a physician can diagnose anal fissures, the tears generally heal by themselves with the proper care. To soften the stool and avoid stressing the injured area (which in turn hastens healing), drink 8 8-ounce glasses of water or more a

Anal Fissures

day and increase your fiber intake. Your doctor may even suggest a bulk-forming laxative, such as a product containing psyllium.

In severe cases your physician may prescribe surgery—a relatively simple outpatient procedure to stitch up the tear.

Complementary and Alternative Treatments

Nutrition and Supplementation

 For fissures, nutritionists recommend a high-fiber diet with whole grains, fruits, and vegetables to prevent constipation. Eat ½ cup of oat bran cereal each day to increase bulk. Grains, such as buckwheat, contain flavonoids, which help strengthen collagen, an important part of the skin's supportive structure.

The following daily supplements are recommended:

- vitamin C with bioflavonoids (1000 mg)
- vitamin E (400 IU)
- flaxseed oil (1 tblsp)
- zinc (30 mg) until healed, then standard dose
- vitamin A (25,000 IU reduced to 10,000 IU daily; do not exceed 8000 IU daily if you are pregnant)

(For an *acute* condition, take supplements until your symptoms subside. If symptoms persist, seek the advice of your healthcare provider. For a *chronic* condition, consult your healthcare provider regarding the duration of treatment.)

Herbal Therapy

 Anal fissures are often caused by constipation. For information on relieving constipation, see "Constipation."

Homeopathy

 Anal fissures may respond to homeopathic treatment. For the stabbing, burning pain that's associated with a fissure, you may get relief by applying a cream made from *Hamamelis* and *Aesculus*. Other homeopathic remedies are available, depending on *your* symptoms and the stage of the condition. Consult a homeopathic professional.

Hydrotherapy

 A hot sitz bath is one of the best ways to heal an anal fissure and to ease its pain. If a bath is not available, apply hot compresses to the area.

Traditional Chinese Medicine

 Acupuncture If the anal fissures are caused by chronic constipation, the acupuncturist may treat the latter problem by working the auricular acupoints associated with the large intestine, the rectum, and the adrenal gland.

In treating the anal fissure itself, the practitioner stimulates the point that correlates to the lower section of the rectum and heart, which promotes healing.

Acupressure To quell constipation (which can cause anal fissures), the practitioner may manipulate acupressure points on the legs, back, and abdomen that correlate with the large intestine, subcortex, and lower section of the rectum.

Chinese Herbal Therapy If constipation is a contributing factor, herbalists may recommend a number of therapies, including Apricot Seed and Linum formula, or Fructus persica (for dry, hard feces), or Bupleurum and *Tang Gui* formula if the problem is difficulty in evacuating the bowels. There are countless herbs that are used to cure chronic constipation; an herbalist will prepare an individualized remedy according to the causes and severity of the condition.

ANEMIA

Signs and Symptoms

- Pallor
- Fatigue
- Weakness
- Exercise intolerance
- Pale mucous membranes
- Rapid heartbeat
- Lightheadedness
- Chest pain

Description

Anemia is characterized by a low number of red blood cells, decreased levels of hemoglobin (a protein found in the blood cells), or reduced amount of blood. Yet, its symptoms appear so gradually that people may not realize they have the condition until their day-to-day activities are affected. In fact, anemia is a chronic condition in many people.

Iron deficiency anemia is one type of anemia. It occurs when the body's iron supply is too low to manufacture the necessary amount of hemoglobin. Primary causes of the deficiency include inadequate intake of foods enriched with iron, poor absorption of iron by the body, and loss of blood.

Women of childbearing age are anemia's most frequent victims. In fact, an estimated 20 percent of women in the United States are anemic. Pregnant women often become anemic because their body's iron stores are being dipped into to make hemoglobin for their fetuses. In non-pregnant women, the cause is monthly menstrual blood loss. Anemia occasionally develops in infants, children and adolescents due to their rapid growth spurts. Iron-deficiency anemia also is caused by blood loss from the digestive tract, which can occur with peptic ulcers, colon cancer, hemorrhoids, or long-term use of aspirin.

Anemia often occurs in people with chronic diseases, such as rheumatoid arthritis, or chronic infections, such as hepatitis, AIDS, or tuberculosis. In these cases, the body may not manufacture enough red blood cells.

Anemia can also occur in people with vitamin B_{12} or folic acid deficiencies. Vitamin B_{12} and folic acid, like iron, help the body form red blood cells and hemoglobin. Vitamin B_{12} deficiency usually occurs when someone's intestines are unable to absorb the vitamin. Folic acid deficiency is generally caused by poor nutrition or chronic alcoholism.

In some cases, anemia is a genetic condition. Sickle cell anemia and thalassemia are two inherited forms of the disease. Neither has a cure. Treatment for both is directed at reducing the severity of symptoms.

➤ *Iron supplements and plenty of rest are the best bets for fighting amemia.*

➤ *When you gently pull down your lower eyelid, the skin that you see should be pink. If it's white, there is a possibility that you may be anemic.*

Conventional Medical Treatment

A blood test can confirm anemia. If you are diagnosed with the condition, your physician will set out to discover the cause. If the cause is an ulcer or cancer, that will be addressed. However, if there is no illness involved and menstruation and/or low iron intake is to blame, you'll need to make a few dietary changes. First, cut down on beverages such as coffee, tea, colas, and other caffeine-rich drinks that leech iron from the blood. Second, add iron-rich foods to your diet, such as beef, pork, lamb, poultry, eggs, and fish; legumes, such as dried peas and beans; and carbohydrates, such as potatoes and brown rice. Drinking vitamin C-rich citrus juice with these iron-filled foods helps your body absorb the mineral. In more severe cases, an iron supplement (ferrous sulfate) may be suggested.

Treatment for Vitamin B_{12} deficiency involves injections that usually must continue for life. Folic acid deficiency can be corrected by eating foods high in folate—such as dark green leafy vegetables—and reducing alcohol intake.

Complementary and Alternative Treatments

Nutrition and Supplementation

Fifty percent of those suffering from iron-deficiency anemia are children; women make up another 20 percent. It is important to start children on the road to healthy eating while they are young. Infants as young as six months should be introduced to foods rich in phytochemicals and antioxidants, such as beets, broccoli, carrots, and applesauce. A quarter cup of "green" juice (made from vegetables high in chlorophyll), diluted 50 percent with water or apple juice, can quickly improve a child's condition.

Anemia caused by vitamin B_{12} deficiency (pernicious anemia) is more serious. Sufferers have difficulty absorbing the vitamin and must take supplements by injection, retention enema, or lozenges dissolved under the tongue. Treatment must be maintained for life unless the underlying cause can be diagnosed and corrected.

All anemics should include iron-rich foods in the diet such as red meat, liver, apples, apricots, bananas, broccoli, leafy greens, raisins, whole grains, and yams. Be sure to get enough vitamin C to help with iron absorption. In addition, B_{12} can be found in mackerel, salmon, and eggs, and in fermented soy products, such as miso and tempeh. Combine these foods with sources rich in folic acid. Avoid beer, candy bars, dairy products, soft drinks, coffee and tea, as these products contain additives that interfere with iron absorption.

Supplementation is effective only when tailored to your specific form of anemia. Anemia is not necessarily a sign of iron deficiency. However, the following daily suggestions below will help improve any anemic condition until a healthcare provider can be consulted.

- blackstrap molasses (1 tblsp twice daily for adults, 1 tsp in milk or formula twice daily for children)—a good source of iron and essential B vitamins

- folic acid (800 mcg twice daily)—essential for red blood cell formation

- biotin (300 mcg twice daily)—aids in red blood cell formation

- vitamin B_{12} injections (2 cc weekly or as prescribed by healthcare provider)—for red blood cell production

- vitamin C (3000 to 10,000 mg)—helps iron absorption

- brewer's yeast (as directed on label)—rich in basic nutrients
- vitamin B complex (50 mg 3 times daily)

(Consult your healthcare provider regarding the duration of treatment.)

Aromatherapy

 Essential oils that may help you cope with anemia include Roman chamomile, lemon, and red thyme.

Ayurvedic Medicine

 Ayurveda classifies anemia according to the basic dosha conditions: vata, pitta, and kapha. For all types, some Ayurvedic practitioners advise eating plain yogurt with a little ground turmeric. Before starting any new regimen to treat anemia, consult your doctor.

Bodywork and Somatic Practices

 Massage increases vitality to improve overall body function, as does Cranio-Sacral Therapy. Oriental bodywork, polarity therapy, and reflexology may also be appropriate.

Herbal Therapy

 Numerous herbs are used to treat anemia. Most do so by promoting better circulation, stimulating digestion, increasing iron absorption, or improving the intake of vitamins and other minerals. Some of the herbs most commonly suggested include dandelion, parsley, nettle, goldenseal, red raspberry, yellow dock, and mullein.

To prepare any of the teas, make a standard infusion: steep 1 teaspoon of dried or fresh herb in 1 cup boiling water for 5 to 10 minutes; strain.

Herbal products are available in health food stores and in some pharmacies and supermarkets. Follow package for specific directions.

Traditional Chinese Medicine

 Acupuncture Acupuncture is often used to treat anemia, a condition referred to in Chinese medicine as "blood deficiency." To counteract this deficiency (which can lead to a weakened *chi*), an acupuncturist works on the points associated with the spleen, the heart, the liver, and the lungs to reinvigorate blood flow to these organs. In doing so, anemia-related symptoms, such as fatigue, dizziness, dry skin, and blurry vision, may be lessened or cured altogether.

Acupressure To improve blood circulation and regulate the *chi* in the vital organs affected by anemia, the practitioner manipulates the acupressure points that correlate with the heart (Large Intestine 4 and Heart 7), lungs (Small Intestine 4 and Lung 9), liver (Stomach 36 and Liver 3), and spleen (Gallbladder 34 and Spleen 4).

Ginseng is used to combat anemia-related lethargy, while angelica and ligusticum are used as a tonic to strengthen and purify the blood.

Chinese Herbal Therapy Return Spleen Tablets are a much-prescribed Chinese anemia remedy, as are Eight Treasure Pills, *Dang Gui Four,* Ten Complete Great Tonifying Pills, and *Tang Kwei Gin* tonic. Kind Mother Decoction is made especially for women who experience anemia due to heavy menstruation. All are available in health food stores; use as directed.

a

ANOREXIA NERVOSA

Signs and Symptoms

- Distorted body image
- Dissatisfaction with body
- Pronounced weight loss
- Low body fat
- Excessive fear of becoming fat
- Reduction in food intake and/or food refusal
- Preoccupation with calories, food, and food preparation
- Loss or absence of menstrual periods (in women)
- Extensive exercise
- Dry, flaky, or cracked skin
- Dry, sparse hair on scalp
- Pale, downy hair on face and body
- Hypothermia
- Depression

Description

Anorexia nervosa is a psychological disorder that most often affects young women between the ages of 12 and 21. In fact, less than 10 percent of all those with anorexia nervosa are males. The problem typically occurs in someone with a distorted body image who desperately wants to lose weight. She may start by eliminating high-calorie foods and snacks from her diet, then progress to skipping meals altogether, or eating smaller portions. Often, a person with anorexia nervosa may eat only a few small items of food a day, such as an apple and a few carrot sticks. To burn off even more calories, many sufferers become obsessive exercisers.

Unfortunately, when the body doesn't have a store of calories to use as fuel for everyday functions (such as breathing, walking, moving), it starts to burn its own muscle cells in order to come up with the calories it needs to survive. Indeed, the anorexic's heart muscle can often become so weak and depleted that it stops beating. Many victims of severe anorexia die of heart attacks—even though they may be in their teens or twenties. Other consequences of anorexia include delayed sexual maturation, gastrointestinal disorders (including constipation), and liver and kidney damage.

Anorexia doesn't have one specific cause. Risk factors include:

- Low self-esteem
- Perfectionist personality
- High expectations, stress due to multiple responsibilities and/or tight schedules
- Ambivalence about independence
- Early puberty

Conventional Medical Treatment

Psychotherapy, rather than drug therapy, is the first line of treatment for anorexia. A mental health professional trained to treat eating disorders encourages the patient to gain weight by increasing daily caloric intake by 300 calories every two weeks. The psychotherapist also tries to determine the psychosocial issues affecting the sufferer's body image, and seek to build her sense of self-worth and a more positive body image. In severe cases, bed rest with supervised meals are called for until patient has gained 10 to 20 pounds. Since the goal in treating anorexia is to encourage the individual to get better on her

ⓐ

own, forced or tube feeding is usually avoided. In instances where the individual is clinically depressed, an anti-depressant may be given.

For More Information
American Anorexia Bulimia Association, Inc.
165 West 46th Street, NW, Suite 1108
New York, NY 10036
212-575-6200
www.aabainc.org

National Eating Disorders Organization
6655 South Yale Avenue
Tulsa, OK 74136
918-481-4044
www.kidsource.com/nedo/index.html

Complementary and Alternative Treatments

Nutrition and Supplementation

 Until recently, anorexia was believed to be solely a psychological disease. Now, however, scientists and nutritionists have identified a number of physical symptoms as well, such as a zinc deficiency and a chemical imbalance similar to the one associated with clinical depression. Because of this combination of psychological and physiological components, it is essential that the anorexic seek counseling with a specialist trained in eating disorders as well as a nutritionist. In the meantime, eat a diet high in fiber, including fresh raw fruits and vegetables. These foods cleanse the body and help your appetite return to normal. Avoid sugar and processed or junk foods, which contain no nourishment at all.

In addition, follow these guidelines daily to help your system adjust to normal eating habits.

Most Important

- multivitamin and mineral complex that supplies these dosages: beta-carotene (25,000 IU), vitamin A (10,000 IU), calcium (1500 mg), magnesium (1000 mg), potassium (99 mg), selenium (200 mcg)

- zinc (50 mg, not to exceed a total of 100 mg from all supplements)—take with copper to prevent copper deficiency

- copper (3 mg)

Also Recommended

- a prodophilus formula (taken as directed on label)—to replace the friendly bacteria lost from vomiting and use of laxatives

- vitamin B complex (100 mg 3 times daily) helps prevent anemia and replaces lost B vitamins

- vitamin B_{12} injections (1 cc 3 times weekly)—increases appetite and prevents loss of hair;

use in lozenge form if injections are not available

- vitamin C (5000 mg in divided doses)—to repair the immune system
- brewer's yeast (start with 1 tsp and work up to 1 tblsp)—supplies balanced amounts of the B vitamins
- kelp (2000 to 3000 mg)—replaces minerals
- vitamin D (600 IU)—helps calcium absorption to prevent bone loss
- vitamin E (600 IU)—increases oxygen uptake for total body healing

(Consult your healthcare provider regarding the duration of treatment.)

Aromatherapy

To lessen anxiety and soothe the nervousness and low spirits that often accompany anorexia nervosa, aromatherapy practitioners suggest any of the following essential oils: bergamot, basil, Roman chamomile, clary sage, lavender, neroli, or ylang-ylang.

Ayurvedic Medicine

Ayurvedic practitioners worry about the lack of nourishment as well as the depression that's often associated with anorexia. They may recommend cardamom, fennel, and ginger root to help stop vomiting and improve digestion, and advise a bland, soothing diet without spices, coffee, or tea.

To soothe and calm the nervous system, practitioners also may suggest massaging the head and feet with warm sesame oil.

Herbal Therapy

Try herbs that stimulate the appetite, such as ginger root, ginseng, and peppermint. Herbal products are available in health food stores and in some pharmacies and supermarkets. Follow package for specific directions.

Remember to consult your doctor before embarking on any new regimen. Anorexia shouldn't be ignored; the disorder can have serious consequences.

Hydrotherapy

Use constitutional therapy several times weekly: apply alternating applications of hot and cold towels to the front and back of the body focusing on the abdomen and lower back. To stimulate the digestive system, apply cold compresses to stomach for 30 minutes before meals.

Traditional Chinese Medicine

Acupuncture Acupuncture can help enhance an anorexia sufferer's general recovery by promoting feelings of well-being and by balancing the body' s *chi,* or energy levels, which have most likely been impaired by the patient' s habitual self-starvation. The length of treatment will vary, depending upon the needs of the individual and the severity of her condition.

Chinese Herbal Therapy Anorexia wreaks havoc with the digestive system and depletes the body of essential vitamins and minerals. Herbs may be used to counteract these imbalances and restore the body to its natural state of being.

Some common prepared formulas include Saussurea and Amomum Stomach Nurturing Pills and Vitality Combination.

Yoga and Meditation

Yoga seeks to enhance emotional control and restore peace of mind. Yoga poses build chi (vital energy), improve body awareness, and stimulate and tone the digestive and the endocrine systems. Specific yoga poses for eating disorders include Bow, Boat, Peacock, Rooster, and Lion. Daily meditation can help you achieve increased emotional control.

ANXIETY DISORDERS

Signs and Symptoms

- Episodes of shortness of breath
- Episodes of panic
- Excessive worrying
- Heart palpitations and/or increased heart rate
- Hyperventilation (breathing too heavily and deeply)
- Excessive sweating
- Numb sensation in hands and/or feet
- Stomach pains and/or gastrointestinal distress
- Chest pains
- Dizziness
- Dry mouth
- Impatience and/or irritability
- Difficulty concentrating
- Possible drug/alcohol abuse to numb feelings
- Headaches
- Fatigue

Description

Your heart beats faster, you breathe more rapidly, you tremble, and your stomach becomes upset. While these symptoms are classic by-products of fear, they also denote anxiety disorders. Unlike ordinary fear, the symptoms of an anxiety disorder stay with you for at least a month. Also unlike fear, you may not know exactly what it is that has you so distressed—or perhaps you do know what has you upset, but the problem is minor compared with the intensity of your emotional reaction. Among the many recognized types of anxiety disorders are panic attacks, obsessive-compulsive disorder, phobias, and post-traumatic stress disorder.

Anxiety disorders have no single cause. In some, the condition can be traced to childhood fears or losses that are reactivated later in life. Psychological stressors, such as chronic chaos at work or an unhealthy relationship, can also cause anxiety disorders. Some experts believe that people with abnormalities of their neurotransmitters are more prone to getting anxiety disorders; others believe anxiety disorders are genetic.

Other associated medical problems, such as thyroid abnormalities, hypoglycemia, and hypoadrenia, can mimic anxiety disorders. So be sure to consult your healthcare provider for a thorough checkup to rule out any physical causes for your symptoms.

Foods to Calm

Low-fat proteins tend to stimulate your mind and body, whereas carbohydrates have a calming effect. Other soothing foods include bread, pasta, and most cereals. If you are prone to nervousness and suspect you have an anxiety disorder, experiment with checking your moods with your diet for a few days to discover what your "comfort foods" are.

Health Notes

➤ A nutritious diet (without caffeine), moderate aerobic exercise, and regular sleep keep the body and mind healthy, strong, and flexible enough to handle most stressful situations.

➤ Anxiety disorders are not always preventable, but it helps to avoid people and situations that make you anxious. If avoidance is impossible, learning to calmly face your stressors is beneficial.

Conventional Medical Treatment

Psychiatric intervention is the conventional way to treat anxiety disorders. Usually this calls for a psychotherapist to work with the patient to uncover what is causing the anxiety. Anti-anxiety medications such as benzodiazepines (Ativan®, Xanax®) or antidepressants (BuSpar®, Buspirone®) may also be prescribed.

For More Information
Anxiety Disorders Association of America
11900 Parklawn Drive, Suite 100
Rockville, MD 20852
301-231-9350
www.adaa.org/Default.htm

Complementary and Alternative Treatments

Nutrition and Supplementation

The focus here is on reducing stress, since that is what triggers anxiety attacks. To that end, avoid consumption of caffeine, alcohol, and refined sugar. Instead, eat small meals throughout the day emphasizing asparagus, avocados, bananas, broccoli, brewer's yeast, brown rice, dried fruits, green leafy vegetables, legumes, raw nuts and seeds, soy products, whole grains, and yogurt. These foods supply essential minerals normally depleted by stress.

Recent studies report on the benefits of DL-phenylalanine (DLPA) in treating anxiety disorders. DLPA is a supplement consisting of D-phenylalanine and L-phenylalanine, a combination more potent than taking either amino acid alone. Use only under the supervision of a healthcare provider. The following daily supplement suggestions will aid in relieving symptoms of anxiety:

Most Important

- calcium (2000 mg)—a natural tranquilizer
- magnesium (600 to1000 mg)—helps relieve anxiety, tension, and nervousness
- vitamin B complex (50 mg)—maintains normal nervous system function; supplemented with vitamin B_1 (thiamine) (50 mg 3 times daily with food)—has a calming effect on the nerves; and vitamin B_6 (50 mg 3 times daily with food)—energizes while it calms
- vitamin C (5000 to 10,000 mg in divided doses)—has a tranquilizing effect in large doses
- zinc (50 mg, not to exceed a total of 100 mg from all supplements)—calms the central nervous system

Also Recommended

- DLPA (600 to1200 mg)—increases the brain's production of endorphins, which helps relieve anxiety and stress (Do not take if you are pregnant, nursing, or suffer from panic attacks, diabetes, high blood pressure, or phenylketonuria, or PKU. Discontinue use if no improvement is noticed within one week.)
- melatonin (start with 2 to 3 mg taken 2 hours or less before bedtime)—a natural sleep aid that should be taken only if your symptoms include insomnia
- pantothenic acid (vitamin B_5) (50 mg 3 times daily)

(For an *acute* condition, take supplements until your symptoms subside. If symptoms persist, seek the advice of your healthcare provider. For a *chronic* condition, consult your healthcare provider regarding the duration of treatment.)

Aromatherapy

The following aromas are noted for their anti-anxiety properties: clary sage, lavender, geranium, bergamot, juniper, lemon, orange, and ylang-ylang. To ease the jitters, you might want to try a few drops of lavender oil on a handkerchief or tissue; inhale occasionally.

Bodywork and Somatic Practices

Massage is a classical technique to restore relaxation and circulation for better mental and emotional well-being.

CranioSacral Therapy/SomatoEmotional Release, Oriental bodywork, reflexology and polarity therapy—each in its own style—may help, and possibly heal, the physical-emotional elements of this problem. The Trager and Feldenkrais methods also may be useful in lowering inner turmoil.

Herbal Therapy

Herbalists offer a variety of herbs for easing anxiety. Valerian, which has been used as a sleep aid and tranquilizer for more than 1000 years, is considered one of the best anti-anxiety herbs. To use the herb as a tea, steep 2 teaspoons of chopped root in 1 cup of boiling water for 15 minutes; let stand for 8 to 12 hours. Strain. The herb is also available in capsule and tincture form. A blend of lavender, oats, linden flower, catnip, and lemon balm is also effective for easing anxiety, say herbalists. To make a tea, combine equal amounts of the herbs, then steep 4 tablespoons of the blend in 4 cups boiling water for 10 minutes. Strain through cheesecloth. Drink up to 6 cups a day.

Other helpful herbal supplements include:

- kava kava (as directed on label)
- St. John's wort (300 mg 3 times daily with food) (Do not use in conjunction with antidepressants. St. John's Wort may act as a mild monoamine oxidase inhibitor (MAOI); consult your healthcare provider regarding potential dietary and medication restrictions.)
- gingko biloba (60 mg twice daily)

Herbal products are available in health food stores and in some pharmacies and supermarkets. Follow package for specific directions.

Homeopathy

See a homeopathic professional for chronic anxiety. For acute, or sudden, anxiety, a practitioner may recommend one of the following treatments, depending on your symptoms:

- *Gelsemium*—for anxiety before taking a test or giving a speech; symptoms may include weakness, diarrhea, racing heartbeat

- *Argentum nitricum*—for anxiety accompanied by a fear of failure; symptoms may include worry, extreme edginess, diarrhea
- *Lycopodium*—for anxiety accompanied by low self-esteem
- *Aesthusa cynapium*—for performance anxiety
- *Aconite*—for fear of flying

Hydrotherapy

A neutral bath (slighter cooler than body temperature) has a positive effect on the body and can help ease muscular as well as mental tension. Simply fill the tub with lukewarm water (94° to 97° F) and soak with as much of your body submerged with water as possible for at least 20 minutes.

Traditional Chinese Medicine

Acupuncture By unblocking and re-channeling energy pathways, acupuncture can promote relaxation, which can be helpful in treating any number of emotional disorders, including panic attacks, generalized fear and anxiety, and even agoraphobia (fear of large spaces). In cases of hysteria, an acupuncturist may target the heart, kidney, brain, stomach, and head points in an attempt to balance the patient's *chi* and redirect negative or disturbing energy patterns.

Because Chinese medicine contends that excessive fear or anxiety damages the kidneys and large intestine (where it may cause irritable bowel syndrome and colitis), acupuncturists will attempt to strengthen these particular organs.

Acupressure Anxiety-related dizziness can be treated by pressing on the *Yin-tang* point that lies in the center of the face between the eyebrows, or by applying pressure to the Liver 3 point that is located on the feet between the first and second toes.

Hysteria may be relieved by massaging the point that lies just below the lowest crease on the center of the thumb (where it meets the palm). To alleviate general nervousness or heart palpitations, a practitioner may manipulate Heart 7 (found on the outside edge of the wrist), Pericardium 6 (on the underside of the forearm), and the corresponding ear points.

Chinese Herbal Therapy Chinese therapists believe that anxiety disorders are the result of a weakened *shen* (what we might call the psyche, spirit, or soul). There are many Chinese herbs that can help combat feelings of anxiety and the symptoms that accompany certain anxiety dis-

orders, such as dizziness, shortness of breath, heart palpitations, and confusion.

Yoga and Meditation

The daily practice of meditation along with deep breathing and three to four yoga poses can quiet the mind and help break anxiety patterns. Be sure to include the Corpse pose.

ARTHRITIS

OSTEOARTHRITIS

Signs and Symptoms

- Pain and tenderness in joints (typically, joints in one to three sites are affected, and the pain worsens after use and goes away with rest)
- Discomfort in affected joint before or during a change in the weather
- Swelling in affected joints
- Weakness and loss of flexibility in affected joints
- If the joints of the fingers are affected, bony knobs may be visible at the knuckles

Description

Of the more than 100 types of arthritis, osteoarthritis is the most common, afflicting 16 million Americans. In fact, osteoarthritis is said to be the most common—and, longest historically recognized—disorder known to humankind.

Osteoarthritis can affect any joint of the body, but it most commonly occurs in the fingers and

weight-bearing joints, such as the hips, ankles, and knees. The disease occurs when the cartilage, which covers the ends of the joints and acts as a cushion between bones, wears away, allowing the bones to rub against each other. For some people, this can be excruciatingly painful. On the other hand, many people with osteoarthritis experience no signs or symptoms of the condition.

Even though osteoarthritis is usually limited to a single location, the afflicted joint can affect the

Relieving Arthritis in The Hands

If you have arthritis in your hands, it may help to squeeze a tennis ball. This strengthens your forearms and hands as well as relieving stiffness. Since an intact tennis ball is difficult to squeeze, make a small cut in it. A 1-inch cut creates moderate resistance, while a 2- to 3-inch cut results in light resistance.

This exercise can be done several times throughout the day (for example, while watching television).

Avoid this exercise if you have a repetitive stress injury of the hand or arm.

ailment. Conventional treatment usually involves exercises and physical therapy to keep the surrounding muscles strong and flexible. Pain and stiffness can be relieved by analgesics and anti-inflammatory drugs (ibuprofen, aspirin). Bed rest and immobilization of the affected joint may be needed for brief periods of time. When all other measures fail to provide relief, surgical joint replacements (knee or hip) have very high success rates.

entire body. Sometimes the muscles surrounding the joint tighten in order to soften the pain or protect the affected joint, while unaffected joints are forced to work overtime to make up for the ailing joint. In cases of osteoarthritis of the knee, the entire lower leg may eventually become deformed.

Although the precise cause of osteoarthritis is not known, wear and tear appears to be the primary culprit. This is why osteoarthritis is also called wear-and-tear arthritis or degenerative joint disease. Thus, the college quarterback and the professional typist—both of whose joints are taxed daily—are at heightened risk of developing osteoarthritis later in life. Osteoarthritis, especially in the hips and fingers, also tends to run in families.

The risk of developing arthritis of the hand increases with age. In fact, by age 75, 85 percent of the population have some symptom of the condition. Often, bony knobs—also called nodes—develop on the knuckles, making fingers look gnarled. Nodes usually appear first on a single finger but can grow to involve all the fingers. While nodes can be tender or slightly painful, they rarely cause any disability. Nearly 90 percent of people with nodes are women over age 45.

Conventional Medical Treatment

An X-ray may be used to detect the presence of osteoarthritis. However, there is no cure for the

Complementary and Alternative Treatments

Nutrition and Supplementation

 (*Note:* The nutrition and supplement information given here is relevant for all arthritics, including those who suffer from osteoarthritis and rheumatoid arthritis, which follows this "Osteoarthritis" entry.) It is important for arthritics to eat a diet high in protein, and to include complex carbohydrates and lots of fresh fruits and vegetables (avoid citrus fruits). Foods that are particularly protective include lentils, soy, and barley (rich in folic acid); asparagus, egg, garlic, and onions (high-sulfur content inhibits inflammation and assists in the repair and rebuilding of body tissues). Also include deep-sea, cold-water fish—such as tuna, salmon, and trout (high in fatty acids that lubricate the joints)—and soy products such as tofu and tempeh (high in the amino acid methionine). Consume up to a gallon of pure drinking water daily and juices from red, yellow, and green fruits and vegetables (not citrus), six to eight times daily (rich in phytochemicals). Be sure to eat fresh pineapple frequently, as it contains bromelain, an enzyme that fights inflammation.

Reduce your fat intake, as extra weight increases stress on joints and bones, and remember to eat foods rich in fiber every day. Some sufferers have an adverse reaction to nightshade vegetables (peppers, eggplant, tomatoes, white potatoes) because they contain solanine. Solanine interferes with enzymes in the muscles, resulting in pain and discomfort. Avoid iron supplements, as iron has been shown to be involved in pain, swelling, and joint destruction. Get your iron from foods such as peas, cauliflower, fish, broccoli, or blackstrap molasses.

People suffering from arthritis can benefit from an individualized supplement program. A specialist takes into consideration type of arthritis, age, weight, and a number of other factors. Also, studies have indicated that people suffering with arthritis have benefited from taking S-adensyl-L-methionine (SAM-e). Neither a hormone nor an herb, SAM-e is a chemical compound found in all living cells. In most people, the body manufactures all the SAM-e it needs from the amino acid methionine found in soybeans, eggs, seeds, lentils, and meat. It appears to regulate more than 35 different mechanisms and helps the body maintain cell membranes and remove toxic substances.

Following are some daily supplements that can benefit all arthritics.

Most Important

- boron (3 mg)—required for healthy bones; recent studies suggest it may even reverse symptoms of osteoarthritis

- sea cucumber (as directed on label)—replenishes the lubricants needed for connective tissues and joints

- N-acetyl glucosamine (as directed on label)—aids in bone, tendon, and ligament formation

- pantothenic acid (500 mg)—essential for steroid production

- bromelain (as directed on label)—inflammation-fighting enzyme

Also Recommended

- calcium (2000 mg)—needed to prevent bone loss

- shark cartilage (as directed by healthcare provider)

- cat's claw (as directed on label)

- magnesium (1000 mg)—needed to balance calcium

- copper (3 mg)—strengthens connective tissue

- zinc (30 mg, not to exceed more than 100 mg total supplement)—necessary for bone growth; often deficient in arthritics

- coenzyme Q10 (60 mg)—aids in the repair of connective tissue

- niacinamide (500 mg 3 times daily)—helps relieve pain and reduce inflammation (*Note:* this vitamin is especially helpful for rheumatoid arthritis sufferers.)

- vitamin E (400 IU)—an antioxidant that protects joints from damage by free radicals; increases joint mobility

- citrulline (as directed on label)—anti-inflammatory properties (*Note:* this vitamin is especially helpful for rheumatoid arthritis sufferers.)

- glutathione or N-acetyl cysteine (250 mg)—strong antioxidants (*Note:* especially helpful for rheumatoid arthritis sufferers.)

- grape seed extract (as directed on label)—a free radical scavenger that also fights inflammation and strengthens connective tissue

- hydrolyzed collagen (as directed on label)— important for joint tissue rebuilding

- S-adensyl-L-methionine (SAM-e) (as directed on label)

- methyl sulfonyl methane, or MSM (as directed on label)—a sulfur compound that aids synthesis of collagen

- capsaicin (as directed on label, topically or orally)—good pain reliever and anti-inflammatory

(For an *acute* condition, take supplements until your symptoms subside. If symptoms persist, seek the advice of your healthcare provider. For a *chronic* condition, consult your healthcare provider regarding the duration of treatment.)

A recent and widely-accepted treatment for arthritis, particularly osteoarthritis, uses glucosamine. This dynamic substance can actually repair damaged or eroded cartilage. Glucosamine is made up of glucose, the sugar that the body burns for fuel, and an amino acid called glutamine. It provides structure to the bone and cartilage as well as to skin, nails, hair, and other body tissues. Glucosamine sulfate is the most popular form used in the United States. This sulfate acts as a liquid magnet, attracting proteoglycan molecules (which fill in the spaces within the cartilage "netting"). This is important because the fluid acts as a shock absorber while it sweeps nutrients into the cartilage. Without this nutritional fluid, cartilage becomes fragile, thin, and malnourished.

Daily dosage depends on your weight. If you weigh less than 120 pounds, take 1000 mg glucosamine. If your weight falls between 120 and 200 pounds, take 1500 mg glucosamine. If you weigh over 200 pounds, take 2000 mg glucosamine. Because everyone's needs are different, you may need more or less than the preceding dosages, but they are good starting points. Vitamin C and manganese help increase the effectiveness of glucosamine. Manganese is safe up to 50 mg per day.

If you decide to take these supplements, you would be wise to have a thorough consultation with your healthcare provider.

Aromatherapy

For temporary relief of stiff, achy joints, try massaging a blend of 15 drops of rosemary oil, 15 drops of Roman or German chamomile oil, and 1 ounce of soybean oil into the affected joints. You might also try a warm bath laced with rosemary and chamomile; soak for about 20 minutes. Other essential oils to try include camphor, peppermint, lemon, or marjoram.

Ayurvedic Medicine

Ayurveda views inflammatory diseases as energy and digestive imbalances, in which the body is unable to eliminate toxic waste. To treat the disorder, ease discomfort, and increase range of motion in affected joints, Ayurvedic practitioners may recommend trying one or more of the following remedies:

- Take *triphala* to cleanse your intestines, aid indigestion, and stimulate the immune system.

- Use *boswellia,* flaxseed, and fish oils to protect your joints and increase joint mobility. You might also try rubbing warm sesame oil into the affected joints.

- Soak in hot water laced with baking soda, eucalyptus, ginger, peppermint, or salt to decrease discomfort and loosen joints.

- Follow a pacifying diet, depending on your Ayurvedic category of arthritis. You might also add hot spices, such as cayenne, to your diet to loosen joints and control pain.

Bodywork and Somatic Practices

Depending on the severity of the pain and degree of immobility, it may be best to start with more gentle techniques such as CranioSacral therapy, reflexology, Feldenkrais, Trager, Chinese Medical Massage (acupressure), polarity therapy, Therapeutic Touch, and Reiki.

Chiropractic

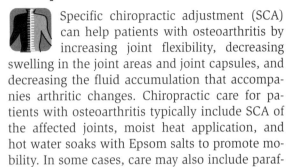

Specific chiropractic adjustment (SCA) can help patients with osteoarthritis by increasing joint flexibility, decreasing swelling in the joint areas and joint capsules, and decreasing the fluid accumulation that accompanies arthritic changes. Chiropractic care for patients with osteoarthritis typically include SCA of the affected joints, moist heat application, and hot water soaks with Epsom salts to promote mobility. In some cases, care may also include paraffin (hot wax) baths.

Herbal Therapy

The effectiveness of herbal remedies for arthritis sufferers varies from person to person, so you may need to experiment a bit. Try one of the following treatments:

- Take a combination tincture of meadowsweet, willow bark, black cohosh, prickly ash, celery seed, and nettle to help temper arthritis symptoms. To make the blend, mix equal amounts of the tinctures; take 1 teaspoonful of the mixture 3 times daily. The blend is safe and can be taken for a period of time.

- Use yucca and devil's claw to reduce inflammation. Other herbs to try include licorice, alfalfa, turmeric, ginger, skullcap, and ginseng.

- Rub a tincture of lobelia and cramp bark over the sore areas to decrease muscle tension.

- Take a combination of 2 parts of willow bark, 1 part of black cohosh, and 1 part of nettle to ease aches and pains.

- Rub cayenne over the affected joints to lessen pain.

Herbal products are available in health food stores and in some pharmacies and supermarkets. Follow package for specific directions.

Homeopathy

Osteoarthritis may respond to homeopathic treatment. However, the selection of a remedy—more than one is available—depends on *your* symptoms and the stage of the condition. Don't try treating this disorder yourself. See a homeopathic professional.

Hydrotherapy

Warm, moist heat packs used for 10 to 20 minutes every 4 hours can bring welcome relief from stiffness and deep pain. Exercises performed in heated water and swimming have also been effective. Drink distilled water to help absorb and eliminate mineral salts and other waste products throughout the skin.

Traditional Chinese Medicine

Acupuncture According to the WHO, acupuncture is a vital addition to the arthritis-fighting arsenal. Acupuncture can be used to help restore the body's energy balance, and it can also help lessen the pain and inflammation that commonly occur in the hands, hips, knees, and spinal joints of osteoarthritis patients. Many doctors now use acupuncture in conjunction with chiropractic techniques when treating osteoarthritis, and it has been used for centuries with Chinese manipulative techniques.

To treat hand and finger pain, the practitioner may focus on Small Intestine 7 (located on the forearm) and the Shang Pa Hsieh sites that lie between the fingers. Additional points may be added, depending on where in the hand the arthritis is located.

More than six different acupoints are stimulated in the treatment of hip pain, and up to 12 points may be manipulated to alleviate arthritis-related knee pain.

Acupressure To lessen the severity of arthritis symptoms, a practitioner may use acupressure on points that correspond to the liver, gallbladder, kidneys, bladder, stomach, and the governing vessel. The practitioner also may massage the points that correspond to the affected area to relieve pain and inflammation.

Chinese Herbal Therapy Chinese herbalists consider osteoarthritis to be a yin-related "external damp" illness, and treat the disease by concocting a remedy that will nourish yin and dispel the damp wind while it alleviates swollen, painful joints.

Asarum Sieboldi may be helpful in relieving joint pain; take 3 to 4 grams daily. Foxnut has analgesic properties and is used to reduce pain and inflammation. It can be taken in pill form (9 to 15 grams per day) or as a 10- to 20-gram daily decoction. Polygonatum cirrhifolium is said to not only cure arthritis, but to combat premature aging.

If the pain shifts from one joint to another, Corydalis Tuber Forumula may be helpful. For fixed pain accompanied by heavy, swollen joints, try Tu-Huo and Loranthus Formula or Stephania and Astragalus Combination (by mail order). Most of these remedies can be found in health food stores.

Yoga and Meditation

 Exercise plays an important role in improving circulation and helping the body eliminate waste. Yoga poses improve flexibility, yet place little stress on joints. Focus on gentle poses, such as the Tree, Triangle, Forward Bend, Spinal Twist, Boat, Bow, Camel, Cow, Locust, Moon Salutation, Chest-Knee, Maha Mudra, and Half Bridge.

RHEUMATOID ARTHRITIS

Signs and Symptoms

- Pain, swelling, redness, and warmth in the affected joint—most commonly affects the smaller joints of your hands and feet, but elbows, knees, and ankles can be affected
- Usually affects joints symmetrically (both hands, for example)

- Overall stiffness and achiness, especially after periods of stillness, such as sleeping or long plane rides
- Symptoms are worse in the early morning and lessen as the day progresses
- General malaise/weakness
- Anemia
- Pain usually occurs during rest and movement

Description

Unlike osteoarthritis, rheumatoid arthritis is an inflammatory, not degenerative, disease. It first appears as an inflammation in a joint's synovium, the membrane that lines and lubricates the joint. Once inflamed, the membrane thickens and become sore and swollen—which in turn may limit the affected joint's movement. In time, this inflammation spreads to other parts of the affected joint, causing even more stiffness and pain. Eventually, the inflammation can spread to organs, such as the heart, lungs, and eyes. Its ability to spread throughout the body makes rheumatoid arthritis a systemic disease—a disease that affects the entire body.

Inflammation is not a harmful state, per se. It's actually your body's normal response to infections and injuries, caused when your white cells battle an invading organism. Typically, the inflammation subsides after the infection is wiped out. However, with rheumatoid arthritis, the autoimmune system seems to fight the body instead of protecting it.

While the disease can strike at any time, it usually occurs between the ages 20 and 50. It affects approximately three times as many women as men.

Unlike illnesses that have a set progression of symptoms, rheumatoid arthritis is unpredictable. What symptoms appear, how often they appear, and what joints and organs are affected vary widely, depending on the individual. In some sufferers, rheumatoid arthritis will flare up occasionally, only to be followed by periods of normal health. Others experience recurring attacks without returning to a state of full wellness in be-

Rheumatoid Research

In an effort to learn more about what causes rheumatoid arthritis, The Arthritis Foundation; the National Institute of Arthritis, Musculoskeletal and Skin Diseases (NIAMS); and the National Institute of Allergy and Infectious Diseases (NIAID) have teamed with a national consortium of 12 research centers in a search for the specific genes that determine susceptibility to rheumatoid arthritis. The research is centered around 1000 families nationwide in which two or more siblings have developed rheumatoid arthritis between the ages of 18 and 60.

tween. Many experience a slow and steady increase in the severity of their symptoms over time.

Some people with rheumatoid arthritis develop small lumps under the skin near the elbow, ears, or nose, or on the back of the scalp, over the knee, or under the toes. Called rheumatoid nodules, these painless and non-problematic bumps range from the size of a pea to the size of a Ping-Pong® ball.

While medical experts have not identified a single cause for rheumatoid arthritis, possibilities include heredity, viral or bacterial infection, and emotional stress.

Conventional Medical Treatment

A series of blood tests, along with a thorough physical exam and medical history, can confirm whether you have rheumatoid arthritis. X-rays may also be helpful. Strategies for treating rheumatoid arthritis differ, depending on whether it is active or in remission. During a flare-up, a combination of rest, heat, and medication is prescribed. Anti-inflammatory drugs—aspirin, in particular—are the first line of treatment and may ease symptoms. There are several other medications used to treat rheumatoid arthritis. Your doctor may prescribe gold salts, penicellamine, methotrexate, azathioprine, or anti-malarials, depending on how

your symptoms progress. Corticosteroids can temporarily relieve pain and inflammation, but they are usually reserved for those with more serious disease.

Physical therapy plays a major role in the treatment of rheumatoid arthritis. It is most effective when swelling and inflammation of the joint are suppressed with medications. Physical therapy can reduce deformity and restore function.

In severe cases, surgical removal of affected joint lining can prevent damage to other joint structures and cartilage. Another surgical procedure fuses the painful, uncushioned bones together but is only performed on the wrist, feet, ankles, and thumbs because it restricts motion. Tendon transfer is another surgical option for repairing damaged tendons and ligaments—it is

Health Note

➤ *Experts believe that practicing stress relief and keeping the immune system strong with a nutrient-dense diet, moderate exercise, and regular sleep can help the body ward off rheumatoid arthritis.*

performed most frequently on the hands. Another option is arthroplasty, or joint replacement, which is usually performed on knees, hips, and shoulders.

For More Information
The Arthritis Foundation
1330 West Peachtree Street
Atlanta, GA 30309
800-283-7800
www.arthritis.org

Complementary and Alternative Treatments

Nutrition and Supplementation

 See "Osteoarthritis" entry.

Aromatherapy

To help reduce inflammation, try drinking ginger-castor oil tea daily at bedtime. (See also "Osteoarthritis" entry.)

Chiropractic

Although chiropractic cannot do a lot to turn back the clock, it can prevent progression of the disease. Specific chiropractic adjustment (SCA) can help patients with rheumatoid arthritis by increasing joint flexibility, decreasing swelling in the joint areas and joint capsules, and decreasing fluid accumulation that results from arthritic changes. For example, if the patient's hands are affected, care includes SCA of the affected joints, moist heat application, and hot water soaks with Epsom salts to promote mobility. In some cases, care may include paraffin (hot wax) baths.

Herbal Therapy

Rheumatoid arthritis and osteoarthritis have many similarities, including herbal remedies. However, there are some subtle variations. For rheumatoid arthritis, take a combination tincture of meadowsweet, willow bark, black cohosh, prickly ash, celery seed, nettle, wild yam, and valerian to help temper arthritis symptoms. To make the blend, mix equal amounts of the tinctures; take 1 teaspoonful of the mixture 3 times daily. The blend is safe and can be taken for a period of time. (See also "Osteoarthritis" entry.)

Herbal products are available in health food stores and in some pharmacies and supermarkets. Follow package for specific directions.

Homeopathy

See "Osteoarthritis" entry.

Traditional Chinese Medicine

Acupuncture To treat rheumatoid arthritis, which commonly affects the wrists, knees, shoulders, ankles, and elbows—acupuncturists may focus on the heart, kidney, back of head, and internal secretion points. They may also target any points that are associated with the afflicted joint.

To help quell arthritis-related foot pain, the practitioner may manipulate Liver 2, Kidney 3, Bladder 60, Liver 3, Stomach 44, and several points on the ear. Arthritic ankle pain is often treated by inserting needles into Stomach 41, Bladder 60, Gallbladder 40, and additional auricular points.

Acupressure For rheumatism-related ankle pain, a practitioner will probably target two points: Large Intestine 4 (in the webbing of the hand between the thumb and forefinger) and Bladder 60 (in the depression behind the outside ankle bone). Several points on the foot and on the ankle itself also may be targeted.

Elbow pain may be relieved by massaging LI 11 (toward the outside of the elbow); knee pain will be helped by manipulating several points on and around the knee itself; shoulder pain is best helped by performing acupressure on several points, including Large Intestine 15 and Gallbladder 21; while wrist pain is alleviated by applying pressure to several acupoints on the wrist. In addition, ear acupuncture may be used to help further relieve the symptoms of rheumatoid arthritis.

Generalized joint pain may be relieved by pressing the two Gallbladder 20 points on the back of the neck.

Chinese Herbal Therapy There are many Chinese herbal arthritis formulas available at health food stores or by mail order, such as Angelica and Loranthes Combination for lower back and knee pain; *Xiao Huo Luo Dan* for stiff joints; *Feng Shih Hsiao Tung Wan* for finger, shoulder, knee, and hip pain associated with rheumatism; and *Tian Ma Wan* for general rheumatic pain.

ASTHMA

Signs and Symptoms

- Wheezing, possibly accompanied by a whistling noise
- Shortness of breath and difficulty exhaling
- Coughing, usually in fits; the coughs may or may not produce mucus
- Tightness in the chest; though the chest feels constricted, it isn't painful
- Constricted throat that is dry and literally feels squeezed shut
- Sleeping difficulty
- Congested nasal passages (more common in those who suffer from chronic attacks)
- Increased pulse rate
- Extreme difficulty in breathing (emergency symptom)

Description

Sufferers describe asthma as a feeling of suffocation, and it's easy to see why. During an attack, the muscles that encompass the body's airways—which include the trachea, bronchial tube, and bronchi—begin to contract around these important air passages, constricting them. If that weren't uncomfortable enough, the inner lining of the lungs and these now-squeezed airways begin to swell, narrowing the airways further and making it increasingly difficult for air to pass through. When irritated, the membranes of the lungs and airways exacerbate the situation further by secreting a thick mucus.

Asthma attacks range widely in severity. They can be so mild that sufferers don't even realize they have the condition, or so severe that victims must be rushed to the hospital or face death by suffocation. Furthermore, a person who had a mild bout two months ago can have a life-threatening assault a year from now.

There are as many as 10 to 20 million Americans of all ages who have asthma—50 percent of them under the age of 10. Up to 10 percent of all children have asthma—twice as many boys as girls—making it the leading cause of chronic illness in children. In fact, asthma is a leading cause of missed school days, responsible for 7.5 million absences among elementary school students each year.

Many of these children will "grow out of" the condition by the time they reach adulthood. Many carry it with them their whole lives. Many more individuals don't even develop asthma until they are well into their third or fourth decade. Asthma is hereditary, and research is currently underway to isolate an asthma gene.

No one really knows why some people get asthma and some don't. However, it seems asthma victims have especially sensitive airways that become constricted, inflamed, and congested after coming in contact with an irritant. Asthma symptoms usually appear within minutes after exposure to an irritant, and the majority of attacks are not life-threatening.

Of course the attack-triggering irritant varies from asthma sufferer to asthma sufferer, but leading instigators include inhaled irritants—typically pollens, molds, animal dander, strong odors, fumes from paint and gas, and smoke. Interestingly, the mites found in house dust are a common inhaled allergen and play a large role in asthma's nighttime attacks. It makes sense, since people typically spend eight hours in bed where they mingle with whatever mites live in their linens.

Unfortunately, the number of people with the condition seems to be growing. One estimate states the number of asthma cases has doubled between 1984 and 1994. For an explanation, one has only to look at a specific inhaled asthma-trigger: environmental pollutants. The increased use of environmental chemicals, such as pesticides and other petrochemicals, has led many

Treating Illness "By The Clock"

Chronotherapy, or "timed" therapy, is designed to track a condition's daily, monthly, or yearly cycle and treat it accordingly. Although not widely used, it has helped many asthma sufferers.

For many female asthmatics, the condition can occur in monthly cycles. A survey of 182 patients at the Medical College of Pennsylvania concluded that nearly half of their asthma-related emergency room visits occurred immediately prior to, or during, menstruation. Increased doses of inhaled steroids during this monthly period has proven beneficial for many female patents.

- Sputum examination (mucus secretions are checked for abnormal cells)

- Histamine challenge (patient is exposed to irritants then checked to see if asthma erupts)

- Exercise challenge (patient works out on a treadmill, rowing machine, or exercise bike to see if asthma occurs)

- Sinus X-ray (to see if patient has a sinus condition that might trigger asthma)

- Skin testing (patient's skin is repeatedly pricked to insert minute amount of any of a number of known allergens; if a welt appears, that signals a possibility the substance will trigger an asthma attack)

If you are diagnosed with asthma, your doctor develops a treatment plan for you based on your symptoms and asthma triggers. Conventional treatment is based on the approach of identifying and evaluating asthma triggers, then working toward controlling, removing, or avoiding those triggers. Thus, if dust or mites trigger your asthma, expect to keep your home and linens scrupulously clean. If animals are the problem, you must avoid petting them or even standing next to them. If an environmental pollutant is to blame, you must—to the best of your ability—avoid it. In addition, medication is often used to prevent or lesson a reaction. These medications include inhaled bronchodilators, oral bronchodilators, inhaled steroids, oral steroids, cromolyn, and nedocromil.

researchers to make a connection between their increased use and the growing number of asthma sufferers.

However, airborne substances aren't the only elements to blame. Other irritants include feathers, aspirin, food additives (such as metasulfites and tartrazine, also known as FD&C yellow no. 5), and nonsteroidal anti-inflammatory medications. There are even people who get a case of asthma from strenuous exercise, extreme emotions (such as fright, anger, or anxiety), a complication of a viral or sinus infection, or a pre-existing food sensitivity, such as an allergy to shellfish.

Conventional Medical Treatment

Do you suspect you have asthma? Visit your doctor, who can make a diagnosis after performing a complete physical and any—or all—of the following diagnostic tests:

- Spirometry/pulmonary function tests (breathing into a machine to measure the lungs' ability to inhale and exhale)

Relaxation Techniques

A faster breathing rate is normal when you are excited or experiencing stress, but if you suffer from asthma, you may also experience breathing difficulties at such times. Relaxation techniques can be extremely helpful. Slow down your breathing rate by taking a "time out" from the stressful situation. Sit still in a quiet place and concentrate on taking slow, even breaths. You may want to close your eyes and focus on something calming. Relaxation often works as well as medication to relax the muscles that have tightened around the airways.

a

Health Notes

➤ *If you're an asthma sufferer, the single most important way to prevent symptoms from occurring is to know your triggers—then control, remove, or avoid them.*

➤ *For women: The estrogen loss three days before a menstrual period, and four days into the period, can trigger asthma attacks.*

➤ *Some people have exercise-induced asthma attacks. Warm up slowly during exercise or dance classes. Consider swimming, which is a recommended exercise. Using an inhaled bronchodilator 30 minutes before exercise can prevent an attack.*

➤ *Avoid all airborne allergens, such as pet dander, dust mites, and mold as well as areas in which there are cockroaches.*

➤ *If you smoke, quit. Avoid secondhand smoke, including industrial smoke, wood burning stoves, and burning leaves.*

➤ *Avoid inhaling fumes from cleaning fluid, fresh paint, insecticide sprays, and perfumed deodorants.*

For More Information
American Lung Association
1740 Broadway
New York, NY 10019
800-LUNG-USA
www.lungusa.org

Asthma and Allergy Foundation of America
1233 Twentieth Street NW, Suite 402
Washington D.C. 20036
800-7-ASTHMA
www.aafa.org

Complementary and Alternative Treatments

Nutrition and Supplementation

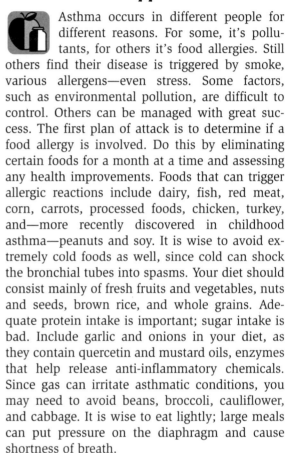 Asthma occurs in different people for different reasons. For some, it's pollutants, for others it's food allergies. Still others find their disease is triggered by smoke, various allergens—even stress. Some factors, such as environmental pollution, are difficult to control. Others can be managed with great success. The first plan of attack is to determine if a food allergy is involved. Do this by eliminating certain foods for a month at a time and assessing any health improvements. Foods that can trigger allergic reactions include dairy, fish, red meat, corn, carrots, processed foods, chicken, turkey, and—more recently discovered in childhood asthma—peanuts and soy. It is wise to avoid extremely cold foods as well, since cold can shock the bronchial tubes into spasms. Your diet should consist mainly of fresh fruits and vegetables, nuts and seeds, brown rice, and whole grains. Adequate protein intake is important; sugar intake is bad. Include garlic and onions in your diet, as they contain quercetin and mustard oils, enzymes that help release anti-inflammatory chemicals. Since gas can irritate asthmatic conditions, you may need to avoid beans, broccoli, cauliflower, and cabbage. It is wise to eat lightly; large meals can put pressure on the diaphragm and cause shortness of breath.

Recent studies in London link adulthood obesity with asthma. The reason isn't completely clear, but researchers believe that lack of exercise, together with poor diet, reduce the normal stretching of the airways, leading to narrowing and difficult breathing.

Recent research indicates that supplementing the diet with simple antioxidants can help asthmatics breathe easier. The study showed that persons who supplemented with both vitamins E and C showed improved pulmonary function after being exposed to two common air pollutants, ozone and sulfur dioxide. Additional daily supplementation can include:

Most Important

- quercetin (500 mg 3 times)—stimulates the immune system

- bromelain (100 mg 3 times)—stabilizes cells to stop inflammation; best taken with quercetin

- flaxseed oil (1000 mg twice daily before meals)—a good source of essential fatty acids necessary for production of anti-inflammatory prostaglandins

- vitamin B_5 (50 mg 3 times)—to reduce stress and benefit the adrenal system

- vitamin A (15,000 IU; do not exceed 8000 IU if you are pregnant)—promotes tissue repair and immunity

- mixed carotenoid complex (10,000 IU)—an antioxidant and precursor of vitamin A

- vitamin B complex (50 mg 4 times daily)—stimulates the immune system, supplemented with vitamin B_6 (½ cc weekly or as prescribed by healthcare provider), and vitamin B_{12} (1000 mcg twice daily between meals)—decreases inflammation that occurs during an attack; lozenge is the best form

- vitamin E (600 IU and up)—a powerful antioxidant

- vitamin C with bioflavonoids (1500 mg 3 times daily)—keeps infection at bay and increases air flow; fights inflammation

Also Recommended

- coenzyme Q10 (100 mg)—helps counter histamine

- kelp (2000 to 3000 mg for 21 days, then reduce to 1000 to 1500 mg)—supplies minerals in balanced amounts

- vitamin D (600 IU)—repairs tissues

- glutathione (600 mg)—depleted in asthma sufferers

- N-acetyl glucosamine (as directed on label)—necessary for the regulation of mucus secretions

(For an *acute* condition, take supplements until your symptoms subside. If symptoms persist, seek the advice of your healthcare provider. For a *chronic* condition, consult your healthcare provider regarding the duration of treatment.)

Aromatherapy

Some therapists recommend a chest rub of eucalyptus, lavender, and Roman chamomile essential oils to reduce asthma symptoms. To ease breathing, place a few drops of cedarwood, eucalyptus, or peppermint on a handkerchief or tissue and inhale. Take care in using the rub or inhalation if your asthma is caused by allergies, and consult your doctor before starting a new regimen.

Ayurvedic Medicine

Ayurveda views asthma as a kapha dosha disorder that begins in the stomach and progresses to the lungs and bronchi. The goal of treatment is to move the excess kapha back to the stomach, then eliminate the excess. An Ayurvedic practitioner may suggest drinking licorice-ginger tea or cinnamon-*trikatu* tea (*trikatu* is a blend of ginger and peppers) or a mixture of onion juice and black pepper. The practitioner may also recommend that you rub brown mustard oil into your chest or ingest a mixture of brown mustard oil and sugar several times a day on an empty stomach.

Before starting any new regimen to treat asthma, consult your doctor.

Bodywork and Somatic Practices

CranioSacral Therapy, Oriental bodywork, and reflexology are good compliments to other treatments.

Chiropractic

Proper chiropractic manipulation of the spine—specifically, manipulation of the nerves that enervate the lungs—may decrease the frequency and intensity of asthmatic reactions. Typically, these adjustments are performed on the thoracic (mid-back) section of the spine. For chronic asthmatics, ongoing chiropractic care should be performed in conjunction with other therapies, such as the use of pocket inhalers or at-home nebulizers.

Herbal Therapy

Several herbs can help clear the airways of the excess mucus that's associated with asthma, say herbalists. Try infusions of elecampane or mullein. To make the elecampane tea, steep 1 teaspoon shredded root in 1 cup cold water for 10 hours; strain. Heat and drink up to 3 times daily. For the mullein tea, steep 1 to 2 teaspoons dried leaves, flowers, or powdered root in 1 cup of boiling water for 10 to 15 minutes. Drink several times daily. Other beneficial herbs include marshmallow, slippery elm, and passion flower.

Herbal products are available in health food stores and in some pharmacies and supermarkets. Follow package for specific directions.

Homeopathy

Asthma may respond to homeopathic treatment. However, the selection of a remedy—more than one is available—depends on *your* symptoms and the stage of the condition. Don't try treating this disorder yourself. See a homeopathic professional.

Hydrotherapy

To decrease symptoms, including congestion, try hot foot baths. As you soak your feet, apply cool water to your head. Alternatively, you can cool your head by using a fan.

Traditional Chinese Medicine

Acupuncture Acupuncture can be quite useful in reducing the severity of asthma symptoms and in keeping the condition under control. In using auricular therapy, the acupuncturist may apply needles to the lung, bronchi, trachea, heart, ping-chuan, and adrenal gland points.

In treating asthma with acupuncture to the body, the therapist takes into account the severity and frequency of the asthma attacks when determining exactly what points to target. Some practitioners also burn moxa cones over specific asthma-related points on the chest.

Acupressure To help relieve asthma symptoms, an acupressurist may work on points on the chest, forearm, neck, clavicle, abdomen, calves, ankle, and the upper and lower back.

Chinese Herbal Therapy An herbalist may prepare a decoction containing cinnamon twigs, ginger, white peony root, licorice, and Chinese dates. They also may prescribe Minor Blue Dragon Formula for asthma; this remedy contains more than a dozen different herbs to relieve the typical runny nose, watery eyes, shortness of breath, and wheezing. Additional Chinese asthma formulas include Rehmannia Eight, Cyperus and Ligusticum Formula, Mahuang Formula, Gingeng and Astragalus, and Fritillaria Extract Tablets. An herbalist determines the individual cause of a patient's asthma before deciding which herbs are the most appropriate.

Yoga and Meditation

Breathing exercises and certain yoga poses are powerful tools for coping with asthma. Practice several of the following poses daily: Stand Sun, Wind Removal, Seated Sun, Cobra, Bow, Shoulder Stand, and Plow.

ASTIGMATISM

Signs and Symptoms

- Blurred areas in the field of vision of one or both eyes
- Distorted vision in one or both eyes, typically when looking at vertical, horizontal, or diagonal lines

Description

Astigmatism is a condition in which one or both eyes has a misshapen cornea. In a normal eye, the cornea is symmetrically curved. In an astigmatic eye, areas of the cornea are steeper or flatter than normal, causing areas of your vision to be blurred. Although astigmatism often occurs on its own, it can also occur in combination with nearsightedness or farsightedness.

Astigmatism is usually present from birth and tends to remain constant, neither improving nor deteriorating with time.

Conventional Medical Treatment

An ophthalmologist or optometrist can diagnose astigmatism with a thorough examination. Corrective glasses or contact lenses are usually prescribed to counteract the unevenness of one or both corneas. Lenses also can be made to address a combination of astigmatism and nearsightedness or farsightedness.

Health Note

➤ If you have astigmatism, schedule yearly eye exams with your ophthalmologist to ensure that your corrective lenses are still effective.

For More Information
National Eye Institute (NEI)
National Institutes of Health
2020 Vision Place
Bethesda, MD 20892-3655
301-496-5248
www.nei.nih.gov

Complementary and Alternative Treatments

Nutrition and Supplementation

 Nutritionists encourage adequate intake of nutrients necessary for healthy eye function. Protein (found in meat, eggs, poultry, and fish) and vitamin A (found in yellow fruits and vegetables) are required for proper eye function.

Include the following daily supplements to maintain healthy eye function:

Most Important

- vitamin C (5000 IU)
- vitamin B complex (100 mg), supplemented with vitamin B_2 (50 mg)
- vitamin A (10,000 to 15,000 IU; do not exceed 8000 IU daily if you are pregnant)
- vitamin E (400 IU)
- zinc (20 to 25 mg)

Also Recommended

- calcium and magnesium (standard dose)
- chromium (300 mcg)
- omega 3 and 6 and DHA capsules (as directed on label)
- grape seed extract (as directed on label)

(Consult your healthcare provider regarding the duration of treatment.)

Traditional Chinese Medicine

 Acupuncture Chinese practitioners believe that most vision disorders are due to impaired liver functioning, so an acupuncturist may treat astigmatism by working to strengthen the liver and restore energy imbalances associated with that organ. Commonly used acupoints in the treatment of astigmatism include Bladder 1, Stomach 1, Liver 4, and Triple Warmer 6.

Studies indicate that stress may actually aggravate or promote astigmatism in children, so acupuncture may be used to relieve anxiety and promote relaxation, thereby reducing the severity of the ailment.

Acupressure To help prevent an astigmatic condition from worsening, an acupressure practitioner may work on points around the eyes, nose, temples, and cheeks.

Chinese Herbal Therapy Consult a qualified Chinese medical practitioner regarding treatment. Frequently, herbs are used to treat liver problems, which are believed to be associated with astigmatism.

ATHLETE'S FOOT

Signs and Symptoms

- Intense itching on the sole of the foot or in between the toes
- Stinging or burning sensation between toes
- Cracked, red skin that may or may not ooze liquid
- Dry scaling and fissuring of skin between toes
- Small, pink, water-filled blister between toes
- Nails that separate from the nail bed
- Foot odor

Description

Also known as *tinea pedis,* athlete's foot is a common fungus infection. Intense itching is the hallmark of athlete's foot. In fact, the condition is so irritating that many sufferers vigorously scratch at the area just for a few moments of relief. Unfortunately, scratching not only worsens the existing infection, it spreads the fungus to new skin. In cases where scratching is especially intense, the skin can become extremely weepy and warm to the touch.

Athlete's foot is caused by mold-like fungi called dermatophytes, a moderately contagious organism that is most commonly spread in locker rooms, public showers, and swimming pools—hence, the name "athlete's foot." It can also be caught by sharing an infected towel or by stepping on a mat after someone with athlete's foot stood there. Athlete's foot infections are rarely dangerous.

Poor hygiene, continually moist skin, and minor skin or nail injuries increase your chances of catching athlete's foot from a contaminated surface. Clean, dry, and intact skin rarely becomes infected.

Conventional Medical Treatment

Athlete's foot is usually diagnosed by a visual exam. Treatment typically involves an over-the-counter anti-fungal cream or liquid that is applied to the area twice a day. In severe cases, a stronger cream or an oral anti-fungal medication is prescribed. In addition, you are instructed to keep your feet dry, wear absorbent socks, wash your feet daily, wear open-toe shoes or sandals whenever possible, and change socks when damp.

Foot Odor

Why do feet sometimes smell really bad? When your feet sweat, your socks and shoes become damp, creating an ideal environment for odor-causing bacteria, which flourish in warm, moist environments. To hide the smell of foot odor, people try everything from charcoal insoles to deodorant powders. Yet these products only mask foot odor, they don't get rid of the guilty bacteria. If you want fresher-smelling feet, you must treat the source of foot odor.

The goal in ridding yourself of foot odor is to make your footwear inhospitable to odor-causing bacteria. The easiest way to do this is to minimize dampness in shoes. As soon as a pair of shoes becomes wet or damp—either with sweat or after a walk in the rain—remove them. Do not put them on again until they are completely dry; it usually takes two or three days for a pair of shoes to dry after being sweat in or rained on. For this reason, it's wise to buy two or three pairs of shoes—this includes workout shoes, which many people wear at the gym on consecutive days.

Socks, too, should be changed the moment they become damp. Moreover, feet should be washed with anti-bacterial soap between sock changings or at the end of each day.

If your feet sweat unusually heavily, visit your healthcare provider to rule out any undiagnosed medical problems.

For More Information
The American Academy of Dermatology
930 North Meacham Road
Schaumberg, IL 60173
888-462-DERM
www.aad.org

Health Notes

➤ *To avoid athlete's foot, wash hands and feet daily, dry skin thoroughly, and go barefoot as often as possible.*

➤ *When wearing your shoes, choose socks that are woven from a blend of cotton and synthetic fibers—past advice about wearing only 100 percent cotton socks has recently been refuted.*

➤ *Buy well-ventilated all-leather shoes. Don't forget to alternate footwear each day.*

Complementary and Alternative Treatments

Nutrition and Supplementation

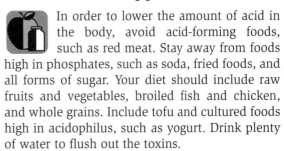 In order to lower the amount of acid in the body, avoid acid-forming foods, such as red meat. Stay away from foods high in phosphates, such as soda, fried foods, and all forms of sugar. Your diet should include raw fruits and vegetables, broiled fish and chicken, and whole grains. Include tofu and cultured foods high in acidophilus, such as yogurt. Drink plenty of water to flush out the toxins.

A daily nutritional supplement regimen such as the one below should help your condition.

Most Important

• a prodophilus formula (1 tsp in water twice daily on empty stomach)—replenishes friendly bacteria

• colloidal silver (apply topically as directed on label)—a natural antibiotic and disinfectant that promotes healing

• garlic (as directed on label)—destroys fungus

Also Recommended

- vitamin B complex (100 mg)—promotes healthy skin

- vitamin C (3000 to 10,000 mg 3 times daily in divided doses)—promotes immune function

- zinc (50 mg daily, not to exceed a total of 100 mg from all supplements)—inhibits fungus and stimulates the immune system

- essential fatty acids (1 tblsp flaxseed oil)— promotes healing of skin disorders

- vitamin A (50,000 IU daily for 1 month, then reduce to 25,000 IU; do not exceed 8000 IU daily if you are pregnant)—heals tissues and stimulates the immune system

- vitamin E (start with 400 IU daily and slowly increase to 1000 IU daily)—promotes healthy skin

- oil of oregano (apply topically as directed on label)

(For an *acute* condition, take supplements until your symptoms subside. If symptoms persist, seek the advice of your healthcare provider. For a *chronic* condition, consult your healthcare provider regarding the duration of treatment.)

Aromatherapy

 Tea tree oil is especially effective for combating athlete's foot and other skin infections. For athlete's foot, apply the essential oil directly to the affected area after thoroughly washing and drying. Dilute with aloe gel or vegetable oil if it's too strong.

Ayurvedic Medicine

 Ayurvedic practitioners recommend cleaning the affected area with tea tree oil, then applying an aloe vera-turmeric mixture for 2 to 3 weeks. *Note:* turmeric stains fabric and skin, so wear old socks.

Homeopathy

 See "Yeast Infections" entry.

Hydrotherapy

 Wash and thoroughly dry the affected areas often.

Traditional Chinese Medicine

 Chinese Herbal Therapy To treat athlete's foot, an herbalist may prepare a decoction of fresh aloe vera juice and licorice, which can be applied directly to the affected area 3 times a day, as needed.

Garlic can also be used to treat athlete's foot. Simply puree 3 to 5 fresh cloves, apply them to the area and wrap in a clean, dry cloth or sterilized gauze. Leave the cloth in place for 1 to 2 hours before removing. Wipe away garlic with another clean, dry cloth (don't use water).

ATTENTION DEFICIT DISORDER (ADD)

Signs and Symptoms

- Difficulty sustaining attention
- Easily distracted
- Fidgeting and physical restlessness

- Has difficulty allowing others to speak without interrupting
- Doesn't appear to listen to others when they speak
- Often talks excessively

- Frequently loses things
- Difficulty following directions
- Shifts from one unfinished task to another
- Inability to play or sit quietly
- Impulsive personality
- Inability to organize thoughts, toys, work space

Description

A few decades ago, a child who couldn't sit still and wouldn't pay attention in class was called "hyper," or worse, a "problem child." Today, the same youngster might be diagnosed with attention deficit disorder (ADD), also known as attention deficit hyperactivity disorder (ADHD). The condition basically describes a person's inability to concentrate—on sitting still, on a lesson given in class, on reading a book, on what someone else is saying, and so on. Demanding that a person with ADD pay attention will not work, nor will punishment. It's not known exactly why a person with ADD has such difficulty focusing.

The cause of ADD is also unknown. Prominent theories include heredity, lead poisoning, allergies to food additives, brain injuries incurred by the child during the mother's pregnancy (perhaps the mother was in an accident, smoked cigarettes, or used drugs or alcohol), oxygen deprivation during birth, or head trauma as an infant. ADD affects many more males than females.

ADD typically appears before the age of seven; however, it isn't limited to children. Some children do outgrow it, but many more do not, meaning many adults are afflicted with the disorder.

Conventional Medical Treatment

If left untreated, ADD can isolate a sufferer, whose behavior may unintentionally frighten people. There is also a connection between untreated attention deficit disorder and parental abuse, failure at school, and low self-esteem. Thus, if you suspect that you or your child may have attention deficit disorder, a trip to your physician is in order. To arrive at a diagnosis of ADD, your doctor conducts a series of physical and neurological examinations as well as behavioral observation. The doctor also requests a detailed history of early childhood development. Treatment for ADD includes behavior modification techniques, avoiding overstimulation, providing a consistent daily routine, and avoiding sugar and food additives, which are believed to contribute to hyperactivity. In more severe cases, a drug may be prescribed to help reduce hyperactivity. Methylphenidate (Ritalin®) is the most common of these, but pemoline (Cylert®) is also used. These medications decrease motor activity and increase attention span in children. Side effects, such as insomnia and weight loss, are rare.

For More Information
National Attention Deficit Disorder Association
P.O. Box 1303
Northbrook, IL 60065-1303
www.add.org

Children and Adults with Attention
Deficit/Hyperactivity Disorders
8181 Professional Place, Suite 201
Landover, MD 20785
800-233-4050
www.chadd.org

Treating ADD with Medication

Controversy abounds on treating hyperactive children with Ritalin® and other medications. If your child has ADD and you'd like to further explore non-medicated methods of care, you may want to read *Ritalin Free Kids: Safe and Effective Homeopathic Medicine for ADD and Other Behavioral and Learning Problems* (Prima Publishing, 1997) by Judyth Reichenberg-Ullman, N.D., M.S.W., and Robert Ullman, N.D. For more information, call 800-632-8676.

Health Note

➤ *If you are pregnant, avoid tobacco, alcohol, and all drugs unless prescribed by your doctor. These practices could cause your child to develop ADD.*

Complementary and Alternative Treatments

Nutrition and Supplementation

Nutritional deficiencies are a factor in many psychological disorders. Many children with learning disorders have an allergic reaction to casein and gluten. Casein is a protein found in milk, so it may be wise to eliminate dairy from your diet. Gluten is found in grains, making wheat, spelt, oats, barley, and rye problematic. Common food allergens are corn, soy, eggs, tomatoes, yeast, and peanuts. Eat instead a diet high in protein that also includes high-fiber fruits and vegetables, plus brown rice, lentils, and potatoes. Obtain protein from fish, poultry, lamb, and non-animal sources, such as beans and legumes, raw nuts and seeds, and tofu. Avoid alcohol, caffeine, canned and packaged foods, carbonated beverages, chocolate, all junk foods, refined and processed foods, saturated fats, and sugar. Also avoid foods containing artificial colors or ingredients, as well as fatty foods.

Enhance brain power with the following daily supplements (if for a child, check with a health professional for appropriate dosages):

Most Important

- calcium (1500 mg)—essential for normal brain and nervous system function

- magnesium (1000 mg)—helps calcium absorption

- vitamin B complex (50 mg 3 times daily with food)—essential for normal brain and nervous system function

Also Recommended

- choline (500 to 2000 mg)—improves brain function; use only under professional supervision

- coenzyme Q10 (as directed on label)—improves brain function

- dimethylglycine (100 mg)—carries oxygen to the brain

- vitamin C with bioflavonoids (5000 to 20,000 mg in divided doses)—a free radical scavenger

- vitamin E (200 to 600 IU)—improves circulation and brain function

- N-acetyl cysteine (as directed on label)—important because of its antioxidant qualities

Herbal Therapy

Red clover, hawthorn berry, lemon balm, and bacopa are recommended for calming the nervous system of an extremely active child. See a qualified herbalist for details on using them.

Traditional Chinese Medicine

Acupuncture Because attention deficit disorder is thought to be caused by heart and liver imbalances, traditional Chinese medical practitioners treat them accordingly. An acupuncturist seeks to correct any energy imbalances in the meridians that correspond to these organs. Practitioners also may use acupuncture to promote relaxation and alleviate stress, which can exacerbate the condition.

Chinese Herbal Therapy Herbal preparations that can be used to calm the central nervous system and balance *chi* include Ginseng and Zizyphus Forumula, Astragalus Combination, and Concha Marguerita and Ligustrum Formula.

Other herbs that may be prescribed with the preceding formulas for ADD are Schisandra, Biota or Arbor Vitae seeds, and Wild Chinese Jujube.

BACK PAIN

Signs and Symptoms

- Constant or intermittent pain, usually in the lower back, that becomes worse with movement

- Pain that appears after lifting something heavy or during a stressful situation, pregnancy, or exercise

- Stiffness or loss of flexibility

Description

When it comes to backaches, not everyone feels the same type or extent of pain. Some are in a state of continual discomfort, others feel a stab of pain when they bend, reach, or lift. The ache can start slowly and grow, or come on suddenly. Certain people experience pain in the upper back, others feel pain shooting down their legs; though most are affected only in the lower back. Bed rest helps some people feel better, yet it doesn't do a thing for others. Some people encounter a single episode of back pain during their entire lives, while others are immobilized by a sore back several times each year.

Just as there are numerous types of back pains, there are also many causes. Disk disorders (such as a slipped disk—also called prolapsed or herniated disk) and compression fractures of the spine are back injuries that can lead to back pain. Two other causes of back pain are weak stomach muscles and obesity, both of which tax the back muscles and make them work harder. A lifetime of bad posture can also stress the back muscles, as can an accident or overuse.

Illness can also cause a sore back, because pain elsewhere in the body can radiate to the back. Some of the most notable illnesses are perforated ulcer, acute pancreatitis, cardiovascular conditions, and appendicitis.

Conventional Medical Treatment

In order to find the cause of your discomfort, your physician or orthopedist performs a thorough physical exam—including an in-depth posture check and a rundown of vital signs—and asks for a complete health history. If a cause doesn't immediately present itself, you may be asked to take a blood test, and radiographs, a bone scan, and/or an X-ray may be requested.

While treatment for your back pain depends on the cause, most physicians do prescribe a combination of some rest on a firm surface (resting in bed for more than two days can cause muscle weakness and slow recovery), exercises to strengthen the abdominal muscles, and stretches to keep back muscles supple. If the pain is severe, you may use an anti-inflammatory, such as ibuprofen or acetaminophen (Tylenol®). If there is no relief, your doctor may prescribe stronger analgesics or muscle relaxants. In many cases, physical therapy treatments may be prescribed. You may also be reminded to bend your knees—not

What's Sciatica?

The sciatic nerve begins at the buttock and runs the length of the back of the leg. If a nerve in the back is pinched, or if a disk is herniated, pain often shoots down the sciatic nerve. This pain can range from moderate to severe and may feel worse when you cough, sneeze, or laugh. Tingling or numbness may also be present. If you experience what seems like sciatica, don't hesitate to see your physician. If a pinched nerve or herniated disk is causing your sciatica, you can get treatment.

Health Notes

➤ If a person's abdominal muscles are weak, the body taps into the back's strength, overtaxing lower back muscles. The result is soreness and pain during movement. The easiest way to avoid back strain is to develop strong stomach muscles by doing sit-ups and abdominal crunches, and make them supple with gentle daily stretching.

➤ Strong abs also improve posture, helping those who slouch to stand or sit correctly, which also helps prevent back strain.

➤ A quick way to analyze whether your posture is contributing to back pain is to stand with your heels against a wall. You should be able to slide your hand in the space behind your lower back, and your calves, buttocks, shoulders, and head should be touching the wall. If this doesn't describe you, your posture could use some work.

➤ When lifting heavy objects, use proper lifting techniques to avoid back injury. When picking up objects, always bend at the knees, using your leg muscles to help lift the load. Bending over directly from the waist puts pressure on the lower back, straining muscles.

➤ Always bend at the knees, not at the waist, when picking up an object (even a pencil) off the floor. Even a slightly incorrect bending movement can pull a back muscle.

➤ Avoid carrying heavy shoulder bags. When you must, alternate shoulders often to evenly distribute muscle use.

➤ Backaches affect approximately 80 percent of the population at some point in their lives. In fact, it's the second leading cause of employee absenteeism in the United States.

your back—when lifting heavy objects and to lift with your leg muscles, while keeping the object close to your body.

For More Information
American Pain Society
4700 West Lake Avenue
Glenview, IL 60025
847-375-4715
www.ampainsoc.org

Complementary and Alternative Treatments

Nutrition and Supplementation

Although back pain is generally alleviated through exercise and stretching, diet plays an important role as well. Animal foods, including all meats and protein products, contain uric acid, which puts strain on the kidneys and can contribute to back pain. Avoid these foods until you are healed. Eliminate oils, fats, sugar, and highly processed foods. Follow a fasting program to eliminate toxins from the body. At the onset of pain, drink 2 large glasses of water. Within minutes, you may feel relief. Muscle aches and back pain are often the result of dehydration. Drink the recommended 8 8-ounce glasses of water daily to keep acidic waste from building up in muscles and other tissues.

To help relieve your pain, follow these daily supplementation guidelines:

Most Important
- DL-Phenylalanine (500 mg 3 times daily) helps alleviate pain; do not take if you are pregnant or nursing or suffer from panic attacks, diabetes, high blood pressure, or PKU
- calcium (1500 to 2000 mg)—for strong bones
- magnesium (700 to 1000 mg)—works with calcium
- vitamin D (400 IU)—aids absorption of calcium and magnesium
- zinc (50 mg, not to exceed a total of 100 mg from all supplements)—promotes a healthy immune system

- copper (3 mg)—helps form elastin needed for healthy nerves

Also Recommended

- manganese (2 to 5 mg; do not take at the same time as calcium)—aids in healing cartilage and tissue in the neck and back

- flaxseed oil (1 tblsp)—repairs muscles and improves their flexibility

- vitamin B complex (50 mg 3 times daily)—relieves stress in back muscles

- vitamin C with bioflavonoids (3000 to 10,000 mg)—essential for formation of collagen, and repair of tissues; relieves back tension

- glucosamine sulfate (as directed on label)—necessary in bone, tendon, and ligament formation

- hydrolyzed collagen (as directed on label)—important for joint tissue rebuilding

- sea cucumber (as directed on label)—replenishes the lubricants needed for connective tissues and joints

- bromelain (as directed on label)—inflammation-fighting enzyme

- shark cartilage (as directed by healthcare provider)—reduces inflammation

(For an *acute* condition, take supplements until your symptoms subside. If symptoms persist, seek the advice of your healthcare provider. For a *chronic* condition, consult your healthcare provider regarding the duration of treatment.)

Aromatherapy

When used for massage or in a relaxing bath, the essential oils of lavender, marjoram, and rosemary can help alleviate back pain and muscle spasms as well as improve muscle tone and general well-being. Other beneficial oils include Roman or German chamomile, coriander, and eucalyptus. Create a blend with the oils or use singularly. For a massage, you must add the oils to a carrier oil.

Ayurvedic Medicine

To calm a simple backache caused by tight muscles, Ayurvedic practitioners recommend applying a ginger powder paste (wash off after several minutes) or taking *kaishore guggulu* with warm water twice.

Bodywork and Somatic Practices

Stress, poor posture, and weak abdominal muscles may all play a role in this condition. Movement re-education will help you avoid unconscious slumping postures, and may restore lost flexibility and vitality. It can also lift the slight depressive state that drags at your energy and well-being. Constant pain can be addressed with manual therapies, such as trigger point myotherapy, Hellerwork, Rolfing, Cranio-Sacral Therapy, massage, and Oriental bodywork.

Chiropractic

Chiropractic adjustment has proven to be extremely effective in preventing, managing, and controlling both acute and chronic back pain, regardless of the cause. For example, for an acute back spasm, or "throwing out" one's back, a chiropractor may use a combination of ice, ultrasound, and specific chiropractic adjustment (SCA) to correct spinal subluxation and decrease back pain. For chronic back pain, a chiropractor may use moist heat and electromuscle stimulation to decrease spasticity and muscle splinting. SCA would then be administered to correct vertebral subluxation.

Herbal Therapy

Several herbs can ease back pain say herbalists. For local pain, rub cayenne cream into the affected area. For general pain relief, drink willow bark tea; willow contains natural salicylate compounds, the primary ingredient in aspirin. If you need a muscle relaxant, use feverfew, alfalfa, burdock, oat straw, slippery elm, or valerian root tea; and to fight inflammation, try yarrow.

To prepare willow or valerian tea, stir 2 teaspoons powdered bark or chopped root into 1 cup boiling water. Let stand for 8 to 10 hours; strain. To make the yarrow tea, steep 2 teaspoons dried herb in 1 cup of boiling water for 10 minutes; strain.

Herbal products are available in health food stores and in some pharmacies and supermarkets. Follow package for specific directions.

Homeopathy

A homeopathic practitioner may advise one of the following treatments for back pain, depending on your symptoms:

- *Arnica*—for easing pain caused by injury or trauma

- *Rhus tox*—for soothing the pain that comes from overexertion or lifting a heavy object (pain that lessens as you move around)

- *Hypericum*—for tail bone pain brought about by a fall; also useful for neck pain resulting from whiplash injury

Hydrotherapy

Apply contrast therapy (alternating hot and cold cloths) to the affected area until pain and stiffness subside. Exercise in warm water to help prevent recurrences. A long neutral bath (slightly cooler than body temperature can help ease muscular tension) or add apple cider vinegar to hot water for a hot compress application. For directions on making a hot compress, see "Hydrotherapy" in the "Introduction to Complementary Therapies" section.

Traditional Chinese Medicine

Acupuncture Numerous scientific studies show acupuncture to be enormously successful in treating all kinds of back pain, largely because it can relieve tense or contracted muscles, pinched nerves, and spinal misalignments at the same time that it restores energy and blood flow to the area and strengthens weakened musculature.

In treating back pain, the acupuncturist usually inserts needles directly into the muscles or ligaments that are in need of treatment, along with related acupoints elsewhere on the body and in the ear.

An acupuncturist may use electrical acupuncture to further relieve back spasms or tight muscles. This simply involves fastening tiny clips (which resemble minute jumper cables) onto the acupuncture needles and stimulating the painful or inflamed area with a very gentle electrical current. These vibrations help improve circulation to the area, which in turn alleviates pain and improves mobility.

If back pain has been caused by an accident or a sports-related injury, treatment will be most effective and require the fewest treatments if it's done as soon as possible after the injury has occurred. Usually, acute back problems can be treated in less than four sessions, while chronic pain may require additional sessions.

Acupressure Acupressure serves two purposes in the treatment of back ailments: it can alleviate symptoms of pain and it can re-open blocked energy channels, which may help prevent pain from recurring.

The Bladder 54 acupressure points just behind the knees are a common site of back-related treatment; pressing these points is thought to unblock stagnant energy patterns in the back and provide pain relief. Lower back pain may be treated by manipulating various points at the base of the spinal column, behind the knees, on the buttocks, on the ankles, and in the ear.

Chinese Herbal Therapy Back pain—and lower back pain in particular—is thought to be caused many times by an imbalance in the kidneys, so a Chinese herbalist attempts to alleviate the symptoms while strengthening the affected organ.

There are several Chinese herbal ointments that can be used topically to relieve back pain, including Traumatic Injury Medicine and *Zheng Gu Shui*. Both of these liniments work by soothing tense muscles and promoting relaxation. Other formulas designed to alleviate the causes of back pain include Rehmannia Eight, and Angelica and Loranthus Combination.

Many times, the practitioner will apply various types of herbal plasters directly onto the painful area.

Yoga and Meditation

 Back pain is a condition that can really be helped by yoga, but you must work with a gifted teacher. If poses are done incorrectly, yoga can aggravate your back condition. Do not try yoga if your back problem involves bulging or herniated disks. To strengthen your back and gain flexibility, try the Half Moon I or the Easy Bridge pose. For a stiff, achy back, try the Reclined Spiral Twist or the Cat and Dog Tilt, or relax in the Corpse pose and meditate.

SYMPTOM:

BAD BREATH (HALITOSIS)

Bad breath doesn't always have a medical cause— often the culprit is something you ate: garlic, onions, shallots, cruciferous vegetables, dairy products, peanut butter, and coffee. All of these foods have the power to cause bad breath. Why? After your stomach and small intestine digest the food, its volatile substances are absorbed into your bloodstream, where they are carried to your lungs to be given off in your breath. Other causes of bad breath include gum disease, sinus problems, or chronic infections of the respiratory tract.

A breath mint can mask odors only as long as the mint is actually in your mouth. Brushing your teeth and tongue thoroughly can help (many people prone to bad breath carry a travel toothbrush and toothpaste to work to brush in the rest room after lunch or a coffee break). If you want to wipe out the odor at the source, your best bet is to nibble on a bit of parsley, which is full of odor-neutralizing chlorophyll. Instead of just masking the odor, the chlorophyll travels the same internal route as the offending food, arriving at the lungs where it neutralizes any unpleasant smells. (As a nice bonus, parsley is also rich in iron and vitamins A and C.) You can also take chlorophyll concentrate or alfalfa tablets to purify the breath. (Follow the directions on the product label.)

For a complementary treatment, try one of these aromatherapy treatments: gargle with 1 to 3 drops tea tree oil in a glass of water, or place 1 drop of peppermint oil on the tongue (do not use in excess or it will burn) and allow it to be absorbed into the mucous membranes. Ayurvedic practitioners recommend chewing on fennel seeds or cloves after meals, or take 1/2 teaspoon of triphala in warm water approximately 1/2 hour before going to bed.

BEDSORES

Signs and Symptoms

- Areas of red, sensitive skin (in early stages)
- Open, ulcerated sores that don't seem to heal (in later stages)

Description

As anyone who has been bedridden for any period of time can tell you, bedsores are one of the unfortunate parts of the experience. Also known as pressure sores or decubits ulcers, they begin as

Vitamin C for Bedsores

Research has shown that bedsores sometimes heal faster when patients receive high doses of vitamin C. Try putting a blend of vitamin C, amino acids, and complex sugars directly on the bedsore. In some patients, this has speeded the healing process.

sensitive, red patches of skin that eventually become sores or ulcers. Bedsores develop on weight-bearing parts of the body—commonly on the hips, shoulder blades, elbows, base of the spine, knees, ankles, and heels—where the bones are near the skin.

Conventional Medical Treatment

For bedsores to heal, you must keep weight off of them. Place cushioning at pressure points to help distribute body weight more evenly, thus keeping pressure from building in one spot. Air mattresses, foam pads and specially-designed pads for heels and elbows are available from medical supply stores. Clean ulcerated areas twice daily with an anti-microbial cleanser to keep sores germ-free and speed healing.

For More Information
American Academy of Dermatology
930 North Meacham Road
Schaumburg, IL 60173
888-462-DERM
www.aad.org

Complementary and Alternative Treatments

Nutrition and Supplementation

 People who suffer from bedsores are usually deficient in a number of nutrients, especially zinc and vitamins A, E,

B_2, and C. Eat a balanced diet of which 70 percent is raw fruits and vegetables. Drink liquids (steam-distilled water, herbal teas, sugar-free juices) around the clock to keep the colon clean. Eliminate animal fats, junk food, processed foods, fried food, and sugar. Get your fiber from oat bran or ground flaxseeds. Fiber prevents constipation and absorbs dangerous toxins.

Supplementing your vitamin and mineral intake is very important. Try the following daily suggestions until healing is complete.

Most Important

- vitamin E (400 IU)—improves circulation
- zinc (30 mg, not to exceed a total of 100 mg from all supplements)—heals tissues
- copper (3 mg)—balances zinc

Also Recommended

- free-form amino acid complex (as directed on label)—supplies protein needed for healing
- mixed carotenoid formula (15,000 IU)—improves skin tissue
- vitamin B complex (100 mg twice daily with meals)—reduces stress and aids in healing
- vitamin B_{12} (2000 mcg twice daily)
- vitamin C (3000 to 10,000 mg in divided doses)—aids in healing, improves circulation, and enhances immune function
- vitamin D (400 to 1000 IU)—essential for healing
- colloidal silver (apply topically as directed on label)—a natural antibiotic that destroys viruses, fungi, and bacteria; promotes healing
- garlic (as directed on label)—a natural antibiotic
- kelp (500 to 1000 mg daily)—provides a balance of minerals
- vitamin A (25,000 IU for 1 month, then reduce to 5,000 IU; do not exceed 8000 IU daily if you are pregnant)—heals skin tissue

(For an *acute* condition, take supplements until your symptoms subside. If symptoms persist, seek the advice of your healthcare provider. For a *chronic* condition, consult your healthcare provider regarding the duration of treatment.)

Aromatherapy

 To clean sores and promote healing, dab a solution of 4 drops of tea tree oil and 1 cup of water over the affected area.

Herbal Therapy

 Herbal therapists recommend external application of the following therapeutic herbs, under appropriate supervision: echinacea, goldenseal, myrrh gum, pau d'arco, slippery elm.

Herbal products are available in health food stores and in some pharmacies and supermarkets. Follow package for specific directions.

Homeopathy

 To help heal bedsores, apply *Calendula* ointment to the affected skin.

Traditional Chinese Medicine

 Acupuncture Acupuncture can be used to improve blood and energy flow to the affected area—including the shoulder blades, buttocks, and hips—which may help bedsores heal faster. Acupuncture also can be used to relieve the pain associated with this condition.

Chinese Herbal Therapy There are many Chinese herbs that can speed healing and lessen the pain of bedsores, including Bletilla Striata, which can be mixed into an ointment with sesame oil and applied to the affected area 2 to 3 times a day. Some herbalists may add powdered amethyst to this preparation to enhance its curative properties.

Additionally, *Lien Chiao Pai Tu Pien* is a skin-healing formula that can be found at health food or herb stores; follow package instructions (and do not use it during pregnancy).

BITES/STINGS

ANIMAL BITES

Signs and Symptoms

- Puncture wounds where each tooth entered the skin
- Pain at the wound sight
- Swelling, redness, and warmth at the site
- Chills/fever
- Lightheadedness

Basic Description

Although animal bites can look different, depending on what bit you, most people know a bite when they see one: two or more puncture wounds where the teeth entered the skin, gashed skin, torn-away chunks of flesh, and perhaps, an accompanying deep scratch or two.

Of the approximately 1000 people who visit emergency rooms each day for animal bites, most were attacked by domestic animals. Dogs are responsible for the majority of these bites, though some are caused by cats. On the other hand, all types of non-domestic animals bite—from large, exotic beasts, such as sharks and bears, to more common creatures, such as raccoons, squirrels, skunks, and chipmunks.

Conventional Medical Treatment

If your new puppy or the family cat bites you, the bite is usually small and shallow. You can take care of this by cleaning the wound with an antiseptic, such as Betadine® or hydrogen peroxide, or by washing the wound with warm water and soap. After cleaning, gently dry the wound with a clean towel or piece of cotton, apply an antibiotic cream (such as Bacitracin® or Neosporin®) and

Health Notes

➤ When walking your dog, you probably come into contact with other dogs and their owners. If, during one of the encounters, the dogs begin snarling at or fighting with each other, don't try to get in between the dogs or pick up your dog—you could accidentally get bitten. Instead, pull back on your dog's leash, and let the other owner do the same. Each of you can then pull off your dogs in different directions.

➤ Do not try to "win over" a frightened or angry dog who is snarling, growling, barking, baring its teeth, or lunging. Even though you are trying to be friendly, by approaching such a dog, you're asking to be bitten.

dress with dry gauze. If the injury is small enough, you can use a Band-Aid® instead of gauze. Keep the wounded area elevated and immobilized.

For larger wounds, press a cloth against the injury to stop the bleeding, then go straight to the doctor's office or emergency room. Your physician will thoroughly clean the wound and remove any damaged tissue. You will probably be placed on antibiotics, and if you haven't had a tetanus shot recently, you will be given a booster.

If you are bitten by an unknown or non-domestic animal, go straight to your doctor's office or the emergency room. Your physician will call animal control, who will attempt to capture the animal and determine if it has rabies. (If the animal does have rabies, it will be killed.) Your doctor may give you a skin biopsy to test whether you have been infected with the rabies virus. To treat rabies, your doctor will inject an antibody directly into the wound and surrounding muscle. Usually five injections are given over a period of 28 days.

Complementary and Alternative Treatments

Nutrition and Supplementation

 See your healthcare provider immediately after being bitten. Then to help speed healing, follow these daily suggestions:

- vitamin C (4000 to 10,000 mg daily for 1 week, then reduce to 3000 mg daily)—fights infection; helps repair collagen and connective tissue
- garlic (2 capsules 3 times daily)—a natural antibiotic
- vitamin A (25,000 IU; do not exceed 8000 IU daily if you are pregnant)—assists in healing the skin
- vitamin E (400 IU)—heals the skin
- vitamin B complex (50 mg 3 times daily)—aids in tissue oxidation

(Take supplements until your symptoms subside. If symptoms persist, seek the advice of your healthcare provider.)

Traditional Chinese Medicine

 Acupuncture Once you've seen a healthcare provider to have the bite treated and get a tetanus shot, if necessary, acupuncture can help to lessen inflammation, hasten healing time, and treat pain.

An acupuncturist can also treat symptoms of shock that may accompany an animal bite; the practitioner focuses on the ear points related to the adrenal gland, back of head, and heart.

An acupuncturist also may prescribe a homeopathic remedy.

Chinese Herbal Therapy Herbs can be used to help strengthen the immune system, which can lessen the chance of an animal bite becoming infected and speed the recovery process. Common immune-boosting formulas are Rehmannia Six, Major Four Herbs, Eight Immortal Long Life Pills, Ginseng and Atractylodes, and Panax Gingseng Capsules.

Chinese herbal preparations designed specifically to treat injuries and traumatic incidents include Pseudoginseng and Dragon Blood Formula and Tian Qi and Eucommia.

INSECT BITES AND STINGS

Signs and Symptoms

- Bumps, swelling, and/or redness at the site of the bite
- Itchiness or pain that develops within three hours of being bitten or stung

Description

Some insects bite, others sting. Either way, the result is one or more small bump-like entry wounds where the bug's salivary fluid or venom entered your skin. Mosquitoes, ants, fleas, ticks, gnats, chiggers, bees, wasps, hornets, yellow jackets, spiders, and scorpions are among the many insects that can bite or sting you.

Conventional Medical Treatment

For most people, insect bites and stings are nothing more than a minor annoyance. If you have a mild insect bite or sting, gently remove the insect from your skin (if it is still there), or scrape the stinger from your skin (use a credit card to avoid touching the stinger). Then wash the area and apply a cold compress or ice to reduce pain and in-

---

Ticked Off

If you look down and see a tiny, black insect on or stuck into your arm or leg or other body part, it's not a scene from a horror film. It's a tick—a very real scene from outdoor America. How do you remove a tick? Don't start pulling on it—you will only make it burrow deeper. Instead, cover the tick and the surrounding skin with toothpaste, cooking oil, car oil, body lotion or anything else that will limit its oxygen. Clear nail polish is good because it forces the tick to withdraw from the skin. After three or four minutes pass, the tick will usually relax its grip. Using a pair of tweezers, grasp the tick as close to its head as possible and firmly pull. Drop the tick into a fire or flush it down the toilet, then wash your skin with soap and water. (If you suspect it to be a deer tick, save the tick for identification by a doctor. Watch yourself closely for the next ten days for signs of Lyme disease. For more information about deer ticks *see* "Lyme Disease" entry.

If the tick's head breaks off below the skin, wipe the area in alcohol and cover it with a bandage. See a doctor as soon as possible to have the head removed.

flammation. You can reduce pain and swelling by applying hydrocortizone cream or calamine lotion to the area.

If you are allergic to bees, wasps, hornets, or yellow jackets (one in ten Americans are) and are stung by one, go immediately to the nearest emergency clinic or hospital emergency room. You will be given a shot of epinephrine to help your body rid itself of the insect venom. If you are planning a backpacking or hiking trip in a remote area, ask your physician beforehand for an emergency kit containing a hypodermic syringe with epinephrine.

If you are bitten by a poisonous spider (the black widow and brown recluse are the most dangerous spiders in the United States) or scorpion, tightly tie a piece of fabric or a bandage one or two inches above the wound to slow the movement of venom. Next, place a bag of ice over the wound. Be sure to keep the wound below heart-

level. Call an ambulance immediately, or have someone drive you to the nearest hospital emergency room, where you will be treated with an anti-venom preparation.

Complementary and Alternative Treatments

Nutrition and Supplementation

 To avoid mosquito bites, eat brown rice, fish, wheat germ, or brewer's yeast before spending prolonged periods outdoors. These foods are rich in thiamine, a vitamin that seems to repel mosquitoes.

To assist the healing process, try these daily suggestions:

- quercetin (as directed on label)—reduces allergic reactions

- vitamin C with bioflavonoids (500 to 2000 mg in divided doses)—an anti-inflammatory that relieves the toxicity of bites

- glutathione and zinc (in topical spray form; use as directed)

(Take supplements until your symptoms subside. If symptoms persist, seek the advice of your healthcare provider.)

Aromatherapy

 The essential oils of tea tree and lavender are effective for treating all types of minor insect bites and stings; apply either oil daily directly to the bite or sting until itching has stopped and the bite is healed.

Ayurvedic Medicine

 Ayurvedic remedies are quite effective in treating the itch and localized swelling caused by insect bites. Try one of the following treatments: Apply a sandalwood paste, *neem* paste, or a blend of sandalwood and turmeric to the affected area. You also might try applying cilantro pulp to the site.

Health Notes

➤ Consider applying a natural insect repellent before going outdoors. Add 6 drops of tea tree oil, eucalyptus, rosemary, cedar, citronella, or rue—or a combination of these herbs—to enough unscented body lotion to coat the entire body. Apply 20 minutes before going outside.

➤ If you are bothered by a yellowjacket or get stung by one, resist the urge to squash it. Crushing the insect releases a chemical that attracts not only other yellow jackets, but wasps as well.

➤ Eating garlic the night before a daytime hike alters the smell of your perspiration, creating an odor that naturally repels insects.

➤ To avoid attracting bees, don't wear perfume, hairspray, scented body lotion, shiny jewelry, or dark colors.

For a natural insect repellent, rub *neem* oil into exposed skin before venturing outdoors. Ayurvedic practitioners say the oil contains a component called salannin that's as effective as the synthetic chemical diethyl toluamide (DEET).

Herbal Therapy

To reduce itching from mosquito bites, dab the bite with tincture of witch hazel. You can also apply aloe gel or lotion.

To avoid being bitten in the first place, herbalists advise using a natural insect repellant, such as the following: Combine 1 cup bay leaf, 4 cups pennyroyal, 2 cups rosemary, and 1 cup eucalyptus in a jar with a tight-fitting lid. Pour in enough oil to cover the herbs by an inch. Fasten the lid and set in a sunny spot for 2 weeks. Strain through cheesecloth, and apply before going outside.

Herbal products are available in health food stores and in some pharmacies and supermarkets. Follow package for specific directions.

Homeopathy

Seek medical attention immediately for any insect sting that produces a pronounced allergic reaction—severe swelling or difficulty in breathing. For other stings, homeopathic practitioners usually advise one of the following approaches, depending on the symptoms:

- *Apis*—every 10 minutes (or sooner) for a bite characterized by redness, stinging, and mild swelling, or one that feels better when cold compresses are applied to the affected area
- *Ledum*—if the site of the sting is pink, not red; also good for mosquito bites

Hydrotherapy

Apply cold compresses to lessen itching and reduce swelling. You can add apple cider vinegar to the water. A clay or mud pack can be useful in drawing poisons from the site.

Traditional Chinese Medicine

Acupuncture Acupuncture can be used to treat the anaphylactic shock that may result from an insect bite or sting. The practitioner targets acupoints in the ear that relate to the immune and nervous system, along with points that correspond to the area that's been stung.

Chinese Herbal Therapy Several herbs can be useful in relieving the irritation and inflammation that accompanies a bug bite or sting. Some common Chinese remedies include aloe vera and angelica anomala, both of which can soothe itchiness.

The Chinese first aid pills *Yunnan Bai Yao* can be ingested or broken open and applied topically to relieve pain, inflammation and itchiness. The oral dosage is 0.2 to 0.5 grams 4 times a day; if using externally, apply the powder from 1 or 2 tablets directly into the affected site, as needed.

SNAKE BITES

Signs and Symptoms

- Two small, parallel puncture wounds
- If the area around the bite begins to swell or change color, or is extremely painful, a poisonous snake may have bitten you
- Nausea and blurred vision are also symptoms of a poisonous snake bite

Description

If you are bitten by a snake, you will certainly know it. Not only will you see the snake—either as it strikes you or as it retreats after striking you—but you will also notice the telltale fang marks on your skin. These look like two small, red puncture wounds about an inch to three inches apart (depending on the size of the snake's jaw). The wound may sting a little (if the snake is not poisonous) or a lot (if it is poisonous). If the area around the wound becomes inflamed or turns red or blue, it was probably inflicted by a poisonous snake.

The majority of snakes in the United States are not poisonous. You can tell whether the one that bit you was poisonous by the physical appearance of the snake. Most poisonous snakes have elliptical, slit-shaped eyes, triangular heads, and a slight indentation on each side of their heads halfway between their eyes and their nostrils. This "pit" is what gives rattlesnakes, copperheads, water moccasins, and other poisonous snakes their collective name of "pit vipers."

Conventional Medical Treatment

If you are absolutely sure that your snake bite was not inflicted by a poisonous snake, you can wash the area thoroughly with mild soap and warm water. Then apply an antibiotic cream and bandage the wound.

If you are bitten by a poisonous snake, it's important that you should remain as quiet, still, and

Health Notes

➤ If you know you're going to be in snake country, wear leather boots that extend up your calf, and stay on busy, non-wooded hiking paths.

➤ If you see a snake, stay at least 6 feet away from it.

➤ When it comes to avoiding snake bites, when you do your hiking is as important as where. That's because snakes, which are cold-blooded creatures, like to bask in the daytime sun to raise their body temperatures. In fact, the majority of snakebites occur mid-morning and late afternoon.

calm as possible. Hold the bitten area lower than heart level. These measures will slow your blood circulation, increasing the time it takes for the snake's venom to reach your heart. Meanwhile, ask someone to call an ambulance or drive you to an emergency room.

To further reduce blood flow, tightly tie a belt, ribbon, string, or scrap of cloth 2 or 3 inches above the bite. If the bite is above heart level, tie the bandage a few inches below the wound. Do not untie the bandage.

You will have to suck out the venom if the bite:

- was inflicted by a poisonous snake that was not a coral snake

- occurred within the last five to ten minutes

- is on the arms or legs

- occurred in an area that is more than 30 minutes from medical help

Make a 1/4-inch deep cut with a razor blade or knife edge (preferably sterilized with flame, alcohol, whiskey, or soap and water) over each fang mark. Make the cut along the length of the limb, not across it. Suck out the venom using your mouth or a suction device. If you use your mouth,

Keeping Snakes Away

If you live in a region where snakes are common, there are a few things you can do to prevent these unwelcome guests from setting up residence in or around your house. By eliminating debris and keeping woodpiles, rocks, and boards to a minimum, you remove favorite places for them to inhabit. If you cannot get rid of woodpiles and other such snake hideouts altogether, at least make sure that they are kept at a distance from your home. It is also helpful to cut weeds and seal all cracks.

immediately spit out the venom. Do not use your mouth if you have open sores in or around your mouth. (This treatment is not recommended unless you are trained to perform it or are more than 30 minutes away from the nearest medical facility.)

Complementary and Alternative Treatments

Nutrition and Supplementation

Although most snakes are not poisonous, it is wise to see your healthcare provider immediately. Then to help fight pain and speed healing, follow these daily supplement guidelines:

Most Important

- calcium (500 mg every 4 to 6 hours until pain eases)—acts as a sedative and relieves pain
- magnesium (1000 mg with the first 500 mg of calcium)
- vitamin B_5 (pantothenic acid) (500 mg every 4 hours for 2 days)— the anti-stress vitamin
- vitamin C with bioflavonoids (2000 mg every hour for 5 to 6 hours, up to a total of 15,000 mg)—relieves pain and fights infection

- vitamin A (10,000 IU; do not exceed 8000 IU if you are pregnant)—promotes tissue healing
- vitamin E (600 IU)—promotes healing
- zinc (30 mg)—boosts immunity
- N-acetyl cysteine (200 to 600 mg)—detoxifies the system
- glutathione (200 mg)—detoxifying agent

(Take supplements until your symptoms subside. If symptoms persist, seek the advice of your healthcare provider.)

Herbal Therapy

To reduce pain and aid in healing, apply a poultice of slippery elm, comfrey, plantain, or white oak bark and leaves.

Traditional Chinese Medicine

Acupuncture In some cases, acupuncture can be used to treat shock that results from a snake bite. To be effective, treatment must be sought immediately, and if possible, used on the way to the hospital.

BLADDER INFECTION (CYSTITIS)

Signs and Symptoms

- Burning sensation during urination
- Frequent urination
- Urge to urinate when the bladder is empty
- Shooting pain in the vaginal canal and/or pubic area

- Cloudy, blood-streaked, or strong-smelling urine
- Pressure or pain in lower abdomen or back

Description

Though bladder infections do strike men, they are more common among women. Known medically as cystitis, this condition is caused by a bacterial infection—usually the bacteria is from the *E. coli* strain. This bacteria is transferred from the hands, anal area, or skin of the genitals to the bladder through the urethra (or urine canal). Also called honeymoon cystitis, the condition also commonly occurs when bacteria is introduced to the urethra through foreplay or sexual intercourse.

Conventional Medical Treatment

While cystitis can be quite painful, it is also very treatable. At the first sign of a bladder infection, visit your doctor, who can diagnose the condition with a urine test. If left untreated, a bladder infection can migrate through the urinary tract to the kidneys, possibly resulting in a kidney infection (pyelonephritis), which is a more serious condition.

The most common medical treatments are antibiotics, such as sulfa drugs. Your doctor will also ask you to increase your intake of water and avoid diuretics, such as caffeinated beverages and alcohol. Symptoms typically abate 24 to 48 hours after beginning medication.

For More Information
Interstitial Cystitis Association
51 Monroe Street, Suite 1402
Rockville, MD 20850
301-610-5300
www.ichelp.org

Complementary and Alternative Treatments

Nutrition and Supplementation

 Fluids are key to ridding yourself of a bladder infection. Drink an 8-ounce glass of water every hour, and 1 quart of pure, unsweetened cranberry juice daily. Cranberry juice adds acid to the urine and prevents bacteria from adhering to the lining of the bladder. Eat natural diuretics, such as celery, parsley, and watermelon, but avoid citrus fruits, which upset the body's pH balance. Avoid alcohol, caffeine, carbonated beverages, coffee, chocolate, refined and processed foods, and simple sugars. All these will have an adverse effect on the bladder.

Avoid taking iron supplements until you have healed. Too much iron aids in bacterial growth. Follow the daily guidelines below to promote the healing process.

Most Important

- colloidal silver (as directed on label)—a natural antibiotic that destroys bacteria and fungi; promotes healing

- garlic (as directed on label)—a natural antibiotic and immune enhancer

Health Notes

➤ *The moment you suspect a bladder infection, begin drinking an 8-ounce glass of water every half hour. This will dilute the urine, making urination less painful.*

➤ *Cranberry juice changes the pH balance of urine, helping to reduce your risk of getting a bladder infection, because it makes the bladder inhospitable to invading microorganisms.*

➤ *Some experts believe you can help prevent bladder infections (and urinary tract infections) by urinating immediately after sexual intercourse.*

➤ *Avoid using feminine hygiene products, such as powders, sprays, and douches. These upset the pH balance of the area, making it more inhabitable to bacteria.*

➤ *Don't use a diaphragm if you get frequent urinary infections. Ask your doctor about other contraceptive options.*

- vitamin C (4000 to 5000 mg daily in divided doses)—aids the healing process

- bioflavonoids (1000 mg)—important in immune function

Also Recommended

- a prodophilus formula (as directed on label, on empty stomach)—restores friendly bacteria

- calcium (1500 mg)—reduces bladder irritability

- magnesium (750 to 1000 mg daily)—balances calcium

- potassium (99 mg)—replaces potassium lost as a result of frequent urination

- vitamin E (600 IU)—combats bacteria

- vitamin A (50,000 IU for 2 days, then 25,000 IU for 2 days, then reduce to 5000; do not exceed 8000 IU if you are pregnant)—speeds healing

(For an *acute* condition, take supplements until your symptoms subside. If symptoms persist, seek the advice of your healthcare provider. For a *chronic* condition, consult your healthcare provider regarding the duration of treatment.)

Aromatherapy

For the pain that accompanies bladder infections, apply a massage oil of bergamot and lavender or chamomile and a carrier oil (such as safflower oil) to the lower abdomen as needed.

You also might try a hot sitz bath to which you've added a few drops of the essential oils of juniper, sandalwood, or German chamomile.

Ayurvedic Medicine

To lessen the burning sensation that accompanies a bladder infection, Ayurvedic practitioners advise drinking coriander tea or a coriander-cumin-fennel tea. They also suggest taking a blend of *shatavari*, *guduchi*, *punarnava*, and *kamadudha* twice daily.

Chiropractic

In cases of chronic cystitis, chiropractic adjustments may be beneficial. Once the nerve interference is corrected by proper alignment, healing can occur. Experts recommend that such chiropractic care be done in conjunction with conventional medical supervision, which may include medication.

Herbal Therapy

A number of herbs are helpful in treating—and preventing—bladder infections. Try one of the following:

- Take urva ursi (also called bearberry) capsules. Urva ursi acts as an anti-inflammatory and diuretic. *Caution:* Do not take this herb for more than one week or if you are pregnant.

- Sip nettle tea to alleviate inflammation. To make the tea, steep 1 teaspoon of dried leaves or root in 1 cup of boiling water for 10 to 15 minutes; strain and let cool. Take 1 tablespoon every hour, but no more than 1 cup (16 tablespoons) a day.

- Wash the perineal area with goldenseal solution before and after intercourse to prevent recurrent infections. To make the solution, boil 2 teaspoons of the herb in 1 cup of water for 15 minutes. Strain and let cool to room temperature.

- Drink cranberry or blueberry juice daily to help combat and prevent infection. Both juices contain compounds that keep bacteria from adhering to bladder walls. If bacteria can't stick to the walls, they can't cause infection there.

- Drink warm yarrow tea at least 3 times daily to flush out the infection. To make the tea, steep 1 teaspoon of the dried herb in 1 cup of boiling water for 15 minutes; strain.

- Sip cool parsley tea to flush toxins from the bladder. To make the tea, steep 1 bunch of parsley in 8 cups boiling water until the water cools; strain. Drink throughout the day.

Herbal products are available in health food stores and in some pharmacies and supermarkets. Follow package for specific directions.

Homeopathy

A homeopathic practitioner may recommend one of the following treatments, depending on your symptoms:

- *Cantharis*—if you feel a frequent urge to urinate, along with a burning pain during urination
- *Sarsaparilla*—if you have pain at the completion of urination
- *Berberis*—for pain (during or after urinating) that seems to extend from the bladder to the urethra
- *Staphasagria*—for pain that follows intercourse or anger

Cystitis can easily develop into a serious infection. If these remedies don't clear up the infection after a few doses, see a medical professional.

Hydrotherapy

Drink at least 8 to 10 glasses of water daily to help prevent cystitis, and if an infection has already started, to flush bacteria and toxins from the system. To calm bladder spasms and pain, take a sitz bath in hot water that's at least waist deep several times a

day. You can add 1 cup of cider vinegar to the bath water, if desired. Hot foot baths several times a day can also help.

Traditional Chinese Medicine

Acupuncture Acupuncture can be used to treat all manner of bladder-related ailments, including cysititis and urinary tract infections. This intervention may help with painful symptoms and may lessen the duration of an infection.

Acupuncture can also be used to tone and strengthen the bladder and kidneys which may help prevent recurrences. The practitioner may focus on the meridians and acupoints associated with these organs.

Acupressure For bladder infections, the most common sites manipulated are Bladder 60, Spleen 6, and Kidney 3 and 6 (all located on or near the ankles), along with Conception Vessel 12 and 16 on the abdomen.

The practitioner may also recommend that individuals who suffer from frequent bladder infections perform this routine on their own at least once a day, which may cut down on the frequency and severity of recurrence.

Chinese Herbal Therapy Gentiana Formula is a bladder infection preparation available in most health food stores. Other formulas that are used to treat or prevent bladder infections are Dianthus Formula, Corydalis Formula, Ginseng and Astragalus, and Hoelen and Polyporus.

BLISTERS

Signs and Symptoms

- Elevated, flesh-colored or pinkish bump that is filled with fluid
- Tenderness at the site

Description

A blister is a flesh-colored, fluid-filled bump on the skin. Blisters may be little larger than the head of a pin, or they may be several inches across.

Use Heat Lamps With Caution

Some people use heat lamps to treat skin ailments that benefit from the heat, such as psoriasis. In most cases, this is a safe practice, since the lamp does not actually come in contact with the skin. Use caution, however. Misuse, that is, overexposure or contact with the heat lamp, can cause blistering as well as burning or even heatstroke.

They can occur on any part of the body, but are particularly common on the feet.

A blister is a superficial injury to the skin that causes the epidermis (top layer of skin) to separate from the dermis (lower layer of skin). Fluid fills this pocket, causing it to swell into a bump.

Ill-fitting shoes are the cause of classic blisters. When the shoe rubs against part of the foot a blister can form. Blisters also can develop when the epidermis is burned—this includes sunburn.

Conventional Medical Treatment

While most blisters don't require medical attention, physicians are quick to tell people not to break the blister. It may be tempting, but breaking the blister can let bacteria enter the wound, resulting in an infection. A broken blister also

Health Notes

➤ *Avoid wearing shoes and clothing that chafe. Also use gloves during blister-causing activities, such as rope climbing.*

➤ *When buying shoes, always have your feet measured. Even once you've reached adulthood, foot size can vary, depending on how much you weigh or how much you have been exercising.*

takes longer to heal. Your best bet is to wash the area with soap and water, apply an antibiotic ointment, cover the wound with a bandage, and avoid applying any kind of pressure to the area until it heals. Most unbroken blisters heal within three to five days.

For More Information
American Academy of Dermatology
930 North Meacham Road
Schaumburg, IL 60618
888-462-DERM
www.aad.org

Complementary and Alternative Treatments

Aromatherapy

 Essential oils of lavender, benzoin, and myrrh are helpful in drying and healing blisters, especially those on the feet.

Herbal Therapy

 There are a number of topical herbal remedies that may help heal blisters. Aloe vera gel can be applied directly to the affected area. You also can use a calendula salve or a cold lavender compress. Or combine 15 drops lavender essential oil with 1 ounce vegetable oil; apply to the blister 3 times a day.

Herbal products are available in health food stores and in some pharmacies and supermarkets. Follow package for specific directions.

Homeopathy

 Bathe broken blisters with *Hypericum* or *Calendula* lotion.

Traditional Chinese Medicine

 Chinese Herbal Therapy Aloe vera can be used to remedy any discomfort caused by blisters, and many pre-made liniments can help speed recovery and lessen pain.

Body Odor

Body odor is usually nothing more than a hygiene issue. Sweat is the most common cause of body odor. Though sweat has no odor of its own, when it is left on the body, the benign bacteria that inhabit it start to decompose, causing the characteristic smell. The easiest way to combat this kind of odor is to shower after perspiring and change into clean clothes.

Sweat can also carry the odors of strong-smelling foods (such as garlic and curry) and beverages (such as coffee and alcohol), and cigarette smoke. For example, if you eat onion soup one night for dinner then wake up the next morning and go to the gym, you'll probably notice that no one is willing to use the treadmill next to you—your onion-perfumed sweat is driving fellow exercisers away. This kind of body odor

is easily treated with one to three sprigs of parsley eaten immediately after a strong-smelling meal. The chlorophyll in parsley neutralizes odors in the stomach before they have a chance to be carried out of the body via perspiration. Eaten daily, parsley can also clear up the body odor of heavy coffee or alcohol drinkers, and smokers. If you can't get your hands on parsley, go to the natural food store and buy chlorophyll capsules. Taking 1 to 3 capsules a day will have the same result as parsley.

If you can't find an explanation for your body's odor, see your physician. Body odor can also be a symptom of zinc deficiency, liver disease, diabetes, kidney failure, constipation, internal parasites, or a gastrointestinal condition.

Boils

Signs and Symptoms

- Large, swollen, pink or red lump under the skin, usually filled with pus
- Pain, itching, and localized warmth in the surrounding skin
- General fever
- General fatigue

Description

A boil is a local infection in one or more hair follicles, usually caused by the staphylococci bacteria. Boils, or *furuncles* as they're also known, are fairly common—it's believed that most people get at least one during their lifetime. While they can occur anywhere, boils are most likely to appear on the face, neck, armpits, buttocks, breasts, or thighs. When a cluster of two or more boils form a connected mass under the skin, it is called a carbuncle.

Typically a boil grows rapidly over several days. As more pus collects within the boil, the area grows more tender and painful. Finally, it comes to a head with a white or yellow center in the nodule. It then bursts, drains, and heals.

Poor hygiene, poor general health, friction between skin and clothing, and disorders such as

Health Note

➤ *Some experts believe that a weak immune system, or an immune system suppressed by illness, is less able to fight off the staphylococci bacteria. Maintain a strong immune system by eating a nutrient-dense diet, drinking 8 to 12 glasses of water daily, and getting regular, adequate sleep.*

acne, dermatitis, diabetes mellitus, or immune deficiency disorders all make you more susceptible to boil-causing staphylococci.

Conventional Medical Treatment

Because a boil usually ripens and drains on its own within 10 to 14 days, medical assistance isn't always needed. Apply warm, moist compresses to accelerate the healing process. When the boil (or carbuncle) is on or near your nose, cheeks, forehead, or spine, however, it can spread more rapidly and can become a brain abscess or spinal abscess. In these instances, prompt medical treatment can help prevent serious complications.

Have a doctor examine any carbuncle or boil that persists longer than two weeks or has redness surrounding it. With boils that last more than two weeks, there's the threat that the infection may spread to the bloodstream or internal organs. In these more serious situations, your physician may prescribe an oral antibiotic or surgically drain the boil.

For More Information
American Academy of Dermatology
930 North Meacham Road
Schaumburg, IL 60618
888-462-DERM
www.aad.org

Complementary and Alternative Treatments

Nutrition and Supplementation

 Follow a fasting program to cleanse the body of toxins that may cause boils. The following daily suggestions are for persons over the age of 18:

- colloidal silver (applied topically as directed on label)—a natural antibiotic and disinfectant that promotes healing

- garlic (as directed on label)—a natural antibiotic that boosts immune function

- vitamin A (75,000 IU daily for 1 month, then reduce to 25,000 IU daily; do not exceed 8000 IU daily if you are pregnant)—an antioxidant necessary for proper immune function

- vitamin E (600 IU)

- vitamin C (3000 to 8000 mg in divided doses)—stimulates the immune system; a powerful anti-inflammatory

- coenzyme Q10 (60 mg)—utilizes oxygen and boosts immune function

- kelp (2000 to 3000 mg)—supplies a balance of minerals

Aromatherapy

 Use hot compresses with essential oils of tea tree or lavender to draw out the infection and speed healing. Once the boil has drained, apply 1 or 2 drops of tea tree oil 3 to 4 times a day until the wound has healed. An antiseptic, tea tree oil is effective in killing bacteria.

Ayurvedic Medicine

 According to Ayruveda, boils could be caused by chronic constipation, a toxic liver, or diabetes. To heal a boil, an Ayurvedic practitioner may suggest applying a ginger-turmeric paste. Be sure to cover the boil with a bandage; turmeric stains fabric and skin.

Herbal Therapy

 To heal a boil, take a combination of tinctures of echinacea, cleavers, and yellow dock. Combine the tinctures in equal amounts and take 1 teaspoonful of the blend 3 times daily. Nettle tea is also beneficial. To make the tea, steep 1 to 2 teaspoons chopped fresh herb in 1 cup boiling water for 10 minutes; strain. Drink 2 cups a day.

Goldenseal may also be beneficial, as it helps cleanse the lymph glands. Take it as directed on the label, and consult your healthcare provider before using it if you have a history of diabetes, cardiovascular disease or glaucoma. *Note:* This herb should not be taken daily for more than 1 week, and should not be taken at all if pregnant.

You also might try adding raw garlic to your diet. Alternatively, you can take a garlic capsule 3 times daily.

An onion poultice may hasten healing. The onion should be wrapped in cloth before it is applied, and should not directly touch the boil.

Herbal products are available in health food stores and in some pharmacies and supermarkets. Follow package for specific directions.

Homeopathy

 Homeopathic practitioners often recommend one of the following treatments for boils, depending on your symptoms: *Silicea* to help a boil come to a head; *Belladonna* if the boil is hot, red, and throbbing, but with very little pus; and *Hepar sulphuris* to help your body reabsorb a boil before pus has formed.

Hydrotherapy

 Use hot compresses for 15 minutes several times a day to help draw out the boil. Or use alternate hot and cold compresses; apply hot for 3 to 5 minutes, then cold for 30 seconds. Apply ice to the boil and a hot compress over the ice.

Traditional Chinese Medicine

Acupuncture Treatment for boils should be focused on the liver meridians.

Chinese Herbal Therapy Since boils and furuncles are usually caused by a staphylococcal infection and tend to recur in individuals with impaired immunity or those under extreme stress, TCM practitioners will typically prescribe herbs to fight the infection and strengthen the immune system.

BRONCHITIS

Signs and Symptoms

- A hacking cough that produces mucus
- Wheezing
- Shortness of breath
- Burning, soreness, and/or feelings of constriction in the chest
- Sore throat
- Fever (in few cases)

Description

Bronchitis occurs when the mucous membranes that line the lung's air passages (bronchi) become inflamed. The condition is actually a common one, affecting most people at least once, if not several times, during their life. However, it's when bronchitis becomes a reoccurring illness that one has to worry.

The same viral infection that causes the common cold is the one most often responsible for causing acute bronchitis. The infection spreads from the head into the bronchi and lungs, changing from a cold to bronchitis. Influenza and strep throat can also cause the bronchi to become inflamed, resulting in bronchitis. If bronchitis does not clear up, it can become pneumonia.

Some people are more susceptible to bronchitis than others: the elderly, infants, smokers, asthmatics, alcoholics, individuals with compromised immune systems, people with lung or heart problems, individuals in poor general health, and people who live in moist, polluted environments.

Conventional Medical Treatment

If you are diagnosed with bronchitis, your physician will encourage you to rest as much as possible, increase your fluid intake, and use a vaporizer to keep phlegm loose enough to be easily coughed up. A physician may even advise aspirin or a nonprescription cough medicine.

If your breathing becomes especially labored, a bronchodialator drug may be prescribed to open narrowed bronchi passages. And if your phlegm becomes gray or green, your physician may put you on an antibiotic. If treated properly, an epi-

Warning to Smokers: More Reasons to Quit

Bronchitis, lung cancer, and other lung conditions aren't the only reasons to quit smoking. Here are seven more:

- One cigarette can increase your heart rate up to 25 beats per minute, increasing blood pressure.
- Cigarettes contain 4000 known toxins.
- Smoking one pack of cigarettes depletes your body of 500 milligrams of vitamin C. That's more of the vitamin than most people get in a day!
- Each year, approximately 3000 non-smokers die of lung cancers attributed to secondhand smoke.
- A non-smoker married to a smoker has a 50 percent greater chance of developing lung cancer than a non-smoker married to a non-smoker.
- In children, secondhand smoke causes an estimated 150,000 to 300,000 cases of respiratory illnesses (including bronchitis, asthma, pneumonia) each year.
- Babies born to women who smoke during and after pregnancy are three times as likely to die within their first two years of life as babies born to non-smokers.

Health Notes

➤ *Cigarette, cigar, and pipe smoke compromise lung health. If you are a smoker, quit. If you don't smoke, avoid being around people who do.*

➤ *A nutrient-dense diet can help keep the body's immune system healthy and strong enough to ward off the illnesses that can deteriorate into bronchitis.*

sode of bronchitis typically clears up within $1\frac{1}{2}$ weeks with no lasting effects.

If you are in one of the high-risk groups, your doctor will most likely prescribe all the above, but may also take a chest X-ray and phlegm culture to determine the seriousness of your condition and to rule out other conditions.

For More Information
American Lung Association (ALA)
1740 Broadway
New York, NY 10019
800-LUNG-USA
www.lungusa.org

National Heart, Lung and Blood Institute
Information Center
P.O. Box 30105
Bethesda, MD 20824-0105
301-592-8573
www.nhlbi.nih.gov

Complementary and Alternative Treatments

Nutrition and Supplementation

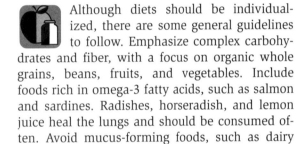

Although diets should be individualized, there are some general guidelines to follow. Emphasize complex carbohydrates and fiber, with a focus on organic whole grains, beans, fruits, and vegetables. Include foods rich in omega-3 fatty acids, such as salmon and sardines. Radishes, horseradish, and lemon juice heal the lungs and should be consumed often. Avoid mucus-forming foods, such as dairy products, wheat, sweet fruits, and processed foods.

Daily supplements that benefit those with bronchitis are as follows:

Most Important

- coenzyme Q10 (60 mg)—improves breathing
- proteolytic enzymes with bromelain (between meals as directed on label)—reduces inflammation
- zinc (1 15-mg lozenge 5 times daily, not to exceed 100 mg total from all supplements)—necessary for tissue repair
- vitamin A (20,000 IU twice daily for 1 month, then reduce to 15,000 IU daily; do not exceed 8000 IU daily if you are pregnant)—heals and protects tissues
- vitamin C with bioflavonoids (3000 to 10,000 mg in divided doses)—reduces histamine levels and enhances immune function
- mixed carotenoid formula (15,000 IU daily)—protects and repairs lung tissue

Also Recommended

- chlorophyll (3 times daily as directed on label)—purifies the blood to improve circulation

- vitamin B complex (100 mg 3 times daily)—activates enzymes needed for healing
- garlic (as directed on label, with food)—reduces infection and rids the body of toxins
- N-acetyl cysteine (200 mg)
- N-acetyl glucosamine (as directed on label)—necessary for the regulation of mucus production

(For an *acute* condition, take supplements until your symptoms subside. If symptoms persist, seek the advice of your healthcare provider. For a *chronic* condition, consult your healthcare provider regarding the duration of treatment.)

Aromatherapy

Both inhalation and steam inhalation therapies with essential oils of eucalyptus, lavender, pine, and rosemary can help clear congestion and ease breathing. For instructions on how to prepare an inhalation, see "Aromatherapy" in the "Introduction to Complementary Therapies" section. Avoid inhalation therapy if you have asthma.

Other beneficial essential oils include benzoin, myrrh, frankincense, bergamot, marjoram and sandalwood.

Bodywork and Somatic Practices

CranioSacral Therapy, Oriental bodywork, and reflexology are good compliments to other treatments.

Chiropractic

Chiropractic manipulation of the thoracic (mid-back) and cervical (neck) sections of the spine relieves pressure on the nerve pathways supplying the lung. This allows more flexible movement of the diaphragm and relieves constricted breathing. It also improves flow of lymph fluid, allowing full immune protection by the lymphatic system and proper enervation to the lungs. In conjunction with proper medical attention, which may include antibiotics, chiropractic is extremely effective in decreasing muscle tightness and spasticity associated with chronic coughing and labored breathing.

Herbal Therapy

Numerous herbs have anti-inflammatory and expectorant capabilities and are helpful in fighting bronchitis. A handful of common remedies follow.

- To soothe a dry bronchial cough, drink a hot mullein-coltsfoot tea several times a day. To make the tea, steep 1 teaspoon each of dried mullein, coltsfoot, and anise seed in 1 cup boiling water for 10 minutes; strain.

- For bronchial spasms, drink thyme 3 three times daily. To prepare the tea, steep 1 teaspoon of thyme leaves in 1 cup of boiling water for 5 to 10 minutes; strain through cheesecloth.

- To quiet a cough, try echinacea tincture. Take 15 to 30 drops 2 to 5 times daily.

- To loosen phlegm and open clogged bronchial tubes, drink coltsfoot tea daily. To make the tea, steep 1 to 2 teaspoons of the herb in 1 cup of boiling water for 10 minutes; strain.

- To soothe inflamed bronchial tubes, sip plain mullein tea. To make the tea, steep 1 to 2 teaspoons of the herb in 1 cup of boiling water for 10 minutes; strain.

- For an expectorant, try aniseed and garlic.

Other therapeutic herbs include horehound, goldenseal, and ginseng. Herbal products are available in health food stores and in some pharmacies and supermarkets. Follow package for specific directions.

Homeopathy

Bronchitis may respond to homeopathic treatment. However, the selection of a remedy—more than one is available—depends on *your* symptoms and the stage of the condition. Don't try treating this disorder yourself. See a homeopathic professional.

Hydrotherapy

Use steam inhalation to help clear congestion. See "Aromatherapy" in "Introduction to Complementary Therapies" section for directions. Adding aromatic oils is optional. A mustard plaster can be applied to the chest to loosen deep congestion.

Traditional Chinese Medicine

Acupuncture Acupuncture is useful in opening up congested bronchial tubes and lessening inflammation, which can ease breathing and relieve the chronic cough that plagues many bronchitis sufferers.

Using auricular therapy, an acupuncturist targets the bronchi, heart, lung, and adrenal gland points. In performing full-body acupuncture, various lung, liver, stomach, and bronchial points are manipulated. If additional symptoms are present (coughing, phlegm, or fever) other points are targeted, as necessary.

Acupressure To relieve bronchial spasms, acupressure targets the lung, spleen, stomach, kidney, bladder, conception vessel, and adrenal points on the forearm, front of the calf, back of the neck, chest, ankles, and upper back (between the shoulder blades and the spine).

Chinese Herbal Therapy Chinese doctors blame internal damp-heat conditions for bronchitis, and thus will most often treat this condition by using herbs to expel the damp-heat and fortify the lungs and bronchial tubes.

For centuries, apricot seed has been used in formulas to treat the coughs and wheezing associated with bronchitis. Use caution with this herb, as apricot seed alone can be toxic in high doses.

Joint fir, or ephedra, is a well-known herbal bronchial dilator, but like apricot seed, is best used in combination.

Multi-ingredient formulas commonly used to treat bronchitis symptoms are Rehmannia Six, Bronchitis Pills (compound), Ginseng and Astragalus, Fritillaria Extract Pills, and Mahuang and Ginkgo Formula.

BRUISES

Signs and Symptoms

- A deep purple area under the skin that becomes brownish, then greenish, then yellowish as it fades and heals
- Tenderness at the site

Description

A bruise gets its deep color from a blood vessel or vessels that break under the skin and leak blood into the surrounding area. As it heals, it becomes paler in color and less painful to the touch. Depending on how many vessels were broken, bruises can be the size of a pencil eraser or 6 or more inches across. A black eye is also bruise—if there is no accompanying eye damage or nose breakage, it can be treated just like any other bruise.

Bruises are caused when enough pressure is placed on the skin to break the blood vessels underneath. A few of the ways this can be accomplished are: by being gripped too tightly, by being struck (by a hand, foot, or object), by falling, or by walking into something.

Why Do Bruises Change Color?

Anyone who has ever gotten a bruise before has watched it turn from blue-black to blue-green, green-brown, yellow-brown, and yellow, before finally disappearing completely. Did you ever wonder what's behind your bruise's color transformation? The answer is blood. As the hemoglobin in the blood breaks down, the blueness of a bruise begins to disappear and is replaced by more and more yellow pigment.

Health Notes

➤ Vitamin C is responsible for mending broken vein walls, making it essential in helping the body heal bruises. People who do not have enough vitamin C in their diet are especially prone to bruising. Eat a diet rich in citrus fruits, strawberries, tomatoes, uncooked peppers, and other raw produce.

➤ People on blood thinning heart medications are often prone to easy bruising because of their blood's inability to clot. If you are on such medicine and are experiencing bruising, see your physician for bruise-preventing and healing advice.

➤ If you notice that you are bruising more easily or frequently than usual, visit your doctor. This may be a sign of a blood disorder.

Conventional Medical Treatment

Unless the bruise is especially large or is accompanied by broken skin or a raised and swollen area, medical attention is rarely necessary. Your doctor also may instruct you to elevate the injured area and ice the site for 30 to 45 minutes several times daily for 2 or 3 days after the injury.

For More Information
American Academy of Dermatology
930 North Meacham Road
Schaumburg, IL 60618
888-462-DERM
www.aad.org

Complementary and Alternative Treatments

Nutrition and Supplementation

 Studies show that people with vitamin C deficiencies bruise easily, most likely because their blood vessels are weak. Avoid a deficiency and guarantee your consumption of bioflavonoids by eating a diet rich in dark-green, leafy vegetables and fresh fruits. To help blood clot, eat leafy greens, such as kale, which is rich in vitamin K. Everyone bruises, but if you bruise frequently for unexplained reasons, see your healthcare provider.

To speed healing of bruises, consider the following daily suggestions:

- vitamin C with bioflavonoids (3000 to 10,000 mg in divided doses)
- vitamin K or alfalfa (as directed on label)
- coenzyme Q10 (60 mg)—essential for construction of body cells
- iron (as directed by doctor)—corrects deficiencies
- grape seed extract (as directed on label)—protects skin tissues
- fish oil or flaxseed oil (as directed on label)—promotes healing

(Take supplements until your symptoms subside. If symptoms persist, seek the advice of your healthcare provider.)

Aromatherapy

 Bruises respond favorably to cool compresses laced with essential oils of lavender, yarrow, hyssop, camphor, or helichrysum (also known as immortelle). Apply several times a day for about 10 minutes.

Herbal Therapy

 Witch hazel and arnica (in cream or tincture form) are two topical preparations that can be used to treat bruises.

Herbal products are available in health food stores and in some pharmacies and supermarkets. Follow package for specific directions.

Homeopathy

 Homeopathic practitioners may recommend one of the following treatments, depending on your symptoms:

- *Arnica*—for bruising from blunt trauma to the muscles—for example, being struck or falling down; Arnica ointment can be applied to bruises, but not when the skin is broken.
- *Ledum*—if a bruise feels cold and improves when a cold compress is applied
- *Bellis perennis*—if there is blood under your skin (hematoma) or if the bruise is from a blow to the breast or pelvic area
- *Ruta graveolens*—if the bruise is from a kick to the shin
- *Hypericum*—if the bruised area is rich in nerves, such as the fingers or toes.

Hydrotherapy

 Apply an ice pack to the bruised areas for 5 minutes on, 3 minutes off, for a total of 16 minutes. To speed healing and reduce swelling, apply contrast therapy (alternating hot and cold cloths) several times a day. You also can try applying a warm compress soaked in strong sage tea. Use the compress for 30 minutes 3 times daily.

Traditional Chinese Medicine

薬 ***Acupuncture*** Acupuncture may help alleviate the swelling surrounding a bruise and regulate blood flow to the area. Different points are targeted, depending upon the location and severity of the bruise.

Chinese Herbal Therapy Herbs that can be used to soothe the bruise and hasten healing include aloe vera and achyranthes; these work by improving circulation. Chinese yam can be mixed with water to form a poultice, and decoction of corydalis can help heal bruises caused by a fall or injury.

BULIMIA

Signs and Symptoms

- Periodic bingeing (eating large amounts of food within a given period of time) followed by purging (self-induced vomiting)
- Concern with weight and figure, though most bulimics remain in the normal weight range for their height
- Teeth scrapes on the knuckles of fingers from induced vomiting
- Discolored teeth or cavities from enamel erosion caused by stomach acid that is vomited up
- Periods of exercise after bingeing
- Overuse of laxatives and/or diuretics
- Feelings of shame or low self-worth following a binge
- Depression

Description

Like anorexia, bulimia is an eating disorder that most often strikes young women. Theories about what causes the condition abound. An imbalance of serotonin levels, a perfectionist attitude, social pressures to be thin, fear of one's sexuality, and mental disturbances are all hypotheses for what causes bulimia.

Because a bulimic's weight is often normal or near-normal, and because binge-eating and purging are often done in secret, bulimia is difficult to diagnose. Families should look for the regular disappearance of large amounts of food from the house (unless the bulimic purchases her own), food wrappers and containers hidden in her bedroom, scrapes over the knuckles—particularly the second and third fingers—caused by induced vomiting, and a change in the color of tooth enamel caused by the corrosive stomach acid. Laxatives or diuretic packages and frequent, excessive exercise workouts are also warning signs.

Conventional Medical Treatment

Though bulimics are less likely than anorexics to waste away to nothing, they are at risk for a variety of serious health problems, including life-threatening dehydration, potassium depletion,

That Full Feeling

A hormone called cholecystokinin-pancreozymin (CCK) may be the reason why bulimics binge. According to preliminary research conducted at the National Institute of Mental Health (NIMH) and Duke University, the chemical, which is found in the small intestine and the brain, controls appetite. When inadequate levels of this hormone are produced—which happen to many bulimics—the body fails to feel full—thus the urge to continue eating.

Health Note

➤ *While there is no recognized way to prevent bulimia, the earlier the condition is identified and treated, the easier it is to reverse.*

cardiac arrhythmia, and tooth decay. Thus, if you suspect the condition in yourself or a loved one, it is important to visit a physician.

After performing a thorough physical examination to assess your overall health, the physician asks about your medical history and interviews you about your attitudes toward food and weight. If a diagnosis of bulimia is made, your physician may suggest a psychotherapist and/or a nutritionist to help you overcome the problem. You also may be referred to a self-help therapy group for people who are fighting bulimia. Relapses are common, though bulimia can be overcome with long-term psychotherapy.

For More Information

American Anorexia Bulimia Association, Inc.
165 West 46th Street, NW, Suite 1108
New York, NY 10036
212-575-6200
www.aabainc.org

National Eating Disorders Organization
6655 South Yale Avenue
Tulsa, OK 74136
918-481-4044
www.kidsource.com/nedo/index.html

Complementary and Alternative Treatments

Nutrition and Supplementation

 Eliminate junk foods and white flour products from your diet, as well as sugar in any form. You may experience anxiety, depression, fatigue, headache, insomnia, and/or irritability for a while after you eliminate sugar.

Many people with eating disorders suffer from a deficiency of zinc, which could actually be a cause of the disease. Heart functioning eventually becomes impaired because a body lacking zinc will start scrounging for it within the body, actually consuming it from muscle tissue and the heart. Because zinc plays such a vital role in appetite regulation, it is essential to supplement the diet with it, in liquid form, if possible. Many bulimics report a suppression, even elimination, of the desire to binge and purge once their zinc levels are supplemented.

Sea vegetables, such as kelp, nori, and dulse, provide important minerals as well as vitamin B_{12} and beta-carotene. Other foods rich in minerals include alfalfa, spirulina, blue-green algae, and barley greens. Water consumption is essential to healing this disease; the malnutrition that often results from bulimia can inhibit the ability to recognize the body's need for liquid and lead to a state of dehydration. Protein supplement drinks also may be recommended to boost protein and calorie intake.

Consult with a health care provider for an individualized rehabilitation program, and follow the daily suggestions below for a healthy start:

Most Important

- zinc (50 mg, not to exceed a total of 100 mg from all supplements)
- copper (3 mg)—needed to balance zinc
- multivitamin and mineral complex (as directed by healthcare provider)
- vitamin A (15,000 IU; do not exceed 8000 IU daily if you are pregnant)
- mixed carotenoid formula (25,000 IU)
- potassium (99 mg)
- selenium (200 mcg)

Also Recommended

- a prodophilus formula (as directed on label)—replaces friendly bacteria and protects the liver
- calcium (1500 mg at bedtime)—has a calming effect

- magnesium (750 mg)—relaxes smooth muscle
- free-form amino acid complex (as directed on label)—counteracts protein deficiency, a serious problem in bulimia
- vitamin B$_{12}$ (1 cc 3 times weekly or as prescribed by healthcare provider)—aids digestion of food and the assimilation of all nutrients; injections are best
- vitamin C (5000 mg in divided doses)—necessary for all cellular and glandular functions

(Consult your healthcare provider regarding the duration of treatment.)

Homeopathy

Bulimia may respond to homeopathic treatment. However, the selection of a remedy—more than one is available—depends on *your* symptoms and the stage of the condition. Don't try treating this disorder yourself. See a homeopathic professional.

Traditional Chinese Medicine

Acupuncture Bulimia can be helped with acupuncture treatments that focus on restoring the body's energy levels, reducing stress, and promoting feelings of relaxation and well-being. Various auricular and body points are targeted, depending on the specific needs of the client.

Chinese Herbal Therapy Because bulimia wreaks havoc on the immune system, various herbs may be prescribed to bring the body back into balance, including angelica, astragalus, and ginseng.

Pre-made immunity-boosting tonics can be found in most health food stores. Popular formulas include Saussurea and Amomum Stomach Nurturing Pills and Vitality Combination.

In addition, an herbalist may prescribe formulas to calm and strengthen the digestive system, which is weakened by repeated bingeing and purging. Common preparations for this purpose include Ginseng Stomachic Pills and Internal Formula.

Additional herbs may be used to combat the sore throat, fatigue, menstrual problems, skin conditions, and dehydration that can accompany bulimia.

BUNIONS

Signs and Symptoms

- Bony protrusion at the base of the big toe
- Pain at the site
- Decreased motion in the toe

Description

A bunion is a bump or bend that develops at the base of your big toe. If your big toe becomes very crooked, it can overlap your second toe. This mild deformity is common and is more likely to occur in women than in men.

b

Shoe Sense

Even if your job requires you to be a slave to fashion, try to avoid wearing high heels all day long. They put increased pressure on the ball of the foot, and the stress can eventually contribute to the development of abnormalities, such as bunions and hammertoes. Flat-soled shoes exert significantly less pressure on the ball of the foot, and going barefoot exerts less pressure still, although in most professions, you probably won't get away with it.

There are individuals who are genetically predisposed to developing bunions. Most people, however, get them from scrunching their feet into tight shoes with a pointed toe area.

Conventional Medical Treatments

A physician usually can diagnose a bunion simply by examining the area, though an X-ray may be necessary in some cases. Once a bunion is diagnosed, you will need trade your foot-pinching shoes for roomy, comfortable footwear. While this won't make the bunion go away, it will relieve the pain and keep it from growing worse. In some cases, bunions can lead to osteoarthritis or bursitis—so if your bunion suddenly becomes more painful, contact your physician. People with severe pain and deformity may need surgery to realign the bones.

For More Information
American Podiatric Medical Association
9312 Old Georgetown Road
Bethesda, MD 20814-1698
1-800-FOOTCARE
www.apma.org

Complementary and Alternative Treatments

Nutrition and Supplementation

 The following daily supplements may help with pain and inflammation:

- D-phenylalanine (500 mg)
- niacinamide (15 mg)
- magnesium (400 mg)
- sea cucumber (as directed on label)—reduces pain and inflammation

Traditional Chinese Medicine

 Acupuncture Because bunions often begin as a simple inflammation of the joint on the big toe, acupuncture can be used to improve blood and energy flow to the area, which can alleviate the pain and swelling associated with this condition, especially when combined with self-massage.

Acupressure To relieve pain in the big toe, apply pressure to Liver 3, which lies on the top of the foot between the big and second toes.

Chinese Herbal Therapy The fresh juice from an aloe vera leaf can be applied topically to relieve the ache and inflammation.

Health Notes

➤ It may seem strange to have a chiropractor treat a bunion. But according to practitioners, postural imbalances can lead to foot problems, including bunions. These imbalances can be addressed with regular spinal manipulations.

➤ Bodywork that emphasizes proper movement, such as the Alexander technique and the Feldenkrais method, prevent bunions by teaching individuals to stand, walk, sit, and move in a manner that doesn't strain any one part of the body.

BURNS

Signs and Symptoms

First-Degree

- Pink or red areas that may or may not be accompanied by swelling and blisters
- Tenderness or pain at the site

Second-Degree

- Mottled, intensely red areas
- Blistering at the site, sometimes accompanied by oozing fluid
- Intense pain
- Swelling

Third-Degree

- Charred black and/or white areas
- Visible bone, fat, nerves and/or muscles
- Victim may be in shock or unconscious
- First- and second-degree burns often accompany third-degree burns
- Severe pain, or if the nerves have been burned, lack of feeling

Basic Description

A first-degree burn is the most minor type of burn. It only affects the outer layer of skin—the burn is at the surface only. First-degree burns can be caused by the sun (sunburns), chemicals, or heated objects or fluids.

With a second-degree burn, the top layer of skin has been burned through and the second layer of skin has also been burned (though not burned through). Second-degree burns also can be caused by the sun (sunburns), fire, chemicals, or heated objects or fluids.

A third-degree burn is an extremely severe burn that damages the top and bottom layers of skin and the underlying layers of fat, nerves, muscles, and even bones. The area will be charred black or white and will be dry and powdery. Third-degree burns are usually caused by fire, though they can also be caused by chemicals or electrical wires.

Conventional Medical Treatment

Unless the first-degree burn is accompanied by more serious burns, or covers large areas of the hands, feet, face, groin, buttocks, or major joint, you can treat it at home. If the second-degree burn is limited to an area 3 inches in diameter or smaller, it can also be treated at home. If the skin

Health Notes

➤ In cases of chemical burns, the skin will continue to be burned as long as the chemical is present. Immediately run cool water over the area.

➤ A first- or second-degree burn (with no presence of third-degree burns) can be treated immediately with cool water. This reduces pain and swelling.

➤ To remove hot wax, tar, or melted plastics from the skin, hold an ice cube against the substance until it hardens. Then gently remove.

➤ Reduce the swelling that often accompanies burns by keeping the burned area elevated.

is unbroken, run cool water over the area or soak it in a cool bath. Either way, keep the area submerged for 2 to 4 minutes. Then cover the burn with a sterile bandage or clean cloth. Minor burns usually heal without further attention. If an infection sets in, see your physician.

If the second-degree burn is larger than 3 inches in diameter, or has occurred on the feet, face, groin, buttocks, hands, or major joint, immediately go to your physician or hospital emergency room.

If any part of the body contains third-degree burns, immediately call an ambulance. If you are a bystander, check to see if the burn victim is breathing. If not, perform cardiopulmonary resuscitation (CPR). (If you are not trained in CPR, find someone who is.) If the person is breathing, cover the burned areas with a cool, moist, sterile bandage or a clean sheet (make sure it is a flat-weave sheet rather than a fuzzy one). *Do not* apply any oils, ointments, or lotions, and *do not* move the victim.

For More Information

National Burn Victim Foundation
246-A Madisonville Road, PO Box 409
Basking Ridge, NJ 07920
908-953-9091
www.nbvf.org

Complementary and Alternative Treatments

Nutrition and Supplementation

Increase your protein intake and consume 5000 to 6000 calories daily to aid in tissue repair and healing. It is important to drink plenty of liquids, preferably water, during the healing process.

Once you have treated the burn locally, these daily supplements should speed healing:

Most Important

- free-form amino acid complex (as directed on label)—promotes the healing of tissues

- potassium (99 mg)—replaces potassium lost from burns

- colloidal silver (as directed on label)—a natural antibiotic and disinfectant that promotes healing

- vitamin A (100,000 IU for one month, then reduce to 50,000 IU (Before taking this high dosage, check with your healthcare provider. It must only be taken under supervision. Do not exceed 8000 IU daily if you are pregnant)—needed for tissue repair; best assimilated if used in emulsion form

- mixed carotenoid formula (25,000 IU)—a precursor of vitamin A and an antioxidant

- vitamin B complex (100 mg with food)—promotes the healing of skin tissue

- vitamin C with bioflavonoids (10,000 mg immediately after a burn, 2000 mg 3 times a day until healed)—an antioxidant essential in the formation of collagen; promotes the healing of burns

- vitamin E (start with 600 IU and increase slowly to 1600 IU)—heals and prevents scarring (You can open a capsule and apply directly to the scar once healing has begun.)

- zinc (30 mg 3 times daily, not to exceed a total of 100 mg from all supplements)—heals tissues

Also Recommended

- selenium (200 mcg)—protects skin from antioxidant damage

- glutathione (200 mg)—protects skin from antioxidant damage

(Take supplements until your symptoms subside. If symptoms persist, seek the advice of your healthcare provider.)

Aromatherapy

For first- and second-degree burns, immediately apply lavender oil to the area. Alternatively, you can fill a bowl with cold water and ice, add 3 to 6 drops of lavender oil, and make a cold compress. Apply the compress to the burned area. Replace as soon as the compress warms, until the pain subsides.

Ayurvedic Medicine

To ease the pain and speed healing of small, minor burns, an Ayurvedic practitioner may suggest applying aloe vera gel, ghee (clarified butter), or coconut oil to the site of the burn. The practitioner may also suggest drinking fresh cilantro juice.

Herbal Therapy

Apply fresh aloe vera directly to small, minor burns (or sunburned skin). Simply slit open an aloe plant leaf, and apply the liquid. You also can use commercially-produced aloe vera gel available in most drugstores. Plantain juice or salve may also be beneficial.

Herbal products are available in health food stores and in some pharmacies and supermarkets. Follow package for specific directions.

Homeopathy

Your homeopathic practitioner may recommend one of the following internal treatments for small first- or second-degree burns, depending on your symptoms:

- *Urtica urens*—for first-degree burns
- *Cantharis*—for second-degree burns
- *Causticum*—for burns that are more than 20 minutes old

You also may apply a lotion containing *Urtica* and *Calendula* to the affected area.

Hydrotherapy

If the skin isn't broken, immediately plunge the burned area into cold water or hold it under cold running water. You can also apply a cold compress until the pain subsides, about 10 minutes.

Traditional Chinese Medicine

Acupuncture Acupuncture may be used to help lessen swelling and promote faster healing. Acupuncture also has an anesthetic component (it releases endorphins and other "feel good" bodily chemicals) and can be used to relieve pain.

Chinese Herbal Therapy Aloe vera may be used topically to soothe the burn and speed healing. Various oils and liniments are available that speed healing and relieve pain, such as Red Flower Ointment and White Flower Ointment.

BURSITIS

Signs and Symptoms

- Pain and swelling in a joint
- Stiffness in the affected joint
- Pain with movement of joint

Description

A bursa is a sac-like membrane filled with synovial fluid that acts as a cushion between the bone and fibrous tissues of the muscles and tendons. It makes movement of joints easy by limiting friction. There are 156 bursae in the body—bursitis results when one of them becomes inflamed. It occurs most commonly in the shoulder.

Bursitis is a repetitive motion injury, meaning that it is generally associated with overuse of a given joint. Thus, any motion that is repeated many times a day—such as swinging a tennis racquet, throwing a baseball, playing an instrument, using a computer, or cutting hair—can cause bur-

Health Notes

➤ *The moment you feel symptoms of bursitis in a joint, rest the area for 2 to 3 days. This is not always an easy task, but you may be able to head off a full-blown case of bursitis.*

➤ *Bodywork that emphasizes proper movement, such as the Alexander technique and the Feldenkrais method, can prevent bursitis by teaching individuals to move without straining any one part of the body.*

sitis. On the other hand, there are cases where there seems to be no definable cause.

Conventional Medical Treatment

Bursitis can disappear within 2 weeks if the joint is given absolute rest. During this "time off," RICE therapy (rest, ice, compression, and elevation) is recommended, and many sufferers wear special braces or wraps to keep the area immobilized. Aspirin can be used to keep inflammation in check. Some physicians inject cortisone into the affected joint.

In extremely severe cases, surgery may be performed to remove the inflamed bursa. Unfortunately, this results in limited motion.

For More Information
American College of Sports Medicine
P.O. Box 1440
Indianapolis, IN 46206-1440
317-637-9200
www.acsm.org

Complementary and Alternative Treatments

Nutrition and Supplementation

 When treating bursitis, consider the following daily supplemental guidelines:

Most Important

- vitamin A (50,000 IU for 2 weeks, then 5000 IU; do not exceed 8000 IU if you are pregnant)—aids in tissue repair and promotes immune function

- vitamin C with bioflavonoids (3000 to 8000 mg in divided doses)—reduces inflammation and is essential to collagen formation

- vitamin E (400 IU)—a free radical scavenger

- calcium (1500 mg)

- magnesium (750 mg)

- zinc (40 mg, not to exceed a total of 100 mg from all supplements)— important to tissue repair

- copper (3 mg)—to balance the zinc

Also Recommended

- vitamin B complex (100 mg twice daily)—important to cellular repair, supplemented with vitamin B_{12} (as prescribed by doctor)—necessary for proper digestion, absorption of foods, and the repair of nerve damage (most effective if taken by injection; otherwise, use lozenge form)

- sea cucumber (take as directed on label)—replenishes the lubricants needed for connective tissues and joints

- bromelain (take as directed on label)—inflammation-fighting enzyme

- hydrolyzed collagen (take as directed on label)—important for joint tissue rebuilding

- glucosamine sulfate (take as directed on label)— aids in healing

(For an *acute* condition, take supplements until your symptoms subside. If symptoms persist, seek the advice of your healthcare provider. For a *chronic* condition, consult your healthcare provider regarding the duration of treatment.)

Aromatherapy

Aromatherapists suggest the essential oils of juniper, Roman or German chamomile, and cypress for treating bursitis.

Bodywork and Somatic Practices

Good bets for gentle, immediate relief and healing include reflexology, Therapeutic Touch, massage, CranioSacral Therapy, Feldenkrais, Trager, and Oriental bodywork. Later, to reduce the likelihood of any further problems, such as repetitive motion syndrome, old injury history, or persistent pain cycles, use trigger point myotherapy, Hellerwork, Rolfing, Aston-Patterning, or Alexander technique.

Chiropractic

Bursitis is sometimes caused by malposition of the joint. Corrective adjustments are beneficial, especially in chronic cases. In acute cases—specifically those caused by repetitive motions and the "overuse syndrome" typically seen in athletes—specific chiropractic adjustment (SCA) can be extremely effective. Chiropractic care may also include physical therapy, such as ultrasound and electromuscle stimulation. A chiropractor may recommend specific exercises to prevent bursitis in the shoulder from progressing to frozen shoulder syndrome, which sometimes happens in serious cases.

Herbal Therapy

For easing the discomfort of bursitis, try willow or meadowsweet tea; both herbs contain salicylate, a natural pain reliever. To prepare the tea, steep 1 teaspoon of either dried herb in 1 cup boiling water for 10 to 15 minutes; strain and drink 3 cups daily.

Alternatively, you might try a blend of tinctures of meadowsweet, horsetail, and willow bark. Combine equal amounts of the tinctures and take 1 teaspoon of the blend 3 times daily.

A combined tincture of lobelia and cramp bark is also therapeutic when rubbed into muscles to calm the tension produced by bursitis.

Homeopathy

Your homeopathic practitioner may suggest *Ruta graveolens* to ease the pain of bursitis.

Hydrotherapy

When pain is acute, apply an ice pack for 20 minutes on, 20 minutes off during the first 24 hours. After that, use contrast therapy (alternating hot and cold compresses) up to 3 times daily. *Caution:* Never use a cold compress for longer than 20 minutes at a time; extended exposure to cold can damage skin.

You also might try soaking in a warm Epsom salts bath for 20 to 30 minutes once a week.

Traditional Chinese Medicine

Acupuncture Acupuncture can help reduce the inflammation and relieve the stiffness that accompanies bursitis, and it may promote the drainage of excess fluid. Acupoints targeted vary, depending on whether the pain is located in the hip, knee, or shoulder.

Acupressure Acupressure can be used to alleviate the pain and inflammation associated with bursitis.

Chinese Herbal Therapy Corydalis Analgesic Tablets might be prescribed to combat bursitis-related pain, and aloe vera can be used as a topical medication. Herb plasters can also be used locally on affected areas.

CANCER

Description

Cancer is a frightening illness to many people, and for good reason. It is the second leading cause of death in the United States, claiming the lives of half a million Americans each year. On the other hand, scientific research has uncovered new findings that have led to more effective methods of treatment and prevention. It has also revealed a great deal about the mysterious nature of the disease.

Cancer is a disease characterized by uncontrolled cell growth anywhere on or in the body. Cells, the body's building blocks, each contain thousands of genes. Cells are perpetually replicating in order to replace themselves as they die. When a new cell is created with an altered genetic code, the change, or mutation, can increase a person's vulnerability to cancer. Cancer is by no means an instantaneous occurrence; rather, damage accumulates slowly over time as vulnerable cells are assaulted by harmful substances, such as chemicals, viruses, and radiation. In certain cases, the vulnerable cell can no longer withstand the assault and becomes cancerous. The affected cell then begins to replicate itself to become a cloned cluster of malignant cells. These abnormal cells have the ability to spread from the affected site to other areas of the body, a process called *metastasis*.

Cancer can be triggered by both genetic and environmental factors. In ovarian and breast cancer, heredity plays a strong role. Some other types of cancer are occasionally passed from one generation to the next, but approximately 75 percent of cancer cases are caused by external influences, such as smoking and tobacco use, poor diet, and exposure to carcinogens, or cancer-causing substances.

Fortunately, many forms of cancer are preventable, or even curable, especially when detected early. A healthy lifestyle is the best line of defense against cancer, whether or not you have a hereditary risk of developing the disease. This includes adopting a healthy diet and incorporating regular exercise in your weekly schedule. Frequent medical screenings are another important element in cancer defense. Perform regular body and skin self-examinations, and contact your doctor immediately if you notice any of the general **CAUTION** signs of cancer: **C**hange in bowel or bladder habits; **A** sore that does not heal; **U**nusual bleeding or discharge; **T**hickening or lump in breast or elsewhere; **I**ndigestion or difficulty in swallowing; **O**bvious change in a wart or mole; **N**agging cough or hoarseness.

There are two main goals of cancer treatment: to cure the disease or, at least, to control it in order to extend and improve the patient's quality of life. Treatment can involve surgery to remove the abnormal growth, radiation to destroy cancerous cells in a specific area, and/or medication taken orally or intravenously to kill cancer cells throughout the body (called chemotherapy). Today, many patients are opting for complementary therapies, which do not involve the use of surgery or drugs. In most cases, these therapies are used in conjunction with conventional cancer treatments, either to relieve discomfort or to augment standard medical approaches. Many of these alternative treatments have provided significant benefits to cancer patients.

Health Note

➤ *According to studies, tomatoes are the richest source of lycopene, a close relative of beta-carotene. It appears to be a strong inhibitor of prostate and colon cancer and heart disease. Cooking lycopene improves the body's ability to absorb it, so tomato juice, paste, and puree are excellent sources.*

Breakthrough Cancer Treatments

The evidence is mounting—herbs may help to prevent cancer when used in combination with traditional cancer treatments, such as chemotherapy and radiation. Cancer researchers say that this combined approach may improve quality of life, and in some cases, prevent the growth of certain cancers. For example:

- *Milk Thistle.* Studies indicate that silymarin, the powerful antioxidant compound found in milk thistle, offered almost complete protection from skin cancer in mice that were exposed to known carcinogens.

- *Green Tea.* Two prominent cancer institutes are studying the effects green tea has on preventing cancer. Green tea, made from the unfermented leaves of the tea plant, contains catechins, substances that may have important anticancer and antibacterial actions.

- *Ginseng.* Studies are underway to determine if this traditional Chinese herb can slow the onset of colon cancer. In a Korean study, subjects taking ginseng supplements demonstrated a decreased risk of stomach cancer. Other studies suggest similar findings.

For More Information
American Cancer Society
1599 Clifton Road, NE
Atlanta, GA 30329
800-ACS-2345
www.cancer.org

National Cancer Institute
Cancer Information Service
Building 31, 9000 Rockville Pike
Bethesda, MD 20892
800-4-CANCER
TTY: 800-332-8615
http://cis.nci.nih.gov

Cancer Treatment Centers of America
3455 Salt Creek Lane
Arlington Heights, IL 60005
800-615-3055
www.cancercenter.com

Complementary and Alternative Treatments

Nutrition and Supplementation

 Note: The following information varies, depending upon any treatment that is being undertaken; always consult with your oncologist or other healthcare providers before making changes to your diet.

Once you understand that as many as 70 percent of all cancers have been linked to lifestyle factors, including nutrition, you can appreciate the benefits of a solid, balanced diet. What you eat plays an important role not only in treating, but in

Chronotherapy

Also called "timed therapy," chronotherapy tracks the cyclical nature of a condition and adjusts treatment accordingly. Although not widely used, it has proven helpful for some cancer sufferers.

Most chemotherapy medications attack cancer cells by interfering with cell division, but these drugs can also invade noncancerous cells and cause harmful side effects, including hair loss, nausea, increased rates of infection, and organ damage.

Doctors have recently begun using programmable pumps to administer medications at times when cancer cells are most susceptible—and normal cells aren't. To determine the best time for treatment, doctors study cell cycles. For example, cell division of the stomach lining usually occurs during the day; chemotherapy for colon cancer can be more effective at night, when healthy cells are less susceptible to damage.

preventing, cancer. Organic whole foods and pure water supply us with essential nutrients that can help keep some cancers from developing. And, if cancer already exists, these foods give your body the best possible support to overcome the disease. Because many people with cancer have problems absorbing the nutrients in their diets, particularly when undergoing certain treatments or taking some medications, consult your healthcare provider to determine whether you should have a comprehensive digestive stool analysis.

To minimize malnutrition, eat a high-calorie diet and aim to obtain 40 percent of your calorie intake from high-quality protein, concentrating on lamb, fish, chicken, soy products and eggs as protein sources. Milkshakes provide a protein-rich drink, and skim milk powder can be stirred into foods, such as casseroles, desserts, and sauces to add extra protein. Ask your healthcare provider about high protein supplement drinks to boost your protein and calorie intake.

Blood that has balanced pH levels inhibits the growth of cancer cells. An ideal range is 7.2 to 7.4. To keep your pH balanced, your diet should include a lot of alkaline-forming foods. These include raw fruits and vegetables, nuts, seeds, legumes, and grains. Emphasize the following fruits: apples, apricots, avocados, bananas, berries, currants, dates, figs, grapes, grapefruit, kiwis, lemons, limes, mangos, melons, nectarines, olives, oranges, papayas, peaches, pears, persimmons, pineapple, quince, raisins, raspberries, strawberries, tangerines, and watermelons.

Recommended vegetables include artichokes, asparagus, beets, broccoli, brussels sprouts, cabbage, carrots, cauliflower, celery, corn, cucumbers, ginger, kelp, seaweeds, sprouts, mustard greens, onions, parsley, bell peppers, potatoes, pumpkin, radishes, spinach, squash, tomatoes, watercress, and yams. An additional advantage to the cruciferous family (broccoli, cauliflower, cabbage, mustard greens, etc.) is that they contain detoxifying agents called indoles. Experts believe these indoles may remove cancer-causing substances from the body.

Other alkaline-forming foods include green beans, limas, peas, soybean products (soy milk, tofu, miso, and tempeh), rice, barley, oats, ama-ranth, almonds, coconuts, and chestnuts. Seeds to eat include radish, sesame, and alfalfa. Eat them in sprouted form whenever possible.

Soy foods contain a number of factors that boost the body's cancer-fighting ability. These substances, called isoflavones, include genestein, diadzen, and glycitein. They carry benefits in a number of areas, including acting as weak estrogens, which protects the body against hormone-dependent cancers, such as breast, endometrium and prostate. Isoflavones may also reduce the formation of blood vessels that feed cancer tumors and reduce the life span of cancer cells.

Foods high in fiber can benefit people with cancer. To get the most fiber from your foods, eat them in their natural state, as most of it is lost when food is processed. Look to fruits, vegetables, and whole grains for your fiber.

Chlorophyll purifies the blood and has powerful anti-mutation factors. Eat barley grass, alfalfa, spirulina, and blue-green algae to get nutrients necessary for detoxifying your system. Also look for "green" phytochemical drinks that contain chlorophyll, made with soy, vegetables, and wheatgrass. These are also valuable for their antioxidant properties.

Don't overlook the value of juice. Freshly squeezed juices provide enzymes and antioxidant nutrients that are easy on the digestive system. Carrot juice is high in beta-carotene and vitamin A, but should be watered down because it is also high in sugar. Add a teaspoon of vitamin C powder to juice to make it a preventive tonic. Drink fruit juices in the morning, and vegetables juices in the afternoon.

Green tea is another valuable beverage. It contains antioxidants as well as substances called polyphenolic catechins. These fight free radicals even better than vitamin E. Green tea is valuable in countering the effects of radiation and keeps pH levels balanced.

Mushrooms have been found to have incredible healing properties. Shiitake, maitake, and reishi mushrooms contain anti-tumor properties. Asians use them to enhance longevity. Research conducted in Japan showed a highly significant rate of tumor elimination in animals fed extracts of these mushrooms. In addition, shiitake mushrooms boost the immune system, and maitake mushrooms help the body cope with the added stress of cancer treatments.

Seaweed softens hardened tumors.

There are certain foods to avoid as well. Do not eat peanuts, junk food, processed foods, excessive saturated fats, salt, sugar, or white flour. Avoid caffeine, alcohol, and all teas except herbal. Never eat hot dogs, smoked or cured meats, or luncheon meat. Eat broiled fish three times weekly as your condition improves. Dairy should be consumed in limited quantities or not at all.

The following daily supplement recommendations are not all-inclusive. Consult a specialist to develop an individualized program.

Most Important

- coenzyme Q10 (100 mg)—improves cellular oxygenation

- dimethylglycine (as directed on label)—enhances oxygen utilization

- melatonin (2 to 3 mg, taken 2 hours or less before bedtime)—aids sleep

- mixed carotenoid formula (25,000 IU)—repairs and rebuilds all cells

- proteolytic enzymes (as directed on label)—a potent free radical scavenger

- selenium (200 mcg)—a free radical scavenger that also aids in protein digestion

- shark cartilage (as directed on label, under supervision of health care provider)—inhibits and even reverses the growth of some types of tumors

- vitamin A (50,000 to 100,000 IU for 10 days, then 50,000 IU for 30 days, then reduced to 25,000 IU; do not exceed 8000 IU daily if you are pregnant)—requirements are higher for people with cancer; use emulsion form for best assimilation

- vitamin E (up to 1000 IU)—fights cancer

- vitamin B complex (100 mg)—necessary for normal cell division and function

- vitamin C with bioflavonoids (5000 to 20,000 mg in divided doses)—a potent anti-cancer agent that promotes the production of interferon in the body

Also Recommended

- N-acetyl cysteine (as directed on label)—detoxifies harmful substances; protects the liver and other organs

- raw glandular complex, plus raw thymus (as directed on label)—stimulates production of T-lymphocytes; helps prevent bladder damage from cancer drugs

- chromium picolinate (at least 600 mcg)—builds and maintains muscle mass

(Consult your healthcare provider regarding the duration of treatment.)

Aromatherapy

You can fight the physical and emotional stress of cancer and its treatments by taking a relaxing bath to which you've added 7 to 12 drops of an essential oil such as lavender, Roman Chamomile, or geranium. To lessen radiation burns and prevent scarring, you might try niaouli, tea tree, or lavender oil. Rosemary may help stimulate hair growth after chemotherapy. Check with your oncologist before starting an aromatherapy regimen.

Bodywork and Somatic Practices

Cancer calls for a full-scale teaming of both conventional medical and complementary therapies. Emotional and spiritual well-being deserve as much attention as the physical body; therefore, initial helpful complementary therapies could include Oriental bodywork, CranioSacral Therapy/SomatoEmotional Release, polarity therapy and reflexology. As care continues, all energy therapies, movement re-education modalities, and most manual therapies can help provide support for the immune system.

Herbal Therapy

Although many claims have been made for herbal cures for cancer, none have been proven. However, several herbs have been shown to ease the side effects of cancer and its treatments. Try ginger for the nausea that often accompanies chemotherapy. If you're concerned about hair loss, you might want to try horsetail. Talk with your doctor before treating yourself with these herbs.

Homeopathy

 Cancer might respond to homeopathic treatment. However, the selection of a remedy—more than one is available—depends on *your* symptoms and the stage of the condition. Don't try treating cancer yourself. See a homeopathic professional.

Hydrotherapy

 Some therapists recommend controlled hyperthermia treatments once or twice weekly and constitutional hydrotherapy several times weekly. For directions, see "Hydrotherapy" in the "Introduction to Complementary Therapies" section. Be sure to consult your doctor before starting any new regimen.

Yoga and Meditation

 With your doctor's approval, establish a daily routine, including several yoga poses, deep-breathing exercises, meditation, and visualization. This relaxing routine can help combat the discomfort and emotional and physical tension associated with cancer treatment. Visualizing your body fighting off the cancer (and winning) also may promote healing, say some specialists.

BLADDER CANCER

Signs and Symptoms

- Blood in the urine
- Pain during urination
- Need to urinate frequently
- Appetite or weight loss
- Low-grade fever
- Pain in the pelvic area or lower back

Description

Bladder cancer is frequently mistaken for a bladder infection, because the two conditions share many of the same symptoms. The presence of blood in the urine and painful urination, though, are telltale signs of bladder cancer.

Bladder cancer strikes three times as many men as women and is usually found in people over the age of 40. Approximately 40,000 new cases of bladder cancer are diagnosed yearly in the United States, and more than 15,000 people die from it each year. It is commonly caused by exposure to artificial chemicals and industrial compounds.

Conventional Medical Treatment

If you suspect that you have bladder cancer, visit your physician immediately. Often the diagnosis is suspected because blood is detected during a routine microscopic examination of urine conducted during an annual physical exam. To confirm the diagnosis, your doctor may perform a CAT scan, or a cystoscopic examination, during which a scope is passed through the urethra into the bladder to collect a sample of the bladder lining, which is then tested for malignant cells. If bladder cancer is diagnosed early, surgery alone is usually successful in removing the growth. After surgery, the patient must be tested every 3 to 6 months for recurring masses. Approximately 70 percent of bladder surgery patients develop another small tumor within five years.

If the cancer is not diagnosed early and is allowed to penetrate the bladder wall or surrounding layer of fat, the cancer will probably require surgery followed by radiation therapy or chemotherapy. During radiation therapy, a focused beam of high-energy radiation is used to destroy cancerous cells. Radiation is targeted only at affected areas and is performed regularly for a set

C

➤ If you smoke, quit. Smoking is believed to cause bladder cancer.

➤ Drink only non-chlorinated water or filtered water. Researchers have found that people who drink chlorinated water double their risk of bladder cancer, compared to people who drink water disinfected by other processes.

period of time. During chemotherapy, the patient must take medication (usually intravenously) that is designed to kill cancer cells.

Complementary and Alternative Treatments

Traditional Chinese Medicine

 Acupuncture Traditional Chinese Medicine regards cancer as an energy imbalance caused by any number of factors, including poor diet, lack of exercise, stress, environmental toxins, or overwork.

Acupuncture may be used to improve the flow of energy along the bladder meridian and by targeting specific acupoints, which may offer pain relief. It also can be used to help reduce the negative side effects of radiation or chemotherapy.

Acupressure This modality works on the same principles as acupuncture, and the same meridians can be manipulated to help alleviate pain and promote overall energy balance. Herbs that strengthen the immune system may often be very beneficial.

Chinese Herbal Therapy Studies in Japan have demonstrated that fresh aloe vera juice contains chemicals that slow the growth of cancer cells and impair their ability to spread.

BONE CANCER

Signs and Symptoms

- A lump or hard mass on the surface of a bone
- Pain in the affected area
- Weakening or fractures of the affected bone
- Appetite or weight loss

Description

Cancer rarely originates in the bone; instead, cancer from another area of the body sometimes metastasizes, or spreads, to a bone. For this reason, and because bone cancer is difficult to detect early, people who have had another type of cancer are routinely screened for bone cancer. The only type of bone cancer that actually begins in the bone is osteosarcoma, an uncommon primary bone cancer that has the same symptoms as secondary bone cancer.

Conventional Medical Treatment

If you feel a lump on a bone, or a bone fractures spontaneously, visit your physician immediately. While your doctor may take X-rays to help produce

➤ Breast, prostate, thyroid, lung, and kidney cancer have a propensity to spread to bone. If you have one of these forms of cancer, make sure you are screened for bone cancer.

➤ If you are diagnosed with bone cancer, consult your physician before engaging in weight-bearing exercise.

a diagnosis, a bone biopsy usually is required to confirm the presence of malignant cells. If the cancer is limited to a small area of bone, a surgeon may be able to remove only the cancerous masses. More severe cases, however, often require amputation of all or a portion of a limb. After surgery, chemotherapy or radiation is usually required. (See "Conventional Medical Treatment" in the "Bladder Cancer" entry for more information on radiation and chemotherapy.)

Complementary and Alternative Treatments

Traditional Chinese Medicine

 Acupuncture Bone cancer can be extremely painful; acupuncture can offer much-needed relief by releasing "feel good" endorphins and enhancing relaxation.

Acupressure This therapy can be used to improve the patient's disposition and enhance feelings of well-being as well as to alleviate pain. Care must be taken when applying pressure, so as not to cause discomfort or damage fragile bones.

Chinese Herbal Therapy See "Bladder Cancer" entry above.

BRAIN CANCER

Signs and Symptoms

Brain cancer is usually asymptomatic until the tumor reaches a certain size. At that point, symptoms include:

- Persistent headaches
- Vomiting
- General weakness, or localized weakness in the arms or legs
- Loss of coordination

- Dizziness
- Change in personality
- Loss of mental abilities, including memory
- Double vision, or loss of vision
- Seizures

Description

Brain cancer is a tumor or tumors that form on the brain itself. Most brain tumors have spread to the brain from other affected parts of the body (such as the breast or the lung) via the bloodstream. Only a small percentage of brain cancer cases originate in the brain.

In its early stages, brain cancer often produces no symptoms, or it displays symptoms that are mistaken for everyday headaches. As a result, the

Bad for the Brain?

Researchers have found that electric utility workers exposed to high levels of magnetic radiation are 2.5 times more likely to die from brain cancer than workers exposed to lower levels. However, studies linking electronic radiation to brain cancer are not limited to utility workers. There is growing concern that the electromagnetic radiation emitted by cellular phones—the fastest-growing consumer electronic device in history—can cause brain cancer. In several recent cases of brain cancer, the victims argued that they developed tumors near the place where the telephone antennas pressed against their heads. The victims all reported using their cellular phones for several hours each day. Many scientists, however, dispute this claim. Although high-level electromagnetic waves are known to cause cataracts and bodily tissue damage, the radiation from cellular phones is very weak. Plus, the radiation absorbed by even a heavy cellular phone user is only a fraction of the amount of radiation to which the brain is exposed each day.

condition is often quite advanced before it is detected. Brain cancer is a very serious condition that can cause extensive neurological damage or death.

The exact cause of brain cancer is unknown, but heredity is suspected to play a role in its development.

Conventional Medical Treatment

If you suspect you have a brain tumor, see a physician immediately. A CAT scan or MRI of the head can usually confirm the presence of a tumor and pinpoint its location. If a tumor is found, the physician may take a CAT scan of the chest and abdomen to make sure the cancer has not affected other areas of the body. If the tumor is localized and is situated in an area where removal is possible (on the outer surface of the brain, for example), surgery may be performed. However, some tumors—particularly those located deep within the brain tissue—cannot be operated on. In these cases, radiation and chemotherapy will be used to destroy cancerous cells. (See "Conventional Medical Treatment" in the "Bladder Cancer" entry for more information on radiation and chemotherapy.)

Health Notes

➤ If you or your child have recurrent or severe headaches, consult your physician. Brain cancer is the second most common type of cancer in infants and children and is as common as ovarian cancer in adults.

➤ Choose organic foods, which are grown without pesticides. Studies report that farm workers who are continually exposed to pesticides have a higher incidence of brain cancer than the general population.

Complementary and Alternative Treatments

Traditional Chinese Medicine

 Acupressure By pressing on certain acupressure points along the body's meridians, a practitioner may be able to reduce cancer-related pain and headaches.

Chinese Herbal Therapy Traditional Chinese Medicine considers any type of tumor formation the result of stagnant blood, so a practitioner may recommend formulas that energize blood flow and strengthen the immune system, such as Ginseng and Astragalus Formula. In cases of brain cancer, an herbalist may prescribe the Chinese formula called Three Yellows.

BREAST CANCER

Signs and Symptoms

- A lump or thickening in the breast or the tissue surrounding the breast
- Tenderness in the breast
- Swelling in the armpit area
- Change in the appearance of the breast (one may be higher than the other, or take on a different shape)
- An area of flattening or indentation of the skin of the breast
- Change in color or texture of the breast
- Change in the nipple (nipple may be retracted, dimpled, itchy, or flaking)
- Clear or bloody discharge from the nipple

Description

Current statistics report that one woman in nine will get breast cancer in her lifetime. This does not mean that a 30-year-old woman is at high risk for developing breast cancer at that point in her life, but rather that she has a one-in-nine chance of developing the condition at some point in her life. In actuality, a woman has a 1-in-5900 chance of having breast cancer at age 30, and a risk of 1-in-800 at age 80. Men rarely develop breast cancer.

Heredity plays a large role in determining a woman's risk for breast cancer. People who have three or more close relatives with the condition, and people whose families have breast cancer in more than one generation are at increased risk. People who have relatives with early onset of breast cancer, cancer in both breasts, or ovarian cancer also have an elevated risk of developing breast cancer. Women who have mutations of the BRCA1 or BRCA2 genes have up to an 85 percent chance of developing breast cancer by age 70. This genetic mutation occurs most often in Jewish women of Ashkenazi descent.

Yet, heredity is not the only risk factor for developing breast cancer. A high-fat diet, excessive alcohol intake, obesity, giving birth to a child after the age of 30 or not giving birth at all, an early onset of menstruation, and menopause after age 52 are all thought to increase breast cancer risk. Exposure to environmental toxins are another suspected risk factor. On the other hand, some women develop breast cancer without being in any of the high-risk groups.

Conventional Medical Treatment

If you notice even a slight change in one or both breasts, visit your physician immediately, since breast cancer can spread to the lymph nodes and to other parts of the body. Your doctor physically examines your breasts and takes a mammogram, or breast X-ray. If the mammogram reveals a mass of tissue, or is unclear, your physician may recommend an ultrasound test. This diagnostic test uses sound waves to create an image of interior breast tissue. It is used not only to pinpoint the location of a mass, but to help determine whether the mass is cancerous. In many cases, a needle biopsy is required to confirm diagnosis. There are two types of needle biopsies. During *fine needle aspiration*, a small needle is inserted into the breast lump. If the lump is a cyst and not a tumor,

fluid will drain from it when pierced with the needle. If the lump is a tumor, cells are removed for examination. During a *core needle biopsy*, actual breast tissue cells are removed for examination.

If the tumor is less than 4 centimeters in size, it can be surgically removed with a *lumpectomy* (removal of the lump), followed by radiation. If the tumor is large, *mastectomy* (removal of the breast and underlying tissue) is necessary. After mastectomy, the breast can be reconstructed either at the time of surgery or at a later date. During breast cancer surgery, lymph nodes from the underarm are removed and examined for the presence of cancer cells. Women with positive lymph nodes require follow-up chemotherapy or hormone therapy with tamoxifen. There are several treatment options for breast cancer, depending on the size of the tumor, lymph node involvement, and whether the tumor cells have positive or negative estrogen receptors. Women should discuss the various options with their physicians.

Hormone therapy is another common method of treating breast cancer. The hormone tamoxifen blocks the effects of estrogen on the breast, which in turns stops the growth of cancerous cells. Unfortunately, tamoxifen has been shown to raise the risk of uterine cancer, so women are screened carefully before being given the drug.

The Dangers of Weight Gain

Gradual weight gain may be detrimental to more than just your figure. According to a recent study, women who continue to gain excess weight after puberty and throughout adulthood are at increased risk of developing breast cancer. The study revealed that a 30-year-old woman who is 10 pounds overweight has a 23 percent greater chance of developing breast cancer than a 30-year-old woman who is not overweight. A 30-year-old who is 20 pounds overweight is at 52 percent greater risk than her peers. Fortunately, researchers believe that overweight women in their 30s can decrease their breast cancer risk by shedding excess pounds.

C

Health Notes

➤ *Breast self-exams are crucial to discovering breast cancer in its earliest stages. Perform the test every month, 7 to 10 days after your menstrual period, or on the same day each month. Start by visually examining your breasts in front of a mirror. Inspect your breasts in four positions: arms at side, arms overhead, hands on hips pressing firmly to flex chest muscles, and bending forward. Look for any puckering, dimpling, or patches of discolored skin. Next, raise your left arm and, using the finger pads of your right hand, gently feel the underarm area for any lump, hard knot, or thickening. Move slowly toward the breast, working in a spiral motion from the outer edges of the breast to the nipple. Check the entire breast area, using light, medium, and firm pressure. Gently squeeze the nipple and check for discharge. Repeat on the right underarm and breast using your left hand.*

➤ *Because self-exams cannot detect very small masses, regular mammograms are an important part of breast cancer screening. The American Cancer Society recommends that women have a first, or baseline, mammogram at age 40 and repeat the test every one to two years. After age 50, women should have a mammogram every year.*

➤ *Fruits and vegetables contain antioxidants and phytochemicals, both of which have been shown to help ward off cancer. Soy foods contain genistein, a phytoestrogen that blocks the cancer-stimulating process in the body.*

➤ *Regular physical activity may help reduce your risk of breast cancer. Some research indicates that regular moderate exercise can have a preventive effect on breast cancer.*

For More Information
Y-ME National Breast Cancer Organization
212 West Van Buren Street
Chicago, IL 60607-3908
800-221-2141 English
800-986-9505 Spanish
www.y-me.org

Complementary and Alternative Treatments

Nutrition and Supplementation

 In addition to following the diet and supplement recommendations listed under the general "Cancer" entry, you would benefit from the consumption of flaxseed oil. The essential fatty acids in this oil have a protective effect against breast cancer. Take 1 tablespoon daily. Use it or extra virgin, cold-pressed olive oil on your salad.

Soybeans and soy products contain phytoestrogens that help prevent many forms of cancer. Since they are high in protein, soy products are perfect replacements for meat.

The maitake mushroom kills cancer cells by enhancing the activity of T-helper cells, and studies indicate the mushroom helps control breast cancer. It also minimizes the side effects of chemotherapy.

Traditional Chinese Medicine

 Acupuncture In China, acupuncture has been used to successfully treat breast cancer in its earliest stage. The thinking is that acupuncture unblocks stagnant *chi* pathways, allowing vital nutrients to nourish the area while harmful toxins and damaged cells are whisked away.

In a 1987 Russian study, acupuncture was also shown to lessen radiation-induced nausea and edema in breast cancer patients and to alleviate pain. The same study found that acupuncture improved lymph flow and normalized hemostasis. Another Soviet study followed three women who were confined to their beds with metastatic breast cancer; after undergoing acupuncture treatments, all three patients reported that their pain was gone and their mobility was fully restored.

An Israeli study demonstrated that *moxibustion* (heated cones or sticks made from the Chinese herb, mugwort, which are used to heat certain acupoints) dramatically improved the post-surgery survival rate of mice that had been injected with breast cancer tumors. Only 40 percent of the mice that received post-op moxibustion treatment died after the surgical removal of the tumor, while the mortality rate for the mice receiving only surgery was 70 percent.

Acupoints that may be manipulated to relieve breast pain include Liver 3, Stomach 18 and 36, Small Intestine 1, Gallbladder 41, and Conception Vessel 17.

Acupressure This modality may be used to improve the flow of *chi* in breast cancer patients, manage pain, and remedy treatment-related queasiness.

Chinese Herbal Therapy In a study done at Penn State University, a daily dose of garlic was shown to minimize the incidence of breast cancer in mice injected with the carcinogen. In fact, breast cancer affected 90 percent of the rats fed a normal (non-garlic) diet, while only 35 percent of the mice who ate garlic for 2 weeks before and after the injection contracted the disease.

In addition, since Chinese medicine regards breast cancer as resulting from one of three conditions (sluggish *chi* due to a liver deficiency, dampness due to a malfunctioning spleen, or stagnant toxins throughout the body), various other herbs may be prescribed to counteract any or all of these conditions. There are many Chinese herb formulations that may be used to minimize the side effects of conventional cancer treatment. Always see a practitioner for a diagnosis first.

CERVICAL CANCER

Signs and Symptoms

Cervical cancer in its early stages usually does not produce symptoms. Later, the most common symptoms are:

- Bleeding from the vagina after intercourse, between periods, or after menopause
- Bloody vaginal discharge

Description

Cervical cancer is one of the most common cancers affecting women. Women between the ages of 30 and 55 have the highest incidence of cervical cancer. Women who have had sexually transmitted disease, and those who have had many pregnancies beginning at a young age, are at greater risk. If you smoke, quit. Cigarette smoking is a suspected risk factor for cervical cancer. Getting an annual pelvic examination and Pap test is the only way to screen for cervical cancer. A Pap test can detect malignant cells before symptoms are present.

Fortunately, cervical cancer is slow to develop. If diagnosed at an early stage, when the cancer is still confined to the outermost layers of cervical tissue, cervical cancer has a cure rate of almost 100 percent. Even in more advanced cases, when the cancer spreads deeper into the cervical wall, the chances of recovery are good. On the other hand, if the cancer is allowed to spread to other organs, the prognosis is not as good.

Conventional Medical Treatment

If you notice any type of unexplained bleeding or discharge, see your gynecologist immediately, who performs a pelvic examination and Pap smear. If the Pap smear reveals abnormalities, your doctor examines your cervix closely (using a

Health Notes

➤ *Women should have their first Pap test when they become sexually active or at age 18, and the test should be performed annually thereafter.*

➤ *Sexually transmitted diseases (STDs) are the most common cause of cervical cancer. To reduce your risk of developing STDs and cervical cancer, always use condoms.*

➤ *If you smoke, quit. Cigarette smoking is a suspected risk factor for cervical cancer.*

device called a colposcope) and takes a tissue sample to check for malignant cells. If cancer is confirmed, your doctor may take X-rays to determine if the cancer has spread to any of the surrounding organs.

Treatment for cervical cancer depends on what stage it is in. If it is caught early, laser surgery, freezing, or cauterization may be used to remove the malignant cells from the outer layer of tissue. If the cancer has advanced into the cervical wall, radiation may be performed. (See "Conventional Medical Treatment" in the "Bladder Cancer" entry for more information on radiation therapy.) Your doctor also may recommend a hysterectomy, an operation in which the cervix and uterus are removed.

Complementary and Alternative Treatments

Traditional Chinese Medicine

 Acupuncture Acupuncture may be used as an adjunct treatment during the early stages of cervical cancer to boost the body's immune system and improve the flow of *chi* to diseased cells.

Acupressure Acupressure may be useful in alleviating the pain of cervical cancer and the

stomach upset caused by conventional treatments.

Chinese Herbal Therapy Garlic has been shown to inhibit the growth of cancer cell while promoting the production of healthy cells, which may account for this herb's popularity in the prevention and treatment of all types of cancer, including cervical. Ginseng also is known for its immunity-boosting, anti-cancer properties.

COLORECTAL CANCER

Signs and Symptoms

In its early stages, colorectal cancer often produces no symptoms. When it reaches later stages, the most common symptoms are:

- Change in bowel movements, including diarrhea, constipation, or change in shape of stools
- Rectal bleeding
- Blood in or on stool
- Abdominal cramps or pain
- Nausea and vomiting
- Appetite and weight loss
- Fatigue

Description

Colorectal cancer isn't always accompanied by noticeable symptoms, and its symptoms are frequently mistaken for hemorrhoids. Colorectal cancer is a highly curable type of cancer, but— primarily because of its lack of symptoms—it accounts for approximately 20 percent of malignant disease deaths in this country. It also can easily spread to surrounding tissues and organs.

One of the most significant risk factors for colorectal cancer is a history of digestive disorders, specifically polyps (small tumors on the inner lining of the colon) and ulcerative colitis. A diet high

Six Tests to Detect Colon Cancer

Colorectal cancer is the third leading cause of cancer deaths in the United States and Canada (for men, it ranks behind lung and prostate cancer, and for women, it ranks behind lung and breast cancer). There are six tests to help identify colon cancer. Preparation for each test may involve special diets, laxatives, or enemas.

- *The occult blood test.* This home test is used to detect tiny amounts of occult (hidden) blood in the stool, often caused by premalignant polyps or early tumors. Several days prior to the test, you must abstain from aspirin and ibuprofen, vitamin C, iron supplements, and red meat. A small card is used to collect minute stool smears for several days before it is mailed to a designated lab. If occult blood is detected, further testing is done.

- *The gloved finger/digital rectal exam.* Most physicians perform this exam as part of a routine physical, but only a small percentage of colorectal tumors can be detected by a digital exam.

- *Sigmoidoscopy.* During this test, the lower portion of the colon and rectum are examined with a flexible, lighted tube that allows the physician to view the inside of the bowel. Approximately 40 to 50 percent of colorectal cancers can be detected by sigmoidoscopy. The procedure can be used to detect both cancers and polyps, and polyps can be removed during a sigmoidoscopy.

- *X-rays with barium enema.* This test is performed on patients at high risk or with a positive occult blood test. An enema is used to cleanse the bowel and coat the inside of the colon, which is then inflated with air and examined with X-rays, which can help detect polyps. Preparation for this test and the exam itself are uncomfortable but not painful.

- *Colonoscopy.* This test is usually performed by an endoscopist at a hospital. The patient may have to take laxatives and/or enemas, as well as a mild sedative, in preparation for a colonoscopy. A flexible scope fitted with a monitor is maneuvered through the colon. Like a sigmoidoscopy, this procedure can detect both cancers and polyps, and polyps can be removed during the process. A colonoscopy can take up to 30 minutes.

- *Genetic screening.* Three major genes for colon cancer can be identified through blood tests. Genetic screening is still in its infancy. Even if you have the colon cancer gene, it's not a guarantee that you will get the disease.

in animal products (including meat, poultry, eggs, and dairy products) is another risk factor. Colorectal cancer risk increases significantly after age 40.

Conventional Medical Treatment

If you notice any symptoms of colorectal cancer, see your physician immediately. Your doctor will probably examine your rectum with a gloved hand, check a stool sample for the presence of blood, and take a blood test. A barium X-ray, CAT scan, colonoscopy, or sigmoidoscopy also may be required to confirm the presence of a tumor.

Surgery to remove the diseased portion of rectum or colon is the most common treatment for colorectal cancer. If the tumor has spread outside the colon, chemotherapy is typically administered following surgery to decrease the chance of recurrence. If the cancer is too widespread for surgery, chemotherapy alone may be prescribed. (See "Conventional Medical Treatment" in the "Bladder Cancer" entry for more information on chemotherapy.)

C

Health Notes

➤ *Studies have found that people who take aspirin at least every other day have lower rates of colorectal cancer.*

➤ *People who consume a low-fat, high-fiber diet have been found to have lower rates of colorectal cancer. Dietary fat—especially saturated fat—is a chief contributor to colorectal cancer. Fiber, on the other hand, helps to rid the body of waste materials faster, increases bulk, and decreases the concentration of carcinogens in the intestine.*

➤ *Obesity is a risk factor for colorectal cancer. If you are overweight, speak to your doctor about a sensible weight-reduction plan.*

➤ *Daily moderate exercise is believed to help prevent colorectal cancer by boosting the metabolism, which in turns helps the body speed waste through the digestive tract.*

Complementary and Alternative Treatments

Nutrition and Supplementation

 In addition to following the nutrition and supplementation recommendations listed under the general "Cancer" entry, you would be wise to include 30 grams of fiber daily in your diet. Fiber facilitates the transit of food through your body. Obtain fiber from fruits, vegetables, and whole grains. At first you may notice an increase in gas, but that problem will clear up quickly. Cabbage juice helps prevent colorectal cancer. Be sure to add a teaspoon of vitamin C to your juice.

Traditional Chinese Medicine

 Acupuncture Obesity increases one's risk for getting colon and rectal cancer; acupuncture can be used to correct overeating and help maintain weight loss.

Acupressure Acupressure can be used to promote blood circulation and improve the flow of energy throughout the body. Pressing on Pericardium 6 (located on the inner forearm about 2 inches above the wrist) can help quell queasiness and vomiting caused by conventional medical treatments.

Acupressure also can be used to help control diarrhea or constipation, which may be especially uncomfortable for an individual with colon or rectal cancer.

Chinese Herbal Therapy The American Cancer Society conducted a study of astragalus and found that the herb repaired immune system functioning in 90 percent of the cancer patients involved in the study. Other research has shown that individuals who take astragalus during chemotherapy recuperate faster and live longer than those who don't.

KIDNEY CANCER

Signs and Symptoms

- Bloody or cloudy urine
- Pain in the lower abdomen or back
- Lump or mass in the lower back
- Appetite and weight loss
- Fever
- Fatigue

Description

There are several types of cancer that can affect the kidney. Renal cell carcinoma, the most common type of kidney cancer, affects the outer layer of kidney tissue. It occurs twice as often in men as in women and most commonly affects smokers between the ages of 55 and 60. Transitional cell carcinoma, a less common type of kidney cancer, affects mostly middle-aged women and is associated with the abuse of analgesic drugs, such as phenacetin. Wilms' tumor, the most common form of kidney cancer in children, usually afflicts children under the age of 7, but has a very high cure rate.

Since kidney cancer is often mistaken for a bladder infection, many people don't seek treatment until the condition is advanced. However, if it is diagnosed and treated before the cancer spreads to surrounding tissues, the recovery rate is high.

Conventional Medical Treatment

If you notice any symptoms of kidney cancer, see your physician immediately. Kidney cancer is usually diagnosed with an X-ray, CAT scan, or ultrasound examination of the abdomen. If these tests reveal any abnormalities, your doctor may take a biopsy of kidney tissue to test for malignant cells.

Treatment for kidney cancer depends on the extent of the cancer. If only a small area is affected, the mass itself may be surgically removed. If the tumor is large, the affected kidney, as well as the surrounding tissue and nearby lymph nodes, may be removed. Surgery is usually followed up with radiation or chemotherapy. (See "Conventional Medical Treatment" in the "Bladder Cancer" entry for more information on radiation and chemotherapy.)

Health Note

➤ *If you smoke, quit. Cigarette smoking is a serious risk factor for kidney cancer.*

Complementary and Alternative Treatments

Traditional Chinese Medicine

Acupuncture Acupuncture can be used to restore energy levels within the kidney meridians as well as ease pain caused by kidney cancer. Auricular points typically targeted to relieve kidney problems are the kidney, bladder, liver, heart, and sympathy areas.

Acupressure This form of deep tissue massage can be used to strengthen the immune system by opening blocked pathways along the kidney meridians, which should increase the individual's energy level and improve disposition.

Chinese Herbal Therapy *Fu Zheng* therapy is often used alongside conventional treatment methods in the fight against cancer, because it bolsters the immune system, and helps protect the body from the damaging effects of radiation and chemotherapy. Individuals who use *Fu Zheng*—an herbal regimen made up of atractylodes, ligustrum, codonopsis, ginseng, ganoderma, and astragalus, among others—have an increased survival rate, due to the therapy's ability to increase T-cell functioning.

Depending upon the specific cause of an individual's kidney cancer, an herbalist may also advocate the use of such kidney tonic formulas as Rehmannia Six, Panax Ginseng Capsules, Cerebral Tonic Pills, and Eight Immortal Long Life Pills. Because certain herbs can actually impair kidney function, they should always be prescribed by a trained professional acupuncturist.

LEUKEMIA

Signs and Symptoms

In its early stages, leukemia often produces no symptoms. When it reaches later stages, the most common symptoms are:

- Anemia (symptoms include fatigue and pallor)
- Increased susceptibility to illness and infections
- Bruising or bleeding easily
- Swollen lymph nodes
- Appetite and weight loss
- Headaches
- Pressure under the lower left ribs from enlargement of the spleen

Description

Leukemia is cancer of the blood. The condition is characterized an overabundance of abnormal white blood cells that are unable to perform their primary function—fight disease. These abnormal cells reach extremely high levels in the bone marrow (where blood cells are formed), lymphatic system, and blood stream. The excess white blood cells interfere with the functions of vital organs, eventually preventing the body from creating healthy platelets and red and white blood cells. The consequences of this lack of healthy cells are many: without healthy white blood cells, the body is unable to fight off infections; without platelets, blood does not clot properly; and without red blood cells, the necessary amount of oxygen is not carried to the body's organs.

Although leukemia is the most common form of childhood cancer, it also affects adults. The condition does occur more often in men than women. Risk factors for leukemia include a family history of leukemia, smoking, and prolonged contact with industrial carcinogens.

Conventional Medical Treatment

If you notice any symptoms of leukemia, see your physician immediately. To diagnose the condition, your physician performs a blood count to determine the levels of white blood cells. If leukemia is suspected, a bone marrow biopsy may be necessary.

Health Notes

➤ People who have had radiation therapy for a previous cancer are at increased risk of developing leukemia.

➤ According to a recent study, women who have between 1 and 20 alcoholic drinks over the course of their pregnancies are twice as likely to have infants with leukemia.

➤ Smoking raises your chances of developing leukemia by as much as 30 percent. If you smoke, quit.

Treatment depends on the severity of the condition. In many cases, chemotherapy or radiation therapy can cause the leukemia to go into remission, causing blood cell levels to return to normal. (See "Conventional Medical Treatment" in the "Bladder Cancer" entry for more information on radiation and chemotherapy.) If the patient has extremely low levels of healthy cells, blood transfusion is sometimes necessary. Very serious cases of leukemia often require bone marrow transplants, during which diseased bone marrow is removed and replaced by healthy donor bone marrow. A combination of chemotherapeutic drugs may also be administered.

For More Information
Leukemia Society of America
600 Third Avenue
New York, NY 10016
800-955-4LSA
www.leukemia.org

Complementary and Alternative Treatments

Traditional Chinese Medicine

 Acupuncture There is some controversy about using acupuncture on people with leukemia, because it does improve blood flow and increase the number of white blood cells produced, which may actually spread the disease (which is characterized by an overabundance of white blood cells). Therefore, leukemia patients would be wise to consult their healthcare provider before undergoing acupuncture.

LIVER CANCER

Signs and Symptoms

In its early stages, liver cancer often produces no symptoms. When it reaches later stages, the most common symptoms are:

- Pain or bloating in the upper right abdominal area
- Jaundice (yellowing of the skin and eyes)
- Itching
- Appetite and weight loss
- Nausea and vomiting
- General fatigue and weakness

Description

Liver cancer is the second most common form of metastasized cancer—cancer that has spread from another affected organ. In fact, only 1 to 2 percent of all cases of liver cancer originate in the liver. When cancer does begin in the liver, it is usually caused by cirrhosis, a hepatitis B infection, or exposure to certain environmental toxins and industrial compounds. Liver cancer occurs in men twice as often as it does in women, and is usually found in people over the age of 50. Alcoholics have a very high risk for developing liver cancer.

Since many people with liver cancer do not have any noticeable symptoms, usually it is not diagnosed until it is very advanced. Liver cancer is a very dangerous condition that is usually fatal; the majority of patients live for less than a year after being diagnosed with liver cancer.

Electrochemical Tumor Treatment

Electrochemical treatment (ECT) is a medical treatment for cancer that is used in more than 500 Chinese hospitals. ECT involves inserting platinum anodes into the center of a cancerous mass and platinum cathodes around the tumor. A direct electrical current is maintained between the anodes and cathodes for anywhere from 30 minutes to several hours. This treatment is most often used to treat cancer of the liver, lungs, skin, and breast. According to Chinese studies, ECT is as effective as radiation and chemotherapy in treating superficial tumors, and it is more effective than these traditional therapies in treating deep tumors.

Conventional Medical Treatment

If you notice even subtle abnormalities in your health, including any of the symptoms of liver cancer, see your physician immediately. To diag-

Health Notes

➤ *If you have been treated for hepatitis B or C, talk to your physician about the risks of developing liver cancer.*

➤ *People with hemochromatosis—a disease that causes the body to hoard iron—are at a higher risk for developing liver cancer. Excess iron can build up to toxic levels in the liver.*

➤ *Research has found that copper—a mineral found in seafood, organ meats, and green vegetables—may inhibit the growth of liver cancer. Copper helps the body use iron efficiently and is believed to support the body's immune function.*

nose liver cancer, your doctor performs a thorough physical examination, takes blood tests, and may order a CAT scan or ultrasound examination. To confirm a diagnosis, a liver biopsy also may be necessary.

Most cases of liver cancer are inoperable. In some cases where the cancer is detected early, chemotherapy or radiation can reduce the size of the tumor to an operable size. After surgery, chemotherapy and radiation are used to kill cancer cells. In advanced cases, when surgery is not an option, chemotherapy or radiation can keep the cancer from spreading to other tissues. (See the "Conventional Medical Treatment" in the "Bladder Cancer" entry for more information on radiation and chemotherapy.) Advanced cases of liver cancers are rarely cured.

Complementary and Alternative Treatments

Traditional Chinese Medicine

 Acupuncture This modality may be used to improve energy flow in the liver meridian and carry toxins out of this diseased organ.

Acupuncture Acupoints that may be stimulated in the treatment of liver cancer are Liver 14 and Conception Vessel 12 on the chest, Liver 3 on the top of the foot, and related points in the ear.

Chinese Herbal Therapy Several studies have shown that a Panax ginseng extract seems to not only inhibit the growth of liver cancer cells, but to stimulate protein synthesis in these cells, causing them to revert to their healthy, pre-cancerous state.

In a U.S. study, 46 people with Stage II primary liver cancer were given *Fu Zheng* herbal therapy along with chemotherapy or radiation. Twenty-nine of the subjects survived for one year and ten survived for three years.

There is also an extract of soy that is used for cancer therapy.

Lung Cancer

Signs and Symptoms

In its early stages, lung cancer often produces no symptoms. When it reaches later stages, the most common symptoms are:

- Chronic, hacking cough that may bring up phlegm
- Blood-streaked phlegm
- Chronic respiratory infections
- Shortness of breath or wheezing
- Chest pain
- Hoarseness
- Appetite and weight loss
- Fatigue and muscle weakness

Description

Lung cancer is the leading cause of cancer death in the United States in both men and women. Approximately 175,000 new cases are diagnosed each year. It most commonly strikes people between the ages of 45 and 70 who are smokers or ex-smokers. People who are regularly exposed to radon or industrial carcinogens are also at increased risk. Approximately twice as many men get lung cancer as women.

Lung cancer usually originates in the lung tissue or bronchial tubes, but in some cases it spreads to the lungs from the breast, colon, prostate, kidney, thyroid, or other organ. Lung cancer can also easily spread from the lungs to surrounding organs.

Lung cancer treatment does not have an extremely high cure rate. That's why prevention is key. Don't start smoking, and if you still smoke, make every effort to quit.

Conventional Medical Treatments

Between 5 and 10 percent of lung cancers are discovered during routine chest X-rays for other illnesses, such as chronic bronchitis or pneumonia. Sputum (phlegm) examinations also frequently uncover cancer cells. Lung cancer is often asymptomatic in its early stages, so if you are a smoker or ex-smoker, your physician may suggest yearly chest X-rays. A CAT scan may be taken to check for very small lesions and to help determine whether the cancer has spread to other sites. Your physician also may want to perform a bronchoscopy to view air passages or take a biopsy of lung tissue.

If the cancer is localized, your physician may recommend lung resection, an operation to remove only the damaged portion of the lung. Chemotherapy and/or radiation are the most common avenues of treatment for people who have many cancerous growths on their lungs. (See "Conventional Medical Treatment" in the "Bladder Cancer" entry for more information on radiation and chemotherapy.)

Health Notes

➤ *If you smoke, quit immediately. Though not all cases of lung cancer are caused by smoking, smokers have by far the highest incidence of lung cancer. Also avoid exposure to secondhand smoke. Non-smoking spouses of smokers have a 30 to 80 percent higher risk of developing lung cancer than people who are not frequently exposed to cigarette smoke.*

➤ *Fruits and vegetables contain antioxidants, substances that help neutralize the cancer-causing free radicals that are created by cigarette smoke. Try to eat four servings of fruit and five servings of vegetables each day.*

➤ *Consume 140 mg or more of vitamin C daily. Studies have shown that people who get less than 90 mg of vitamin C a day had a 90 percent higher risk of developing lung cancer than those who get 140 mg or more.*

➤ *People who ingest 55 to 200 mcg of selenium daily have a 46 percent lower rate of lung cancer than the general population. Selenium is an antioxidant found in whole grains, asparagus, garlic, eggs, and mushrooms. Studies have also found that rates for all types of cancer are 10 percent higher in areas with selenium-poor soil.*

Complementary and Alternative Treatments

Nutrition and Supplementation

In addition to following the nutritional and supplement recommendations listed under the general Cancer entry, try eating shiitake or maitake mushrooms or take a maitake supplement. These mushrooms kill cancer cells and are particularly effective in controlling lung cancer. They also minimize the side effects of chemotherapy.

Recent research shows that taking N-acetyl cysteine and glutathione supplements can be helpful.

Traditional Chinese Medicine

Acupuncture In addition to studying the efficacy of electroacupuncture as a tool in diagnosing lung cancer, as has been done at the University of California at Los Angeles and the University of Southern California, therapists also use acupuncture—with and without electrical stimulation—to treat the cough, shortness of breath, and chest discomfort often symptomatic with lung cancer.

Acupressure To quiet a cancer-related cough, have a practitioner work on the following acupressure body points: Lung 1, 5, 7, and 9; Conception Vessel 17 and 22; Stomach 36; Spleen 6, and Kidney 6.

Chinese Herbal Therapy Chinese herbs have long been used to combat lung cancer. Herbal remedies might include dandelion, Job's tears, achyranthes, bletilla, ophiopogon, and Japanese honeysuckle. Yet, perhaps the most famous liver cancer curative is pseudoginseng, which quells the internal bleeding often associated with lung cancer.

Many other herbs have been tested. A long-term study conducted by the Beijing Institute for Cancer Research found that 91.5 percent of the small-cell lung cancer patients who were given the traditional Chinese kidney tonics Six Flavor Tea or Golden Book Tea as an adjunct to radiation and chemotherapy experienced substantial tumor shrinkage, as opposed to 46.9 percent who used the conventional therapy alone. A large number of the patients who drank Chinese medicinal tea also lived considerably longer than their chemo-only counterparts.

LYMPHOMA

Signs and Symptoms

- Painless swelling of lymph nodes
- Itching all over the body
- Chronic or intermittent fever and chills
- Fatigue and weakness
- Appetite and weight loss
- Coughing and shortness of breath

Description

Lymphoma is a term for cancers of the lymphatic system, which includes the spleen, the lymph nodes, and lymphatic vessels. Hodgkin's disease is a type of lymphoma that typically affects young

men under the age of 30. All other types of lymphatic cancers are grouped under the term non-Hodgkin's lymphoma. The types of non-Hodgkin's lymphoma vary from non-aggressive (those that remain in the lymphatic system) to aggressive (those that spread, either quickly or slowly, to other organs of the body). Non-Hodgkin's lymphoma usually affects men over the age of 40.

When detected early, Hodgkin's disease is easily treated and has a high cure rate. In fact, close to 90 percent of all cases are cured. Non-Hodgkin's lymphoma, while not as easy to cure, is often successfully treated.

The exact cause of lymphoma is unknown, though the disease is suspected to have a hereditary component.

Conventional Medical Treatment

If you suspect you have lymphoma, see your physician immediately. To diagnose the condition, your doctor gives you a thorough physical examination, as well as blood and urine tests. If lymphoma is suspected, your doctor may perform a chest X-ray or tomography scan of your abdo-

Health Notes

➤ Occupational exposure to solvents, phenoxy herbicides, and metal fumes increases your risk of developing lymphoma.

➤ Ultraviolet rays are now considered a risk factor for non-Hodgkin's lymphoma. Always wear a sunscreen of SPF 15 or greater when outdoors, and avoid exposure to sunlight when the sun is at its strongest, between 11 a.m. and 3 p.m.

➤ People with celiac disease have higher rates of lymphoma. If you have celiac disease, talk to your physician about the risk of developing lymphoma.

men. A lymph node biopsy or bone marrow biopsy may be used to confirm diagnosis.

Radiation is the most common avenue of treatment for Hodgkin's disease; if the cancer is widespread, chemotherapy is often used. In cases of non-Hodgkin's lymphoma, chemotherapy is the preferred treatment, but radiation is sometimes used. Surgery is rarely used as a treatment option for lymphoma. (See "Conventional Medical Treatment" in the "Bladder Cancer" entry for more information on radiation and chemotherapy.)

Complementary and Alternative Treatments

Traditional Chinese Medicine

Acupuncture Acupuncture can be very effective in clearing toxins from the lymphatic system and in helping manage lymphoma-related pain and/or treatment-related nausea.

Acupressure This form of massage can be useful in draining toxic lymph nodes and improving the flow of *chi* throughout the entire lympathic system.

Chinese Herbal Therapy Herbs can be used as tonics to repair damage that chemotherapy and radiation may inflict on the body's immune system. Popular immunity-fortifying herbs include formulas such as Rehmannia Six and Cerebral Tonic Pills, along with added angelica, astragalus, Chinese yam, codonopsis, cordyceps, ginseng, and gotu kola.

ORAL CANCER

Signs and Symptoms

- Small white or red lump or thickened patch of skin in the mouth—usually located on the side or bottom of the tongue, on the floor of the mouth, inside the cheeks, on the gums, on the roof of the mouth, or on the palate

- A sore in the mouth that does not heal
- Pain while eating or drinking

Description

Oral cancer is cancer of the mouth or upper part of the throat. It is a common form of cancer among people who drink excessively and among people who use tobacco products—cigars, cigarettes, snuff, and chewing tobacco. Industrial carcinogens also are believed to contribute to oral cancer.

An oral tumor begins as a small, painless lump in the mouth. As the cancer progresses, the lump becomes red and painful; at this stage the tumor is easily mistaken for a canker sore. It may also grow in size. People with the condition may also have difficulty swallowing or notice that small wounds in the mouth will not heal. If left unchecked, the cancer may spread to the nearby lymph nodes in the neck.

When detected at an early stage, oral cancer is highly curable. However, since the lump rarely causes discomfort, and because it may be the only symptom, oral cancer is often allowed to progress untreated. In fact, an estimated 25 percent of people with oral cancer die because of delayed detection and treatment.

Conventional Medical Treatment

If you notice an abnormal growth in your mouth, or experience any of the symptoms of oral cancer, see your dentist or physician immediately. Either can take a tissue sample from the tumor to examine for cancerous cells. If the tumor is small and the cancer has not spread to other tissues, surgery alone is usually successful in removing the cancer. Surgical options include laser surgery and cryosurgery (freezing the tumor with liquid nitrogen). If the tumor is large or if the cancer has spread to the lymph nodes, a combination of surgery and radiation or chemotherapy may be required. (See "Conventional Medical Treatment" in the "Bladder Cancer" entry for more information on radiation and chemotherapy.) If a signifi-

➤ *A diet that contains four or more servings of fruit a day can reduce oral cancer rates by 20 to 80 percent. Studies have shown that the antioxidants beta-carotene and vitamin E can help eliminate precancerous oral lesions.*

➤ *If you smoke, quit. Cigarette and cigar smoking are among the highest risk factors for oral cancers.*

➤ *If you drink, imbibe sensibly. Drinking two or more alcoholic beverages per day significantly increases your odds of developing oral cancer.*

cant amount of tissue is removed from the mouth, reconstructive surgery may be necessary.

Complementary and Alternative Treatments

Traditional Chinese Medicine

 Acupuncture Acupuncture can be used to block energy pathways and stimulate the release of endorphins, both of which can help alleviate any pain caused by oral cancer.

Acupressure To relieve the stomach upset caused by radiation or chemotherapy, an acupressure technician may apply a firm touch to Pericardium 6 (on the inside of the forearm).

Chinese Herbal Therapy Aloe has been shown to reduce the spread of cancerous tumors and have a protective effect on the skin during radiation treatments. A common Chinese herbal formula prescribed to cancer patients is Three Yellows, while single herbs that may be added to treat mouth cancer include akebia, balloon flower, and Chinese black cohosh.

OVARIAN CANCER

Signs and Symptoms

In its early stages, ovarian cancer rarely produces symptoms. When it reaches later stages, the most common symptoms are:

- Mild pain or swelling in the abdomen or lower back
- Mild indigestion, diarrhea, or constipation
- Pain during intercourse
- Bleeding from the vagina between periods or after menopause

Description

Ovarian cancer is the fifth leading cause of cancer death in women, resulting in approximately 12,000 deaths each year. More women die of ovarian cancer than any other cancer of the reproductive system. Ovarian cancer is virtually asymptomatic during its early stages, so by the time it produces any noticeable symptoms, the cancer is usually well established. On the other hand, when the disease is caught early, the survival rate is good.

The majority of women with ovarian cancer have already gone through menopause. Women with a family history of ovarian, breast, or uterine cancer are at increased risk. Women with late menopause and women who were never pregnant are also at increased risk.

Conventional Medical Treatment

A pelvic examination can reveal a growth on the ovary. In fact, when ovarian cancer is caught early, it is usually detected during a routine pelvic examination. Additional tests may be required to confirm diagnosis and determine the extent of the cancer. Either a *laparoscopy* (during which a surgeon makes a small incision in your abdomen to look directly at the ovaries) or a *biopsy* (during

Health Notes

➤ A diet high in animal fat puts women at increased risk for ovarian cancer.

➤ Selenium is believed to help protect the body from ovarian cancer. Selenium is an antioxidant found in whole grains, asparagus, garlic, eggs, and mushrooms.

➤ Feminine powders and other hygiene products that contain talc put women at greater risk for developing ovarian cancer.

➤ Taking the oral contraceptive pill reduces a woman's lifetime risk for developing ovarian cancer by as much as 50 percent, and this effectiveness increases with duration of use.

the Stomach points on the calf, the Bladder points near the spine, and the Conception Vessel point on the stomach. Additional auricular points may also be targeted during a session, depending upon the individual's specific symptoms.

Acupressure This modality can be helpful in alleviating the abdominal pain associated with ovarian cancer. The practitioner manipulates points related to Stomach 36 (near the knee), Spleen 6 (near the ankle), and Conception Vessel 6 and 12 (on the torso).

Chinese Herbal Therapy Studies in Japan and China indicate that licorice—long renowned for its immunity-enhancing properties—may also be useful in inhibiting the growth of tumors, as it has been found to stimulate the body's production of interferon. See also other "Cancer" entries above.

which a tissue sample is taken from the ovaries) can confirm the presence of cancer. Ultrasonography or a CAT scan of the abdomen, kidneys, and uterus can determine if the cancer has spread to other tissues.

Treatment for ovarian cancer depends on how developed the cancer is, though surgery is always required. If the cancer is detected early, the diseased ovary is typically removed. In more advanced cases, the ovaries, fallopian tubes, uterus, and nearby lymph glands may be removed. To eliminate any remaining cancer cells after surgery, radiation or chemotherapy is usually prescribed. (See "Conventional Medical Treatment" in the "Bladder Cancer" entry for more information on radiation and chemotherapy.)

Complementary and Alternative Treatments

Traditional Chinese Medicine

 Acupuncture More than eight acupoints may be stimulated in the treatment of the abdominal pain and bloating that often accompany ovarian cancer, including

---

PANCREATIC CANCER

Signs and Symptoms

In its early stages, pancreatic cancer often produces no symptoms. When it reaches later stages, the most common symptoms are:

- Abdominal pain that may radiate to the back
- Appetite and weight loss
- Nausea and vomiting
- Change in bowel movements, including constipation and diarrhea
- Jaundice (yellowing of the skin and eyes)
- Blood in the stool (indicative of intestinal bleeding)

Description

Approximately 28,000 new cases of pancreatic cancer are diagnosed each year. Since symptoms are rare during the early stages, pancreatic cancer is usually not diagnosed until it has reached advanced stages. In fact, pancreatic cancer is ranked behind only lung cancer, colorectal cancer, and breast cancer as the most common causes of cancer death. Weight loss is one of the most pronounced symptoms of pancreatic cancer—most people who have the disease lose 25 pounds or more once the cancer has become established.

Smoking is the primary risk factor for pancreatic cancer. People who have had diabetes or are over the age of 60 are also at increased risk, as are people who consume high-fat diets or are exposed to industrial carcinogens. The disease strikes men more often than women, and men of African-American or native-Hawaiian decent are especially susceptible.

Conventional Medical Treatment

If you have any of the symptoms of pancreatic cancer, see your physician, who feels your abdomen for signs of tenderness or swelling. If pancreatic cancer is suspected, your doctor may take an ultrasound, CAT scan, or X-ray. A biopsy of pancreatic tissue may be necessary to confirm diagnosis.

Treatment for the condition depends on the extent of the cancer. If the tumor is small and limited to the tissues of the pancreas, the mass alone can be surgically removed. If the cancer has spread to the intestine, your physician may need to remove a portion of the affected intestine as well. Follow-up for either of these surgeries usually includes chemotherapy or radiation. If the cancer has spread extensively to surrounding tissues or nearby organs, chemotherapy may be the only option. (See "Conventional Medical Treatment" in "Bladder Cancer" entry for more information on radiation and chemotherapy.)

Complementary and Alternative Treatments

Traditional Chinese Medicine

 Acupuncture An acupuncturist may be able to help lessen the abdominal and back pain caused by pancreatic cancer. Up to 10 body points may be stimulated during the session, including those associated with the bladder, small intestine, and governing vessel.

Acupressure Acupoints that may be pressed in an attempt to alleviate back pain are Bladder 60, Kidney 3 and 6, and Conception Vessel 6. If the pain is concentrated in and around the abdomen, acupoints on the torso will probably be added.

Chinese Herbal Therapy Immune-strengthening herbs may be used to improve the body's abilities to fight pancreatic cancer, including garlic, astragalus, aloe vera, and morinda root. Additional herbs may be prescribed to combat abdominal discomfort and other cancer-related symptoms.

There is also an extract of soy that is used for cancer therapy.

Health Notes

➤ Eat a low-fat, high-fiber diet. High fat intake—especially of saturated fat—has been shown to increase the risk of pancreatic cancer.

➤ If you smoke, quit. According to one study, an individual's risk for developing pancreatic cancer decreases by 48 percent within two years of giving up cigarettes.

PROSTATE CANCER

Signs and Symptoms

In its early stages, prostate cancer often produces no symptoms. When it reaches later stages, the most common symptoms are:

- Increased frequency of urination
- Difficulty beginning or ending urination
- Pain during urination or ejaculation
- Weakened urine stream
- Blood in urine or semen
- Hip or lower back pain
- Appetite and weight loss

Description

Prostate cancer is a common affliction of men over the age of 50, yet few men affected even know they have it. In its early stages, the disease usually has no symptoms, making early detection difficult. When symptoms do appear, they are sometimes ignored as symptoms of beginning prostate enlargement, a common, non-threatening condition that affects middle-aged men. Prostate cancer also eludes detection because it develops slowly. Unfortunately, if left untreated, prostate cancer can result in death. In fact, it is the third most common cause of cancer death and the second most common cause of cancer death among men.

Elderly men are, of course, at greatest risk; less than 1 percent of all cases are in men under 50. Men with a family history of prostate cancer are also at increased risk. Other risk factors include a history of sexually transmitted disease, regular exposure to industrial carcinogens, and a high-fat diet.

Conventional Medical Treatment

If you have any symptoms of prostate cancer, see your physician, who may perform a rectal examination to check for signs of the condition. If the prostate feels enlarged, the doctor may want to conduct further tests—X-ray, blood test, urine

Health Notes

➤ *Beans, lentils, peas, and dried fruits contain hormone-like compounds called isoflavonoids, which some researchers believe may protect against prostate cancer by enhancing natural estrogen activity.*

➤ *Eat a low-fat, high-fiber diet. Research has found a connection between a high-fat diets and prostate cancer.*

➤ *Men over the age of 40 should have yearly rectal examinations to screen for prostate cancer.*

➤ *Some medical organizations, such as the American Cancer Society, recommend annual prostate specific antigen (PSA) blood tests to screen for prostate cancer. The test is not universally recommended, however, because it is not always a reliable indicator; other disorders of the prostate can also cause PSA levels to rise.*

analysis, or prostatic ultrasound. A biopsy of prostate tissue also may be required to confirm diagnosis.

Treatment for prostate cancer depends on the extent of the disease. If the cancer is small and limited to the prostate gland, the tumor itself may be surgically removed. If the cancer has spread throughout the prostate, the entire gland may have to be removed. In either case, follow-up radiation is usually given. If the cancer has spread to other tissues, your physician may administer a combination of chemotherapy and radiation. In some cases, an *orchidectomy*—removal of the testicles—is necessary to eliminate the male hormones that promote the growth of prostate cancer. The drugs leuprolide and flutamide may also be administered to further suppress male hormones. (See "Conventional Medical Treatment" in "Bladder Cancer" entry for more information on radiation and chemotherapy.)

Complementary and Alternative Treatments

Nutrition and Supplementation

In addition to following the nutrition and supplementation recommendations listed under the general "Cancer" entry, you should consume foods high in zinc (50 to 100 milligrams). Zinc nourishes the prostate gland and can be found in foods, such as mushrooms, pumpkin seeds, seafood, sunflower seeds, and whole grains. Eat cultured products, such as yogurt, in moderation. Eliminate red meat from your diet; there is a direct correlation between the consumption of red meat and prostate cancer.

Traditional Chinese Medicine

Acupuncture In the case of prostate cancer, acupuncture may be used to help improve energy flow to the prostate gland in an attempt to lessen swelling and make urination easier.

Acupressure Acupressure should *never* be performed directly on the prostate gland in individuals with prostate cancer, as it may disturb the tumor and cause the disease to spread. However, it is perfectly fine to use acupressure on non-related sites (including Pericardium 6 and various auricular points) to counteract nausea caused by conventional treatments.

Chinese Herbal Therapy *Fu Zheng* (a Chinese herbal therapy that includes ganoderma, atractylodes, ginseng, astragalus, ligustrum, and codonopsis) has proven effective in bolstering an immune system weakened by prostate cancer. In fact, the purpose of *Fu Zheng* is to strengthen both *chi* and blood; hence, the name *fu* (meaning "fortify") and *zheng* (meaning "constitution").

Chinese specialists consider cancer to be caused by damp-heat conditions, and prescribe herbs to help bring the body back into balance.

SKIN CANCER

Signs and Symptoms

The general warning signs of skin cancer are: change in the color, size, or shape of a mole or a wound that does not heal. Following are the signs and symptoms of the three most common types of skin cancer:

Basal Cell Carcinoma

- Pearly or waxy flesh-colored bump, usually on the face, ear, or neck
- Flat, flesh-colored or brown scar-like lesion, usually on the chest or back

Squamous Cell Carcinoma

- Firm, red, wart-like nodule with a scaly or crusted surface, usually on face, ears, neck, hands, or arms
- Flat lesion with scaly or crusted surface that sometimes ulcerates, usually on face, ears, neck, hands, or arms

Melanoma

- Dark bump anywhere on the skin that is changing in size
- A mole or dark spot of skin that is asymmetrical in shape and has irregular borders
- A new or existing growth that bleeds and does not heal

Description

The three most common types of skin cancer are basal cell carcinoma, squamous cell carcinoma, and melanoma. Basal cell carcinoma is the most common and least aggressive form of skin cancer; it rarely spreads to other parts of the body. Squamous cell carcinoma is a slightly less common, but more aggressive skin cancer; if not treated early on, it can spread to other tissues and organs. Melanoma is the fastest-growing and most deadly form of skin cancer. Melanoma originates in the body's pigment cells and spreads inward into internal tissues and organs. Melanoma can occur on any skin surface: face, back, arms, palms, soles of feet, toes, and mucous membranes.

While many people think of skin cancer as a superficial, non-threatening disease, it has the potential to metastasize to surrounding tissue or be carried by blood or the lymphatic system to internal organs. Fortunately, if it is detected early, skin cancer is highly treatable.

Ultraviolet light plays a primary role in most cases of skin cancer. People with a fair complexion, light eyes, blonde or red hair, or many freckles are at increased risk. One or more incidences of severe sunburn during childhood also greatly increases your risk of developing skin cancer as an adult.

Conventional Medical Treatment

At least once a month, check your skin for any changes in existing moles or for the presence of new moles. If you notice anything out of the ordinary, see your physician or a dermatologist. To diagnose skin cancer, your dermatologist conducts a physical examination. A biopsy of the affected skin may be necessary to confirm diagnosis. Your doctor also may order an X-ray or CAT scan to determine whether the cancer has spread to other parts of the body.

If a skin growth is determined to be cancerous or precancerous, surgery is usually required to remove the affected tissue. If the cancer has spread to surrounding skin or muscle, those tissues may have to be removed as well. There are a number of surgical procedures used to treat skin cancer, including laser therapy, cryosurgery (freezing the area with liquid nitrogen), or Mohs' chemosurgery (where one layer of tissue is removed at a time). In some cases, immunotherapy, topical

Health Notes

➤ Protect yourself against ultraviolet rays, regardless of the weather or season. Try to stay indoors between 10 a.m. and 3 p.m., when UV rays are at their strongest. Always use a sunscreen with SPF of 15 or higher when outdoors. Wear a hat and long-sleeved clothing for extra protection.

➤ Several studies have shown that antioxidants (such as selenium, beta-carotene, vitamin C, vitamin B_6, and vitamin E) help lower risk for skin cancer by up to 25 percent—even in the presence of other risk factors, such as sun exposure.

➤ Selenomethionine (SeMet), a form of selenium, has been shown to reduce sun-related skin damage. A dosage of 100 micrograms daily is recommended during the summer to protect against skin cancers; 200 micrograms daily is recommended for those with a personal or family history of skin cancer.

➤ St. John's wort makes skin more sensitive to ultraviolet rays. Do not go into the sun unprotected if you are taking St. John's wort or are using a skin care cream that contains the herb.

➤ Never use artificial tanning beds or tanning lamps. These emit ultraviolet radiation that can cause skin damage and skin cancer.

➤ The prescription creams Retin A® and Renova® both contain trentoin, a vitamin A derivative that destroys precancerous skin lesions. However, both preparations cause skin to be more sensitive to ultraviolet light.

chemotherapy, or radiation therapy are used after surgery. (See "Conventional Medical Treatment" in "Bladder Cancer" entry for more information on radiation and chemotherapy.)

For More Information
Skin Cancer Foundation
P.O. Box 561
New York, NY 10156
800-SKIN-490
www.skincancer.org

Complementary and Alternative Treatments

Nutrition and Supplementation

You need a low-fat, high-antioxidant diet filled with foods such as carrots, sweet potatoes, squash, broccoli, cabbage, turnips, and citrus fruits. Avoid direct sunlight and *never, ever* visit tanning booths.

The following daily supplements should help treat your skin. This list is not all-inclusive; consult with a medical expert for an individualized treatment plan.

- dimethylglycine (as directed on label)—improves cellular oxygenation

- coenzyme Q10 (100 mg)—improves cellular oxygenation

- essential fatty acids (as directed on label, 3 times daily before meals)—protects cells

- proteolytic enzymes (as directed on label)—free radical scavengers that reduce inflammation

- selenium (200 mcg)—protects against UV damage

- vitamin A (50,000 to 100,000 IU for 10 days; do not exceed 8000 IU daily if you are pregnant)—destroys free radicals; use emulsion form for best assimilation

- mixed carotenoid formula (15,000 IU)—carotenoids are precursors of vitamin A

- vitamin B complex (100 mg)—required for cell division and function

- vitamin C with bioflavonoids (5000 to 20,000 mg in divided doses)—a potent anti-cancer agent

- vitamin E (up to 1000 IU)—promotes healing and tissue repair; use emulsion form

(Consult your healthcare provider regarding the duration of treatment.)

Traditional Chinese Medicine

Acupuncture Although acupuncture is not effective in the treatment of skin cancer itself, it is very helpful in alleviating the headaches, nausea, and lethargy that often accompany traditional treatment methods, such as chemotherapy and radiation.

Acupressure This modality may prove useful in improving the energy level and outlook of people suffering from skin cancer, and it can certainly be helpful in alleviating discomfort caused by the disease itself or by aggressive medical treatments.

Chinese Herbal Therapy Many Chinese herbs have been proven effective against skin cancer. Aloe vera, meanwhile, has been shown to have a protective effect against radiation-induced skin disturbances (a troubling side effect of conventional cancer treatment).

Scientists at the University of California at Los Angeles found that garlic extract inhibited the growth of melanoma cells by more than 50 percent, and that it actually caused the diseased cells to revert back to their healthy, pre-cancerous state. Many other studies have also shown that garlic is a potent remedy for skin cancer as well as a possible deterrent.

Herbalists also may advocate Gentiana Formula and *Dang Dui* and Arctium Combination to help skin heal faster. Japanese wax privet is known to enhance immunity and counteract the gastrointestinal ravages of chemotherapy and radiation.

STOMACH CANCER

Signs and Symptoms

In its early stages, stomach cancer often produces no symptoms. When it reaches later stages, the most common symptoms are:

- Pain or discomfort in the upper or middle abdominal region, which is sometimes made worse by eating
- Change in bowel movements, including diarrhea or constipation
- Bloated feeling after meals
- Vomiting after meals
- Vomiting blood
- Black or blood-streaked stools
- Appetite and weight loss
- General weakness and fatigue

Description

Stomach cancer, sometimes called gastric cancer, is a difficult condition to diagnose, since its early symptoms are mild. In fact, an estimated one out of every four people with malignant stomach tumors will have symptoms identical to those associated with a peptic ulcer.

Stomach cancer affects twice as many men as women and usually strikes people over the age of 50. Indeed, it is rare for someone under the age of 40 to have stomach cancer. People who have a sibling or parent with stomach cancer are two to four times more likely to develop the condition. Stomach cancer is especially common in Asian countries, such as Japan. Certain dietary factors may play a role, including high-salt intake, high intake of preservatives, such as nitrates, and low levels of fiber in the diet.

Conventional Medical Treatment

If you have any of the symptoms of stomach cancer, see your physician immediately. If stomach cancer is suspected, your doctor may perform an endoscopy (during which a flexible scope is fed into the stomach through the mouth), a CAT scan, or an ultrasound. A stomach tissue biopsy will be necessary to confirm the diagnosis.

Treatment for stomach cancer depends on how advanced the cancer is. Individual tumors that are confined to the stomach are removed surgically. If the cancer has affected a majority of stomach tissue, the stomach may have to be removed. Chemotherapy or radiation are generally employed (sometimes in combination) following surgery. (See "Conventional Medical Treatment" in "Bladder Cancer" entry for more information on radiation and chemotherapy.) If the cancer has

Health Notes

➤ *The antioxidants beta-carotene, vitamin E, and selenium can reduce the risk of stomach cancer. These nutrients are thought to prevent carcinogens from damaging cells.*

➤ *Cruciferous vegetables, such as cauliflower, broccoli, brussels sprouts, and cabbage, can lower the risk of stomach cancer. Aim for one or two servings daily.*

➤ *Eat one or two meals that include garlic, shallots, onions, or scallions every day. These vegetables are known to block carcinogens that can cause stomach cancer.*

➤ *Excess salt irritates the stomach lining and causes the cells to reproduce more often, which can result in stomach cancer. Restrict your intake of sodium to 500 to 2000 mg per day.*

spread to nearby organs, chemotherapeutic drugs are given, sometimes along with radiation.

Complementary and Alternative Treatments

Traditional Chinese Medicine

 Acupuncture Acupuncture can be used to improve the flow of blood and *chi* along the stomach meridian. It also can be an effective way to control pain.

Acupressure Acupressure can be used to stimulate the body's endorphins to help relieve stomach pain. It also can be used to bolster immunity and emotional well-being.

Chinese Herbal Therapy Garlic has been found to help prevent stomach cancer among subjects studied in China, according to a recent report by the National Cancer Institute. The recommended dose is 3 to 5 fresh cloves a day (it can also be taken in capsule form).

Ginseng is another herb reputed to have anticancer properties. According to a Korean study, rats who were given a carcinogen along with ginseng extract in their diets experienced a much lower incidence of gastrointestinal tumors (3.4 percent) than the ginseng-free control group (44 percent). Interestingly, the rats with a high-salt diet experienced the highest incidence of stomach cancer (61.9 percent).

TESTICULAR CANCER

Signs and Symptoms

- Change in the size or shape of a testicle
- A painless lump or swelling in a testicle
- Pain or tenderness in the affected testicle
- A feeling of heaviness in the affected testicle

Description

Testicular cancer usually originates in the testicles (rather than spreading to the testicles from other tissues)—specifically in the testicle cells responsible for producing sperm. In its early stages, testicular cancer is usually detected as a pea-sized lump or mass. When detected and treated early, testicular cancer is highly curable. Approximately 85 percent of men diagnosed with testicular cancer will survive five years or more.

Testicular cancer is most common among Caucasian men between the ages of 15 and 35. Men of Scandinavian descent and men who had undescended testicles at birth have higher rates of this cancer, as do men who live in rural environments and unmarried men of high socioeconomic status.

Conventional Medical Treatment

If you notice a change in the size or shape of a testicle, see your physician, who may perform a physical examination of the testicles and possibly a scrotal ultrasound. A biopsy of the affected testicle also may be necessary to confirm diagnosis.

Testicle Self-Exam

Early detection and treatment are the keys to a successful recovery from testicular cancer. The best way to screen for testicular cancer is to perform a regular self-examination. Starting at age 13, men should examine themselves on a monthly basis. The best time to perform a self-exam is after a bath or shower, when the testicles are relaxed. Place your index and middle fingers under one testicle while placing the thumb on top. Roll the testicle from side to side while feeling for lumps or other abnormalities. A normal testicle feels uniformly smooth, although one is usually larger than the other. Both testicles should be examined.

Health Notes

➤ *Chlorine-based chemicals may increase the risk of testicular cancer. If the water in your neighborhood is chlorinated, drink only bottled water or purchase a filter to purify the water.*

➤ *Eat at least four fruits and five vegetables daily to lower your risk of developing testicular cancer.*

In addition, your physician may perform a CAT scan of the torso to determine whether or not the cancer has spread to nearby organs.

Surgical removal of the affected testicle is the most common form of treatment. If both testicles are affected, both may be removed. Surgery is usually followed by radiation or chemotherapy to eliminate any remaining cancer cells. (See "Conventional Medical Treatment" in "Bladder Cancer" entry for more information on radiation and chemotherapy.)

Complementary and Alternative Treatments

Traditional Chinese Medicine

Acupuncture Electroacupuncture biofeedback is being studied as a diagnostic tool for the early screening of testicular and other types of cancer. Electroacupuncture biofeedback devices have been used in this country for the past 15 years and are currently undergoing testing by the FDA.

Acupressure Acupressure may be used to reduce discomfort caused by the disease and lessen stomach upset brought on by chemotherapy and other conventional treatments.

Chinese Herbal Therapy Fu Zheng herbal therapy may be used to enhance immunity and ward off testicular cancer.

THROAT CANCER

Signs and Symptoms

In its early stages, throat cancer often produces no symptoms. When it reaches later stages, the most common symptoms are:

● Hoarseness
● Sore throat
● Pain or difficulty swallowing
● Swelling in the neck
● Chronic coughing
● Blood in the phlegm

Description

Hoarseness is a symptom of many upper respiratory and throat conditions, but it is often the only symptom of early-stage throat cancer. Hoarseness occurs because many throat cancers begin as tumors on the vocal cords or around the larynx. If throat cancer is detected and treated during its early stages, it has a high cure rate. If it is ignored or undetected, the cancer can spread to other areas of the throat and to the head or upper respiratory tract, complicating treatment.

Throat cancer affects more men than women. Smokers are at greatest risk for developing throat cancer, but heavy drinkers are at high risk as well. Throat cancer rarely occurs in people under the age of 50.

Conventional Medical Treatment

If you suspect that you have throat cancer, see your physician immediately. To diagnose the condition, your doctor may perform an *indirect laryngoscopy* (during which your throat is examined with a mirror) or a *direct laryngoscopy* (during which you are anesthetized and your throat is examined with a fiberoptic scope). A biopsy of the

Health Notes

➤ *If you drink alcohol, imbibe it sensibly. Studies have shown that people who drink two or more alcoholic drinks a day are at increased risk for developing throat cancer.*

➤ *When taken in high dosages, vitamin C has been shown to decrease the risk of throat cancer. Aim for 200 to 300 mg of vitamin C with bioflavonoids 3 times a day.*

➤ *Researchers report that people who take vitamin E supplements reduce their throat cancer risk by one-half. Vitamin E helps prevent cancer by reducing cell oxidation and it fights the disease indirectly by boosting the immune system.*

affected area may be necessary to confirm diagnosis.

If the cancer is limited to a small, operable area, individual tumors may be surgically removed. Radiation treatment generally follows such surgery. If the cancer is widespread or is in an inoperable region of the throat, chemotherapy or radiation may be administered. (See "Conventional Medical Treatment" in "Bladder Cancer" entry for more information on radiation and chemotherapy.) In severe cases, the vocal cords and larynx must be removed. To help regain speech after serious surgery, speech therapy or a surgically-inserted prosthesis may be necessary.

Complementary and Alternative Treatments

Traditional Chinese Medicine

Acupuncture Acupuncture has many applications in the treatment of throat cancer. Acupuncture has also been used to alleviate pain and improve the ability to swallow in patients with cancer of the esophagus. Commonly targeted sites include Small Intestine 17, Large Intestine 4 and 11, and Lung 11, along with auricular points that relate to the pharynx, esophagus, larynx, and tonsils.

Acupressure Points that may be pressed to alleviate throat pain include Lung 11 (at the corner of the thumbnail) and Gallbladder 20 at the top of the neck.

To help quiet a cancer-related cough, an acupressurist may focus on several body points, including Lung 1, 5, 7, and 9; Conception Vessel 17 and 22; Spleen 6; Kidney 6, and Stomach 36.

Difficulty swallowing—a common throat cancer symptom—can be helped by pressing Conception Vessel 17 and Governing Vessel 13.

Chinese Herbal Therapy See earlier "Cancer" entries.

UTERINE CANCER

Signs and Symptoms

In its early stages, uterine cancer often produces no symptoms. When it reaches later stages, the most common symptoms are:

- Heavy periods or vaginal bleeding between periods
- Vaginal bleeding after menopause
- Vaginal discharge, ranging from watery and pink to thick and brown

Description

Uterine cancer is the most common form of gynecological cancer, affecting an estimated 31,000 to 35,000 women each year. It usually develops after menopause. Endometrial cancer—cancer that begins in the endometrium (the lining of the uterus)—accounts for the vast majority of uterine cancer cases. Uterine sarcoma, which begins in the wall of the uterus, is a very aggressive but relatively rare form of uterine cancer. If uterine cancer is detected and treated early, it is highly curable.

A high level of estrogen is the chief risk factor for uterine cancer; estrogen stimulates endometrial cells to grow more quickly than normal, resulting in a precancerous condition called *endometrial hyperplasia*. Excess estrogen in the body may be the result of estrogen-only hormone replacement therapy and an overabundance of fat cells (which stim-

ulate estrogen production). High-risk groups for uterine cancer include women who reach menopause after age 52, women on long-term tamoxifen therapy, women who have never given birth, women with irregular periods, and women with a family history of uterine cancer.

Conventional Medical Treatment

Routine Pap smear tests rarely detect uterine cancer before any symptoms appear, but a yearly pelvic exam is an important screening procedure. Most tumors are discovered after they have grown and begin producing non-menstrual bleeding. If you notice any abnormal bleeding, see your physician immediately. A biopsy of endometrial tissue is necessary to confirm the presence of cancerous cells.

Most cases of uterine cancer require surgical removal of the uterus, ovaries, and fallopian tubes. In premenopausal women, an ovary may be left to forestall menopausal symptoms and osteoporosis. Radiation is generally administered following surgery, and if the tumor has spread, chemotherapy also may be indicated. (See "Conventional Medical Treatment" in "Bladder Cancer" entry for more information on radiation and chemotherapy.) If the cancer has spread to other parts of the body, progesterone therapy may be used to limit the spread of the cancer.

Health Notes

➤ *Several studies have found a correlation between a sedentary lifestyle and uterine cancer. As a preventative measure, exercise moderately at least 3 times per week.*

➤ *Estrogen is contraindicated if uterine cancer has spread beyond the uterus.*

➤ *Eat a low-fat, high-fiber diet. Uterine cancer has been linked to excessive amounts of saturated fat in the diet.*

➤ *Use of birth control pills containing progesterone is associated with a lowered risk of uterine cancer.*

➤ *If you are postmenopausal and with your uterine intact, and decide to take hormone replacement therapy, be sure to take a combination of estrogen and progesterone. Estrogen alone dramatically increases the risk of uterine cancer.*

➤ *Women with "apple" body shapes have a higher incidence of uterine cancer than women with "pear-shaped" bodies. Fat cells in the midsection are more metabolically active than those elsewhere and can alter blood levels of sex hormones, resulting in increased risk of uterine cancer.*

Complementary and Alternative Treatments

Traditional Chinese Medicine

Acupuncture In one Russian study, acupuncture was shown to be effective in relieving the pain and edema that often result from radiation treatments. Another study found that laser acupuncture decreased radiation edema by 22 to 37 percent.

Acupressure This modality is considered useful in balancing *chi* and reducing fatigue (typical acupoints targeted for this purpose are Large Intestine 4 and 10, Conception Vessel 6, Stomach 36, Lung 9, and Kidney 3).

Chinese Herbal Therapy Aloe vera has been scientifically proven to reduce the production and spread of cancerous tumors—including those in the uterus—and to fortify the immune system, as have ginseng, licorice, and garlic.

Because uterine cancer has been associated with feelings of depression and emotional loss, an herbalist also may choose to treat the disease by prescribing herbs to remedy these psychological imbalances.

CANKER SORES

Signs and Symptoms

- Small, white or yellow sores with red borders that appear on the inside of the mouth—on the tongue, gums, soft palate, or the inside surfaces of the cheeks and lips

- Sores may appear singly or in clusters

- Pain at the site

Description

Most people know that they have a developing canker sore when they notice a slight stinging sensation somewhere inside their mouth—usually on the cheek or tongue, but sometimes on the gums or soft palate. A few hours later, a sensitive red bump appears. By the next day, the bump becomes an ulcerated and painful sore.

Also known as *aphthous* ulcers, these sores—which strike women slightly more often than men—usually make their first appearance when you are between the ages of 10 and 40. The sores may never come back again, or they may recur periodically over the course of your life. While canker sores are ordinarily more of an annoyance than a health hazard, extremely severe attacks can be accompanied by fever, listlessness, and swollen glands.

At this time, the specific cause of canker sores is unknown, though there appears to be a heredi-tary disposition toward them. (If your mother or father suffers from recurrent bouts of canker sores, you may, too.) There also seems to be a connection between canker sores and physical irritation—from braces or dentures, for example. Food allergies are also a suspected cause of the condition. Some women even get canker sores before their menstrual periods. Some people are susceptible during times of extreme stress or fa-

Health Notes

➤ *Cancel any dental appointments if you have even one canker sore or an outbreak of them. Fluoride solution and the prodding of the instruments used during a professional teeth cleaning can aggravate the condition.*

➤ *If you suspect that an ill-fitting pair of dentures or orthodontic device (such as a retainer or braces) is causing canker sores, contact your dentist or orthodontist. A minor adjustment can help prevent further problems.*

➤ *To ease the pain of canker sores, try sucking on an ice cube. The cold temperature will temporarily numb the area.*

tigue; others are prone due to deficiencies of vitamin B_{12}, iron, or folic acid.

Conventional Medical Treatment

With good mouth hygiene (make sure to brush your teeth and tongue regularly and floss daily), canker sores usually disappear within 7 to 10 days. Refrain from touching or picking at the sores, since these habits can cause irritation or even a secondary infection. While the sores heal, you also may want to avoid spicy and acidic foods (such as tomatoes), which can easily irritate them. To relieve pain, consider trying over-the-counter topical analgesics, such as benzocaine (Orajel®).

If the sores become infected or last for more than 2 weeks, contact your physician or dentist, who may prescribe antibiotics.

For More Information
American Dental Association (ADA)
211 East Chicago Avenue
Chicago, IL 60611
312-440-2500
www.ada.org

Complementary and Alternative Treatments

Nutrition and Supplementation

 Nutrition plays a vital role in the treatment of canker sores. Avoid meat, tomatoes, oranges, and citrus fruits. Avoid sugar and processed foods. Eat foods containing live cultures (for example, *Lactobacillus acidophilus*), such as plain, unsweetened yogurt.

Follow these daily nutritional guidelines:

- L-lysine (500 mg 3 times daily on empty stomach)—deficiency may cause outbreak of sores in and around mouth; do not take longer than six months
- vitamin B complex (50 mg 3 times daily)—promotes healing and builds immunity, supplemented with vitamin B_3 (50 to100 mg 3 times daily)—deficiency has been linked to canker sores
- vitamin C with bioflavonoids (3000 to 8000 mg in divided doses)—fights infection and boosts the immune system; use buffered form
- zinc (1 15-mg lozenge every 3 waking hours for 2 days, not to exceed a total of 100 mg daily)
- vitamin A (50,000 IU daily for 2 weeks, then reduce to 25,000 IU daily; do not exceed 8000 IU if you are pregnant)—speeds healing (Put a few drops of vitamin A oil directly on the sore.)
- glutathione and zinc (oral spray form, as directed on label)
- coenzyme Q10 (chewable form, as directed on label)

Ayurvedic Medicine

 Ayurvedic practitioners suggest drinking cranberry juice to ease the stinging, biting soreness associated with canker sores. They also advise avoiding hot, spicy foods and alcoholic beverages—all of which can exacerbate the condition.

Hydrotherapy

 To quiet pain and speed healing, rinse your mouth with warm salt water (dissolve 1 teaspoon of salt in 1/2 cup water) several times daily until the symptoms subside.

Traditional Chinese Medicine

Acupuncture Because practitioners generally attribute canker sores to a damp-heat condition, they typically treat with acupuncture therapy for damp-heat syndrome.

Acupressure To help alleviate the pain of canker sores, a practitioner may apply pressure to

Large Intestine 4 (between the thumb and index finger), Stomach 36 (right below the kneecap), and various ear points.

Chinese Herbal Therapy To soothe a canker sore and speed healing time, take 4 to 9 grams of akebia daily until symptoms subside. Applying fresh aloe vera juice directly to the canker sore also can help reduce pain.

Other herbs used to treat canker sores and mouth ulcers are Superior Sore Throat Powder Spray, which may be used up to 3 times a day.

CARPAL TUNNEL SYNDROME

Signs and Symptoms

- A tingling or numb sensation in the hand, usually in the thumb and the first three fingers
- Burning pain in the fingers that may radiate to the wrist and arm
- Symptoms usually worsen during activities that involve grasping, turning, or twisting, or repetitive motion such as keyboarding at the computer

Description

A relatively unknown condition as recently as the 1980s, carpal tunnel syndrome (CTS) has become a common health problem. Fortunately, the condition can be prevented, and it can be easily treated with specific nutritional and physical therapies.

The carpal tunnel is a nerve passageway that runs through the wrist to the thumb and first three fingers (not the pinkie) and the nine tendons that flex the fingers. This passageway and the median nerve above it are vulnerable to compression through repeated motions of the hands and wrists. Continued compression presses the median nerve against the eight carpal bones of the hand. When the median nerve becomes pinched or irritated, this ultimately leads to soreness, tenderness, and weakness. One or both hands may be affected.

The condition can be caused by work that re-quires repetitive motion of the hands or wrists, such as twisting, grasping, turning, or vibration. While carpal tunnel syndrome is known for affecting many who work regularly at the keyboard of a computer, they are not the only ones at risk. The condition can affect anyone who uses their hands for their work, including gymnasts, musicians, meat cutters, small parts assembly workers, tennis players, canoeists, and knitters, as well as those who use vibrating machinery, such as chainsaws and jackhammers. Pregnant women are especially susceptible to a temporary form of CTS, because of decreased circulation in their hands. Women who take birth control pills and menopausal women are also vulnerable to this condition, as are people with hypothyroidism, Raynaud's disease, and diabetes.

Conventional Medical Treatment

Medical treatment usually begins with immobilization of the hand with a splint to encourage the natural healing process. The splint must be worn during the day at work and is often worn during the night as well. Anti-inflammatory medications (such as corticosteroids), pain killers, or muscle relaxants—given as an injection or orally—are sometimes prescribed to treat specific symptoms or as a second course of treatment if the splint alone does not accelerate healing. Physical therapy can also help the patient rebuild strength and range of motion.

Health Notes

➤ *When doing any repetitive motion work, be sure to take a break every thirty minutes.*

➤ *To avoid carpal tunnel syndrome while typing or keyboarding, keep your lower arm and wrist straight, not flexed, and parallel to the ground. If it makes you feel more comfortable, use a wrist splint while typing, or buy a keyboard wrist-support pad or one of the new "ergonomically correct" modular-shaped keyboards. If possible, use a desk or computer table with a lower tray or area for your keyboard.*

➤ *When possible, don't use your hands to twist or grasp—instead use tools made for this purpose, such as jar openers, key turners, and electric can openers.*

➤ *If you are working at a desk, adjust your chair so that your feet are comfortably resting on the floor and you can sit up straight.*

➤ *Strengthen your hands by doing palm presses: Lean your body slightly forward and gently push your palms downward on a table top.*

If the condition does not improve with treatment, you may have to wear a cast. In serious cases that do not respond to any other treatments, surgery is often advised. While surgery for carpal tunnel syndrome is typically successful, the condition may return if the motions that caused the condition are repeated.

For More Information
National Institute of Arthritis and Musculoskeletal and Skin Diseases
Bld. 31, Room 4C05
31 Center Drive MSC 2350
Bethesda, MD 20892-2350
301-495-4484
www.nih.gov/niams

Complementary and Alternative Treatments

Nutrition and Supplementation

Avoid salt and foods containing sodium, as they promote water retention. Eat fresh pineapple daily for up to 3 weeks; pineapple contains bromelain, which reduces pain and swelling. Large amounts of oxalic acid promote joint problems, so eat in moderation foods such as eggs, fish, spinach, asparagus, beets, and vegetables of the cabbage family.

These daily supplements will help prevent and treat CTS:

Most Important

- coenzyme Q10 (30 to 90 mg)—tissue oxygenation

- lecithin capsules (1200 mg 3 times daily before meals)—improves nerve function

- vitamin B complex (50 mg 3 times daily)—essential to nerve function, supplemented with vitamin B_6 (100 mg twice daily for 12 weeks; nerve damage may result if you exceed this amount)—a diuretic, and vitamin B_1 (50 mg 3 times daily for 12 weeks)—increases the uptake of vitamin B_6

Also Recommended

- grape seed extract (as directed on label)—an anti-inflammatory

- kelp (as directed on label)—beneficial to nerves

- evening primrose oil (as directed on label)—contains essential fatty acids vital to nerve function

- glucosamine sulfate (as directed on label)—to reduce inflammation

- bromelain (as directed on label)—inflammation-fighting enzyme

(For an *acute* condition, take supplements until your symptoms subside. If symptoms persist, seek the advice of your healthcare provider. For a *chronic* condition, consult your healthcare provider regarding the duration of treatment.)

C

Aromatherapy

Aromatherapists recommend the essential oils of marjoram, lavender, and eucalyptus. See a qualified therapist for instructions.

Ayurvedic Medicine

Ayurvedic practitioners may advise using a turmeric-salt paste or an Indian *bdellium* paste to reduce swelling and inflammation caused by carpal tunnel syndrome. (Be aware that turmeric will stain fabric and skin.) Practitioners may also recommend cool compresses and gentle stretching to improve circulation.

Bodywork and Somatic Practices

Any manual therapy that can open the restricted connective tissue will be most effective in reducing pain, inflammation, and immobility. Look into sports massage, trigger point myotherapy, Trager, Hellerwork, Rolfing, CranioSacral Therapy and Oriental bodywork. Therapeutic Touch can help reduce inflammation. Further on in the healing process, use Feldenkrais, Alexander technique, Trager, and Aston-Patterning for postural alignment and enhanced structural efficiency.

Chiropractic

Chiropractic manipulation and physical therapy modalities are effective in decreasing the pain and treating the cause of carpal tunnel syndrome. The chiropractor may also recommend the use of splints (braces) to prevent impingement on the nerves by the carpal bones. Splints are often recommended for night use, to immobilize the wrist in the sleeping position (many people curl their wrists up as they sleep, particularly when sleeping on their side) and promote healing.

Herbal Therapy

Several herbs may benefit those suffering from carpal tunnel syndrome. Try gingko biloba for improved circulation and nerve function, skullcap for easing muscle spasms, and butcher's broom as an anti-inflammatory.

Hydrotherapy

Some therapists advise using contrast therapy (alternating hot and cold compresses) on the affected wrist to soothe pain and decrease swelling and inflammation. Others recommend applying an ice pack to the joint morning and evening for 10 minutes on, 10 minutes off; apply the cold for a total of 40 minutes during each session.

Traditional Chinese Medicine

Acupuncture Acupuncture can be extremely helpful in opening blocked energy pathways in the hand, arm, and wrist, improving circulation to the affected area. Acupuncture also may be used to stimulate the release of endorphins (the body's natural "feel good" chemicals), which can alleviate the pain caused by carpal tunnel syndrome.

In addition to working on acupoints on the hand, wrist, and forearm, the practitioner also may treat acupoints related to the neck, back, and shoulders to correct any posture problems that may be contributing to the disorder.

Acupressure Acupressure is often used to treat the pain and numbness caused by carpal tunnel syndrome. Points usually targeted include Pericardium 6 and 7, Triple Warmer 5, and Small Intestine 6 on the wrist, along with related points on the ear.

Yoga and Meditation

Gentle yoga poses can help relax the neck and upper back. Tension in those areas can cause pain, swelling, and inflammation in the wrist tendon. Avoid poses that stress the wrist or neck, such as hand stands or neck stands. Also avoid any poses that twist the arm or wrist. Beneficial poses include Supported Downward Facing Dog and Half Locust.

CATARACTS

Signs and Symptoms

- Blurry or distorted vision in one or both eyes, which sometimes worsens in bright light
- Appearance of "halos" of light around bright lights or lighted objects
- Impaired night vision

Description

The lens, one of the eye's primary focusing mechanisms, is located just behind the pupil. A normal lens is transparent, allowing light into the eye. Cataracts, however, renders a lens cloudy, making it difficult for the necessary light to enter. Although cataracts typically start in only one eye, both eyes usually become affected with time, causing either largely diminished sight or total blindness. Cataracts usually develop gradually—many people don't realize that they have the condition until they struggle to pass a vision test.

Cataracts is one of the world's most common vision problems. In fact, approximately 16 million people worldwide are blind because of cataracts.

Age plays a significant role in the formation of cataracts—many people develop some clouding of the lens after age 60. Yet age isn't the only cause. Diabetes mellitus, family predisposition, long-term use of corticosteroid drugs, and overexposure to ultraviolet rays can all lead to cataracts. An eye injury can also cause cataract formation later in life. In rare instances, infants are born with cataracts or develop the condition shortly after birth.

Conventional Medical Treatment

An ophthalmologist tests for cataracts with a complete eye examination, a slit-lamp examina-

Less Weight, Better Eyesight

According to a recent study, overweight men are more likely to develop cataracts than their lean peers. Researchers found men with a body mass index (BMI) of 27.8 (or about 20 percent above normal weight for their height) or greater had more than twice the incidence of cataracts than men with a BMI of less than 22 (or normal for their height). Even being slightly overweight increases one's risk of developing cataracts—those whose BMI was between 22 and 27.8 were 1.5 times more likely to get cataracts than those whose BMI was under 22.

The researchers' explanation for these findings is that BMI strongly affects glucose levels, which increase risk of cataract formation. Higher BMI also increases uric acid concentrations in the blood and the risk of gout, both of which have been linked to cataract development.

Health Notes

➤ *Cataracts are often caused by ultraviolet light. To protect your eyes from UV rays when outside, always wear sunglasses that specify at least 99 percent protection from UVA and UVB rays and a brimmed hat. In addition, always avoid tanning salons, tanning lamps, and other forms of ultraviolet radiation.*

➤ *Eat four or more servings of vegetables a day. In one study, adults who ate less than 3¹/₂ servings of vegetables each day were five times more likely to develop cataracts than people who ate four or more.*

➤ *Antioxidants such as beta-carotene and vitamins C and E may help prevent cataracts. Riboflavin and niacin are also believed to play a role in cataract prevention.*

tion, and perhaps, ultrasonography to further evaluate the opacity of the lens. If the diagnosis is cataracts, glasses and contact lenses may be able to offer temporary help.

If your lack of vision begins to interfere with everyday activities, your physician may recommend cataract surgery. Under general or local anesthesia, the clouded lens is removed from the eye and, in most cases, replaced with an artificial one. The surgery, done on an outpatient basis, typically takes one hour. More than 98 percent of all cataract operations result in improved vision.

For More Information
American Society of Cataract and Refractive Surgery
4000 Legato Road, Suite 850
Fairfax, VA 22033
703-591-2220
www.ascrs.org

National Eye Institute (NEI)
National Institutes of Health
2020 Vision Place
Bethesda, MD 20892-3655
301-496-5248
www.nei.nih.gov

Prevent Blindness America
500 East Remington Road
Schaumburg, IL 60173
800-331-2020
www.preventblindness.org

Complementary and Alternative Treatments

Nutrition and Supplementation

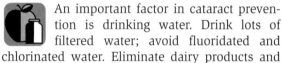 An important factor in cataract prevention is drinking water. Drink lots of filtered water; avoid fluoridated and chlorinated water. Eliminate dairy products and saturated fats, which promote the formation of free radicals and can damage the lens. Use only cold-pressed oils. Medical journals report an association between cigarettes and cataracts, probably because smoking generates free radicals.

Nutritionists recommend the following daily supplements:

Most Important

• copper (3 mg)—important for proper healing and, along with manganese, retards the growth of cataracts

• manganese (10 mg taken separate from calcium)

• glutathione (as directed on label)—helps maintain a healthy lens; slows the progression of cataracts

• vitamin A (25,000 to 50,000 IU; do not exceed 8000 IU if you are pregnant)—vital for normal vision

• mixed carotenoid formula (as directed on label)—a precursor of vitamin A

• vitamin B_1 (thiamine) (50 mg)—important for intracellular eye metabolism

- vitamin C with bioflavonoids (3000 mg 4 times daily)—a free radical destroyer

- vitamin E (400 IU)—helps arrest and reverse cataract formation

- zinc (30 mg, not to exceed a total of 100 mg from all supplements)—protects against light-induced damage

Also Recommended

- selenium (400 mcg)—destroys free radicals

- riboflavin (50 mg)—a deficiency has been linked to cataracts

(Consult your healthcare provider regarding the duration of treatment.)

Traditional Chinese Medicine

 Acupuncture In treating cataracts, the acupuncturist usually pinpoints Bladder 1, Stomach 1, Large Intestine 4, and Triple Warmer 6, along with related auricular points and associated points, following a complete diagnosis.

Acupressure Cataracts can be treated by firmly massaging the acupressure points around the eye socket and on the cheeks, forehead, and temple.

Chinese Herbal Therapy The herbal formula Dendrobium Moniliforme Night Sight Pills also may be prescribed for cataracts. Because Traditional Chinese Medicine attributes most eye disorders to liver dysfunction, an herbalist may also prescribe tonics to strengthen this organ and improve the flow of *chi* within the liver meridian.

CAVITIES

Signs and Symptoms

- Pain in a specific tooth—a dull ache or shooting stab when the tooth is exposed to hot and cold temperatures and sugary substances

- In advanced cases, a dark spot will appear on the tooth (though it may be on a surface that you cannot see)

Description

A cavity is a hole in the tooth's protective enamel layer. Cavities are the result of tooth decay, a process triggered by bacteria in the mouth, sugary food, and a vulnerable tooth surface. The bacteria in your mouth help with digestion by converting a portion of the sugars and carbohydrates you consume into acid. This acid and bacteria can combine with mucus and food particles to form a sticky deposit called dental plaque, which clings to the surfaces of your teeth. If it is not brushed away, the acid in plaque erodes the outer enamel surface of the tooth. These points of erosion are called cavities, or *dental caries*. In time, the acid can move further into the tooth, invading the interior dentin material, and in severe cases, tunneling through the tooth to the root.

Of course, this process does not happen overnight. A cavity takes time to develop. It can take a year or more for a cavity to develop in permanent teeth, or less than a year in primary teeth (children's first set of teeth).

Too Young For Tooth Care?

Your child is ready for at-home dental care even before her first tooth appears. A major cause of decay in primary teeth is what pediatricians and dentists call "nursing bottle syndrome." Infants who frequently fall asleep with bottles or while nursing often develop cavities on the inner surface of the front teeth. This is caused by the pooling of milk or juice in the baby's mouth. To prevent this type of tooth decay, avoid feeding an infant immediately before bedtime. If your child falls asleep while feeding, remove the bottle from her mouth. Once an infant's first tooth appears, parents can use a soft dampened cloth to clean swab the teeth after meals; when the baby has several teeth, use a soft toothbrush—without toothpaste—to gently brush the tooth. Don't have your child use toothpaste until she is old enough to learn how to rinse and spit after brushing. Children should be taken to see a dentist when they reach age three.

Conventional Medical Treatment

If you feel pain in a tooth, schedule a visit with your dentist. The dentist physically examines the tooth and may take X-rays before diagnosing a cavity. Standard cavity treatment involves drilling away the decayed portion of the tooth, then plugging the resulting hole with silver amalgam, gold inlay, or tooth-colored plastic resin. This "plug" is known as a filling.

If the cavity is so deep that it has burrowed into the tooth's root, you must get a root canal. In a root canal, the dentist removes the tooth's nerve and vascular tissue as well as the decayed portion of the tooth. The resulting canal is then sterilized and filled with a dental cement.

For More Information
American Dental Association (ADA)
211 East Chicago Avenue
Chicago, IL 60611
312-440-2500
www.ada.org

Health Notes

➤ *People with deeply-grooved molars are at higher risk for cavities. If you are one of these people, talk to your dentist about having a preventative sealant applied to your molars to help keep plaque and bacteria from settling in the crevices.*

➤ *Sweets aren't the only foods that contribute to cavities. Because they contain simple sugars that stick to the teeth, starchy foods are especially damaging. To minimize your chance of developing cavities, try eating carbohydrates only with meals, when other foods increase saliva production and help clear away simple sugars. And, of course, always brush your teeth or rinse your mouth with water after eating.*

➤ *The bacteria in plaque do not feed on artificial sweeteners. So if you are in a situation where you can't brush your teeth after a meal, chew a piece of sugarless gum that contains xylitol. This artificial sweetener can help reduce the risk of enamel decay by interfering with the bacteria's sugar metabolism.*

➤ *Floss every day to remove plaque from between your teeth. Also, visit your dentist for a yearly professional cleaning.*

Complementary and Alternative Treatments

Nutrition and Supplementation

 A healthy diet is very important for building strong teeth. Include calcium-rich foods in your meals, especially broccoli, dark leafy greens, milk, yogurt, sardines and canned salmon (with bones), and sesame seeds. Eat raw fruits and vegetables to keep your saliva from becoming too acidic.

Avoid refined sugars, white flour products, excessive amounts of sweets and carbonated soft drinks (which are high in sugar). Substitute desserts made with fresh fruit or yogurt. Use honey instead of sugar to sweeten desserts and beverages.

Experts recommend the following daily supplements for adults:

- calcium (1500 mg)—essential for strong, healthy teeth

- magnesium (750 mg)—balances with calcium

- vitamin A (5000 IU)—important for tooth formation

- vitamin B complex (50 mg)—maintains healthy gums

- vitamin D (400 IU)—aids in calcium absorption and helps heal gums

- vitamin C (3000 mg)—protects against infection (Do not use in chewable form.)

Aromatherapy

 The essential oils of caraway, clove, niaouli, and nutmeg can help quiet the throbbing pain of a toothache caused by cavity. Using the tip of your finger, apply a single drop of one of these essential oils to the gum surrounding the painful tooth. If the oil is irritating to your gum, dilute it with 1 or 2 drops of safflower oil. Use the oil just until you're able to see a dentist for treatment.

Ayurvedic Medicine

 Ayurvedic practitioners recommend having cavities treated by a dentist as soon as possible. Until you can see your doctor, however, applying one of the following remedies directly to the affected tooth may bring pain relief: paste or oil made from sesame seeds, or a blend of powdered ginger, ground cardamom, and licorice extract.

Hydrotherapy

 Some hydrotherapists suggest using either a hot-water bottle or an ice pack on the jaw near the tooth to lessen pounding dental pain. Others advise using a charcoal compress. To make the compress, simply combine 1 tablespoon of activated powdered charcoal and enough water to make a paste. Apply the mixture to a piece of gauze and place the gauze over the affected tooth. Bite down to hold the compress in place and to allow the charcoal to ooze around the tooth.

CELIAC DISEASE

Signs and Symptoms

- Abdominal pain or cramps
- Bloating
- Diarrhea
- Foul-smelling, grayish stools that may float and may be larger than normal
- Gas
- General weakness and fatigue
- Weight loss
- In children, failure to grow or muscle weakness

Description

Celiac disease is a type of malabsorption syndrome. During digestion, food is broken down into nutrient molecules that can be absorbed by the bloodstream. In people with malabsorption syndrome, nutrients are not released into the bloodstream but are instead eliminated in the stool. As a result, the body does not get the nutrients it needs from food.

Also called celiac sprue, celiac disease is a relatively uncommon ailment, affecting approximately 1 person in 1000. It is caused by a sensitivity to gluten, a substance found in wheat, rye, oats, and barley. With extended exposure to gluten, the intestinal lining loses the tiny folds through which nutrients are absorbed and stops producing adequate amounts of digestive enzymes.

While the precise cause of gluten sensitivity is unknown, celiac disease is believed to be hereditary. The disease is diagnosed most often in children, though it can appear in adults with no prior sensitivity to gluten.

Conventional Medical Treatment

To diagnose celiac disease, your physician may take a stool sample and a barium X-ray of your small intestine. You may also have to have a biopsy (tissue sample) taken from the lining of your small intestine. Celiac disease is usually treated with a strict gluten-free diet. When carefully followed, a gluten-free diet allows the villi of the small intestines to resume their normal shape and absorption ability. Within two to four months,

Health Notes

➤ *People with celiac disease who do not eat a gluten-free diet are at increased risk of developing intestinal lymphoma.*

➤ *According to a recent study, celiac disease occurs in 5 percent of people with Type 1 diabetes.*

Gluten-Free Diet Tips

A gluten-free diet can be challenging to adhere to, since most bread and pasta products contain gluten. However, many health food stores sell gluten-free breads, and corn and rice pasta products. Some direct-mail companies, such as The Gluten-Free Pantry (800-291-8386), specialize in gluten-free bakery and cooking products. Gluten in the form of wheat flour and other "fillers" are often used in processed foods and canned foods, such as soups. Read labels carefully.

you should resume normal digestion and will begin to regain weight.

For More Information
Celiac Disease Foundation
13251 Ventura Boulevard, Suite 3
Studio City, CA 91604
818-990-2354

Gluten Intolerance Group of North America
15110 10th Ave SW, Suite A
Seatle, WA 98166
206-246-6652
www.gluten.net

Complementary and Alternative Treatments

Nutrition and Supplementation

 The number one enemy of celiac is gluten in any form. Avoid all products containing barley, rye, wheat, oats, hydrolyzed vegetable or plant protein, textured vegetable protein, malt, modified food starch, binders, fillers, and "natural flavorings." Do not eat hot dogs, gravies, luncheon meat, beer, mustard, catsup, non-dairy creamer, white vinegar, curry powder, or seasonings. Be sure your nutritional supplements do not contain gluten. Gluten-free products are available at health food stores, or call 800-633-3826 and ask for a gluten-free product catalog.

Because lactose intolerance often occurs with celiac disease, eliminate milk and dairy products from your diet. For optimum health, breastfeed your child for a longer period of time and postpone introducing cow's milk and grains into the diet until the child is older. Do not eat sugary products, processed foods, bouillon cubes, chocolate, or bottled salad dressings.

Although it may sound as though there aren't any foods left to eat, you can and should eat foods rich in folic acid, such as green leafy vegetables, lentils, seeds, nuts, and beans. Be sure to include raisins, strawberries, raspberries, fresh vegetables, sunflower seeds, and rice bran. Pay close attention to your intake of iron and B vitamins; people with celiac disease are often deficient in these nutrients.

Because celiac disease affects the intestine, your body is unable to absorb many vital nutrients. Make sure your healthcare professional checks your digestion and nutrient absorption. Supplementation is necessary, and the daily guidelines that follow should help manage your symptoms. (*Note*: To avoid any digestive problems you should gradually build up to these amounts. Always do so under the supervision of your healthcare professional.)

Most Important

- complete multivitamin and mineral complex
- free-form amino acid complex (as directed on label)—supplies protein in a form your body can assimilate
- vitamin B complex (as prescribed by healthcare provider)—necessary for proper digestion; injections are best because they bypass the digestive system

Also Recommended

- zinc (1 15-mg lozenge 5 times daily, not to exceed a total of 100 mg from all supplements)—promotes healing
- copper (3 mg)—to balance with zinc

- evening primrose oil (as directed on label)—provides essential fatty acids needed for intestinal health
- magnesium (750 mg daily)—a deficiency is common in people with celiac disease
- calcium (1500 mg)—works with magnesium
- vitamin C (2000 to 5000 mg in divided doses)—boosts the immune system
- L-glutamine (2 g)—supports intestinal immune system
- a prodophilus formula (as directed on label)

(For an *acute* condition, take supplements until your symptoms subside. If symptoms persist, seek the advice of your healthcare provider. For a *chronic* condition, consult your healthcare provider regarding the duration of treatment.)

Traditional Chinese Medicine

 Acupuncture Acupuncture can be used to help remedy typical symptoms, including gastrointestinal discomfort, abdominal distention, lethargy, irregular bowel movements, and slack muscle tone in the stomach region. The practitioner typically targets points that relate to the small intestine, large intestine, and stomach.

Acupressure This method of treatment can help relieve the constipation or frequent bowel movements that often accompany celiac disease. It also can ease abdominal discomfort and increase the patient's energy level.

Chinese Herbal Therapy Herbs that are sometimes used to treat the disorder include trifoliate orange (for digestive upset and abdominal bloating), fennel (to regulate and enhance digestive functions), and nutmeg (to tone the small intestine).

An herbalist also may prescribe over-the-counter herbal formulas, such as Ginseng Stomachic Pills or Aplotaxis Carminative Pills.

CHICKENPOX

Signs and Symptoms

- An extremely itchy rash that progresses from small, red spots to fluid-filled sores, which rupture and develop scabs
- Fever
- Fatigue

Description

Chickenpox is one of the most common childhood diseases. It is a highly infectious illness, characterized by a body-wide rash that strikes about two weeks after exposure to the varicella zoster virus (a member of the herpes zoster family). The virus can be spread through infected res-

Health Notes

➤ Trim your child's fingernails to minimize scratching and to reduce the risk of infection and scarring.

➤ Since sun exposure can cause healing chickenpox wounds to scar, the patient should avoid going outdoors or apply a sunscreen of SPF 15 or higher when going outdoors.

➤ Never give aspirin to a child with chickenpox, because it can increase the child's risk of developing Reyes syndrome—a rare, but possibly fatal, condition.

The Chickenpox Vaccine

For generations, chickenpox was considered an unpleasant, but ultimately unavoidable, childhood illness. However, a vaccine for chickenpox has been developed that is 95 percent effective in preventing the illness. The vaccine is recommended primarily for those who will be hit hard by a bout of chickenpox, specifically people over the age of 12 who have not had chickenpox and young children with weak immune systems who have not had the illness. Although the vaccination is available to all children, many pediatricians question the need to immunize against a condition that is not generally not life-threatening. And since the vaccine has only been used since the mid-1990s, its long-term side effects are still not known. Contact your pediatrician for advice on whether to vaccinate your child against chickenpox.

piratory droplets or by touching open chickenpox sores. At first, the rash consists of small, itchy red bumps that appear on the torso. After a day or two, these bumps fill with fluid. In another day or two, the sores drain and scab over. During the first five days, however, new sores continue to appear, covering the body with a variety of bumps, fluid-filled sores, and small scabs. The condition is contagious until the last of the bumps have scabbed over.

Since you become immune to the virus after you've had it, and since most people get the illness during childhood, it is rare to see an adult with chickenpox. On the other hand, adults suffer more seriously from the virus than children do. The fever, rash, and fatigue that accompany adult chickenpox can force the frail and elderly into the hospital. Also, people with adult chickenpox often develop pneumonia as well. A pregnant woman can pass chickenpox to her unborn child, increasing the risk that the child will be born with a congenital malformation.

Conventional Medical Treatment

A physician can diagnose the condition with a physical exam, but an office visit usually isn't necessary. A phone call to your doctor to confirm the symptoms is typically enough. To prevent spreading the condition, keep the affected person away from other people until the rash disappears. Keep the skin clean with tepid baths, and apply calamine lotion directly to sores to reduce itching. Cool oatmeal baths with over-the-counter oatmeal powders can also help relieve itching.

For children or adults with severe cases of chickenpox, or those with suppressed immune systems, acyclovir (an antiviral medication) may be prescribed.

For More Information

The American Academy of Pediatrics
141 Northwest Point Boulevard
Elk Grove Village, IL 60007-1098
847-228-5005
www.aap.org

National Institute of Allergies and Infectious Diseases
Building 31, Room 7A50
31 Center Drive MSC 2520
Bethesda, MD 20892 -2520
301-496-5717
www.niaid.nih.org

Complementary and Alternative Treatments

Nutrition and Supplementation

There isn't much you can do in the way of nutrition to improve your comfort or health during a bout of chickenpox. The best you can do is drink pure vegetable broth and freshly made juices with protein powder and brewer's yeast added. These will supply you with nutrients and help keep your skin in healthy condition while it heals. When your fever lowers, your appetite will return to normal. Be kind to your body and start slowly, eating a diet of mashed bananas, avocados, fresh applesauce and/or yogurt. Do not eat cooked or processed foods.

Chickenpox compromises the immune system, so it is important to supplement nutrients specifically targeted at building immunities. The following daily adult supplementation program should help. Parents should consult with a health professional for appropriate dosages for children.

- mixed carotenoid formula (15,000 IU)—stimulates the immune system

- vitamin A emulsion (100,000 IU for 1 week, then 75,000 IU for 1 week; do not exceed 8000 IU daily if you are pregnant)—an immunostimulant that aids in the healing of tissues; the emulsion form is easier to assimilate

- vitamin C (1000 mg 4 times daily)—stimulates the immune system and helps reduce fever

- zinc (30 mg, not to exceed a total of 100 mg from all supplements)—enhances immune function

Aromatherapy

To reduce the intense itching associated with chickenpox and speed healing of the blisters, create a soothing blend of essential oils. For the blend, mix 1 teaspoon each of distilled water and witch hazel and 3 drops each of German chamomile, lavender, and tea tree oil. Sponge on the blisters as needed.

Hydrotherapy

To calm the maddening itch of chickenpox, try a lukewarm bath to which you've added 1 to 2 cups of baking soda or powdered uncooked oats (oats specially prepared for the bath are available in drugstores). Soak for 15 minutes, than gently pat dry; don't rub, or you'll increase itching.

You also can quiet itching by applying cool, moist compresses to affected areas.

Traditional Chinese Medicine

Acupuncture An acupuncturist typically treats adult chickenpox as a damp-heat condition. With children, the illness is usually allowed to run its course.

Chinese Herbal Therapy In most cases, a Chinese herbal therapist treats chickenpox with the herbs bupleurium, burdock, and peppermint, which help reduce the swelling and itching that accompany the condition.

CHLAMYDIA

Signs and Symptoms

- Men may experience painful or frequent urination, discharge from the penis, or redness at the tip of the penis
- Women may not experience any symptoms, or may have slight abdominal discomfort, vaginal discharge, or painful, frequent urination

Description

Chlamydia is the most common sexually transmitted disease in the United States. It is caused by *Chlamydia trachomatis,* an organism that is transmitted through vaginal or anal sex. Symptoms generally appear one to three weeks after exposure to the bacteria, if they appear at all. In fact, many people do not even realize that they are carrying the disease, because chlamydia is sometimes asymptomatic in men and frequently asymptomatic in women. If left untreated, however, chlamydia can lead to chronic inflammation of the urethra and epididymis in men and pelvic inflammatory (PID) disease in women, both of which can cause sterility.

Chlamydia can also lead to secondary infections. For instance, if infected fluids come in contact with the eyes, they can cause eye infections. A pregnant woman can transmit chlamydia to her unborn child, causing the baby to develop chlamydial pneumonia or conjunctivitis. Chlamydia can also cause ectopic pregnancies and premature birth.

Conventional Medical Treatment

A family physician, gynecologist (for women), or urologist (for men) can diagnose chlamydia with a secretions test. In women, secretions are taken from the cervix and tested for the presence of *chlamydia trachomatis*. Since chlamydia is often asymptomatic, women should have this test performed during annual gynecological exams. In men, semen or urethral secretions are tested for the organism. Chlamydia is easily treated with antibiotics, and symptoms usually disappear within two weeks. Both partners should be

Chlamydia Screening

All sexually active women under 20 should have a yearly chlamydia screening.

Women 20 and older should have a yearly chlamydia screening if:

- they have new or multiple sex partners
- they don't consistently use condoms or diaphragms with foam
- they have a cervical infection, vaginal discharge, or bleeding during intercourse, or
- they are pregnant or considering pregnancy.

Health Notes

➤ *The National Institute of Medicine reports that chlamydia is the most common sexually transmitted bacterial disease in the United States. However, many women suffer no symptoms and the disease often goes undetected.*

➤ *Once chlamydia is detected, treatment is simple. A course of antibiotics can clear the condition up in a week. Chlamydia can also be treated with a single antibiotic injection.*

➤ *The only sure way to prevent chlamydia is abstinence or monogamy with an uninfected person. If you are a sexually active adult who is not in a monogamous relationship, you should use condoms to reduce your risk of contracting a sexually transmitted disease.*

➤ *The rate of chlamydia is growing most rapidly among adolescent women. Sexual education—including information about sexually transmitted diseases and how to prevent them—should be combined with strategies to help young women resist pressure to have sex before they're ready.*

➤ *Chlamydia can cause complications during birth and can be transmitted to newborns in the form of eye infections and pneumonia. Pregnant women, and those considering pregnancy, should consider being tested for chlamydia.*

treated for the condition, regardless of who is infected.

For More Information
American College of Obstetricians and Gynecologists
409 12th Street, SW, PO Box 96920
Washington, DC 20024-6920
800-673-8444
www.acog.org

Centers for Disease Control and Prevention (CDC)
1600 Clifton Road
Atlanta, GA 30333
800-311-3455
www.cdc.gov

Planned Parenthood Federation of America
810 Seventh Avenue
New York, NY 10019
212-541-7800
www.plannedparenthood.org

Complementary and Alternative Treatments

Nutrition and Supplementation

 Make the bulk of your diet fresh vegetables and fruits. Eat brown rice, whole grains, white fish, turkey, and raw seeds and nuts. Avoid junk foods and processed foods, and drink sugar-free juices and herbal teas.

The following daily supplements are recommended for treating chlamydia:

• vitamin E (600 IU)

• vitamin B complex (50 to 100 mg 3 times daily with meals)—necessary for proper functioning of the liver

• vitamin C (1500 mg, 4 times daily)—use buffered form

• zinc gluconate (50 mg)

• copper (3 mg)—to balance with zinc

• a prodophilus formula (as directed on label)—replaces friendly bacteria destroyed by antibiotics

Aromatherapy

 Research suggests that the essential oil of red thyme, a gentle anti-infective, may be effective against chlamydia. Consult your doctor before self-treating.

Cholesterol

Traditional Chinese Medicine

Acupuncture In conjunction with conventional medical treatment, acupuncture can be used to lessen the severity of chlamydia-related pain, fever, and urinary dysfunction and to bolster the immune system.

Acupressure Acupressure may be employed to help strengthen immunity, relieve pain, and improve the patient's mood by reducing stress and anxiety.

Chinese Herbal Therapy Garlic may be recommended as a general immunity-fortifying tonic, while gentiana, angelica, bupleurum, and coptis (also called mishmi bitter) may be prescribed to counteract specific symptoms and to keep the disease from compromising fertility and progressing to full-blown PID.

SYMPTOM:

CHOLESTEROL

Cholesterol is a waxy substance that the body needs to help maintain proper nerve function and healthy cells as well as other body functions. There are many types of cholesterol. Low-density lipoprotein (LDL), sometimes called "bad" cholesterol, is what people are referring to when they talk about the dangers of cholesterol. An overabundance of LDL in the bloodstream can cause buildups on the walls of arteries, leading to hardening of the arteries and atherosclerosis (both of which increase the risk of heart disease and stroke). High-density lipoprotein (HDL), on the other hand, is referred to as "good" cholesterol. HDL removes LDL from the bloodstream and the walls of arteries.

While your liver actually manufactures all the cholesterol your body needs, many foods in the typical American diet increase the body's total cholesterol level. Dietary cholesterol is found mainly in animal products, including meat (red meat, poultry, fish, and shellfish), eggs, dairy foods (milk, cream, butter, cheese, and yogurt), and lard. Smoking and excessive alcohol consumption also contribute to high levels of LDL. Regular aerobic exercise, on the other hand, is shown to increase the amounts of HDL in the body.

To determine your blood cholesterol level, visit your physician, who performs a blood test. As your doctor may tell you, healthy LDL and HDL levels differ, depending on age, heredity, gender, and general health. If you do have high levels of LDL, your doctor will probably recommend a cholesterol-restricted diet and exercise program to help lower LDL and raise HDL. In very serious cases, prescription drugs may be used to lower unsafe cholesterol levels.

In the arena of complementary and alternative treatments, the first place to start is your diet. Nutritionists often recommend adding more fiber to the diet. Fiber mops up excess cholesterol and gets it out of the blood. Apples, which are high in pectin, do this job especially well. Old-fashioned oat and buckwheat cereals do the same. It's a good idea to consume small amounts of essential fatty acids (found in nuts, flaxseeds, and fish—especially salmon), which have a similar action in the digestive system. Other important foods are those high in folic acid and B6, such as whole grains, fruits, and vegetables, and soy products, such as tofu and tempeh, which are rich in lecithin.

A deficiency in several vitamins and minerals can adversely affect cholesterol levels. Niacin (vitamin B3) is essential to keeping cholesterol under control. Get your niacin from leafy greens, wheat germ, beans, and tuna. Follow a daily supplement program as outlined below to help manage your cholesterol level:

Most Important

- *chromium picolinate (400 to 600 mcg)—lowers total cholesterol levels*

- *coenzyme Q10 (100 mg)—improves circulation*

- *garlic (as directed on label)—lowers cholesterol levels*

- *vitamin B complex (50 to 100 mg)—prevents homocystein from forming, supplemented with vitamin B3 (300 mg)—lowers cholesterol (do not take if you have gout, high blood pressure, or a liver disorder)*

- *vitamin C with bioflavonoids (3000 to 8000 mg)—lowers cholesterol*

- *vitamin E (200 IU and slowly increase to 1000 IU)—improves circulation; the emulsion form is easily assimilated*

- *tocotrienols (as directed on label)—a form of vitamin E, acts as an antioxidant*

Also Recommended

- *gugulipids (as directed on label)—lowers cholesterol*

- *rice protein supplement (as directed on label)—lowers serum cholesterol*

(Consult your healthcare provider regarding the duration of treatment.)

Ayurvedic practitioners consider high cholesterol levels to be a condition caused by excess kapha. To keep cholesterol levels down, they may advise drinking cinnamon-trikatu tea (trikatu is a combination of ginger and two types of peppers) twice daily and following a diet that avoids fried foods and high-fat dairy products. They also may recommend taking Indian bdellium or the combination formulas Abana and Geriforte. Ayurvedic products are available at many health food stores and Indian pharmacies.

You also may wish to consider Traditional Chinese Medicine. A TCM practitioner will most likely recommend acupuncture to improve the flow of blood throughout the body—especially to the heart—in an effort to open clogged arteries and enhance the elimination of dietary cholesterol. Numerous scientific studies have shown that garlic and ginger can lower serum cholesterol, while ginseng and licorice can reduce blood cholesterol levels while enhancing the body's immune functions. There are specific Chinese herbal formulas with these and other natural ingredients that help normalize cholesterol levels.

Yoga and meditation also can play a role in managing cholesterol. According to research, an elevated stress level also can raise your cholesterol level. So one key to controlling cholesterol is reducing stress. To relax and relieve tension, try deep-breathing exercises, meditation, and three or four yoga poses daily. Yoga practitioners recommend that you be sure to include at least one of these relaxation poses: Baby, Corpse, or Wind Removal. Other therapeutic poses include Sun Salutation, Shoulder Stand, Peacock, Cobra, Spinal Twist, Locust, Lotus, and Bow.

CHRONIC FATIGUE SYNDROME

Signs and Symptoms

- Constant, overwhelming fatigue
- Muscle pain and soreness
- Difficulty concentrating
- Forgetfulness
- Confusion
- Irritability
- Continuous low-grade fever
- Tender, swollen lymph nodes at the neck or armpits
- Generalized headaches
- Lightheadedness or fainting
- Sleep disorders
- Sore throat without evidence of a bacterial infection
- Joint pain that moves from joint to joint without causing swelling or redness

Description

Chronic fatigue syndrome is a condition characterized by extreme, persistent fatigue. The fatigue usually appears suddenly, and is not alleviated by rest. The weakness usually worsens after physical activity and is severe enough to impair your normal daily activities. The syndrome usually strikes young people, and is more prevalent in women than in men.

The cause of chronic fatigue syndrome is unknown, but underlying diseases and viral infections are not thought to be the cause. Many experts believe that the syndrome is caused by nervous system dysfunction, immune system impairment, or low blood pressure.

Conventional Medical Treatment

In order to diagnose chronic fatigue syndrome, a doctor must first rule out other diseases and mental conditions with similar signs, such as psychiatric illness (for example, clinical depression), hypothyroidism, extreme stress, nutritional deficiencies, sleep deprivation, and exposure to the Epstein-Barr virus, which causes infectious mononucleosis. There is currently no test to diagnose chronic fatigue syndrome. Diagnosis is based upon the presence of at least four of the above symptoms lasting for at least six months.

Once a positive diagnosis has been made, the only course of action is to treat the individual symptoms. You will be urged to adopt lifestyle changes, such as incorporating energy-increasing exercise and a nutritious diet into your day. Therapy with a psychologist or professional counselor may be recommended to help you overcome depression, and specific behavioral changes may be suggested to help you sleep. You also may be ad-

Health Notes

➤ *If you have chronic fatigue syndrome and frequently experience lightheadedness, rise slowly from your seated and reclined positions. If you feel lightheaded while standing, ease yourself gently into a seated position to prevent from fainting.*

➤ *Exercise helps ease the symptoms of chronic fatigue syndrome. One study reported that 55 percent of chronic fatigue sufferers who walked or swam for 30 minutes a day, 5 days a week, felt that their condition had improved three months later.*

Chronic Fatigue: Treating the Mind

For many years, doctors have been treating Chronic Fatigue Syndrome (CFS) as a physical illness. Now they are learning to treat the psychological aspects of the disease as well. Here are some interesting facts about the psychological component of CFS:

- Between 50 and 70 percent of CFS patients experience depression, anxiety, or other psychological problems, usually after the onset of the illness.

- According to several experts, treatment protocols should include the options of antidepressant medication and cognitive-behavioral therapy, a form of psychotherapy, to help patients better understand the disease and its symptoms.

CFS suffers can receive counseling from a psychiatrist or psychologist who is both familiar with the disorder and trained in cognitive-behavioral therapy. Other options include a pain specialist or rheumatologist.

vised to break your daily tasks into small portions for easier completion.

For More Information
Chronic Fatigue and Immune Dysfunction Syndrome Association of America
P.O. Box 220398
Charlotte, NC 28222-0398
800-442-3437
http://204.255.5.29

Complementary and Alternative Treatments

Nutrition and Supplementation

Good nutrition is essential to treating CFS. Concentrate on quality protein sources, such as fish, chicken and lamb, and on complex carbohydrates, as they are a steady source of energy. Good foods include whole grains, vegetables, fruits, nuts, and seeds. Boost your immune system with the enzymes provided in juice, especially those "green" juices that contain high levels of chlorophyll. Other beneficial juices are those that contain aloe vera, cucumber, or lemon. Drink a glass of water every two to three waking hours to flush out toxins and help reduce muscle pain. Six 10-ounce glasses daily is not too much. Drink your liquids at room temperature or warmer; cold can shock CFS sufferers.

Avoid caffeine, processed foods, soft drinks, fried foods, and white-flour products, such as bread and pasta. The daily supplement guidelines suggested below will help balance your system:

Most Important

- a prodophilus formula (as directed on label)—replaces friendly bacteria and fights candida, which often occurs with CFS

- coenzyme Q10 (100 mg)—enhances the immune system

- lecithin capsules (1200 mg 3 times daily with meals)—promotes energy

- vitamin C with bioflavonoids (5000 to 10,000 mg)—increases the energy level; use the buffered form

- magnesium and malic acid formula (as directed on label) —reduces body aches and pains

- proteolytic enzymes (as directed on label, 6 times daily on an empty stomach)—improves absorption of nutrients, especially protein

- vitamin E (800 IU for 1 month, then slowly reduce to 400 IU)

Also Recommended

- vitamin B complex (as prescribed by doctor)—essential for increasing energy levels and promoting brain functions; injections are best

- glandular support supplement (adrenal, liver and thymus) (as directed on label)—enhances immune system

183

- maitake and shiitake mushroom supplements (as directed on label)—boosts immune system
- pantothenic acid (100 mg)—enhances immune system functioning
- N-acetyl cysteine (200 mg)—enhances immune system functioning

Ayurvedic Medicine

 Ayurveda views chronic fatigue syndrome as a pitta disorder and treats it by improving digestion and eliminating toxins and allergens. An *Ayurvedic* practitioner may suggest taking *acidophilus, ashwaganda, amla, bala, triphala,* or *lomatium,* according to your needs.

Ayurvedic products are available at many health food stores and Indian pharmacies.

Bodywork and Somatic Practices

 If the body is not overly sensitized, Aston-Patterning, massage, or shiatsu may offer some much-needed pain relief and improve vitality. Excess sensitivity may make CranioSacral Therapy, Feldenkrais, reflexology, Therapeutic Touch, Trager, Reiki or polarity therapy better bets.

Hydrotherapy

 Energize your immune system by taking a hot bath to which you've added hay flower or Epsom salts. Your goal is to raise your body temperature to about 102°F, so soak for 20 to 45 minutes. Follow with at least 1 hour in bed.

Traditional Chinese Medicine

 Acupuncture Acupuncture has proven to be very effective in the treatment and remission of chronic fatigue syndrome.

In most cases, the practitioner begins by attempting to strengthen the immune system and increase the flow of energy in all of the meridians. The acupuncturist also works on balancing patients' *chi* and improving their overall outlook.

Acupressure Some acupressure points that may be manipulated for the relief of symptoms are Conception Vessel 6 on the abdomen; Large Intestine 4 and 10 on the hand and arm, respectively, Lung 9; Stomach 36; Kidney 3; and Gallbladder 20 and 21 on the neck and shoulders. Pressing these points is thought to help combat mental confusion, depression, lethargy, and dizziness, while strengthening the immune system.

Chinese Herbal Therapy Herbs that may lessen the effects of chronic fatigue syndrome include wild Chinese jujube, solomon's seal, ginseng, and cordyceps. Astragalus has been shown to boost the production of disease-fighting white blood cells, while codonopsis may help restore the body's energy level and boost vitality.

In addition, a variety of herbal formulas may be prescribed to treat CFS. These include Astragalus Ten Formula, Ginseng and Atractylodes Formula, Tang Gui and Ginseng Eight, and Minor Bupleurum Formula. Depending on the patient's specific symptoms, the acupuncturist may recommend other herbs, as needed.

Yoga and Meditation

 Exercise, especially yoga with its gentle, easy-going movements, can actually energize the body. To get the most from an exercise session, be sure to include about 5 minutes of breathing exercises, 15 minutes of meditation, and several yoga poses, such as the Mountain, Half Moon, Rag Doll, and Gentle Sun Salute.

CIRRHOSIS

Signs and Symptoms

Cirrhosis often reveals no symptoms until the condition is quite advanced. At this stage, symptoms include:

- Nausea and vomiting
- Appetite and weight loss
- Fatigue
- Sleep disturbance
- Jaundice (yellow coloring of the skin and eyes)
- Darkened urine
- Bruising
- Red, spiderlike blood vessels just beneath the skin
- Lack of interest in sex
- Itching
- Swollen legs, feet, or abdomen
- Muscle wasting

Description

Cirrhosis is a serious, often fatal, liver disease that occurs when liver tissue is continuously damaged. As healthy tissue is replaced with scar tissue, the liver loses its ability to perform its functions, which include detoxifying the blood, storing vitamins and minerals, manufacturing blood clotting substances, and producing bile. A primary result of the condition is that the body becomes poisoned with blood toxins that the liver would usually eliminate. These toxins can have adverse effects on the entire body, including the brain.

Cirrhosis is most often caused by alcoholism—after years of filtering alcohol out of the blood, the liver becomes irreversibly damaged. Other causes of cirrhosis are hepatitis, hemochromatosis (a hereditary disease that causes the body to store excess iron), and Wilson's disease (a hereditary disease that causes liver storage of copper).

Conventional Medical Treatment

If you suspect you have cirrhosis, see your doctor immediately. The disease is diagnosed through observation of symptoms, a blood test, or a liver biopsy. A biopsy, in which a sample of liver tissue is examined microscopically, is the most accurate means of diagnosis.

Health Notes

➤ Your nails may show signs of cirrhosis long before any other symptoms appear. Be on the lookout for banding patterns on fingernails or toenails.

➤ To prevent cirrhosis, curb your intake of alcohol. If you have trouble limiting your alcohol consumption to fewer than two drinks per day, talk to your physician.

➤ Some people's bodies hoard iron. This condition, known as iron overload disease or hemochromatosis, can lead to cirrhosis. Always consult your physician before taking iron supplements.

➤ Vaccinate your children against hepatitis B, which can lead to cirrhosis. Adults at risk of contracting hepatitis B, especially health care workers, should also receive the vaccine.

Since the liver is a resilient organ, the first step to treatment is to discontinue the habits that caused the damage in the first place. If cirrhosis is detected at an early stage and no further damage occurs, the liver should be able to continue to function, albeit in limited capacity. If the cirrhosis is in an advanced stage, your physician treats individual symptoms, such as water-retention and bloating, and strongly recommends a salt-restricted diet and mild diuretics. Liver transplant is the only option for those with severe cirrhosis. Liver transplants are very serious, risky procedures, so they are typically restricted to young or middle-aged people who are in otherwise good health.

For More Information
American Liver Foundation
75 Maiden Lane, Suite 603
New York, NY 10038
800-GO-LIVER
http://sadieo.ucsf.edu/alf/alffinal

Complementary and Alternative Treatments

Nutrition and Supplementation

Experts recommend a mix of high-quality animal and vegetable proteins as well as high-fiber foods such as whole grains, legumes, and fresh vegetables. Use high-quality cold-pressed vegetable oils, and include in your diet almonds, brewer's yeast, grains and seeds, and goat's milk products. To make up for the vitamin K deficiency, eat plenty of green leafy vegetables. Detoxify with fresh vegetable juices such as beet and carrot, and "green" drinks as well as legumes. Avoid all fried foods and hydrogenated/saturated fats. Limit your intake of fish to twice weekly, and do not eat it raw or undercooked. Eliminate candy, milk, white rice, sugar products, pepper, salt, spices, and stimulants of any kind.

Brewer's yeast, rice, and molasses are beneficial. Sesame seeds are especially good for maintaining liver health. Carrots and wheat grass are also good for the liver.

It is extremely important to avoid any substances that are toxic to the liver, including alcohol, insecticides (choose organic produce), drugs, oral contraceptives, food preservatives, and aspirin substitutes (acetaminophen). People with cirrhosis should also avoid taking more than 10,000 IU of vitamin A daily.

Follow this daily supplement regimen to treat cirrhosis of the liver:

Most Important

- vitamin B complex (100 mg, 3 times daily), supplemented with vitamin B_{12} (1000 mcg twice daily)—prevents anemia and protects against nerve damage; use lozenge form
- folic acid (200 mcg)—corrects deficiencies
- evening primrose oil (500 mg twice daily with meals)—prevents imbalance of fatty acids

Also Recommended

- vitamin C (3000 to 8000 mg in divided doses; use a buffered form)
- vitamin E (400 IU)
- liver extract (70 mg)—promotes regeneration of liver tissue and prevents anemia
- L-methionine, L-cysteine, L-glutathione, L-carnitine, and L-arginine (as directed on product label)—aid in detoxification
- coenzyme Q10 (100 mg)—promotes oxygenation
- digestive enzymes (as directed on product label)—lessens strain on the liver
- free-form amino acid complex (as directed on label)—a good source of protein that is easy on the liver
- garlic (as directed on label)—detoxifies the liver and bloodstream

(Consult your healthcare provider regarding the duration of treatment.)

Aromatherapy

The essential oils of thyme (linalol), geranium, rosemary, and rose are sometimes used in treatment of cirrhosis of the liver. Consult a qualified therapist for instructions.

Ayurvedic Medicine

As an overall liver tonic and treatment for cirrhosis, Ayurvedic practitioners advise taking a *kutki-guduchi-shanka-pushpi* herbal formula twice daily after meals and washed down with a little aloe vera juice.

Hydrotherapy

Try soaking in a neutral (body temperature) bath for an hour or two to lower excess body fluid.

Traditional Chinese Medicine

Acupuncture Acupuncture can help strengthen and restore energy balance to the liver, kidney, and heart, which are impaired by excessive drinking. It can also curb alcohol cravings and symptoms of withdrawal, making the individual's recovery more comfortable. Because of the complexity of the disease and its underlying causes, the practitioner may focus on up to 25 acupuncture points on the body, along with related auricular points.

Chinese Herbal Therapy In cirrhosis, Chinese herbs are used to help cleanse and strengthen the liver and associated organs, and to improve circulation within the meridians.

Formulas that may be given in cases of cirrhosis include Bupleurum and Tang Gui, Ginseng and Longan, or Bupleurum and Dragon Bone.

COLD, COMMON

Signs and Symptoms

- Nasal congestion
- Runny nose
- Hacking, dry cough
- Sore throat
- Sneezing
- Headache
- Slight fever and chills
- Fatigue
- Body aches

Description

Everyone has had a cold at some point in their life. The early symptoms are familiar: a tickle in your throat, achiness, and perhaps some nasal congestion. Soon after, you notice the telltale runny nose, low-grade fever, and cough. In no time, you have developed a full-blown cold. The symptoms usually disappear in 7 to 10 days.

Despite what others have told you, common colds are not caused by walks in the rain, exposure to cold air, or going outside with wet hair. Colds are actually caused by one of approximately 200 different viruses. Your symptoms may differ, depending on which virus has infected you—one time you may be bothered by nasal congestion, the next, by fits of coughing.

The virus is usually very contagious. You can contract the illness by inhaling infected droplets that enter the air when a sick person sneezes or coughs. You can also catch a cold by touching an infected surface, then touching your eyes, nose, or mouth. Shaking hands with a person who has been coughing or sneezing into her hand is another common way to get a cold. Symptoms typically appear a day or two after contact with the virus.

Conventional Medical Treatment

While a doctor can easily diagnose a cold with a physical exam, colds are usually self-diagnosed. Thus, formal medical treatment is rarely necessary. Plenty of home rest is a common prescription, as is drinking large amounts of fluid. A humidifier or vaporizer is a good way to keep mucus loose.

Medication is usually not necessary to treat a cold, though adults can take aspirin for aches and pains. Children need to take a substitute pain reliever such as Children's Tylenol® or Children's Motrin®, since aspirin is not recommended. Nonprescription cough syrups and throat drops may ease coughing, and decongestants can relieve nasal congestion. Understand, however, that these remedies do not make colds go away more quickly, they simply alleviate cold symptoms.

It is imperative that you see a physician if you are pregnant, have a compromised immune system, are sick more than 2 weeks, or begin cough-

Can Painkillers Prolong a Cold?

Over-the-counter painkillers—such as aspirin or acetaminophen—may provide temporary relief from cold symptoms, but according to a recent study, they may also cause your cold to linger. A recent study at Johns Hopkins University School of Public Health followed 56 healthy volunteers who intentionally caught colds. Each volunteer was then given either a placebo, aspirin, acetaminophen, or ibuprofen. Those who took aspirin or acetaminophen produced fewer antibodies to fight the virus, suffered from more nasal congestion, and remained ill longer than the others.

Health Notes

➤ *Because cold viruses can survive for several hours on surfaces, such as phone receivers, subway poles, keyboards, and hands, make it a practice to wash your hands several times during the day and avoid touching your face.*

➤ *Organisms found on toothbrushes can cause recurring colds. Change your toothbrush at the first sign of a cold, again when you start to feel better, and again when you are well.*

➤ *Low humidity dries and cracks mucous membranes, reducing their ability to keep cold viruses out of the body. A humidifier adds moisture to indoor air and prevents mucous membranes from drying out and weakening.*

➤ *Studies show that stress can weaken the immune system, making it easier to catch colds. Keep stress to a minimum and aim for at least eight hours of immunity-boosting sleep a night.*

➤ *Moderate exercise boosts the immune system's ability to fight colds. A study found that women who walked briskly for 45 minutes a day, 5 days a week, had about half the rate of colds and the flu as women who didn't exercise. However, if you have a high temperature, muscle aches, hacking cough, chills, or diarrhea, do not exercise.*

➤ *Do not ask your doctor for antibiotics to treat a cold—antibiotics are meant to treat bacterial infections only. In fact, taking antibiotics too often may lead to the development of illnesses with greater antibiotic resistance.*

ing up a thick, gray-green secretion from the lungs.

For More Information
American Medical Association (AMA)
515 North State Street
Chicago, IL 60610
312-464-5000
www.ama-assn.org

National Health Information Center
P.O. Box 1133
Washington DC 20013-1133
800-336-4797
http://nhic-nt.health.org

Complementary and Alternative Treatments

Nutrition and Supplementation

 If you're predisposed to getting many colds during the winter, lower your intake of acidic foods and eat more fruits and vegetables. The antioxidants will help the body fight sickness on its own.

If you already have a cold, cut down or eliminate the gluten (especially wheat) from your diet as well as dairy foods, meat, and sugar. Concentrate on plant foods that supply antioxidants, phytochemicals, and chlorophyll. Fresh, organic juices supply all of these.

Vitamin C and bioflavonoids (always found together in nature) cooperate to protect cells against infection. Take advantage of this dynamic duo by eating grapes, oranges, prunes, cherries, lemon juice, apricots, peppers, papaya, cantaloupe, tomatoes, and broccoli.

If your cold is severe and you feel fatigued, by all means rest. However, if all you have is a stuffy nose, remain active. Activity loosens mucus and fluids. As long as you don't have a fever, take a brisk walk; you'll feel better afterward.

The following daily supplements will help prevent and/or treat the common cold:

- vitamin A (15,000 IU; do not exceed 8000 IU if you are pregnant)—helps heal inflamed mu-

cous membranes and strengthens the immune system

- beta-carotene (15,000 IU)—an antioxidant and precursor of vitamin A
- vitamin C (5000 to 20,000 mg in divided doses)—fights viruses; take 1000 mg per hour to bowel tolerance (If your bowels start to loosen, take 500 mg every other hour.)
- zinc (1 15-mg lozenge every 3 waking hours for 3 days, then 1 lozenge every 4 hours for 1 week; do not exceed a total of 100 mg of zinc per day from all supplements)—boosts the immune system
- free-form amino acid complex (as directed on label)—supplies protein
- kelp (1800 to 3600 mg)—a rich source of balanced minerals
- garlic extract (as directed on label)—boosts immunity

(Take supplements until your symptoms subside. If symptoms persist, seek the advice of your health-care provider.)

Aromatherapy

 To head off a cold before it really takes hold, use the essential oils of ravensare and niaouli, which have antiviral properties, in a diffuser. For a delightful scent, plus an antiseptic effect, add the essential oils of lemon, eucalyptus, pine, or fir to the mixture.

If you're already congested, try a scented steam inhalation to ease breathing and kill bacteria. Add several drops of one of the following essential oils to the steaming water: lavender, eucalyptus, tea tree, peppermint, rosemary, pine, or thyme.

Ayurvedic Medicine

 According to Ayurveda, colds (and the flu) are kapha-vata disorders in which the body has too much moist kapha (a runny nose) as well as too much vata (the chills).

To treat your stuffy head, annoying postnasal drip, and cough, Ayurvedic practitioners may advise drinking ginger-cinnamon or ginger-fennel tea frequently while symptoms last. They also may suggest drinking hot water and ginger several times a day to flush toxins from your system. Using lots of ginger, cayenne, and black pepper in cooking is beneficial as well, practitioners say.

Bodywork and Somatic Practices

Stay away from massage and try Oriental bodywork, reflexology, polarity therapy, Therapeutic Touch, and Reiki.

Homeopathy

Treating a cold with homeopathy is often difficult. Unless you get a very clear picture of the remedy needed for your particular symptoms, you can "chase it" with remedies for a week. If you find a good match, the cold can be resolved pretty quickly.

- *Aconite*—for a cold that comes on very suddenly, sometimes with a high fever, after exposure to cold air or following an emotional shock

- *Allium cepa*—for a cold accompanied by a profuse, watery, nasal discharge that burns the nose and upper lip

- *Arsenicum album*—for a cold accompanied by chills, restlessness, and a burning, watery nasal discharge after sneezing

- *Belladonna*—for a cold that comes on suddenly and intensely, with very high fever and a throbbing headache; face is flushed and hot; skin is hot and dry; very sensitive to noise and movement

- *Ferrum phosphoricum* when you feel like you're "coming down with something," but there are no clear symptoms

- *Kali bichromicum*—for a late-stage cold accompanied by sinus pressure and thick postnasal drip

- *Mercurius*—for a cold accompanied by a bitter, yellow-green nasal discharge; raw, ulcerated nostrils; coated tongue; bad breath; sensitivity to extremes in temperature

- *Nux vomica*—for a head cold with a runny nose during the day and a stopped-up nose at night; symptoms worse outdoors

- *Pulsatilla*—for a "ripe" head cold with bland, thick, yellow-green mucus; nose often clears outdoors

Hydrotherapy

Steam inhalation is one of the best ways to relieve the sinus or nasal congestion from a cold. For instructions on preparing an inhalation, see the "Hydrotherapy" section in the "Introduction to Complementary Therapies."

Soaking in a hot foot bath (102° to 110°F) at night and drinking plenty of water throughout the day also can help relieve discomfort.

Traditional Chinese Medicine

Acupuncture This modality can be used to strengthen *chi* and redirect energy along the body's meridians. Practitioners tend to focus on using acupoints related to the organs most affected by the common cold, such as the lungs, digestive system, and endocrine glands. Acupuncture is also helpful in relieving many cold-related symptoms, including congestion, coughing, fever, muscle aches, and lethargy. Commonly used sites are Large Intestine 4, Lung 7, Kidney 7, and Governing Vessel 14.

An acupuncturist may manipulate many other points as well, depending on specific symptoms. People who are plagued by frequent colds may want to visit an acupuncturist prior to the cold and flu season as a preventive measure.

Acupressure Acupressure treatment can be very helpful in relieving the stiff, achy muscles that often accompany a cold. It also can counteract lethargy and fever and help the immune system work more efficiently.

Points that may be manipulated are Large Intestine 4 (on the hand), Governing Vessel 14 (at the base of the neck), and Bladder 12 (on either side of the spine near the shoulder blades). Various lung, kidney, and stomach points also may be targeted, along with ear points relating to the organs affected.

Chinese Herbal Therapy Chinese patent remedies often used to treat colds include Lonicera and Forsythia Formula, which should be taken at the first sign of illness to lessen the duration and severity of symptoms, and Ilex and Evodia Formula, which combats everything from fever and sore throat to chills and stiff muscles.

COLD SORES

Signs and Symptoms

- Red, painful area of skin, usually around the outside edge of the mouth, that is covered by one or more small, fluid-filled blisters that eventually drain and form a hard, yellow scab

Description

Also called fever blisters, cold sores typically form around the lips, though they sometimes appear in the mouth or on the cheeks, nose, or fingers. The sores are caused by the herpes simplex virus, which can be transmitted through kissing, sharing eating utensils, drinking from the same glass, drying your face with the same towel, or sharing the same face makeup as a person with the virus. After infection, the cold sore may take up to 20 days to appear. Once it develops, the sore can take 7 to 10 days to heal.

Some people develop antibodies to the virus after contracting it for the first time, and they never get cold sores again. Others have repeated episodes of cold sores, usually on or near the original site. Recurrences are usually milder than the initial infection and are sparked by sun exposure, extreme stress, menstruation, or an illness that is accompanied by a fever. Herpes simplex can cause serious illness in some children.

Conventional Medical Treatment

Physicians or dermatologists can diagnose a cold sore by examining the area. They may also take a blood test or a culture of material from your sore in order to establish the presence of herpes simplex virus.

Treatment consists of icing the area to relieve pain and keeping your hands off the sores. The virus can spread from your hands to your cornea, which in turn, can lead to blindness. You should also avoid contact with infants or anyone who has atopic dermatitis. In particular, avoid people who are using an immune system suppression medication, such as cancer patients and organ transplant patients, or those with AIDS, since herpes simplex virus can cause a life-threatening condition in people with suppressed immune systems.

Depending on the severity of the outbreak, your physician may prescribe an anti-viral ointment or oral medication.

For More Information
American Academy of Dermatology
930 Meacham Road
Shaumberg, IL 60173
888-462-DERM
www.aad.org

Health Notes

➤ *Nuts (which contain the amino acid arginine), caffeine, and baked goods are thought to trigger cold sores.*

➤ *In some people, the sun can trigger an outbreak of cold sores. Always wear a sunscreen with SPF of 15 or higher when going outside, and avoid the sun between the hours of 11 a.m. and 3 p.m. when rays are at their strongest.*

➤ *Avoiding alcohol, which is an immunosuppressant, can help prevent cold sores.*

➤ *The body often gives warning signals, called* prodromes, *before cold sore (and herpes) eruptions. Anyone with prior cold sore outbreaks should be on the alert for a puckering, drawing, tingling, or sudden numbness of the skin—common prodromes.*

Complementary and Alternative Treatments

Nutrition and Supplementation

Arginine, an amino acid, encourages the growth of the herpes virus. Avoid foods that contain arginine, including most grains, nuts, chocolate, and legumes. Lysine, another amino acid, balances arginine and inhibits the herpes virus. Lysine can be found in most meats and dairy products.

Take the following daily supplements to treat cold sores:

Most Important

• vitamin B complex (100 to 150 mg twice daily)—important for healing

• vitamin C (3000 to 6000 in divided doses; use a buffered form)

• vitamin E (400 IU)

• vitamin A (50,000 IU; do not exceed 8000 IU if you are pregnant)—vital for healing tissue in mouth and lip area

• *Lactobacillus acidophilus* (as directed on label)—balances bacteria

• zinc and vitamin C lozenges

• L-lysine (4 grams for 4 days in individual doses, then 500 mg 3 times a day for 2 weeks)—fights the virus that causes cold sores

(For an *acute* condition, take supplements until your symptoms subside. If symptoms persist, seek the advice of your healthcare provider. For a *chronic* condition, consult your healthcare provider regarding the duration of treatment.)

Aromatherapy

Any of the following essential oils can accelerate the healing of cold sores: bergamot, eucalyptus, geranium, lavender, lemon, melissa, rose, or tea tree. Apply a single drop twice daily, about 12 hours apart.

Homeopathy

Cold sores may respond to homeopathic treatment. Try these remedies, depending on your symptoms:

• *Arsenicum album*—when the lips burn intensely; you feel chilled

• *Hepar sulfuricum*—for cold sores that are sensitive to cold and painful to the touch

• *Natrum muriaticum*—for cold sores on or near the lips; lips are dry and cracked; can come on after sun exposure

• *Rhus toxicodendron*—if condition is marked by several small, itching blisters filled with yellowish fluid; lips are swollen and inflamed; condition worsens after exertion or exposure to dampness

Traditional Chinese Medicine

 Acupuncture Because practitioners generally attribute cold sores to a damp-heat condition, they typically treat with acupuncture therapy for damp-heat syndrome.

Chinese Herbal Therapy Because Chinese medicine views recurrent herpes outbreaks as a damp-heat imbalance or the result of excess stomach heat, herbs may be prescribed to treat these conditions as well.

Yoga and Meditation

 Since stress can bring on an attack of cold sores, use deep-breathing exercises, meditation, and yoga on a daily basis to release tension. Choose a variety of poses and do three or four each day, being sure to include at least one of the following relaxation poses: Baby, Corpse, or Knee Squeeze.

COLIC

Signs and Symptoms

- Extended periods of loud, sharp wailing and crying in an infant
- Legs drawn up toward the abdomen
- Clenching of fists and curling of toes
- Flushed face
- Cool feet and hands
- Distended stomach

Description

Colic is a condition that affects children younger than three months old. It is marked by crying that continues for hours, several days a week, for several weeks. While pediatricians know that colic affects the digestive system, they still don't know the exact cause. Some theories attribute these painful attacks to allergies, gas, heartburn, overfeeding, or foods that a breastfeeding mother has eaten (especially those with a high-carbohydrate content that might lead to excessive fermentation in the baby's intestines). The baby responds to this pain with severe crying that is often interrupted by wails and screams.

The length of an episode varies from infant to infant. The crying may last only a half hour, or it can continue for several hours until the baby falls asleep from exhaustion or finds relief by passing gas or having a bowel movement.

Though a large number of colicky babies outgrow the condition by three months of age, others have the condition until they are six months old—or even older.

Conventional Medicine Treatment

A pediatrician can diagnose colic after a thorough physical examination. Unfortunately, there is no proven medical treatment for colic. Often, the only advice you get from your doctor is to burp your child after every feeding and—if that doesn't work—to switch to another type of formula (if you are bottle feeding).

For More Information
The American Academy of Pediatrics
141 Northwest Point Boulevard
Elk Grove Village, IL 60007-1098
847-228-5005
www.aap.org

Health Notes

➤ *Creating a calming environment can pacify a colicky baby. Try swaddling the baby in a soft, plushy blanket and giving her a pacifier. Rocking, singing to, or holding a baby over your heart can sometimes lull a colicky baby into a calmer state.*

➤ *Many parents report improvement by changing a baby's position. Time-tested moves include holding a baby upright, or laying him stomach-down on your lap and massaging his back.*

➤ *Placing a warm hot-water bottle against a baby's stomach can loosen cramped abdominal muscles, which may be the reason for colic.*

➤ *Some parents and doctors report luck with gently inserting a rectal thermometer into the baby's rectum, which often spawns an expulsion of gas or a bowel movement, making the baby feel better.*

➤ *While having a colicky baby is extremely taxing for the parent, many parents believe strongly in the importance of continuing to hold the baby while she's crying (as opposed to putting her down in a crib, swing, or bouncing seat), so that the baby feels the parent's physical presence and is not "alone."*

Complementary and Alternative Treatments

Nutrition and Supplementation

 It is estimated that as many as 50 percent of children and babies have difficulty digesting cow's milk, yet many commercial baby formulas contain the substance. Substitute cow's milk with goat's milk or a non-allergic formula.

Breastfed babies may be allergic or sensitive to gas-forming foods in the mother's diet, such as beans, garlic, onions, wheat, and cabbage. Other foods the breastfeeding mother should avoid include caffeine, chocolate, spices, tomatoes, and oranges.

Aromatherapy

 Aromatherapists say any of the following essential oils can help relieve an infant's discomfort from colic: Roman chamomile, fennel, lavender, marjoram, or peppermint. See a qualified therapist for specific advice.

Bodywork and Somatic Practices

 Infant massage has a gas and colic routine as well as a full round of lower torso massage strokes.

Homeopathy

 Colic may respond to homeopathic treatment. However, the selection of a remedy—more than one is available—depends on *your* child's symptoms and the stage of the condition. Don't try treating this disorder yourself. See a homeopathic professional.

Traditional Chinese Medicine

Acupressure Pressing gently on Large Intestine 4 (located on the fleshy part of the hand between the thumb and forefinger) and Conception Vessel 12 (above the navel, between the bottom ribs) may help ease the symptoms of colic.

Chinese Herbal Therapy An herbalist may recommend giving the child a tea made of fennel, ginger, scallions, and citrus peel to help calm the abdominal spasms that characterize this ailment. Depending on what the doctor determines to be the specific cause of the colic, other herbs may be prescribed as well.

COLITIS

Signs and Symptoms

- Abdominal pain
- Diarrhea that contains either blood or pus
- Painful, urgent bowel movements
- Fever
- Fatigue and muscle weakness
- Weight loss
- Joint pain, skin problems, and eye problems

Description

Colitis, or ulcerative colitis as it is also known, is one of the two chronic disorders known as inflammatory bowel syndrome (the other is Crohn's disease). The exact cause of ulcerative colitis is still unknown, but the condition most commonly affects people of Jewish descent between the ages of 15 and 35 and those who have a family history of the disease.

Ulcerative colitis occurs when tiny ulcers and small abscesses develop on the interior walls of the colon, causing moderate to severe inflammation of the intestinal lining. This inflammation causes diarrhea and abdominal pain. Sometimes the ulcers bleed, streaking the diarrhea with blood. Ulcerative colitis usually affects only a small segment of the intestine, though the entire colon can be effected.

Most individuals with colitis have remission periods—during which they do not experience symptoms—that alternate with flare-ups. In some people these painful flare-ups are brought on by stress; in others the cause of flare-ups is less predictable. In the majority of cases, the condition is more a discomfort than a serious health risk. But the approximately 15 percent of sufferers whose entire colons are affected are at increased risk of developing colon cancer.

Conventional Medical Treatment

After taking a detailed history of your symptoms, a physician may perform a barium X-ray, colonoscopy, or sigmoidoscopy to arrive at a diagnosis. Treatment for ulcerative colitis is generally limited to symptomatic periods and typically includes an anti-inflammatory medication, such as sulfasalazine or corticosteroids. An estimated 20 to 25 percent of colitis patients do not respond to medication and need colostomy surgery to remove the affected portion of the colon. If you have had colitis for eight years or more, your physician may suggest an annual colonoscopy to check for cancerous growths.

Health Notes

➤ Eat many small, low-fat/high-protein meals throughout the day instead of three large meals, which can tax the colon. Avoid fried foods, which are high in fat and also cause diarrhea.

➤ During an attack of colitis, avoid nuts and seeds, because they can irritate an inflamed colon.

➤ A high-fiber diet helps move food through the small intestine without overburdening the colon. Fiber should be accompanied by 6 to 8 glasses of water or other liquid each day in order to aid digestion.

➤ Foods with pectin fiber, such as apples and carrots, can soothe the inflamed walls of the colon and boost intestinal efficiency.

C

Crohn's and Colitis Foundation of America
386 Park Avenue South, 17th Floor
New York, NY 10016-8804
800-932-2423
www.ccfa.org

National Digestive Diseases Information
Clearinghouse
2 Information Way
Bethesda, MD 20892-3570
301-654-3810
www.niddk.nih.gov

Complementary and Alternative Treatments

Nutrition and Supplementation

Nutritional needs vary and often depend on other factors, so it is important to consult a holistically-trained healthcare provider to assess your needs. They also can perform a detailed nutritional evaluation, including a comprehensive digestive stool analysis. However, there are some general rules that are important to overall well-being.

Wholesome, natural foods are best, and a diet high in complex carbohydrates also will provide adequate fiber. Include fresh fruits to alleviate constipation. Vegetables and raw juices also help maintain health. The remainder of your diet should consist of legumes and whole grains. Eat brown rice, lentils, or barley to get fiber, and remember that green leafy vegetables are high in magnesium, which aids in regular bowel movements. Protein is best obtained from vegetable sources, but baked or broiled fish, chicken, turkey, and lamb will supply you with acceptable levels. If you eat dairy products, buy the low-fat versions, which are easier to digest. Avoid red meat, sugar, carbonated beverages, and anything containing caffeine—all of which irritate the colon.

Don't skimp on spices; they often aid digestion. Cayenne and horseradish quicken digestion, while basil and dill work to calm an upset stomach.

Food preparation is also important to your diet. Eat food raw as often as possible. If you must cook, steaming is preferable to boiling. Avoid irradiated foods and foods prepared in the microwave. As always, drink plenty of liquids, at least 8 8-ounce glasses of water daily.

These daily supplement suggestions will help prevent and/or treat an attack of colitis:

Most Important

- proteolytic enzymes (as directed on label)—vital for proper digestion of proteins

- a prodophilus formula (as directed on label)—balances intestinal bacteria

- free-form amino acid complex (as directed on label twice daily on an empty stomach)—supplies needed proteins

- L-glutamine (500 mg twice daily on an empty stomach)—maintains the absorption surfaces of the intestines; for better absorption, take with water or juice, 50 mg vitamin B_6, and 100 mg vitamin C

- vitamin B complex (50 to 100 mg in divided doses)—essential for proper digestion and the breakdown of fats, protein, and carbohydrates

Also Recommended

- flaxseed oil (as directed on label)—protects the lining of the colon

- garlic (as directed on label)—has a healing effect on the colon

- Multimineral complex with calcium, chromium, magnesium, and zinc (as directed on label)—minerals are not easily absorbed in colitis victims; calcium is needed for the prevention of cancer, which can occur as a result of constant irritation

- vitamin C with bioflavonoids (3000 to 5000 mg in divided doses)—boosts immune function and heals mucous membranes; use in buffered form

(For an *acute* condition, take supplements until your symptoms subside. If symptoms persist, seek the advice of your healthcare provider. For a *chronic* condition, consult your healthcare provider regarding the duration of treatment.)

Aromatherapy

Try the essential oils of black pepper, Roman chamomile, lavender, neroli, and rosemary to relieve the symptoms of colitis. For specific instructions, see a qualified aromatherapist.

Ayurvedic Medicine

According to Ayurveda, colitis comes about when vata pushes pitta into the colon. The result is inflammation, gas, diarrhea, and abdominal tenderness. Ayurvedic practitioners may recommend fish oils, flaxseed oil, and the herb *boswellia* to lower inflammation. They may also encourage taking *Lactobacillus acidophilus* (a good bacteria that's found in yogurt) to boost intestinal flora and using generous amounts of cumin and ginger, which are soothing seasonings, in cooking. Drinking cumin-ginger tea is helpful, too.

Bodywork and Somatic Practices

Gentle manual therapies can help reduce inflammation, spasms and constipation. Try Oriental bodywork, Cranio-Sacral Therapy, reflexology, and massage. Movement re-education, manual deep tissue techniques, and energy work can also make a difference.

Hydrotherapy

A warm sitz bath with water to the waist or daily contrast therapy (alternating hot and cold compresses) can help relieve discomfort. During an attack, try a hot moist compress on the abdomen.

Traditional Chinese Medicine

Acupuncture The acupuncturist typically attempts to treat the symptoms of colitis (diarrhea, fever, gas, abdominal pain, weight loss) and the cause (be it stress, food allergies, or autoimmune dysfunction) simultaneously.

Different acupoints are targeted, depending on the individual's specific complaints. The bladder and stomach meridians are usually the primary focus, along with points related to the colon.

Acupressure To relieve the symptoms of colitis, a practitioner typically works on Stomach 36 and 40, Spleen 6, and related points in the front and back of the ear. If diarrhea is a problem, Stomach 25 and Conception Vessel 6 may be added to the routine.

Acupressure also can help reduce fever, abdominal cramps and bloating.

Chinese Herbal Therapy Chinese medicine holds that colitis and other irritable bowel syndrome ailments are caused by sadness and anxiety, which results in blocked or stagnant *chi*. To tone the liver, kidneys, and blood, an herbalist may prescribe Ginseng Stomachic Pills or Bupleurum, Inula and Cyperus Forumula (both multisymptom preparations) may be used to treat colitis-related gas, loss of appetite, loose stools, and poor digestion.

Herbs also may be prescribed to strengthen the immune system, minimize allergic reactions, and alleviate stress and tension.

Yoga and Meditation

The following yoga poses can improve blood flow to the intestines and help release the overall tension that accompanies colitis: Chest-Knee, Plow, Locust, Elevated Lotus, and Half Twist.

C

CONJUNCTIVITIS

Signs and Symptoms

- Burning, itching, watering, and redness in one or both eyes
- Yellowish discharge in the eye that forms a crust at the lashline during sleep
- Light sensitivity

Description

Conjunctivitis is an inflammation of the conjunctiva—the transparent membrane that lines the eyelids and the eyeball. Conjunctivitis is caused by a highly contagious viral or bacterial infection or by an allergic reaction in the eye. Infants that are born with blocked tear ducts sometimes develop conjunctivitis (surgery can correct this condition). Regardless of the cause, the symptoms for conjunctivitis are the same.

When caused by a bacterial or viral infection, conjunctivitis is highly infectious and can spread quickly. When an infected person touches a doorknob, telephone, keyboard, or other surface after rubbing her eye, the virus or bacteria is transmitted to that surface. If another person touches the infected surface then later rubs his eye, he may develop conjunctivitis. Symptoms usually appear within two days after contact with the bacteria or virus.

Conventional Medical Treatment

If you think you have conjunctivitis, visit a doctor for a checkup. Your doctor may analyze the eye discharge to see what type of conjunctivitis you have, and, thus, determine a treatment strategy. To treat bacterial conjunctivitis, your doctor may prescribe antibiotic eye drops. If your conjunctivitis is caused by an allergy, an antihistamine may

help. Viral conjunctivitis is typically not treated with medication.

For More Information
National Eye Institute (NEI)
2020 Vision Place
Bethesda, MD 20892-3655
301-496-5248
www.nei.nih.gov

Health Notes

➤ *Apply warm compresses to the affected eye (or eyes) to soothe itching or irritation.*

➤ *If you have conjunctivitis, keep your hands away from your eyes. If you do happen to touch them, wash your hands before touching anything else.*

➤ *To prevent a recurrence of conjunctivitis, discard all the cosmetics and eye creams you used while affected. Also, be sure to change any towels and pillowcases you used during that time.*

Complementary and Alternative Treatments

Nutrition and Supplementation

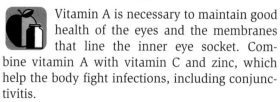 Vitamin A is necessary to maintain good health of the eyes and the membranes that line the inner eye socket. Combine vitamin A with vitamin C and zinc, which help the body fight infections, including conjunctivitis.

Nutritionists recommend the following daily supplements for treating conjunctivitis:

- vitamin C (2000 to 6000 mg in divided doses)
- vitamin A (50,000 IU for 1 month, then reduce to 25,000 IU daily; do not exceed 8000 IU daily if you are pregnant)
- zinc (50 mg)—use lozenge form

(For an *acute* condition, take supplements until your symptoms subside. If symptoms persist, seek the advice of your healthcare provider. For a *chronic* condition, consult your healthcare provider regarding the duration of treatment.)

Homeopathy

 Conjunctivitis may respond to homeopathic treatment. However, the selection of a remedy—more than one is available—depends on *your* symptoms and the stage of the condition. Don't try treating this disorder yourself. See a homeopathic professional.

Hydrotherapy

 Apply alternating hot and cold compresses several times daily to temper the itching, inflammation, and gritty feeling that accompanies conjunctivitis. Use the hot com-

presses for 2 to 3 minutes; follow with cold compresses for 20 minutes.

Traditional Chinese Medicine

 Acupuncture Because practitioners generally attribute conjunctivitis to a damp-heat condition, they typically treat with acupuncture therapy for damp-heat syndrome. The acupuncturist typically focuses on various points along the liver meridian, along with the eye, liver, and related organ points on the ear.

Acupressue Acupressure can be helpful in relieving inflammation and calming irritation. Points that may be targeted are Liver 3 on the foot, Stomach 36 near the knee, and related eye points on the temple and ear.

Chinese Herbal Therapy The herbalist begins by assessing whether the conjunctivitis is caused by an allergy, infection, poor nutrition, or stress. Soaked, big, chrysanthemum flowers laid on eyes will soothe and cool. Patent medicines prescribed may include *Ming Mu Shang Ching Pien* or *Niu Huang Shang Quing Wan.*

SYMPTOM:

CONSTIPATION

Constipation is an uncomfortable condition marked by difficulty passing solid waste from the body. People with constipation typically have bowel movements less than three times a week. Their stools are usually hard and difficult, if not painful, to pass. Constipation can sometimes cause abdominal bloating.

Constipation begins in the intestines. In the colon, water is absorbed from digested food matter, leaving behind a stool. Muscular contrac-

tions then move this stool through the colon. When too much water is absorbed from the stool, or when stool moves through the colon too slowly, constipation usually results. Many illnesses, including hypothyroidism, colon cancer, irritable bowel syndrome, and diverticulitis, can affect this part of the digestive process. Medications—such as those used to treat hypertension, depression, and Parkinson's disease—can also cause constipation. A sedentary lifestyle, low liq-

uid and fiber intake, emotional stress, and travel can also lead to constipation.

Constipation can normally be treated with dietary measures. Drinking 8 to 10 8-ounce glasses of water a day can help soften the stool. Fiber also helps—try to get 25 or more grams a day from fresh fruits and vegetables and whole grains. (See "Nutrition and Supplementation" in the "Introduction to Complementary Therapy" section for information on a whole-foods diet.) Foods helpful in relieving constipation include: rhubarbs, walnuts, flaxseed, avocados, almonds, watercress, apples, grapes, mangoes, dates, endive, parsley, turnips, and dandelion greens. You can use the following spices in cooking or as condiments to aid in digestion and help prevent constipation: turmeric, ginger, garlic, cardamon, cinnamon, cayenne, cumin, black pepper, rosemary, oregano, and thyme. Avoid red meats, dairy products, and caffeinated beverages.

Regular, moderate, physical activity boosts the metabolism, which helps the intestines work more efficiently to quickly dispose of waste. Avoid taking stimulant laxatives to ease constipation; these drugs stimulate intestinal muscles and can lead to decreased digestive function. Instead, take bulk laxatives, such as guar gum, pectin, and psyllium seeds or husks.

Herbal therapists recommend the following herbal remedies to treat constipation: fenugreek (standard infusion, several cups a day), fennel (standard infusion), and aloe vera juice (1/4 cup in the morning and evening). You can also make a laxative tea by steeping 2 teaspoons cascara sagrada or rhubarb root, 2 teaspoons slippery elm, 1 teaspoon licorice, and 1 teaspoon ginger in 6 cups boiled water; take 1 to 4 tablespoons of the tea in the morning and evening.

Some other complementary treatments you can try follow. Aromatherapy can reduce the stress and tension that are sometimes the underlying cause of constipation. Make a massage blend by combining 6 drops marjoram, 6 drops rosemary, 3 drops black pepper or fennel, and 1 ounce vegetable oil; massage this blend into the abdominal area in a clockwise motion. According to Ayurvedic practitioners, people with vata constitutions often suffer from constipation and need to lubricate the digestive tract with warm foods, oil, ghee, and grains. An Ayurvedic practitioner may recommend a vata-clearing, warm sesame oil enema. People with kapha constitutions suffer from sluggish digestion and need to speed digestion with spices and fresh salads. Practitioners may sometimes recommend triphala (a combination of three herbs that strengthens the digestive tract and has a laxative effect.

Another type of complementary treatment is bodywork. For example, some babies who are constipated respond very well to infant massage. Many pregnant women who suffer from the constipation that may occur during pregnancy find massage an effective source of relief. Swedish massage, CranioSacral therapy, polarity therapy, reflexology, and Oriental bodywork can give some immediate relief. If tilted pelvis, weak muscles, or general skeletal misalignment are causing your constipation, deep-tissue work and movement re-education may be helpful.

If you have still have trouble passing solid waste after three days, are in extreme pain, or notice blood in the stool, call your physician immediately.

CORNS AND CALLUSES

Signs and Symptoms

- A thickened layer of skin wherever friction or constant pressure occurs
- Occasional pain or tenderness in the affected area

Description

Corns and calluses are similar ailments. A corn is a spot of hard, thickened skin less than a quarter-inch in diameter that is typically found on the foot or toes. A callus is a larger tract (up to one inch across) of hardened, dead skin found on the hands, feet, or other areas where friction occurs.

Your body develops corns and calluses to prevent tender underlying tissue from being damaged by constant friction or pressure. A pair of ill-fitting shoes can cause your toes to develop corns. Daily use of rope, shovels, barbells, or other hand tools can provoke calluses on your hands.

Conventional Medical Treatment

Corns and calluses usually cause only minor discomfort and are easily treated. Avoid activities or footwear that cause friction in the affected area for a few weeks, and your skin will return to normal. Over-the-counter solutions may help dissolve the thickened skin. If a corn or callus appears ulcerated or infected, see a podiatrist, dermatologist, or family physician. If you have diabetes, see a medical professional to prevent an infection or other complications.

For More Information
American Academy of Dermatology
930 Meacham Road
Schaumberg, IL 60173
888-462-DERM
www.aad.org

Health Notes

➤ *Calluses cause you to shift your weight away from the affected area, changing the way you walk and causing leg and foot fatigue. You can avoid callus strain by using a moleskin pad or by filing the callus with a pumice stone.*

➤ *Only wear shoes that fit properly. Also, do not wear high heels or limit the amount of time you spend in them. Heels of over 2 inches force your toes toward the front of shoes, causing uncomfortable crowding and friction.*

➤ *Donut-shaped corn pads can help remove pressure from the corn.*

Complementary and Alternative Treatments

Aromatherapy

 Aromatherapists recommend the essential oils of lemon and carrot for treating corns and calluses.

Ayurvedic Medicine

 To remove corns and calluses, some Ayurvedic practitioners may advise applying a turmeric-aloe paste followed by mustard oil.

C

Hydrotherapy

Try one of the following treatments to subdue the pain and inflammation associated with corns and calluses:

- Soak your foot in a pan of hot water; dry. Then rub lemon juice into the corn or callus. Repeat daily until symptoms subside.
- Add Epsom salts to a pan of hot water and soak your foot. Dry throughly.

- Apply contrast therapy (alternating hot and cold compresses).

Traditional Chinese Medicine

Chinese Herbal Therapy Aloe vera juice may be massaged into the corn or callus to soften the hardened skin and lessen any pain or inflammation.

SYMPTOM:

COUGHS

Coughing is a protective reflex, whereby the body expels undesired material from the respiratory tract. Coughing can be caused by a speck of microscopic dust, a bit of pollen, or a piece of food that "went down the wrong pipe." When it occurs occasionally and is unaccompanied by other symptoms, coughing is usually nothing to worry about. Taking a drink of water or sucking on a cough drop usually provides adequate relief from any discomfort caused by the cough.

While most coughs are not dangerous, a cough that continues for more than a day, or one that is accompanied by other symptoms is cause for concern. Coughing is a common symptom of many different illnesses, including bronchitis, pneumonia, asthma, influenza, tuberculosis, and even lung cancer, among others. If you think your cough is caused by an underlying illness, call your doctor for advice or an appointment. In addition to a list of your symptoms, your physician will want to hear the cough and know how often your coughing spells occur. If a serious illness is suspected, your physician may want to take a phlegm sample or a chest X-ray.

CRAMPS, MUSCLE

Signs and Symptoms

- Sudden, sharp pain in muscles
- Soreness or tenderness that worsens during movement
- Visible muscle spasm
- Tightness or stiffening in the muscle

Description

A muscle cramp occurs when muscle tissue suddenly contracts, creating a sudden spasm of pain. The muscle may stay cramped for several minutes before returning to its normal position. After cramping, the affected muscle may also be sore and tender to the touch.

Muscle cramps are generally caused by over-

Health Notes

➤ To prevent cramping, always warm up before engaging in any physical activity, and cool down afterward. Stretch all involved muscle groups sufficiently and perform only gentle movements (such as walking) for 5 or 10 minutes before and after use.

➤ Since dehydration makes muscle fibers less flexible and more prone to cramping, be sure to drink at least 8 8-ounce glasses of water daily, or more if you regularly engage in physical activity.

use. Someone who spends long periods of time writing with a pen may experience a cramping sensation in the thumb and first two fingers of the hand. An athlete may get a cramp in a calf muscle after running harder than usual. While physical activity is the primary cause of cramps, dehydration can make the condition worse. Water helps keep muscle tissue supple; when muscle tissue becomes dehydrated, it loses its flexibility and thus is more prone to cramping.

Conventional Medical Treatment

Muscle cramps can usually be treated at home. Gently and continuously massage the affected muscle to relieve the tightness. Once it has loosened up, gently stretch it. If your muscle cramp does not respond to home treatment and lasts for more than an hour, contact your physician. You also should contact your physician if you suffer from frequent muscle cramping. Severe cramps in your shoulders, chest, or arms can be signs of a heart attack.

For More Information
American College of Sports Medicine
P.O. Box 1440
Indianapolis, IN 46206
317-637-9200
www.acsm.org

National Arthritis and Musculoskeletal and Skin Diseases Information Clearinghouse
Bld. 31, Room 4C05
31 Center Drive MSC 2350
Bethesda, MD 20892-2350
301-495-4484
www.nih.gov/niams

Complementary and Alternative Treatments

Nutrition and Supplementation

Eat lots of dark-green and leafy vegetables, such as kelp, brewer's yeast, and alfalfa.

Muscle cramps can be caused by electrolyte (mineral) depletion from overexertion during exercise. To avoid muscle cramps, make a mineral cocktail: combine 16 ounces pure water, the juice of 2 lemons, 1 tablespoon raw honey, and 1/4 to 1/2 teaspoon natural sea salt (available at health food stores); drink during exercise, or whenever you perspire. (*Caution*: If you are on a salt-restricted diet, consult with your healthcare provider before taking this cocktail.) Quality water flushes out toxins stored in the muscles. Drink 1 glass every 3 hours throughout the day.

The following daily supplements are good for preventing or treating muscle cramps:

- magnesium (as magnesium glycinate) (750 mg)

- calcium (as calcium citrate or lactate, not carbonate form) (1500 mg)

- vitamin E (start with 400 IU and slowly increase to 1000 IU daily)—improves circulation; especially beneficial if cramping is due to varicose veins

- vitamin C with bioflavonoids (3000 to 6000 mg)

- vitamin D (400 IU)—necessary for calcium uptake

- potassium (99 mg)—aids in relieving muscle cramps

- omega-3 oils (fish or flaxseed) (as directed on label)—anti-inflammatory

Aromatherapy

Ease your aching, cramping muscles with a delightfully soothing rosemary-lavender massage. To prepare the blend, combine 3 drops each of German chamomile, rosemary, and ginger; 8 drops of lavender; and a 1/2 ounce of almond or avocado oil. Massage the oil into the affected muscles after a relaxing, warm bath. For a different blend, try Roman chamomile, bay, peppermint, and safflower oils. Other beneficial oils include marjoram and clary sage.

Ayurvedic Medicine

In Ayurveda, muscle cramping and spasms are caused by excess vata, which is increased by cold, too much exercise, or poor blood circulation. An Ayurvedic practitioner may suggest massaging the affected muscle with oil of *shatavari* to relax the muscle fibers. He also may encourage you to soak your feet in hot mustard tea.

Bodywork and Somatic Practices

Acupressure and shiatsu are excellent modalities to address cramps.

Chiropractic

Specific chiropractic adjustment (SCA) can be especially helpful in decreasing muscle cramps through active stimulation of the nerves supplying the muscles. Electromuscle stimulation and either moist heat or cold applications can decrease muscle cramps. (Moist heat application is typically used for chronic cramping; cold application, such as ice, is typically used for acute episodes.) The chiropractor may also perform or prescribe cross-friction. A nutritional consult should be obtained in cases of chronic cramping. For example, patients who experience chronic charley horses (cramping of the calf muscles) may be deficient in electrolytes.

Hydrotherapy

Try one or more of the following treatments:

- Apply hot *or* cold packs to the affected muscle for 20 minutes several times daily, until symptoms subside. Some people prefer the hot moist heat; others do best with cool compresses.

- Take a hot bath—either immersion or sitz—for 20 to 60 minutes as needed.

- Use alternating hot and cold compresses twice daily. Apply a hot compress for 3 minutes; replace it with a cold compress for 30 seconds. Repeat the sequence twice. You can add vinegar to the hot pack if desired.

- Take a relaxing hot shower

- Try a neutral (body temperature) bath

Traditional Chinese Medicine

Acupuncture Acupuncture can be used to relax the muscle and improve the circulation of blood to the affected area. Different acupuncture points and meridians are accessed, depending on the specific muscle(s) that need(s) to be treated.

Acupressure Acupressure can be extremely helpful in relieving muscle cramps and spasms. The practitioner usually applies pressure directly to the affected area, and also massages related acupressure points to increase the flow of blood to the area and balance the person's *chi*.

Chinese Herbal Therapy Muscle cramps may be treated with a decoction of corydalis (4 to 10 grams daily). Muscle soreness can be alleviated with *Zheng Gu Shui,* an external liniment designed to relieve pain and relax muscles.

Yoga and Meditation

 Gentle, regular stretching using yoga poses can help ward off cramps, especially in the hamstring and calf muscles.

Try the following poses: Head to Knee, Hero, Posterior Stretch, Spinal Twist, and Standing Angle.

CROHN'S DISEASE

Signs and Symptoms

- Severe abdominal pain and cramping, especially after eating
- Chronic diarrhea, which may contain blood
- Weight loss
- Fatigue
- General weakness
- Low-grade fever
- Abdominal tenderness, especially around the navel or on the lower right side of the abdomen
- Joint pain

Description

Also known as ileitis or regional enteritis, Crohn's disease is one of the two chronic disorders known as inflammatory bowel syndrome. (The other is colitis.) Crohn's disease is a chronic inflammation of the intestine, primarily affecting the lower part of the small intestine (ileum) or the colon. Over time, the inflammation thickens the walls of the intestine, making it unable to absorb nutrients from food.

While the cause of Crohn's disease is unknown, the disease most commonly affects people of Jewish descent between the ages of 15 and 35 who have a family history of Crohn's disease or ulcerative colitis. It almost always begins in young adults. Some sufferers experience only one or two bouts of symptoms followed by a lifetime of remission, while others alternate between symptomatic and asymptomatic periods. In some cases, people experience symptoms continuously. The severity of symptoms also varies from person to person. Some people's symptoms are mild, while others avoid eating in order to lessen the pain felt when food enters the intestines.

Conventional Medical Treatment

After taking a detailed history of symptoms, your physician may perform a barium X-ray, colonoscopy, ileoscopy, enteroscopy, or tissue or mucus biopsy to diagnose Crohn's disease. Currently, there is no cure for Crohn's disease. Treatment, which is generally limited to symptomatic peri-

Can Measles Cause Crohn's Disease?

There is an ongoing debate in the medical community as to whether measles contribute to the development of Crohn's disease. Two separate studies report that people who were exposed to the measles virus in utero have a higher incidence of Crohn's disease. Another study found measles DNA in the inflamed intestinal tissue of individuals with Crohn's disease. On the other hand, various studies report that there is no connection between the two conditions.

ods, usually includes anti-inflammatory medications, such as sulfasalazine and corticosteroids. Your healthcare provider also may recommend a regimen of supplements to supply the nutrients your body cannot get from food.

Up to 70 percent of Crohn's patients require one or more operations to treat complications of the disease, namely obstruction, abscesses, or perforation. In severe cases where the disease is limited to the colon, a colostomy often is performed to remove the affected portion of the large intestine. Although this treatment is effective, it leaves the patient with an ileostomy—an intestinal opening through the abdominal wall—and requires the patient to wear a disposable bag which collects accumulated stool.

Researchers are developing and investigating less aggressive treatments, including:

- long-term antibiotic treatment
- a new corticosteroid, budesonide, that appears to cause fewer side effects than other corticosteroids
- agents that neutralize certain *cytokines*—proteins believed to cause intestinal inflammation
- a separate cytokine, Interleukin 10, that is believed to suppress intestinal inflammation

Controlling Crohn's Disease with Diet

Crohn's disease may go into remission for long periods when patients eliminate foods they cannot tolerate from their diet. As reported in the medical journal, *Lancet,* researchers from Cambridge, England conducted a controlled study of 20 patients with inactive Crohn's disease. Ten of the patients were placed on a carbohydrate- and fiber-rich diet; the remaining 10 were placed on stricter diets which eliminated specific foods. Seven out of 10 of the patients on the stricter diet were able to remain in remission for six months; none of the patients on the high-carbohydrate, high-fiber diet were able to remain in remission this long. In a later trial, researchers found that 51 of 77 patients on the stricter diet remained in remission for over four years. Although the diet was a demanding one, patients were so happy with the general improvement in their condition that they were willing to comply.

- fast-acting immunosuppressive drugs, like methotrexate.

In addition, researchers are investigating supplementation with zinc. Zinc helps neutralize free radicals, those molecules responsible for cellular damage and which may be a contributing factor in intestinal inflammation.

For More Information

Crohn's and Colitis Foundation of America
386 Park Avenue South, 17th Floor
New York, NY 10016-8804
800-932-2423
www.ccfa.org

National Digestive Diseases Information Clearinghouse
2 Information Way
Bethesda, MD 20892-3570
301-654-3810
www.niddk.nih.gov

Health Notes

➤ *Japanese studies show that a diet rich in animal and dairy protein may contribute to the development of Crohn's disease, while a plant-based diet rich in soy foods may prevent development of the disease.*

➤ *Avoid foods high in sugar or salt. Several studies point to high sugar and salt intake as factors that contribute to Crohn's disease.*

➤ *While a liquid diet is advised during a flare-up of Crohn's disease, a high-fiber diet is recommended during remission to help regulate digestion.*

Complementary and Alternative Treatments

Nutrition and Supplementation

Many people with Crohn's disease are histamine-intolerant, so eliminate from your diet all dairy foods (including cheese), fish, hard sausage, and yeast products. Forgo foods that irritate the digestive tract, including alcohol, caffeine, carbonated beverages, chocolate, corn, eggs, meat, pepper, tobacco, white flour, foods with artificial additives or preservatives, fried/greasy foods, margarine, and all animal products (except white fish from clear waters).

Diets high in refined carbohydrates have been linked to Crohn's disease, so don't eat foods such as boxed dry cereals or anything containing sugar. Instead, eat a diet centered around non-acidic fresh or cooked vegetables such as broccoli, cabbage, carrots, garlic, and spinach. Steam, broil, boil, or bake your food. Chewing a couple of papaya seeds daily will enhance your digestion. During an attack, eat steamed vegetables, well-cooked brown rice, oatmeal, and organic baby foods. You need a steady intake of liquids; fresh juices, herbal teas, and steam-distilled water work best.

It is important to have your healthcare provider check your digestive function by doing a comprehensive digestive stool analysis so that an optimal dietary program can be implemented.

This daily supplement guideline should help treat and/or prevent Crohn's disease:

Most Important

- liver extract formulas (as directed on label)—necessary for proper digestion

- vitamin B complex (as prescribed by a doctor)—helps prevent anemia, supplemented with vitamin B_{12} (as prescribed by a doctor)—a deficiency inhibits absorption

- folic acid (as prescribed by a doctor)—needed for cell formation

- flaxseed oil (as directed on label, 3 times daily)—necessary for repair of the digestive tract; essential in Crohn's disease

- vitamin K (as directed on label)—vital to colon health

- zinc (50 mg, not to exceed total of 100 mg from all supplements)—aids in healing; use in lozenge form

- vitamin C with bioflavonoids (1000 mg 3 times daily)—improves immunity; use buffered form

- bromelain (100 mg twice daily, before meals)—improves quercetin absorption

- N-acetyl glucosamine (as directed on label)—improves intestinal health

Also Recommended

- free-form amino acid complex (1/4 tsp twice daily)—essential in the healing of the intestine

- garlic (as directed on label)—combats free radicals

- quercetin (500 mg twice daily, before meals)—slows histamine release

- vitamin D (400 IU)—prevents bone disease from developing as a result of malabsorption

- L-glutamine (2 g)—for intestinal health

- a prodophilus formula (take as directed on label)

- gamma oryzanal (as directed on label)—protects intestinal lining

(For an *acute* condition, take supplements until your symptoms subside. If symptoms persist, seek the advice of your healthcare provider. For a *chronic* condition, consult your healthcare provider regarding the duration of treatment.)

Traditional Chinese Medicine

Acupuncture Acupuncture can be very effective in alleviating the pain, diarrhea, and fever that characterize this ailment. Crohn's disease is treated in much the same way as colitis, but the acupuncturist will also concentrate on points related to the small intestine, mouth, esophagus, and stomach, as symptoms warrant.

Acupressure This modality can be used to remedy the diarrhea, fever, gas, abdominal discomfort, and other symptoms are the hallmark of Crohn's disease. Specific points will be targeted, depending upon the patient' s complaints.

Chinese Herbal Therapy In addition to the herbs mentioned for colitis, Crohn's disease also may warrant the use of herbs that promote digestion and tone the stomach and small intestine.

CROUP

Signs and Symptoms

- A loud, barking cough in a child
- Labored breathing, especially when inhaling
- Hoarseness
- Wheezing or whistling sound while breathing
- Mucus in the airways
- Cold symptoms

Description

Croup is a highly contagious viral infection of the larynx, windpipe, and bronchial tubes. As these important airways narrow from inflammation and mucus buildup, the affected child finds it difficult to breathe. Since the larynx, or voice box, is affected, the cough caused by croup has a forced, barking sound that has been compared to the barking of a seal.

The condition, which strikes boys more than girls, usually occurs in children between the ages of three months and five years. Croup usually lasts for five or six days.

Conventional Medical Treatment

Following a doctor's diagnosis, most cases of croup can be treated at home with measures similar to those used to treat the common cold.

Keeping the environment warm and humid (with a humidifier or vaporizer) is important to make the child comfortable and to loosen phlegm that is trapped in the airways. During an attack of croup, it can help to sit with a child in a bathroom with the door closed and run the shower at full blast with very hot water to create a "room-sized" vaporizer. Drinking large amounts of clear, warm liquids—such as sodium-free broths, warmed fruit juice, and herbal teas—is another way to keep phlegm loose.

Health Notes

➤ *Avoid dairy products, which can increase mucus. Instead of cow's milk, try soy milk.*

➤ *If your doctor recommends ibuprofen for pain relief, and your child has difficulty swallowing pills, liquid ibuprofen is available at most pharmacies.*

➤ *Many croup sufferers find breathing is easier when their head, neck, shoulders, and upper back are propped up by pillows.*

➤ *A mucus suction bulb, available at pharmacies, can help make breathing easier by keeping the nostrils clear of dried mucus. A nasal saline spray can loosen nasal mucus to make suction easier.*

For someone suffering from croup, sitting is usually a more comfortable position than laying down, and breathing is easier when the child is calm rather than agitated or crying. As with any respiratory ailment, children with croup must be protected from strong chemical fumes, cigarette smoke, and exhaust.

If your child's croup hasn't disappeared in six days, or if he is drooling, has difficulty swallowing or bending his neck forward, exhibits a high-pitched squeak when inhaling, has bluish-colored lips, or has a heart rate that exceeds 160 beats per minute, contact your doctor or go to a hospital emergency room immediately.

For More Information

American Medical Association (AMA)
515 North State Street
Chicago, IL 60610
312-464-5000
www.ama-assn.org

National Health Information Center
P.O. Box 1133
Washington DC 20013-1133
800-336-4797
http://nhic-nt.health.org

Complementary and Alternative Treatments

Nutrition and Supplementation

Warm chicken broth simmered with garlic, thyme, and oregano can help soothe the throat and fight infection. Help thin mucus by drinking plenty of fluids, especially herbal teas and steam-distilled water.

Nutritionists recommend the following supplements for treating croup (talk to your health practitioner about specific dosages):

- vitamin C (dosage varies according to age of child)—boosts the immune system

- zinc and vitamin C lozenges (dosage varies according to age of child)—promotes immune function

- vitamin A (2000 IU)—heals mucous membranes

- vitamin E (dosage varies according to age of child)—oxygenates cells

- N-acetyl cysteine (200 mg)—aids in breaking down mucous

(Use supplements until symptoms subside. If symptoms persist, seek the advice of your healthcare provider.)

Homeopathy

Croup may respond to homeopathic treatment. However, the selection of a remedy—more than one is available—depends on *your* child's symptoms and the stage of the condition. Don't try treating this disorder yourself. Seek advice from a homeopathic professional.

Consult your doctor if the cough worsens or your child appears to have trouble breathing.

Traditional Chinese Medicine

Acupuncture Acupuncture can be used to open any blockages in the lung meridians and quiet coughing spasms. The practitioner works on acupoints relating to the lungs and associated organs, such as the heart, the bronchial tubes, and the adrenal glands. Acupuncture can also help calm an anxious child and promote sleep.

Acupressure Although acupressure cannot cure croup, pressing on the Lung 5 acupoint (located near the right elbow) can help control coughing spasms.

Chinese Herbal Therapy Herbal cough medicines are available that may help soothe a croup-related cough.

Cuts, Wounds, Scratches

Signs and Symptoms

- Bleeding and pain
- Tears and abrasions in the outer layers of the skin and possibly the underlying tissue
- Redness and swelling at the wound site (if infected)
- Fever and swollen lymph nodes (if infected)

Description

A cut, scratch, scrape, or wound is an injury to the body's largest organ system, the skin. From a medical standpoint, such injuries are interesting because they allow you to watch the body's self-repair system at work. Most simple injuries heal within two weeks, but one of the biggest dangers is infection.

Most cuts affect only the outer layers of skin, though deep cuts can damage muscles, tendons, and nerves. A laceration is a cut with jagged edges and is often deeper and more damaging than a cut, increasing the risk of infection and scarring. A scrape (also called an abrasion) happens when skin is rubbed against a rough surface, tearing the small blood vessels.. Because scrapes and abrasions sometimes cover a wide area, they are easily contaminated by dirt and bacteria. A puncture wound, such as one caused by a nail or fishhook, creates a deep, narrow hole. Such wounds may not bleed heavily, but may cause internal injury and carry a great risk of tetanus or other infections.

Conventional Medical Treatment

Most simple cuts and scrapes can be taken care of adequately at home. The first steps are to stop the bleeding and clean the injury. For cuts and lacer-ations, allow the blood to flow a little, because that will help carry dirt out of the wound. Then wash the wound with mild antibacterial soap and clean water. If antiseptic wipes are used, use a clean section of the wipe with each cleansing stroke. Stop the bleeding by applying firm but gentle pressure on the cut using clean hands, cloth, or gauze. If the blood soaks through the material used, remove it and replace with clean material. Apply pressure steadily for 10 minutes; your goal is to compress the bleeding vessels long enough to allow the blood to clot. To help slow the bleeding, raise the injured area above the heart. Close small cuts with an over-the-counter bandage or sterile gauze and tape. These dressings help keep the area moist, allowing the cells to regenerate more rapidly and with less scarring.

It's important to attend to scrapes because infections are common. Wash your hands thoroughly before touching the area. Remove dirt completely by washing the area with an antibacterial cleanser and cool, clean water; scrub gently but thoroughly. Use tweezers that have been sterilized in alcohol to remove any dirt that remains. Then rinse and wash the area again. Apply antibiotic ointment and an adhesive bandage, keeping the dressing loose enough so that some air can flow under it. Change the bandage daily and watch for signs of infection, which may not appear for at a day or two. See a doctor if the area is red, tender, or oozing, or has not healed within two weeks.

For puncture wounds, wash the site thoroughly with soap under a strong stream of water. Apply an antiseptic solution and bandage the hole with a sterile gauze pad. Don't tape the hole closed; sealing the wound can increase the likelihood of infection.

More serious wounds may require medical treatment. Seek medical attention if:

- the blood is spurting
- the bleeding can't be controlled following 30 minutes of pressure, or if the wound covers a

Health Notes

➤ *Be prepared to give first aid for cuts, scrapes, and wounds. Keep a first-aid kit handy at home, in the car, or anywhere else you spend time, and make sure the contents are clean and up-to-date.*

➤ *When you administer first aid, be calm and reassuring. Some people, particularly small children, become quite agitated at the sight of blood or from the pain of a small wound. Have the person sit or lie down to lessen the risk of injury that could result from fainting.*

➤ *Antibiotic ointments are the best bet. Many commonly used over-the-counter remedies, such as iodine, may actually retard the healing process.*

➤ *If the cut was caused by a metal object, ask your doctor about a tetanus shot.*

➤ *To limit the risk of infection and to keep scarring to a minimum, keep the edges of the wound together with an over-the-counter bandage until the healing process is complete. Avoid stretching exercises that could widen the scar. Several topical treatments (Mederma Skin Care for Scars® or Clinicel® silicone cushions) may help scar tissue appear softer and smoother.*

➤ *Wear sunscreen to protect newly healed skin from direct sunlight.*

- the cut is deep and to the facial area (to minimize scarring), or to the chest, stomach, back, head, or hand

- numbness or weakness is felt beyond the area of the wound

- signs of infection appear (these include pus, fever, extensive redness, and swelling)

- the cut isn't healing well within two weeks

- the functions of joints or fingers are impaired

- the wound was caused by a metal object and you haven't had a tetanus shot within five years

- the wound was caused by a human or animal bite

Complementary and Alternative Treatments

Aromatherapy

 The essential oils of lavender, tea tree, rosemary, and myrrh are ideal for treating superficial wounds. Simply clean the wound, then place a drop of one of these oils directly on the affected area to prevent infection and speed healing.

Ayurvedic Medicine

 To help heal minor cuts and scratches, clean the affected skin, then apply a paste of turmeric and aloe vera gel. Turmeric imparts a yellow stain to fabric and skin. Then loosely bandage the area.

large area or is more than 1/4 inch deep (Such a wound should be stitched or taped within a few hours by a medical professional.)

- you suspect internal bleeding (symptoms include weakness, perspiration, and pain that seems greater than the visible injury)

- embedded dirt cannot be removed

- the edges of the cut are jagged or gape open

Homeopathy

 Homeopathic practitioners advise, as a first step, using soap and warm water to wash minor cuts, scrapes, and wounds. Then apply *Calendula* ointment to prevent infection and help healing. Alternatively, you can wash the cut or scrape with a blend of 20 drops each of *Calendula* and *Hypericum* tinctures and 1/2 cup water. Then, soak a sterile gauze pad with the mixture and place it over the affected area. Change the dressing several times daily until the cut has healed.

Traditional Chinese Medicine

Acupuncture Acupuncture can help improve the flow of blood to the affected area, which reduces swelling and speeds healing, while carrying infection-causing toxins away from the injury. Acupuncture also can be used to block pain and/or release endorphins, which can help eliminate pain.

Chinese Herbal Therapy There are several Chinese herbs used as external washes or ointments to cleanse, soothe, and hasten the healing of cuts, scratches, and other skin irritations.

More serious wounds can be treated with *Yunnan Bai Yao* (a formula containing pseudo-ginseng). This preparation has antiseptic and clotting properties.

DANDRUFF

Signs and Symptoms

- Flakes of skin on the scalp, face, or ears that may vary in size and appearance—from dry and white to greasy and yellow
- Itchy flaking at the affected area

Description

While everyone's scalp naturally sheds dead skin, dandruff flaking is excessive, with large clumps of dead skin cells lifting off the scalp. Some people mistake a dry scalp caused by harsh detergent shampoos or hot, dry environments for dandruff. But this dryness is nothing more than dehydrated skin. Dandruff, on the other hand, is actually a mild form of seborrheic dermatitis (see "Dermatitis"), a skin condition that has no known cause. Some people are born with a tendency toward the condition and can never get rid of it, while others may experience one or more separate episodes in their lives.

Conventional Medical Treatment

Over-the-counter dandruff lotions and shampoos that contain salicylic acid, sulfur, selenium or tar can effectively treat most people's dandruff. If these treatments fail to improve your condition, visit your dermatologist, who may prescribe a product with a stronger concentration these ingredients or a topical steroid lotion.

For More Information
American Academy of Dermatology
930 North Meacham Road
Schaumburg, IL 60173
888-462-DERM
www.aad.org

Health Notes

➤ While it may be tempting to scratch away excess dead skin from your scalp, this can damage the skin. The best way to remove flakes is to brush your hair with a natural bristle brush to loosen flakes, then rinse with warm water or shampoo.

➤ Dandruff is more prevalent during the winter than during any other season. If you have dandruff, be aware that you may experience an increase in flaking when the cool weather hits.

Complementary and Alternative Treatments

Nutrition and Supplementation

Avoid sugar, fried foods, dairy, flour, chocolate, and nuts.

Deficiencies in essential fatty acids, selenium, and the B-complex vitamins have been linked to dandruff, so follow the daily guidelines below to balance nutrients.

Most Important

- flaxseed oil (as directed on label)—relieves itching and is vital for healthy scalp
- kelp (1000 to 1500 mg)—provides minerals, especially iodine, for increased hair growth
- selenium (200 mcg)—helps control dry scalp
- zinc (30 mg)—repairs tissue and acts as an antioxidant
- vitamin B complex (100 mg twice with meals)—essential for healthy skin and hair

Dandruff

- vitamin E (400 IU and more)—improves circulation

Also Recommended

- vitamin A (up to 20,000 IU, not to exceed 8000 IU if you are pregnant)—prevents dry skin and heals tissue

- mixed carotenoid formula (15,000 IU)—a precursor of vitamin A

- vitamin C with bioflavonoids (3000 to 6000 mg in divided doses)—prevents tissue damage and heals the scalp

- glutathione (as oral supplement, 250 mg daily; in shampoo form, 3 times weekly)—strong antioxidant

(For an *acute* condition, take supplements until your symptoms subside. If symptoms persist, seek the advice of your healthcare provider. For a *chronic* condition, consult your healthcare provider regarding the duration of treatment.)

Aromatherapy

Banish embarrassing and itchy dandruff by rubbing a few drops of the essential oils of rosemary, lemon, and niaouli into your scalp after washing and drying your hair. Or try this anti-dandruff blend: 4 drops of cedarwood, 2 drops of juniper or lemon, and 2 teaspoons of safflower oil. Use several times a week until symptoms subside. Tea tree and patchouli oils are also helpful.

Ayurvedic Medicine

Ayurveda views dandruff as a problem of either fungal infection or poor blood circulation to the scalp. Whichever the case, treatment is simple. Before washing your hair, massage your scalp with sesame oil, which has disinfectant properties.

Fenugreek also has anti-dandruff properties. Use it often in cooking or take a teaspoonful (mixed with a little honey) daily.

Bodywork and Somatic Practices

To provide good lymph and blood circulation, massage may help. (Avoid massage if there are rashes, open cuts, or sores.) CranioSacral Therapy rids the body of stress, strengthens the immune system, and balances fluid and energy flow throughout the body. However, best results come from addressing the body holistically, as in a variety of Oriental bodywork therapies, reflexology, or Reiki. Therapeutic Touch lowers inflammation and irritability and allows the body to heal more swiftly.

Herbal Therapy

To treat pesky dandruff with herbs, you have several options. Try one or more until you find the herbal treatment that keeps your dandruff at bay.

- Drink several cups of nettle tea or take evening primrose capsules daily.

- Rinse your just-washed hair with a strong nettle, sage, and rosemary infusion. To make the infusion, steep equal amounts of dried herbs (about 1 teaspoon each) in boiling water for 10 minutes. Strain and let cool to room temperature. Or use fresh sage and rosemary: steep 1 ounce each of the fresh herbs in 2 cups of water for 24 hours; strain. Use daily.

- Rub burdock seed oil into the scalp to help clear up dandruff caused by seborrhea.

Other helpful herbs include chaparral, dandelion, and red clover. Herbal products are available in health food stores and in some pharmacies and supermarkets. Follow package for specific directions.

Homeopathy

Dandruff may respond to homeopathic treatment. However, the selection of a remedy—more than one is available—depends on *your* symptoms and the stage of the condition. Seek the advice of a homeopathic professional.

Hydrotherapy

Apply contrast therapy (alternating hot and cold water) daily when washing your hair.

Traditional Chinese Medicine

Acupuncture To treat dandruff, an acupuncturist may work points related to the lungs and/or the digestive sys-

tem, both of which are thought to affect the condition of the hair and scalp. Acupuncture also can be used to regulate overactive oil glands caused by hormonal imbalances.

Chinese Herbal Therapy Dang Gui and Arctium Combination and Tang Gui and Gardenia Formula may be recommended for chronic dandruff, especially if it is thought to be caused by seborrheic dermatitis.

DEPRESSION, CLINICAL

Signs and Symptoms

- Persistent feelings of despair, helplessness, hopelessness, or gloom
- Low self-esteem
- Desire to be alone
- Episodes of excessive worry and anxiety
- Irritability
- Lack of interest in once-pleasurable activities
- Abnormal sleeping patterns (insomnia, waking in the early morning, sleeping during the daytime)
- Weight loss or gain
- Fatigue
- Lack of interest in appearance and grooming
- Diminished concentration and decision-making ability
- Inappropriate guilt
- Suicidal thoughts or behavior
- Decreased energy level
- Slowed speech

Description

While everyone feels sad or disappointed at some points during their life, not everyone becomes depressed. Clinical depression is more than a blue mood, it is a psychiatric illness that affects every aspect of a person's life. In fact, depression can take such a toll on a person's spirit that many sufferers are unable to keep up at work, socialize with friends, maintain their households, or even venture out of their home.

Depression strikes women more often than men, and it may strike a person several times during a lifetime. Experts believe that approximately 80 percent of the people who have one episode of depression will have a second. After having a second episode, the chances of having a third, and a fourth episode increase to greater than 90 percent. Without treatment, a single episode of depression generally runs its course between six months and one-and-a-half years.

Although the exact cause of depression is still unknown, researchers believe that certain brain chemicals, called neurotransmitters, play an important role. These chemicals, which help transmit electrical signals between brain cells, are believed to regulate moods. Studies have shown that a high percentage of people with depression have reduced levels of norepinephrine, serotonin, and dopamine—three neurotransmitters. Experts also believe that genetics play a large role in developing the condition.

Mental health experts also see a tendency toward depression in people who lack self-esteem, have adopted submissive or dependent personality traits, or feel a lack of control over their personal surroundings.

Conventional Medical Treatment

If you exhibit four or more symptoms of depression for more than two weeks, contact your physician, who performs a physical examination to rule out any physical ailments. If no physical causes are detected, you are then referred to a psychologist, psychiatrist, or counselor.

While you may feel self-conscious about seeking help for depression, keep in mind that it could take several months or years to overcome clinical depression without professional treatment. Expert treatment, on the other hand, may help you recover and feel better in a matter of weeks. In fact, according to a recent study, 80 percent of those who seek treatment for depression overcome the problem within two to eight weeks. Another reason for seeking professional help is that some people are unable to recover from the illness without assistance. Statistics show that over 50 percent of all victims of suicides are clinically depressed.

Traditional treatment for the condition usually consists of drug therapy and counseling. Commonly-prescribed anti-depressant medications include ricyclics, monoamine oxidase inhibitors (MAOIs), and selective serotonin re-uptake inhibitors (SSRIs). These medications are prescribed to regulate the brain's neurotransmitters, thus addressing any physiological causes for depression. Counseling is typically used in conjunction with drug therapy, to help the sufferer learn how to deal with emotions, attitudes, and personality traits that may have contributed to the depression.

Health Notes

➤ When you're depressed, even regularly performed duties can seem daunting. To avoid feeling overwhelmed, break your tasks into small steps. Also, do not set difficult goals or take on a great deal of responsibility while depressed. Expecting too much from yourself can create feelings of frustration.

➤ When you're depressed, you may want to be alone. However, spending too much time alone can be detrimental to your condition. To prevent yourself from becoming isolated, seek support from people who understand what you're going through, such as sympathetic friends, members of a therapy group, or even an on-line support group.

➤ Make a daily effort to participate in activities that make you feel good. Try moderate exercise, going to a movie, playing an instrument, or attending a concert.

➤ Put off major life decisions—such as getting married, changing jobs, or becoming pregnant—until after your depression has lifted.

For More Information

National Foundation for Depressive Illness
P.O. Box 2257
New York, NY 10116
800-239-1265
www.depression.org

National Mental Health Association
1021 Prince Street
Alexandria, VA 22314-2971
800-969-NMHA
TTY: 800-433-5968
www.nmha.org

Complementary and Alternative Treatments

Nutrition and Supplementation

To prevent chemical and nutritional imbalances that can contribute to depression, avoid fast foods, alcohol, artificial sweeteners, wheat products, simple carbohydrates (like sugar), white flour products, and caffeine. Focus instead on fresh vegetables as well as foods high in protein. Complex carbohydrates are especially important, as deficiencies can cause low serotonin levels, which leads directly to depression. Salmon is high in essential fatty acids, and foods such as turkey and salmon will lift your spirits because they are high in protein and tryptophan, an amino acid necessary to produce serotonin.

Key nutrients for optimizing emotional health include all the B-complex vitamins, essential fatty acids, and magnesium and niacin. Vitamin C is essential for the production of serotonin. S-adensyl-L-methione (SAM-e) has proven effective in treating depression. It isn't an herb or hormone. In fact, it is a chemical compound found in all living cells. In most individuals, the body manufactures all the SAM-e it needs from the amino acid methionine found in soybeans, eggs, seeds, lentils, and meat. Although studies haven't indicated that SAM-e is significantly more effective than prescription anti-depressants, it is less toxic. The following daily guidelines help control depression:

Most Important

- L-tyrosine (up to 50 mg per pound of body weight)—raises dopamine levels, which influences mood and alleviates stress; take at bedtime with 50 mg vitamin B_6 and 100 to 500 mg vitamin C for best absorption. *Caution*: Do not use this supplement if you are currently taking an MAO inhibitor.)

- zinc (30 mg, not to exceed total of 100 mg from all supplements)—a deficiency in people with depression

- vitamin B complex, supplemented with vitamins B_5, B_6 and B_{12} (as directed by your healthcare provider)—necessary for brain and nervous system functioning; injections are recommended for severe cases

- folic acid (400 mcg)—a deficiency in people with depression

Also Recommended

- lecithin (as directed on label)—important in brain function and neurotransmission; do not take if you suffer from bipolar (manic) depression

- calcium (1500 to 2000 mg)—has a calming effect

- magnesium (1000 mg)—works with calcium

- essential fatty acids (as directed on label)—assist in the transmission of nerve impulses

- vitamin C (2000 to 5000 mg in divided doses)—helps prevent depression

- S-adenosyl-L-methionine (SAM-e) (as directed on label)

- St. John's wort (300 mg 3 times daily with food)—raises serotonin levels (Recommended for the treatment of mild to moderate depression. St. John's Wort should not be used in conjunction with other antidepressants, especially selective serotonin reuptake inhibitors (SSRIs). May act as a mild monoamine oxidase inhibitor (MAOI); consult your healthcare provider regarding potential dietary and medication restrictions.)

(Consult your healthcare provider regarding the duration of treatment.)

Aromatherapy

Inhaling a favorite, delightful scent can boost your spirits and relax your mind. Place several drops of an appealing essential oil on a tissue or handkerchief; inhale deeply whenever you please. Some wonderful scents to try include grapefruit, lime, mandarin, bergamot, rose, jasmine, lavender, melissa, and ylang-ylang.

You also can use these scents on your pillowcase and in your bath water.

Ayurvedic Medicine

Ayurveda views depression as being of three types: vata depression, which is associated with nervousness and insomnia; pitta depression, which is associated with anger and fear of failure; and kapha depression, which is associated with weight gain and drowsiness. For each type of mild depression, there are several treatments. For specific remedies, see a qualified Ayurvedic practitioner.

Bodywork and Somatic Practices

CranioSacral Therapy has been used to address mild depression that may appear for "no reason" or is not troublesome enough for medication, but drags down vitality. Oriental bodywork and reflexology are also effective.

Herbal Therapy

Many herbs are well-documented for the treatment of mild depression. Perhaps the best known is St. John's wort, which can stimulate serotonin reuptake. To make a tea using this herb, steep 1 to 2 heaping teaspoons of the dried herb in 1 cup of boiling water for 10 minutes; strain. Alternatively, you can take St. John's wort in capsule or tincture form. (St. John's wort is recommended for the treatment of mild to moderate depression, and should not be used in conjunction with other antidepressants, especially selective serotonin reuptake inhibitors (SSRIs). This herb may act as a mild monoamine oxidase inhibitor (MAOI); consult your healthcare provider regarding potential dietary and medication restrictions.

Other helpful herbs include lavender, lemon balm, oat straw, Siberian ginseng, and licorice.

Herbal products are available in health food stores and in some pharmacies and supermarkets. Follow package for specific directions. Consult your doctor if you can't shake the blues after several weeks.

Homeopathy

Depression may respond to homeopathic treatment. However, the selection of a remedy—more than one is available—depends on *your* symptoms and the stage of the condition. Seek the advice of a homeopathic professional.

Hydrotherapy

Some therapists recommend constitutional therapy several times weekly. For directions, see "Hydrotherapy" in the "Introduction to Complementary Therapies" section. Neutral baths (slightly lower than body temperature) also are suggested.

Traditional Chinese Medicine

Acupuncture In cases of manic depression (see next entry), acupuncture can help balance the patient's mood swings (without interfering with the person's ability to feel sadness or joy, as with conventional medication), control feelings of anger and irritability, and alleviate insomnia and hysteria. The acupoints targeted depend on the symptoms the patient presents at the time of the visit, and on the severity of his or her condition.

Acupressure Acupressure may help regulate the patient's moods and induce a state of calm. To treat mania, the practitioner may press the point located on the center of the bottom crease of the thumb.

Points manipulated during treatment for clinical depression are Heart 7, Spleen 6, and the Yin Tang point, which is centered between the eyebrows.

Yoga and Meditation

 A daily routine of yoga and meditation can help you relax and reflect on your lifestyle. Spend about 30 minutes medi-

tating and 20 minutes doing yoga poses such as Dancer, Knee Squeeze, Lion, Windmill, Shoulder Stand, Sun Salutation, Plow, and Bow.

DEPRESSION, MANIC (BIPOLAR DISORDER)

Signs and Symptoms

People with manic depression alternate between manic symptoms and depressive symptoms.

Manic Symptoms:

- Irritability
- Being easily distracted
- Feelings of euphoria
- Increased energy and activity levels
- Restlessness and racing thoughts
- Rapid speech
- Decreased need for sleep
- Increased sexual drive
- Socially-obnoxious, provocative and/or intrusive behavior
- Substance abuse

Depressive Symptoms:

- Feelings of despair, helplessness, hopelessness, or gloom
- Low self-esteem
- Desire to be alone
- Episodes of excessive worrying and anxiety
- Irritability
- Lack of interest in once-pleasurable activities
- Abnormal sleeping patterns (insomnia, waking in the early morning, sleeping during the daytime)
- Weight loss or gain
- Lack of interest in appearance and grooming
- Diminished concentration and decision-making ability
- Inappropriate guilt
- Suicidal thoughts or behavior
- Decreased energy level
- Slowed speech

Description

Manic depression, *bipolar disorder*, and *manic-depressive illness* are all terms for a mental illness that involves randomly alternating episodes of extreme mania and depression—along with normal periods of behavior in between. For instance, three weeks of mania might precede a month of depression, which is then followed by six months, to many years of normal behavior. Or the periods might come in a totally different order. During a manic phase, a person may be highly animated and talkative, sleeping little, and engaging in frenzied activity. During a depressive state, the same individual may show symptoms of clinical depression, including a change in appetite, sleep disturbances, low self-esteem, and feelings of sadness or worthlessness. Sometimes the mood switches are dramatic and rapid, but most often they are gradual.

According to the National Institute of Mental Health, approximately two million Americans suffer from manic depression, most of whom display symptoms in adolescence or young adulthood. If they are not treated, these symptoms can appear on and off over a lifetime.

Like clinical depression, the exact cause of manic depression is unknown. Also, the illness has been known to run in families. And like clinical depression, an imbalance of neurotransmitters seems to play a role.

Conventional Medical Treatment

If your physician suspects you have manic or bipolar depression, you will be referred to a psychiatrist. The most widely used treatment is lithium, which helps prevent reccurrence of manic

'Tis The Season

Researchers reported that in the majority of sufferers, bipolar disorder is influenced by the time of year. Mania most frequently occurs during the spring or summer, while depression occurs more often in the fall or winter. Experts believe that the increased sunlight during spring and summer elevates mood, while the decreased light during fall and winter depresses mood.

and depressive episodes. For those who cannot tolerate lithium, a combination of anti-convulsants (valproate or carbamazepine) to treat the mania and anti-depressants (fluoxetine/Prozac® or sertraline/Zoloft®) to treat the depression may be used. Therapy also is recommended for people with this condition.

Electroconvulsive therapy (ECT), in which electricity is used to stimulate convulsions, can be helpful in extremely severe cases that do not respond to any medications. ECT is thought to alter the rate at which the brain produces chemicals that affect central nervous system cells. ECT produces fast results—the patient usually feels better within three days of receiving the therapy. There are side effects, including temporary memory loss, headaches, and muscle aches. ECT must be administered separately for each manic-depressive episode.

For More Information

National Depressive and Manic Depressive Association (NDMDA)
730 North Franklin Street, Suite 501
Chicago, IL 60610
800-826-3632
www.ndmda.org

National Foundation for Depressive Illness
P.O. Box 2257
New York, NY 10116
800-239-1265
www.depression.org

Health Notes

➤ *Bipolar disorder is often mistaken for schizophrenia, substance abuse, or post-partum depression. Help your doctor make an accurate diagnosis by presenting a thorough description of all your symptoms.*

➤ *Rapid cycling refers to having four or more yearly cycles of mania and depression. Classic anti-depressant drugs, such as tricyclics and monoamine oxidase inhibitors, can cause an increase in the incidence of rapid cycling in those with bipolar disorder.*

➤ *Many mental health experts report that daily exercise, increased exposure to morning sunlight, and a strict sleep schedule of six to eight hours per day helps lessen the frequency and intensity of manic and depressive episodes in people with bipolar disorder.*

National Mental Health Association
1021 Prince Street
Alexandria, VA 22314
800-969-NMHA
TTY: 800-433-5968
www.nmha.org

Complementary and Alternative Treatments

Nutrition and Supplementation

Bipolar depression is a condition that requires medical supervision. Natural therapies can be used to complement drug therapy, specifically as an adjunct to lithium medication. Some substances, such as 5-hydroxytryptophan and St. John's wort, are useful because of their ability to increase serotonin levels. (St. John's wort is recommended for the treatment of mild to moderate depression, and should not be used in conjunction with other antidepressants, especially selective serotonin reuptake inhibitors (SSRIs). The herb may act as a mild monoamine oxidase inhibitor (MAOI); consult your healthcare provider regarding potential dietary and medication restrictions.

High vanadium levels are associated with manic depression. Experts recommend foods low in vanadium, such as fresh fruits and vegetables. Foods with moderate amounts of vanadium may also be included in the diet; these include grains, dairy products, meats, and seafood. Avoid prepared foods, such as white bread, peanut butter, and commercial breakfast cereals.

Phosphatidylcholine, found in soy lecithin, increases the level of the neurotransmitter acetylcholine, which helps elevate mood.

Nutritionists recommend the following daily supplements for people with manic depression:

- soy lecithin or phosphatidylcholine (10 to 25 g) —*Caution*: Phosphatidylcholine can cause depression in some individuals; discontinue use if this occurs.)
- vitamin C (3 to 5 g)
- vitamin E (400 IU)

(Consult your healthcare provider regarding the duration of treatment.)

Acupressure Manic depression-induced insomnia may be helped by applying pressure to Heart 7, Spleen 6, Kidney 3, and related ear points.

Chinese Herbal Therapy Many Chinese herbs can be helpful in regulating the symptoms of manic depression. Because Chinese practitioners believe that mania is caused by an overstimulated heart, herbs may be given to balance the heart and calm the spirit. In addition, the combination formulas of Bupleurum and Dragon Bone, Concha Marguerita and Ligustrum, Cyperus and Ligusticum, and Ginseng and Zizyphus may be recommended.

DERMATITIS

Signs and Symptoms

- A rash of small, red bumps and thickened skin; the bumps are often filled with fluid
- Itching at the affected site
- Scaling at the affected area

Description

Dermatitis is a condition in which a limited area of skin becomes red, thickened, and covered with a rash of small, red bumps. The area may itch mildly or severely. The term dermatitis means "inflammation of the skin" and refers to specific ailments, such as eczema, allergic contact dermatitis, irritant contact dermatitis, atopic dermatitis, stasis dermatitis, diaper rash, and seborrheic dermatitis—all conditions with similar symptoms.

Dermatitis can be caused by exposure to a skin irritant, such as a new skin care cream or piece of jewelry. Extreme anxiety, stress, or excessive perspiration can also cause a reaction. Some people experience a recurring form of the disease, which comes unexpectedly, goes away when treated, and shows up again sometime later.

Conventional Medical Treatment

If you suspect you have dermatitis, visit a dermatologist, who can diagnose the condition with a physical exam. Most cases are treated with a hydrocortisone cream, which is applied to the area to reduce inflammation and itching. You will also need to keep the afflicted skin clean (your derma-

Health Notes

➤ *To help prevent an outbreak of dermatitis, wear rubber or vinyl gloves when working with any type of harsh household solution, such as cleaning fluid or window cleaner.*

➤ *If you have sensitive skin, avoid fragranced bath products, such as bubble bath or perfumed bath salts.*

➤ *Hot showers and baths aggravate dermatitis. If you have the condition, bathe in lukewarm water. When drying yourself, do not rub at the skin with a towel. Blot away moisture instead.*

➤ *Scratching an area affected with dermatitis can damage the skin. To prevent further itching, avoid wearing skin-irritating wool and acrylic fabrics. If you find it nearly impossible to keep from scratching, try cutting nails short until your condition improves.*

The Eyes Have It

The skin of the upper and lower eyelids is thin and sensitive, making it especially prone to dermatitis. While your eyes may rarely come directly in contact with an aggravating substance, this skin is so sensitive that the touch of a finger or a strand of hair can cause a reaction. For instance, many nail polishes contain toluene, which is a strong irritant. Rubbing an eye with a painted fingernail can cause a reaction. Many hair styling products also contain irritants, meaning that a stray strand of hair falling across the eye can cause irritation, as can a stray hairspray particle that lands on or near the eye. Eye creams and facial cleansers are other common sources of eyelid dermatitis. Dermatitis of the eyelid is easily treated, but many people who experience dermatitis of the eyelid have several episodes throughout their lives, each caused by a different or recurrent use of the same aggravating agent.

tologist may advise using a non-perfumed soap), and dry. If your dermatitis was caused by a skin irritant, you will certainly want to avoid further contact with the substance or object. Most cases of dermatitis disappear within three days to a week of treatment.

For More Information
American Academy of Dermatology
930 North Meacham Road
Schaumburg, IL 60173
800-462-DERM
www.aad.org

National Arthritis and Musculoskeletal and Skin Diseases Information Clearinghouse
31 Center Drive, MSC 2350, Building 31, Room 4C05
Bethesda, MD 20892-2350
301-495-4484
www.nih.gov/niams

Complementary and Alternative Treatments

Nutrition and Supplementation

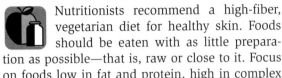

Nutritionists recommend a high-fiber, vegetarian diet for healthy skin. Foods should be eaten with as little preparation as possible—that is, raw or close to it. Focus on foods low in fat and protein, high in complex carbohydrates. Foods such as potatoes, yams, carrots, dark green vegetables, and peppers are high in vitamins A and C, beta-carotene, and chlorophyll. Water is also essential to good skin condition, and you should drink at least 5 8-ounce glasses of pure water daily. Also 2 or 3 8-ounce servings of fresh juice provide a healthy supply of nutrients.

Foods to avoid include dairy products, sugar, fats, and fried or processed foods. Check for food allergies, beginning with gluten (wheat, oats, barley, rye), which often contributes to dermatitis. Try a gluten-free diet for six weeks, and then slowly introduce gluten back into your diet. If your condition improved on the gluten-free regimen, you'll know to completely remove it from your diet.

Nutritionists suggest the following daily supplements:

Most Important

- vitamin B complex (50 to 100 mg 3 times with meals)—necessary for circulation and aids in cell reproduction
- kelp (1000 mg)—contains minerals that promote healing of tissues
- flaxseed oil (1 tbsp)—promotes lubrication of the skin
- vitamin E (400 IU or more)—relieves itching
- zinc (30 mg)—aids healing; use in lozenge form

Also Recommended

- free-form amino acid complex (as directed on label)—supplies protein necessary for repair of all tissues

- vitamin A emulsion (100,000 IU daily for 1 month, then 50,000 IU for 2 weeks, then 25,000 IU; do not exceed 8000 IU daily if you are pregnant)—promotes smooth skin and helps prevent dryness
- vitamin D (400 to 1000 IU daily)—heals tissues
- vitamin C (2000 mg)—important for skin repair

(For an *acute* condition, take supplements until your symptoms subside. If symptoms persist, seek the advice of your healthcare provider. For a *chronic* condition, consult your healthcare provider regarding the duration of treatment.)

Aromatherapy

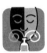

To relieve itchy skin, add 10 drops of German chamomile to warm bath water, then soak for about 10 minutes. Pat dry. (Rubbing your skin will make it itchier.) After bathing, apply lotion or almond oil to which you've added the essential oils of German chamomile, lavender, and bergamot. Other beneficial essential oils include geranium, hyssop, peppermint, and myrrh.

Herbal Therapy

Evening primrose oil is a highly effective treatment for the intense itch that accompanies dermatitis. Take 4 500 mg capsules twice daily until symptoms subside.

Burdock and dandelion teas are also quite helpful in relieving inflammation and itching. Simmer 1 tablespoon of the dried root of either herb in 1 cup of boiling water for 10 minutes; strain. Drink a cupful several times daily.

Other beneficial herbal remedies include: tinctures of nettle, red clover, and cleavers (combine in equal amounts and take ½ teaspoonful daily), or nettle and cleavers teas (drink daily). You also can wash the affected area with a chickweed infusion, or apply a calendula salve to affected skin.

Herbal products are available in health food

stores and in some pharmacies and supermarkets. Follow package for specific directions.

Homeopathy

Dermatitis may respond to homeopathic treatment. However, the selection of a remedy—more than one is available—depends on *your* symptoms and the stage of the condition. Don't try treating this disorder yourself. See a homeopathic professional.

Hydrotherapy

Cold compresses can help quiet itching and pain. Apply 20 minutes on, 20 minutes off while symptoms last. Remember not to use cold for more than 20 minutes at a time; prolonged exposure can damage skin.

Alternately, try a lukewarm (94° to 98° F) bath to which you've added 1 cup of baking soda; soak for 30 to 60 minutes and pat dry.

Traditional Chinese Medicine

Acupuncture This modality is very effective in lessening the itchiness and inflammation associated with dermatitis and related conditions, such as eczema.

Acupressure Acupressure can be used to enhance immunity, thereby reducing the chances of allergic reactions, such as contact dermatitis or eczema. To stimulate the immune system, an acupressurist may target Bladder 47 and 23. Eczema may be treated by pressing on Liver 3, Stomach 36, and various ear points.

Chinese Herbal Therapy Aloe vera is an herb traditionally used to treat dermatitis and eczema. Dang Gui and Arctium Combination can be used to treat chronic dermatitis. Any constitutional diagnosis can be treated by a practitioner/acupuncturist.

Yoga and Meditation

Dermatitis flares up when stress levels rise. To control stress and release tension, use deep breathing, meditation, and yoga in a daily routine. Be sure to include at least four yoga poses in your program. One should be a relaxation pose, such as the Baby, Corpse, or Wind Removal. Breath of Fire breathing can also be helpful.

DIABETES

Signs and Symptoms

- Increased thirst and urination
- Fatigue
- Weight loss despite an increased appetite
- Recurrent skin infections
- Frequent vaginitis (in women)
- Nausea and vomiting
- Blurred and/or weakened vision
- Loss of consciousness or confusion
- Numbness in hands or feet

Description

Diabetes mellitus is a condition characterized by high blood glucose levels. The condition can be caused by a failure of the pancreas to produce sufficient insulin or by the body's resistance to the action of insulin. Insulin is a hormone produced by the pancreas, which enables the body to regulate the amount of sugar (glucose) in a person's blood.

According to the Centers for Disease Control and Prevention, more than 15 million Americans have diabetes—and approximately half of them suffer from the disease unknowingly. Many people are unaware that they have the condition because mild diabetes can continue for years with virtually no symptoms.

There are two types of diabetes. Insulin-dependent diabetes (Type 1) most often strikes children and young adults. In Type 1 diabetes, the pancreas produces little to no insulin. In non-insulin dependent diabetes (Type 2), the pancreas does produce insulin, but the person's body is unable to process it. Most people who suffer from Type 2 diabetes are over the age of 40; many are overweight or even obese.

Diabetes and the Computer Age

Computer programs are available to track every aspect of your condition, such as fluctuations in blood sugar levels, weight, and blood pressure as well as changes in optimum diet and exercise requirements. Before downloading software from the Internet or going to a computer store to buy a program, call the manufacturer of your blood glucose monitor and ask about compatible programs.

Some programs download the information from your blood glucose meter while others need you to type in your current blood sugar level. There are programs that focus solely on tracking fluctuations in your blood sugar readings over a space of time—some of these can even fax this data directly to your physician. There are even "lifestyle" programs that help you create a daily or weekly diet and exercise plan based on your glucose readings.

Health Notes

➤ *Diabetes symptoms are so mild in some people that they mistake them for normal signs of aging. For this reason, the American Diabetes Association, the Centers for Disease Control, and the National Institutes of Health recommend that all adults age 45 and older get blood sugar testing every three years.*

➤ *Diabetes can have an impact on your sexuality. Nerve and blood vessel damage caused by chronic high blood sugar leads to loss of skin sensation and overall lack of libido. In men, diabetes can cause impotence, while in women, it can cause poor vaginal lubrication and pain during sex.*

➤ *Diabetes can affect your skin. To protect your skin watch your blood pressure, keep skin clean and dry, avoid hot showers and baths, use moisturized superfatted soaps and mild shampoos, moisturize your skin, treat cuts immediately, monitor the condition of your feet, and keep your diabetes well controlled to avoid yeast infections.*

➤ *If you have diabetes, always carry a sugar-rich snack, such as a candy bar or a soft drink, in your bag in case your blood sugar levels fall unexpectedly and you don't have access to food.*

➤ *If you are taking a vacation in a high-altitude destination, be aware that your blood glucose meter might give you different readings. The device uses oxygen, which is in shorter supply at high altitudes. Talk with you doctor and the meter's manufacturer before you leave home.*

➤ *Drinking can pose a danger to people on medications that lower blood sugar. Whatever you do, don't drink on an empty stomach. Eat a high-fiber complex carbohydrate along with any alcoholic beverage.*

Diabetes

There is no one definitive factor known to cause diabetes. Heredity does play a part: Approximately two-thirds of all people with diabetes have one or more family members with the disease. Environmental toxins, autoimmune disorders, and viruses (such as mumps or hepatitis) are believed to cause Type 1 diabetes. Obesity significantly raises your risk for Type 2 diabetes.

If not treated, both types of diabetes can result in serious complications. Vision problems, caused by a weakening of the capillaries that supply blood to the eye, are common among people with diabetes and can result in blindness. Kidney disease, also caused by a deterioration of the small blood vessels is another common malady. In addition, people with diabetes are at high risk for developing coronary artery disease, heart attack, stroke, high blood pressure, skin infections, and gangrene (because of poor circulation in the legs).

For More Information
American Diabetes Association
1710 North Beauregard Street
Alexandria, VA 22311
800-DIABETES
www.diabetes.org

Juvenile Diabetes Foundation
120 Wall Street
New York, NY 10005-4001
212-785-9500
www.jdf.org

National Institute of Diabetes and
Digestive and Kidney Diseases
31 Center Drive, MSC 2560
Bethesda, MD 20892-2560
301-654-3810
www.niddk.nih.gov

Conventional Medical Treatment

To diagnose diabetes, your physician takes urine and blood samples and tests both samples for high blood sugar levels. If you are diagnosed with diabetes, you will need to adjust your insulin levels. Since insulin cannot be taken orally, people with Type 1 have to receive daily insulin injections. Your doctor will teach you how to give yourself the necessary insulin injections. At first, this might sound unpleasant, but it quickly becomes part of your daily routine. Some people with Type 2 diabetes are able to control the condition through diet and exercise. Others may require an oral hypoglycemic medication to stimulate the production of insulin.

For either type of diabetes, a diet of complex carbohydrates (brown rice and whole grains), fruits, vegetables, lean protein, and dairy products is also prescribed. Moderate exercise is also a necessity for people with diabetes. Because obesity exacerbates diabetes, overweight individuals are advised to regulate their weight through a sound regimen of low-fat foods and moderate physical activity.

Complementary and Alternative Treatments

Nutrition and Supplementation

 Many healthcare providers who support complementary approaches suggest that people with diabetes follow the same diet as heart disease patients since the disorders are so closely related. Eat many high-fiber vegetables raw, steamed, baked, or stir fried with little or no oil. Adding fresh vegetable, rather than fruit, juices to your diet lowers the need for insulin, as they lower the levels of fat in the blood. Snack on foods such as almonds, nut butters, rice bran crackers, and hummus or other legumes. Diabetics should avoid foods such as pasta, potatoes, rice, corn, bananas, raisins, and sweet fruits and vegetables, such as carrots, until insulin levels stabilize. These foods are high in carbohydrates, and carbohydrates stimulate insulin production. Protein should be obtained through fish, lean meats, low-fat dairy products, soy foods, and legumes. If you suspect a food allergy, eliminate the suspect food from your diet for six weeks and assess any improvement in your condition.

Perhaps the most important mineral for diabetes is vanadyl sulfate. It was discovered in the late 1800s and was used to control the disorder before the development of insulin. Follow the directions on the label. The following daily supplements also improve diabetic condition:

Most Important

- chromium picolinate (400 to 600 mcg)—improves insulin's efficiency

- L-glutamine (500 mg twice daily)—reduces the craving for sugar

- taurine (500 mg twice daily)—helps the body release insulin

- quercetin (100 mg 3 times daily)—helps prevent polyols from forming in the membranes of the eye lens (This condition, which damages the lens, results from excess glucose accumulation.)

- vitamin B complex (50 mg 3 times daily, not to exceed 300 mg from all supplements)

- biotin (50 mg)—improves metabolism of glucose

- vitamin B$_{12}$ (as directed on label)—prevents diabetic neuropathy; injections are best

- zinc (50 to 80 mg, not to exceed a total of 100 mg from all supplements)—deficiency has been linked to diabetes; use lozenge form

Also Recommended

- coenzyme Q10 (80 mg)—stabilizes blood sugar levels

- magnesium (750 mg)—balances the pH level

- manganese (5 to 10 mg)—a deficiency is common in people with diabetes; take separately from calcium

- vitamin A (15,000 IU; do not exceed 8000 IU if you are pregnant)—maintains eye health

- vitamin C (3000 to 6000 mg)—a deficiency may lead to vascular problems in people with diabetes

- vitamin E (400 IU or more)—improves circulation

- multienzyme complex (as directed on label)—aids digestion

- lipoic acid (as directed on label)—treats diabetic neuropathy

- phosphatidyl serine (as directed on label)—aids in treatment of diabetic neuropathy

- acetyl-L-carnitine (as directed on label)—aids in treatment of diabetic neuropathy

Aromatherapy

To relieve diabetes symptoms, some aromatherapists suggest using the essential oils of juniper, geranium, and eucalyptus. See a qualified therapist for details.

Ayurvedic Medicine

Ayurveda considers diabetes a kapha disorder of low agni (digestive fire) and offers a variety of treatments, including the following that can be undertaken with the guidance of a qualified practitioner: Take turmeric daily to control blood sugar (you can take it alone or in combination with ground bay leaf and aloe vera gel); follow a pacifying diet by avoiding too many sweets; and participate in a supervised *pancha karma* program. Consult your doctor before starting a new regimen; diabetes must be carefully monitored.

Bodywork and Somatic Practices

Reflexology, polarity therapy, and Oriental bodywork therapies can be helpful in balancing energy and reducing stress.

Herbal Therapy

Garlic can aid in stabilizing blood sugar. Ask your healthcare provider if garlic capsules are right for you.

Many herbs are known to affect blood sugar levels, which in turn can cause significant variation in the need for insulin. Such variation could ultimately result in insulin shock or diabetic coma. Therefore, persons with known diabetic conditions should take precautions and try herbal preparations only under close medical supervision.

Traditional Chinese Medicine

Acupuncture Acupuncture can be used to help control stress, which in turn impacts the patient's blood sugar level. Acupuncture also can be used to fortify overall immunity and strengthen organs that may otherwise be compromised by diabetes. Usually the practitioner works on points associated with the bladder, kidneys, spleen, pancreas, and related organs and meridians.

Acupressure Acupressure may be used to control diabetes-related symptoms, such as fatigue, cramps, and menstrual problems. In addition, ap-

plying pressure to Bladder points 18, 19, 20, and 23 can help stimulate liver and pancreas functioning, making the body better able to cope with the disease.

Chinese Herbal Therapy Ginseng has been shown to regulate blood sugar levels and is often used to treat diabetes. Major Four Herbs Formula and Rehmannia Six Combination also may be used, but a full diagnosis is needed.

Yoga and Meditation

Yoga, mediation, and breathing exercises can improve blood circulation and enhance digestion, therefore helping you cope with diabetes. Establish a daily routine of at least four poses, such as the Chest-Knee, Sun Salutation, Peacock, Locust, and Leg Lift. Yogic exercises can also be helpful; see a trained therapist for instructions on yogic exercises.

DIAPER RASH

Signs and Symptoms

- A pink or reddish rash covering the groin, and/or buttocks and thighs of an infant or toddler that can progress to peeling of the skin, open sores, and infection

Description

Diaper rash is a form of dermatitis caused by irritation from the constant wetness of a soaked diaper, exposure to a chemical irritant (such as a skin lotion or a laundry detergent) or by ammonia formation beneath the diaper. Ammonia forms when bacteria in the baby's stool reacts

with the baby's urine. The condition is believed to affect 35 percent of all babies.

Conventional Medical Treatment

Fungal and yeast infections are often mistaken for diaper rash, so if you're unsure whether your baby has diaper rash, visit your pediatrician. The doctor will conduct a physical exam to diagnose the condition. Treatment typically includes keeping the area dry and clean and exposed to air as much as possible, changing the baby's diaper frequently, and using zinc oxide diaper cream. With treatment, the condition generally improves within a week. In severe cases, some pediatricians suggest applying a cortisone ointment.

Health Notes

➤ *If you use cloth diapers and do not have them cleaned by a diaper service, always wash them with a mild detergent, and then rinse twice. Do not use bleach. The residue from soap and bleach can irritate a baby's skin.*

➤ *Avoid plastic diaper covers. These trap moisture against the skin, contributing to diaper rash.*

➤ *Bulky or multilayered diapers become misshapen and heavy when wet, chafing against the skin and causing irritation. Change your child as soon as his diaper becomes wet or soiled.*

➤ *If you use disposable diapers and your child experiences recurring diaper rash, you may want to try another brand of disposable diaper. You may find that your baby tolerates one kind better than another.*

➤ *After each diaper change, wash the skin with a mild unperfumed soap or commercial baby wipe and thoroughly dry the area. If possible, leave the skin open to the air for 5 to 10 minutes after each diaper change.*

➤ *Commercial baby wipes often contain alcohol or propylene glycol which can irritate some babies' skin. If your baby is sensitive to these ingredients, look for alcohol-free wipes or use a dampened washcloth. Dry thoroughly.*

➤ *To help prevent diaper rash, try protecting the skin with a diaper cream or zinc oxide ointment. Apply the cream to dry skin only. Discontinue use if a rash develops. Avoid lanolin products, which can irritate skin.*

➤ *If the rash is mainly in the skin creases, this may indicate a yeast infection.*

For More Information
American Academy of Dermatology
930 North Meacham Road
Schaumburg, IL 60173
800-462-DERM
www.aad.org

The American Academy of Pediatrics
141 Northwest Point Boulevard
Elk Grove Village, IL 60007-1098
847-228-5005
www.aap.org

Complementary and Alternative Treatments

Aromatherapy

 To prevent diaper rash, apply an easy-to-make, anti-rash lotion containing essential oils every time you change the baby's diaper. To make the lotion, mix 2 drops each of lavender and German chamomile with 4 teaspoons of safflower oil or carrier lotion.

Homeopathy

 Diaper rash is best treated by a homeopathic practitioner who will recommend a course of treatment. The practitioner may also suggest washing the affected area with a *Calendula* lotion, then dusting it with a *Calendula* powder.

Hydrotherapy

 Change the diaper and wash the area frequently. Expose the area to air whenever you can.

Traditional Chinese Medicine

 Chinese Herbal Therapy An external wash made from chrysanthemum can be used to soothe diaper rash, as can licorice. Internal herbal preparations should be used on infants and children only under a doctor's supervision.

d

DIARRHEA

Diarrhea is a common symptom of many intestinal disorders—viral gastroenteritis, malabsorption syndrome, colitis, irritable bowel syndrome, lactose and gluten intolerance, yeast allergies, and food poisoning.

Some medications, such as antibiotics and antacids, can even cause diarrhea. Surgery on any part of the gastrointestinal tract can result in post-operative diarrhea. A juice fast (a diet consisting of nothing but vegetable and fruit juices) or eating certain fruits or spicy foods can cause diarrhea in some people. Intestinal parasites can also cause this condition.

Diarrhea is characterized by a sudden increase in the number of bowel movements you have, and a change in their consistency. Someone with diarrhea typically has more than three soft-to-watery bowel movements a day. Bowel discomfort, cramping, and a sense of urgency to have bowel movements commonly accompany the condition.

Diarrhea can usually be treated at home with an over-the-counter medication, such as Kaopectate® or Pepto-Bismol®, taken according to package directions.

Nutrition plays an important role in treating diarrhea. The condition may be related to food allergies, especially to milk and gluten (in grains). Foods helpful in preventing diarrhea include: pomegranate, carrots, natural yogurt (containing Lactobacillus acidophilus) apples, and carob. Bananas contain potassium and magnesium, both of which tone the intestines and colon. In addition, take these daily supplements: vitamin C (standard dose), Lactobacillus acidophilus capsules (follow directions on the package label), niacin (standard dose), and carob powder (2 tablespoons mixed with some applesauce).

Herbal therapists recommend the following preparations for treating diarrhea: cayenne pepper capsules (follow directions on product label), ginger tea (standard infusion), and slippery elm powder (mix 1 tsp with pineapple juice). Herbs that soothe the digestive system include: chamomile (standard infusion), marshmallow root (standard decoction), catnip (standard infusion), and fenugreek (standard infusion). You also can make a soothing tea by combining equal parts raspberry, catnip, and chamomile. Use standard infusions.

In cases when you have bowel movements hourly—or even more often—and are losing a lot of fluid, you run the risk of becoming dehydrated. If this is the case, drink extra glasses of water or a sports drink, such as Gatorade®, to replace lost fluids, and call your doctor for further advice.

You may have to go on a three-to-five- day regimen of antibiotics if bacteria is the suspected cause of your condition. Check with your health-care provider.

If your diarrhea is extremely severe and accompanied by other symptoms, such as a change in the quality of your skin (cool, clammy, and pale), chills, fever, muscle weakness, or profuse sweating, or if your fecal matter is tinged with blood, proceed without delay to your doctor's office, a clinic, or a nearby hospital emergency room.

DIVERTICULITIS

Signs and Symptoms

- Sudden onset of diarrhea and/or constipation (people often alternate between the two conditions during a single episode)
- Severe cramps in the abdomen, particularly on the lower left side
- Nausea and vomiting
- Fever with chills

Description

Some people develop multiple small pouches in the lining of their intestines (usually in the colon), that protrude through the muscle of the intestinal wall. These pouches, called diverticula, produce no pain or other symptoms, unless they become inflamed or infected. When a diverticular pocket and the surrounding tissue becomes inflamed, the condition is called diverticulitis.

Diverticulitis is caused when undigested food or fecal matter lodges in the pouch, causing irritation. This compromises blood flow to the area, making the area susceptible to an invasion by bacteria, thus hampering the bowel's ability to remove waste. This, in turn, results in constipation, diarrhea, and cramping.

Studies have shown that diverticulitis can run in families, but it is most common among the elderly, whose intestinal lining starts to weaken. Researchers also believe that diet plays an important role: people who eat a low-fiber diet are at increased risk of developing the condition.

Conventional Medical Treatment

If you have symptoms of diverticulitis for more than two days, or if the pain is extremely severe, contact your physician immediately. A rectal exam and colonoscopy or CAT scan may be needed to diagnose the condition, since diverticulitis is often confused with irritable bowel syndrome.

Common treatment includes bed rest, stool softeners, a liquid diet, and antibiotics. If you happen to suffer from two or more diverticulitis attacks over a period of one to two years, your physician may suggest surgical removal the involved segment of intestine.

In severe cases, one of the inflamed pouches can rupture, spilling undigested food, bacteria, and fecal matter into the abdominal cavity. This results in *peritonitis*, a medical emergency that requires intravenous antibiotic therapy and hospitalization.

For More Information
National Institute of Diabetes and Digestive and Kidney Diseases
31 Center Drive, MSC 2560
Bethesda, MD 20892-2560
301-654-3810
www.niddk.nih.gov

Another Reason to Lift Weights

When you think of weight training, chances are you think of improving your physique. However, a recent Danish study has found that moderate lifting may also decrease an individual's chance of developing diverticulitis. Weight lifting increases lean muscle mass, which boosts the metabolism. Researchers found that this boosted metabolism cut the intestinal digestion time in half, thus helping the intestines do their job more efficiently. This improved digestive efficiency results in a decreased chance of developing diverticulitis.

Diverticulitis

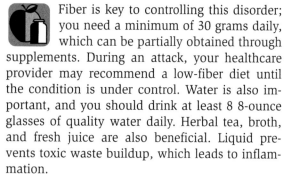

> ### Health Notes
>
> ➤ *Several studies have found a correlation between a low-fiber diet and the incidence of diverticulitis. To help prevent diverticulitis, eat a diet high in fiber-rich raw fruits and vegetables as well as whole grains.*
>
> ➤ *If you must use a laxative, opt for bulk-forming types such as wheat or oat bran, or psyllium seeds. Laxatives that stimulate the intestinal muscle weaken the intestinal wall, which can lead to diverticulitis.*

Complementary and Alternative Treatments

Nutrition and Supplementation

Fiber is key to controlling this disorder; you need a minimum of 30 grams daily, which can be partially obtained through supplements. During an attack, your healthcare provider may recommend a low-fiber diet until the condition is under control. Water is also important, and you should drink at least 8 8-ounce glasses of quality water daily. Herbal tea, broth, and fresh juice are also beneficial. Liquid prevents toxic waste buildup, which leads to inflammation.

Your diet should contain high levels of protein from vegetable sources and fish. Eliminate dairy products, sugar products, red meat, fried and processed foods, and spices. During an attack, avoid seedy foods, such as berries. (Once your condition stabilizes, however, you can resume eating them.) Try to get vitamin K through diet by eating plenty of green leafy vegetables.

Nutritional supplementation is also important. During an attack, switch to liquid forms for better assimilation. Otherwise, follow these daily suggestions:

Most Important

- fiber (as directed on label)—helps prevent constipation
- vitamin B complex (100 mg 3 times daily)—for proper digestion
- proteolytic enzymes (as directed on label)—aids digestion and reduces inflammation of the colon
- a prodophilus formula (as directed on label)—heals intestinal wall

Also Recommended

- flaxseed oil (1 tblsp daily)—protects the cells lining the colon wall
- garlic (as directed on label)—aids digestion and destroys unwanted bacteria
- L-glutamine (500 mg twice daily, with water or juice)—fuels the intestinal cells
- vitamin K (100 mcg)—a deficiency has been linked to intestinal disorders
- vitamin A (25,000 IU; do not exceed 8000 IU if you are pregnant)—protects and heals the colon lining
- vitamin C (3000 to 8000 mg in divided doses)—reduces inflammation; use a buffered form
- vitamin E (up to 800 IU)—a potent antioxidant
- gamma orizanol (as directed on label)—aids in healing the intestinal wall
- N-acetyl glucosamine (as directed on label)—aids in healing the intestinal wall

(For an *acute* condition, take supplements until your symptoms subside. If symptoms persist, seek the advice of your healthcare provider. For a *chronic* condition, consult your healthcare provider regarding the duration of treatment.)

Aromatherapy

Massage the lower abdomen with a combination of 2 drops each of peppermint, Roman chamomile, and rosemary oil, mixed with 1 teaspoon of olive oil to relieve discomfort and a feeling of fullness.

Bodywork and Somatic Practices

 See "Colitis" entry.

Herbal Therapy

 Diverticulosis, the formation of small pouches in the intestinal walls, is a precursor of diverticulitis, a condition in which the pouches become infected because they're filled with debris. Your best bet, then, is to treat diverticulosis so you don't develop diverticulitis. Many of the following remedies are helpful for both conditions:

- Take psyllium (a high-fiber seed) or wheat bran with lots of fluids daily to keep your bowels moving comfortably and to help prevent diverticulitis.

- Use generous amounts of raw garlic, an anti-infective, in dishes such as salads. Or take 3 garlic capsules 3 times daily.

- Drink slippery elm tea to calm inflamed intestines. To make the tea, simmer 2 teaspoons of powder in 1 cup of water for 15 minutes. Drink up to 3 cups daily until symptoms subside.

Other beneficial herbs include licorice, pau d'arco, chamomile, goldenseal, red clover, and yarrow. Herbal products are available in health food stores and in some pharmacies and supermarkets. Follow package for specific directions.

Hydrotherapy

 Some therapists suggest constitutional therapy applied several times a week to treat this disorder. For directions, see the "Hydrotherapy" section in "Introduction to Complementary Therapies" section.

Traditional Chinese Medicine

 Acupuncture Acupuncture can be used to alleviate the intestinal pain and inflammation caused by diverticulitis. It also can be used to remedy constipation, which is a major factor in developing the condition. Points that may be utilized include Bladder 21 and 25, Stomach 25, and Gallbladder 34, along with related intestinal and conception vessel points.

Acupressure To improve digestion and relieve constipation, an acupressurist may work on Stomach 36 (below the knee) and Large Intestine 11 (near the elbow). Additional points that may be targeted are Large Intestine 4, Stomach 44 and 25, and Liver 3.

Chinese Herbal Therapy There are countless herbs that can be used to prevent or treat chronic constipation, the leading cause of diverticulitis, including aloe vera (up to 1 gram of the condensed juice a day—equivalent to the fresh juice from 15 leaves).

Formulas that may be prescribed for constipation include Apricot Seed and Linum, Bupleurum and Tang Gui, Aplotaxis Carminative Pills, and Ginseng and Astragalus, among others.

DIZZINESS

Dizziness is a symptom that can accompany many different types of maladies, from low blood pressure and anemia to motion sickness to anxiety attacks to more serious ailments, such as cardiovascular and respiratory disorders.

The sensations of imbalance, lightheadedness, and faintness that commonly define dizziness often are accompanied by weakness, mental confusion, slowed thinking, and blurred or double vision. This feeling may come upon you abruptly or gradually. The actual dizziness itself may be mild enough to let you attend to your day or severe enough that you literally can't think straight. If you find yourself in the grips of an overwhelming bout of dizziness, try lying down until the feeling passes; dizziness is often aggravated by physical motion, such as standing up quickly or turning your head.

Dizziness is actually caused by inadequate blood flow to the cerebrum and spinal cord. Without a generous supply of blood, these areas don't get the oxygen they need. As uncomfortable as the sensation is, individual episodes of dizziness are generally brief.

Many people mistake vertigo *for dizziness, but* vertigo *is an altogether different sensation— one of revolving in space or of your surroundings spinning around you. This perceived motion often results in nausea, vomiting, a staggering gait, ringing of the ears, or hearing loss (the inner ear is responsible for perceiving motion). Conditions that involve vertigo include severe migraines, head trauma, multiple sclerosis, seizures, herpes zoster, middle ear infection or surgery, Ménière's disease, brain disorders, and drunkenness. Sometimes people experience dizziness and vertigo at the same time, as in post-concussion syndrome.*

SYMPTOM:

EARACHE

An earache is a symptom of many different conditions, most of them disorders of the external and middle ear. An obstruction in the ear canal, a tumor of the ear, an ear infection, trauma to the ear (being struck by a hand or an object on the outer ear), a perforated eardrum, and wax blockage of the ear can all cause earaches. Earaches can also be caused by conditions affecting other parts of the body, including the common cold, frostbite, temporomandibular joint syndrome, and migraine headaches.

To help your physician determine what is causing your earache, describe the type of ache you are experiencing. Is the pain dull, stabbing, throbbing, constant, or intermittent? Is your ear hot or cold to the touch? In addition, make a list of any accompanying symptoms that you are experiencing. Your physician also will want to know how long your ear has been hurting and if you experienced an event that may have caused the earache. After examining the ear itself and considering related symptoms and the type of pain, your physician can make a diagnosis. In the majority of cases, earaches disappear when the underlying condition is treated.

EARDRUM, PERFORATED/RUPTURED

Signs and Symptoms

- Earache
- Partial hearing loss
- Bleeding or discharge from the ear

Description

The eardrum is a thin, sensitive membrane that receives sound waves from the outside world and transfers them through the bones of the middle ear. If something tears the smooth, sound-receiving surface of the eardrum, the result can be a particularly painful and serious condition. Such trauma can also permanently damage your hearing.

Ruptured eardrums actually occur more frequently than you might think. The pressure caused by a severe ear infection can tear the eardrum; so can everyday activities, such as cleaning your ears too vigorously with a cotton swab. In fact, doctors speculate that cotton swabs are a more common cause of eardrum tears than ear infections. Other traumatic events, such as a strong slap·on the ear, a nearby explosion, or flying with an ear infection or cold can produce a change of air pressure in the ear that are violent enough to perforate the eardrum.

Conventional Medical Treatment

If you have any symptoms of a perforated eardrum, visit your doctor as soon as possible. Although small fissures can usually heal by themselves, larger tears often cannot. If left untreated, these wounds can, in the long-term, result in hearing loss and a higher susceptibility to middle ear infections.

How Air Travel Can Damage Your Ears

When an airplane ascends, positive pressure develops in the middle ear, causing the eardrum to bulge outward in an attempt to reduce the pressure. If the pressure becomes too great, the eardrum may rupture. The pressure in the middle usually reaches equilibrium with cabin air pressure during the flight. However, the problem occurs again when the plane descends and negative pressure develops in the middle ear, causing the eardrum to bulge inward. To ease the pain created by all this bulging of the eardrum, passengers can equalize middle ear pressure by yawning, swallowing, or chewing. These activities help open the eustachian tube long enough to allow the pressure to equalize. The chance of rupturing an eardrum during flight is usually low, but risk increases when symptoms of upper respiratory tract infection, ear infection, or common cold are present.

To determine the condition of your eardrum, your physician examines your ear canal with an otoscope, an instrument containing a light and a magnifying lens. If the tear is small, usually your ear is allowed to heal by itself. Small tears usually take two or three months to heal, during which time you must keep your ear dry. If the tear is large, surgery may be required. If there is a threat of infection, your physician may prescribe antibiotics.

For More Information
American Academy of Otolaryngology
One Prince Street
Alexandria, VA 22314
703-863-4444
www.entnet.org

Complementary and Alternative Treatments

Traditional Chinese Medicine

 Acupuncture Acupuncture can be used to help internal inflammation and swelling after the perforation or rupture has occurred.

Chinese Herbal Therapy Kidney tonics may help the ear heal as best it can.

Health Notes

➤ Sometimes, a change in ear pressure can be mistaken for earwax build up. Do not self-diagnose and attempt to remove it yourself. Ear canals are self-cleaning, and because earwax in normal amounts is healthy, it is not necessary to remove normal amounts of earwax.

➤ If earwax is excessive, do not poke around in your ear with a cotton swab or a bobby pin. Instead, put 2 drops of hydrogen peroxide into the ear once a week—this should soften wax and allow it to drain. When you use swabs in the ear canal, not only do you run the risk of leaving infection-causing fibers inside the ear canal, you may also damage the thin tissue of the canal, and will probably only succeed in packing the wax against the eardrum.

Ear Infection (Otitis Media)

Signs and Symptoms

- Earache
- Feeling of fullness in the ear
- Hearing loss
- Pus secretions from the ear
- Fever and chills
- Nausea and diarrhea

Description

Ear infections are caused by a strain of bacteria or a virus that infects the ear. They can vary in their severity, from mild cases, with a small amount of fluid buildup in the middle ear, to more serious cases, where blood or pus blocks the auditory canal. Symptoms may include an array of flu-like symptoms or nothing more than a dull ache. Ear infections can also vary in frequency of occurrence—some people get them only once in their life, while others have recurring infections almost every year. Ear infections are common in infants and young children, because the mechanism to drain fluid from the middle ear is not yet well developed.

Ear infections can originate either in the outer ear (*otitis externa*) or the middle ear (*otitis media*). Infections of the middle ear are more common. If left untreated, ear infections can result in a ruptured eardrum or even hearing loss.

Conventional Medical Treatment

If you experience sharp pain inside your ear, or if you have had a dull ache for more than two or three days, see your doctor immediately. To diag-

Health Notes

➤ Babies who are breastfed for one year or more have fewer ear infections throughout childhood than babies who are fed formula.

➤ If you have children and you smoke, quit. Infants and children who have one or two smoking parents have an increased risk of ear infections.

➤ The use of antibiotics to treat ear infections is controversial. Some studies have shown that the majority of ear infections heal in the same amount of time whether they are treated with antibiotics or not.

➤ Children with allergies may be at higher risk for recurrent ear infections. Check with your MD to see if your child has an allergy.

nose the condition, your doctor examines your ear with an otoscope, an instrument containing a light and a magnifying lens.

Antibiotics are the common method of treatment for ear infections—an antibiotic regimen can usually clear up an infection within a week. Long term, low dose antibiotics (3 to 6 months) may be prescribed for children with recurrent infections.

For More Information

The American Academy of Pediatrics
141 Northwest Point Boulevard
Elk Grove Village, IL 60007-1098
847-228-5005
www.aap.org

Complementary and Alternative Treatments

Nutrition and Supplementation

Breastfeeding enhances immunity. Bottle-fed babies have a higher incidence of otitis media (middle ear infection) than breastfed babies. Breast milk is one of the few sources of GLA (gamma linoleic acid), an essential fatty acid that reduces inflammation.

Babies introduced to cow's milk and solid foods too early are more prone to developing allergies. Allergy-prone children have a higher incidence of otitis. Possible food allergens are peanuts, eggs, wheat, soy, dairy products, and citrus fruits. During an ear infection, eliminate dairy products for 30 days. Feed your baby soy milk, rice milk, or nut milk.

Some experts believe that excessive antibiotic treatment contributes to chronic ear infection. The following supplements may help (dosages will vary according to age and weight of child; follow your doctor's recommendations):

Most Important

- vitamin A
- vitamin C (50 mg every 2 to 3 hours; for total daily dosage, multiply 50 mg by the child's age)
- manganese
- zinc
- vitamin E with selenium

Also Recommended

- quercetin
- germanium
- a prodophilus formula (if antibiotics are administered)
- evening primrose oil
- thymus extract
- N-acetyl-L-cysteine—will help ear to drain (*Caution*: This supplement may cause diarrhea in some children.)

(For an *acute* condition, take supplements until your symptoms subside. If symptoms persist, seek the advice of your healthcare provider. For a *chronic* condition, consult your healthcare provider regarding the duration of treatment.)

Aromatherapy

To quiet the pain of an ear infection, massage around the outer ear with essential oils of lavender or chamomile. To lessen pain while drawing out infection, use a hot compress laced with lavender or chamomile oil on the affected ear. *Caution*: Do not put essential oils in the ear.

Ayurvedic Medicine

Ear infections always require the attention of a qualified healthcare professional. However, you may be able to open and drain the eustachian tubes, and thus alleviate some pain, by massaging the lymph nodes in front of the ears. You also may be able to ward off recurrences by taking the herb gotu kola. Ayurvedic practitioners often use *neem* oil to fight the infection.

Bodywork and Somatic Practices

CranioSacral Therapy can be a very gentle, effective therapy for the problem. Try it in combination with Reiki, Therapeutic Touch, or reflexology.

Chiropractic

In cases of ear infection, the upper cervical vertebrae located near the eustachian tube may be pinching the tube in some way, creating a clog in which fluid and bacteria accumulate. Specific chiropractic adjustment (SCA) to these vertebrae may relieve that pinching. Many parents see a decrease in the frequency and severity of their children's ear infections when these children receive ongoing chiropractic care. Use chiropractic in conjunction with standard medical treatment, which may involve the use of medication to relieve pain and promote drainage of fluid.

Homeopathy

Homeopathic remedies are safe and effective for external as well as middle ear infections, and many are also appropriate for recurrent infections. The best approach is to see a homeopathic practitioner who may recommend one of the following remedies, depending on your symptoms:

- *Belladonna*—for an ear infection with intense pain that extends down to your neck; your ear is red, and you may have a sore throat and sudden high fever

- *Aconite*—if the onset is sudden after you've been exposed to cold

- *Chamomilla*—if the infection is accompanied by extreme irritability and the pain is worse when you bend over (in a child, this type of earache is often associated with teething and may seem to improve when the child is carried)

- *Pulsatilla*—for an earache following a cold that produces heavy congestion; accompanied by thick discharge from the ear

Hydrotherapy

Use hot compresses to help draw out the infection and reduce pain. Or apply alternating hot and cold compresses to increase circulation, decrease pressure in the ear area, and increase the absorption of inflammatory deposits.

Traditional Chinese Medicine

Acupuncture Acupuncture may be used to enhance kidney functioning, which Chinese medical experts associate with ear problems. The acupoints targeted in the treatment of otitis media are the kidney, internal ear, and internal secretion points in the ear itself, along with related points on the body. Acupuncture—alone or with moxibustion—also may be used to help relieve the pain and fever associated with this condition.

Acupressure An ear infection-related fever may be reduced by pressing on Governing Vessel 14, Large Intestine 4, Large Intestine 11, and related ear points.

Chinese Herbal Therapy Because Chinese medicine views ear infections as being caused by kidney disorders, herbal practitioners attempt to enhance kidney function and balance *chi* in the kidney meridian.

Herbal formulas traditionally used for this purpose include Panax Ginseng Capsules, Gentiana, Rehmannia Six, Eight Immortal Long Life Pills, Polygonum Tablets, and Planetary Formula's Twin Kidney Tonics, and Energetics Yin and Energetics Yang, which should be taken simultaneously.

EARWAX BLOCKAGE

e

Signs and Symptoms

- Partial hearing loss
- Ringing in the ear
- A feeling of fullness in the ear
- Earache

Description

The ear canal is lined with glands that produce *cerumen*, or earwax. Together with small hair follicles, this wax works to prevent dust and other foreign particles from entering the ear. As new wax is produced, older wax normally works its way out through the ear canal and into the outer ear. From here, it falls out of the ear during sleep or in the shower. Some people, on the other hand, produce new wax faster than the old wax leaves the ear canal, thus creating a backup of cerumen.

Health Notes

➤ When showering, wash the outside of the ear with mild soap and water. Also, be sure to rinse ears well with warm water after shampooing and conditioning hair; shampoo and conditioner buildup in the ear can make it difficult for wax to leave the ear.

➤ Individuals who are prone to wax blockage can prevent buildup by dropping two drops of hydrogen peroxide into the ear canal once a week. Hydrogen peroxide keeps wax soft enough to migrate out of the ear canal.

➤ Never place a cotton swab or other object into the ear canal when cleaning ears. This can increase chances of wax blockage since it pushes the wax further into the canal.

Conventional Medical Treatment

Wax blockage can usually be treated with home care. A few drops of over-the-counter wax softener can be dropped into the ear canal two or three times a day. After two or three days, the wax will begin to soften, allowing it to move out of the ear canal. If home care doesn't work, visit your doctor, who may gently scoop away the wax with a curette or use a suction device to vacuum away the wax.

Complementary and Alternative Treatments

Ayurvedic Medicine

 To remove a buildup of stubborn wax, Ayurvedic practitioners may suggest a two-step process: First, soften the wax by placing a few drops of warm garlic oil in the ear. Then, after several hours, flush the ear with warm water or a solution of vinegar and lukewarm water.

Homeopathy

 Earwax blockage may respond to homeopathic treatment. However, the selection of a remedy—more than one is available—depends on *your* symptoms and the stage of the condition. Don't try treating this disorder yourself. See a homeopathic professional.

Traditional Chinese Medicine

Chinese Herbal Therapy Asarum Sieboldi can be used to loosen and clear earwax. Simply mix the powdered herb with vinegar and roll into a tiny ball, then place the concoction inside the ear canal and let it dissolve.

e

SYMPTOM:

EDEMA

The swelling of body tissues due to excessive fluid retention is called edema. Fluid normally moves freely between the blood vessels and the body tissues through a process called osmosis. This movement is controlled not only by pressure within the blood vessels, but by the lymphatic system. If too much fluid builds up outside the veins, the lymph system simply transports the excess fluid back into the blood vessel. However, certain illnesses, conditions, and substances alter the pressure in the vessels or decrease the effectiveness of the lymphatic system, allowing fluid to continue to build up in the tissues.

Edema is a symptom of a variety of conditions, including premenstrual syndrome, kidney failure, malnutrition, preeclampsia (in pregnant women) and localized trauma. A sodium-rich meal consumed the day before can cause fluid retention. Certain drugs, such as steroids, also can cause edema. Edema of the legs and hands can be a symptom during normal pregnancy.

Edema can be so subtle that no one but you is aware of it, or it can be so dramatic that the affected area (or entire body) swells grossly. The extent of tissue affected depends on the cause of the condition—allergies can cause facial tissues to swell, heart conditions can result in swelling of the lower legs, malnutrition can cause edema in the abdominal cavity, and premenstrual syndrome can cause the entire body to swell.

If your bloating is caused by a non-threatening condition, such as premenstrual syndrome or a high-sodium meal, home care can help reduce swelling. Elevate your feet 6 to 12 inches above the heart, several times daily to help reduce swollen legs. Walking or other moderate exercise is an excellent way to improve your circulation, which in turn flushes excess liquid from the body.

Because edema may be caused by many other, potentially serious, conditions, consult your healthcare provider immediately if swelling is severe, persists for more than a few days, or if you are pregnant. Because edema is a symptom and not an illness, your physician will first identify and treat the underlying condition. In many cases, once the underlying disorder is addressed and treated, the edema disappears. To help your body release excess liquid, your doctor may recommend a diuretic.

Because fluid retention may be associated with allergies, conduct a food allergy test before doing anything else. Other helpful nutritional therapies include eating foods high in fiber; raw foods, such as apples, garlic, grapes, and onions; protein-rich foods, such as eggs, broiled white fish, and broiled skinless chicken or turkey; and natural diuretics, such as celery, carrots, parsley, and cilantro. Add kelp to your diet to supply you with necessary minerals. Avoid dairy products, meat, alcohol, caffeine, chocolate, fried foods, gravies, salt, and white sugar.

The following daily supplements may also be helpful in treating edema:

- *free-form amino acid complex (as directed on label)—improves protein assimilation; protein deficiency has been linked to water retention*

Edema

- *calcium (1500 mg)—replaces minerals*
- *magnesium (1000 mg)—works with calcium*
- *bromelain (as directed on label)—helps digestion*
- *potassium (99 mg)—very important if you're taking diuretics*
- *vitamin C (3000 to 5000 mg in divided doses)—helps balance and control edema*

(For an acute condition, take supplements until your symptoms subside. If symptoms persist, seek the advice of your healthcare provider. For a chronic condition, consult your healthcare provider regarding the duration of treatment.)

For a complementary treatment, try aromatherapy; the essential oils of fennel, juniper, geranium, and rosemary can be helpful in treating edema. For chronic swelling of hands and feet from prolonged sitting or standing, Ayurvedic practitioners advise taking punarnava guggula twice daily. They also suggest raising your feet on a stool when you're sitting and using a pillow under your feet when you're lying down. Bodywork and somatic practices such as reflexology, polarity therapy, massage, Cranio-Sacral therapy and Oriental bodywork can offer relief, as can the more vigorous bodywork techniques of Trager, Aston-Patterning, Feldenkrais, and Alexander.

Herbal therapists recommend natural diuretics, such as dandelion and parsley, which can help remove excess fluid from the body. To benefit from dandelion, take 1 teaspoonful of dandelion tincture 3 times daily or drink dandelion tea 3 to 5 times daily. To make the tea, steep 2 tablespoons fresh leaves in 1 cup of boiling water for 10 minutes; strain. To benefit from parsley, use generous amounts of parsley in cooking and drink parsley tea 3 times daily. To make the tea, steep 2 teaspoons leaves in 1 cup of boiling water for 10 minutes; strain. Herbal products are available in health food stores and in some pharmacies and supermarkets. Follow package for specific directions. Caution: *Don't use diuretics during pregnancy. Also, consult your doctor before beginning an herbal treatment for edema; swollen ankles, hands, or face can be a sign of a serious internal illness.*

A form of hydrotherapy called contrast therapy may be helpful for swollen ankles. Plunge your feet first into hot water then into cold. Repeat several times. Or try applying alternating hot and cold compresses. You also might try soaking in a neutral bath (slightly lower than body temperature) for about 60 minutes.

Traditional Chinese Medicine offers various therapies for edema. Acupuncture can be used to relieve the swelling and discomfort associated with edema. It can also improve the circulation of blood and chi throughout the body, which can help speed the elimination of excess fluids. Acupuncture body points used to treat edema usually include those that correspond to the bladder, kidney, heart, and liver, along with related auricular points. Chinese Medical Massage can be very effective in relieving blockages and draining excess fluid out of the body. The specific points will vary, according to which areas of the body are retaining fluid. Chinese herbal therapy for edema may include the Chinese patent formulas Rehmannia Eight, Poria Five Herb Combination, Stephania and Astragalus Formula, and Coix Combination.

EMPHYSEMA

Signs and Symptoms

- Shortness of breath that worsens with time
- A chronic, mild cough that may produce small amounts of phlegm
- Decreasing tolerance of physical activity
- An enlarged chest
- Weight loss

Description

Healthy lungs contain 300 million alveoli, elastic air sacs where oxygen enters the blood and carbon dioxide is removed from it. Emphysema develops when the alveoli membrane are destroyed. Though this process occurs slowly and does not affect all alveoli to the same extent, it does impair the lungs' ability to function, which increases the amount of time it takes for air to enter or exit the lungs. This results in shortness of breath.

Also called chronic obstructive pulmonary disease (COPD), emphysema commonly affects long-term, heavy cigarette smokers, but cigar and pipe smokers are also at increased risk. Smoking causes irritation and breakdown of the alvioli.

Smokers are not the only people who develop emphysema, however. Occupational exposures to chemicals, dusts, and fumes can also put a person at risk. Some people are genetically predisposed to the condition, due to a deficiency of the enzyme alpha-1 antitrypsin, which protects the integrity of the elastic fibers in the walls of the alveoli. People with low levels of alpha-1 antitrypsin usually develop severe emphysema sometime in their 20s or 30s.

Conventional Medical Treatment

If you suspect you have emphysema, see your physician immediately. To diagnose emphysema,

Health Notes

➤ *Cold air can exacerbate emphysema. To warm the air as it enters your lungs, try wrapping a soft scarf around your nose and mouth during cold weather or buy a cold air mask (available at your local pharmacy).*

➤ *A dry environment can irritate the lungs. A humidifier can help prevent the air from becoming too dry.*

➤ *To help make breathing easier, avoid other respiratory irritants that may cause shortness of breath or tightness in the chest, such as certain perfumes, dust, fumes from paint, and automobile exhaust.*

➤ *Due to the weakened state of their lungs, people with emphysema should avoid exposure to people with respiratory infections, such as colds, flu, bronchitis, or pneumonia.*

➤ *If you are an active smoker, quit immediately. The first step toward preventing or managing emphysema is learning to live smoke-free.*

your doctor takes an inventory of your symptoms, reviews your medical history, and performs a lung function test and chest X-rays.

There is no cure for emphysema. Therapy can help you learn how to use your lungs as efficiently as possible, thus keeping the disease from progressing. You may also be taught breathing techniques to get the most of the limited airflow. To increase your lungs' efficiency, engage in regular, non-strenuous exercise, such as walking or leisurely cycling. Your physician may prescribe a bronchodilator or anti-inflammatory medication, such as theophylline, sympathomimetics, anticholingergics, or corticosteroids.

In severe cases, home oxygen therapy—where pure oxygen is pumped through a tube from a portable tank—may be necessary. Surgery is also an option in severe cases. Relatively new surgical options include lung transplantation and volume reduction surgery, where up to 30 percent of the most diseased portions of lungs are removed.

For More Information:
American Lung Association
1740 Broadway
New York, NY 10019
800-LUNG-USA
www.lungusa.org

National Heart, Lung, and Blood Institute
National Institutes of Health
P.O. Box 30105
Bethesda, MD 20824-0105
301-592-8573
www.nhlbi.nih.gov

Complementary and Alternative Treatments

Nutrition and Supplementation

Before breakfast, drink a mixture of one teaspoonful of pure, cold-pressed olive oil and apple juice to provide essential fatty acids and help eliminate toxic waste.

Experts recommend a raw-foods diet with emphasis on vegetables and raw fresh vegetable juices. Garlic and onions should be part of the daily diet. Frequent use of spicy foods, such as chili peppers, ginger, and horseradish, helps keep lungs clear of mucus.

Avoid gas-forming foods, such as legumes and cabbage; any foods that require a great deal of chewing; and fried or greasy foods and salt. Also eliminate foods that form mucus, including meat, dairy products, wheat, tobacco, junk foods, and processed foods. Daily supplements include:

- vitamin B_6 (50 mg)—helps remove cadmium (from smoking) from the body
- chlorophyll (as directed on label)—helps you breathe easier
- coenzyme Q10 (60 mg)—improves lung oxygenation
- vitamin E (1000 IU)—an oxygen carrier; use emulsion form
- vitamin C (5000 to 10,000 mg, in divided doses)—aids in healing inflamed tissues
- vitamin A (100,000 IU daily for 1 month, then 50,000 IU until relief, then 25,000 IU; do not exceed 8000 IU daily if you are pregnant)—repairs lung tissue
- N-acetyl cysteine (250 mg)—repairs and protects lung tissue
- glutathione (250 mg)—repairs and protects lung tissue

(Consult your healthcare provider regarding the duration of treatment.)

Aromatherapy

Rub your chest with diluted essential oils of cedarwood, eucalyptus, peppermint, or pine for easier breathing. You also can place a few drops of one of the essential oils on a tissue or handkerchief and inhale deeply.

Bodywork and Somatic Practices

Try Oriental bodywork or reflexology. Soothing, restorative results will also come from Trager, CranioSacral Therapy, polarity therapy, Aston-Patterning, and Therapeutic Touch.

Herbal Therapy

To ease coughing and other discomforts of emphysema, choose one of the following herbal remedies: For excess mucus, try coltsfoot, thyme, or mullein tea before each meal. To make any of the teas, steep 1 to 2 teaspoons of the dried herb in 1 cup boiling water for 10 minutes; strain. If you're bothered by constant coughing, try either of two tea blends: equal amounts of coltsfoot, mullein, and licorice; or equal amounts of marshmallow, mallow, coltsfoot, mullein, violet, and red poppy flowers. To make either of the teas, steep 1 to 2 teaspoons of the blend in 1 cup of boiling water for 10 minutes.

You also might try eating hot, spicy meals laced with generous amounts of cayenne or ginger.

Other helpful herbs include comfrey, fennel seed, fenugreek , rosemary, and rose hips.

Herbal products are available in health food stores and in some pharmacies and supermarkets. Follow package for specific directions.

Hydrotherapy

 Steam inhalations are very effective for loosening and expelling mucus. Add a few drops of a favorite essential oil, if you wish.

Under professional supervision, you also might try constitutional therapy or hot compress applications. For directions on these therapies, see "Hydrotherapy" in the "Introduction to Complementary Therapies" section.

Traditional Chinese Medicine

 Acupuncture Acupuncture may be used to tone the lungs and improve circulation to the area, making it easier to breathe. This modality also can help relieve coughing spasms and curb nicotine cravings in emphysema sufferers who are trying to kick the tobacco habit.

Acupressure Manipulating various lung, conception vessel, and bronchial points can help quiet coughs and ease breathing.

Chinese Herbal Therapy Chinese herbs can be very effective in treating many symptoms of emphysema. Herbal formulas used to treat chronic bronchitis (as emphysema is sometimes called) are Pulmonary Tonic Pills, *Ping Chuan*, Bronchitis Pills (compound), Special Medicine for Bronchitis (also called *Hsiao Keh Chuan*, available in pill or liquid form), Shedanchuanbeye Extract, and Fritillaria Extract Pills. Cordyceps is often used alone or with a formula to tonify the lungs.

Yoga and Meditation

 Any yoga pose that expands the lungs and relaxes the chest can help alleviate the discomforts of emphysema. Performing a daily routine of at least four poses—Fish, Camel, Bow, and Warrior—can be particularly beneficial.

ENDOMETRIOSIS

Signs and Symptoms

- Pelvic pain that may begin just before menstruation and last until several days after
- Sharp pain during sexual intercourse
- Premenstrual spotting
- Heavy menstrual periods
- Infertility
- Pain and straining during bowel movements

Description

The uterus is lined with a tissue called the endometrium. When cells from this lining escape from the uterus and implant themselves on other organs in the pelvic region—usually the fallopian tubes, uterine ligaments, or the ovaries—they cause a painful condition called endometriosis.

During the menstrual cycle, the wayward cells act exactly as they would if they were still in the uterus, first thickening and then bleeding as menstruation begins. But since these displaced cells have left the uterus, there is nowhere for the blood to go. As a result, blisters form that irritate the surrounding tissue, which may, in an effort to contain the blister, create an encompassing cyst. The cyst may then become either a scar or an adhesion of abnormal tissue that binds organs together. If they are located on the ovaries or fallopian tubes, scars or adhesions can interfere with conception.

The condition is not uncommon—it is estimated that between 8 and 30 percent of women of childbearing age suffer from the condition. While most sufferers have no symptoms, others have symptoms that become increasingly painful and debilitating as the disease progresses. Women with endometriosis are more likely to have an ectopic pregnancy, a pregnancy that occurs outside the uterus (usually in the fallopian tubes).

Endometriosis often runs in families and usually strikes women between the ages of 25 and 40 who have not had children. Although its exact cause is uncertain, some experts believe endometriosis occurs when menstrual flow backs up into the fallopian tubes, spilling blood and shedding endometrial cells into the pelvic cavity.

Conventional Medical Treatment

If you suspect you have endometriosis, see your gynecologist immediately. Your physician may be able to feel patches of endometriosis during a pelvic examination, but a *laparoscopy* is the only way to confirm you have the condition. A *laparoscope*—a slim, lighted instrument that is inserted into the abdomen through a small incision—allows the physician to examine your pelvic organs. Considered a minor procedure, a laparoscopy is

usually performed on an outpatient basis with local or general anesthesia. Since ovarian cancer and endometriosis produce nearly identical symptoms—and because some of the hormones prescribed to treat endometriosis can make ovarian cancer grow faster—a laparoscopy is strongly recommended.

Many sufferers find that using birth control pills diminishes the intensity of their symptoms. If oral contraceptives do not help, a testosterone derivative called danazol may be prescribed to cease menstruation. However, most women find danazol difficult to tolerate because of frequent side effects, such as weight gain, excessive hair growth, and acne. During this period, displaced cells and their resulting growths sometimes shrink. Surgery is also an option for removing or destroying growths—*electrocautery* (using an electric current to destroy the cells) or laser surgery are two common options. Unfortunately, recurrences are common. In extremely severe cases, removal of the uterus and ovaries is the recommended treatment.

Gonadotropin–releasing hormone (GNRH) is now the treatment of choice if contraception or surgery fails. It is given by injection, nasal spray, or via an implant replaced every 28 days. Because GNRH suppresses estrogen, side effects include hot flashes, vaginal dryness, and irregular vaginal

Health Notes

➤ *Reduce your stress levels. Some studies suggest that emotional stress may contribute to endometriosis.*

➤ *Exercise lengthens the menstrual cycle and reduces circulating estrogen levels, which helps control the pain and symptoms of endometriosis.*

➤ *Avoid drinking alcoholic beverages if you suffer from endometriosis. Alcohol elevates estrogen levels, thus worsening the symptoms of endometriosis.*

bleeding. GNRH is given only for a six-month cycle because of the risk of bone loss associated with the low estrogen. As with all of the treatment options, recurrence after stopping medication is common.

Endometriosis does not always require treatment. Those who do not develop any symptoms rarely require medical care. And since menopause usually remedies mild to moderate endometriosis, post-menopausal women who are not on estrogen replacement therapy usually need no treatment. However, estrogen replacement therapy sometimes reactivates endometriosis.

For More Information

American College of Obstetricians and Gynecologists
409 12th Street, SW
Washington, DC 20090-6920
800-673-8444
www.acog.org

Endometriosis Association
8585 North 76th Place
Milwaukee, WI 53223
800-992-ENDO
www.endometriosisassn.org

Complementary and Alternative Treatments

Nutrition and Supplementation

 Your diet should include at least 50 percent raw fruits and vegetables. Whole grains, nuts, and seeds are recommended, as are "green" drinks made from dark green leafy vegetables.

Experts recommend limiting the amount of meat and diary products in the diet because these foods increase arachidonic acid which increases inflammation. It is also important to eliminate caffeine and alcohol, dairy products, fried foods, red meats, sugar, salt, junk food, and fast foods. Foods containing phytoestrogens can be beneficial and include soybean products, such as tofu, miso, and tempeh, and legumes, such as lentils, pinto beans, lima beans, yellow split peas, alfalfa sprouts and peanuts. Cruciferous vegetables, such as broccoli, kale, cabbage, and turnips, are also indicated.

One of the functions of the liver is to remove excess hormones from the system, so keep the liver healthy with liver-cleansing foods, such as beets, carrots, and lemons.

Essential fatty acids help reduce the inflammation associated with the excess buildup of the endometrial tissue outside the uterus. Essential fatty acids suppress prostaglandins that increase the cramping that often accompanies endometriosis. Foods sources include salmon, nuts, seeds, and flaxseed oil; evening primrose oil is another source.

Daily supplements include:

Most Important

- vitamin B complex (50 mg)—balances hormones, supplemented with vitamin B_6 (50 mg 3 times daily) (*Caution*: doses over 100 mg are not recommended for long-term use, as side effects may result)

- vitamin C (2000 mg 3 times daily) (*Caution*: high doses may cause diarrhea)—use buffered form

- vitamin E (800 to 1200 IU)

- evening primrose oil (1500 mg)

- vitamin K (200 mcg)—clots blood

- iron (as directed by healthcare provider)—a deficiency is common with endometriosis

Also Recommended

- vitamin A (5000 IU)

- folic acid (400 mcg)

- magnesium (1000 mg at bedtime)

- calcium (1500 mg)—supplies minerals

- selenium (400 mcg)

- flaxseed oil (1 tblsp)

- potassium (3 to 4 times a day; see package for dosage instructions)

(Consult your healthcare provider regarding the duration of treatment.)

Aromatherapy

The essential oils of cypress, geranium, and rose can help calm the symptoms of endometriosis.

Ayurvedic Medicine

Ayurveda considers endometriosis a vata imbalance. As such, treatments are the same as those for premenstrual syndrome. See the "Premenstrual Syndrome" entry.

Herbal Therapy

Herbalists make several recommendations for treating the tension, pain, and cramping that accompany endometriosis. Valerian can help soothe frayed nerves and ease pain so you're better able to cope with the disorder. Cramp bark or black haw can often lessen cramping and painful spasms. Black cohosh and wild yam are helpful for balancing hormones. Alfalfa can restore iron supplies if they are low.

Herbal products are available in health food stores as well as some pharmacies and supermarkets. Follow package for specific directions. For specific formulas and advice, talk with a qualified herbalist, and consult your doctor before starting an herbal regimen.

Homeopathy

Endometriosis may respond to homeopathic treatment. However, the selection of a remedy—more than one is available—depends on *your* symptoms and the stage of the condition. Don't try treating this disorder yourself. See a homeopathic professional.

Hydrotherapy

Try alternating hot and cold sitz baths to increase circulation to the pelvic area; improved blood flow can lessen pelvic congestion and pain.

Traditional Chinese Medicine

Acupuncture This treatment may be used to help lessen the abdominal cramps and lower back pain that often accompany endometriosis. Points utilized may include Stomach 29, Liver 8, and various spleen and bladder points.

Acupressure Acupressure can be very helpful in relieving cramps, backaches, ovarian pain, and other symptoms associated with endometriosis. The points targeted will depend on the patient's specific complaints, although Conception Vessel 6, Spleen 6, and Stomach 36 are often involved, as are various bladder points.

Chinese Herbal Therapy The Chinese herbal formulas White Phoenix Pills, Bupleurum and Tang Gui, Ginseng and Tang Gui Ten, Rehmannia Six, Rehmannia Eight, and Corydalis may be helpful in alleviating the dysmenorrhea caused by endometriosis.

A practitioner typically prescribes tonics to improve the flow of blood and *chi*, and to strengthen any organs that are thought to be causing the disorder (which can vary from person to person).

Yoga and Meditation

The Locust and Boat poses can tone the muscles of the spine and pelvic area. Twisting poses and the Cobbler's pose can also be helpful. Do once or twice a day.

EPILEPSY

Signs and Symptoms

- Recurring seizures, ranging from repetitive twitching movements in a particular area of the body to convulsions of the entire body
- Staring spells wherein the individual is unaware of his or her surroundings
- Loss of consciousness

Description

Epilepsy is a disease characterized by seizures. These seizures occur as a result of abnormal electrical activity in the brain. The type, frequency, and duration of the seizures differ, depending on the person. Seizures may appear for no dis-

Diet as Medicine?

There is new hope for epileptic children in the form of a controversial diet. The ketogenic diet forces the body to metabolize fats and produce substances called ketone bodies, which seem to inhibit seizures. Children who are on the diet must begin by fasting for two or three days, which forces the body to completely use up any stored food. The fast is followed by a two-year diet made up almost entirely of fats. While the body burns dietary fat, it produces the seizure-inhibiting ketones. The diet is doctor-supervised and is recommended for children under age 14 who have failed to respond to at least two epilepsy drugs, suffer at least three seizures a week, and have parents willing to make a two-year commitment. Studies show that more than two-thirds of the children who undertake the diet remain seizure-free, usually without having to take medication.

cernible reason, or they may be triggered by an allergen, a flashing light, noise, drugs, alcohol, stress, menstruation, nutritional imbalances, emotional distress, hunger, or other factors. Some people are conscious during a seizure, while others are not. Some epileptics experience extreme fatigue and confusion after a seizure, while others are able to continue their regular activity after an attack. Some individuals notice warning signs—a tightening of the stomach, a certain sound, or a specific odor—a few seconds to three minutes before an attack that alerts them to an impending seizure.

Seizure disorder, as epilepsy is also known, affects an estimated 1 out every 100 people. In approximately 75 percent of the reported cases, the disorder begins in childhood.

An exact cause can be determined in only about 30 percent of cases. The most frequently identified causes are: genetics (a family history of epilepsy); severe head trauma (including car accidents, gunshot wounds, and sports-related accidents); brain tumor; stroke; poisoning; alcoholism; infection (including meningitis, encephalitis, and lupus); maternal complications (injury or illness during pregnancy); and oxygen deprivation in newborn infants.

Conventional Medical Treatment

To diagnose epilepsy, your doctor takes a detailed medical history, including a history of any seizures, and he or she may perform one or more tests. The most common examination is called an *electroencephalogram* (EEG), wherein a machine tracks the electrical impulses of your brain. Other tests, such as a CAT scan, MRI, serum test, or video monitoring, may be necessary to confirm diagnosis.

Treatment for epilepsy varies according to the

Epilepsy

Health Notes

➤ *Flashing lights, strobe lights, or flashing images can bring on a seizure in some epileptics. People who are sensitive to these impulses should avoid video games, music videos, and night clubs or concerts that use special light effects.*

➤ *Some epileptics experience seizures as a result of loud, percussive noise. Because you can't predict when you may be exposed to such noises, carry earplugs with you at all times.*

➤ *Reduce overall stress levels. Some experts believe there may be a connection between extreme stress and seizures.*

➤ *Alert your doctor and pharmacist to the fact that you take epilepsy drugs. Common medications—birth control pills, erythromycin (an antibiotic), and some asthma, ulcer, and heart medications—can interfere with epilepsy drugs, either lessening or intensifying effects.*

➤ *Research shows that the artificial sweetener aspartame has been associated with seizures in some epileptics.*

➤ *Talk to your doctor before taking nutritional supplements. Dosages of folic acid higher than 400 mcg per day may increase seizure activity in people with epilepsy.*

For More Information
Brain Research Foundation
120 South LaSalle Street, Suite 1300
Chicago, IL 60604
312-759-5150

The Epilepsy Foundation of America
4351 Garden City Drive
Landover, MD 20785
800-EFA-1000
www.efa.org

Helping Seizure Victims

Many of us are not sure how to help a seizure victim. The Epilepsy Foundation recommends the following first aid measures:

- Cushion the person's head.
- Loosen any tight-fitting articles of clothing around the neck, such as a buttoned-down collar or necktie.
- Turn the person onto one side.
- Never place *anything* in the person's mouth.
- Check for a medical I.D. bracelet or necklace marked "Epilepsy" or "Seizure Disorder."
- Do not hold down or restrain the person.
- Remain for a time after the seizure ends to offer help.

Call for emergency help if:

- the seizure lasts more than five minutes.
- the person is carrying medical identification showing a different condition, or is not wearing any medical identification.
- the recovery is very slow.
- a second seizure follows the first.
- the person has difficulty breathing during recovery.
- the person is pregnant.
- there are any signs of injury.

severity of the disorder and the individual. Some people are able to control the condition without medication, while others may require a prescription anti-convulsant drug to reduce the frequency and severity of seizures. Examples of medications used to control seizures include carbamazepin (Tegretol®), phenytoin (Dilantin®), phenobarbitol, and ethosuximide (Zarontin®). Treatment is individualized and often patients need more than one medication to control seizure activity.

Complementary and Alternative Treatments

Nutrition and Supplementation

 Your diet should contain cultured milk products, such as yogurt and kefir, as well as eggs, green leafy vegetables, raw cheese, raw milk, and soybeans. Drink fresh juices made from carrots, green leafy vegetables, red grapes, and seaweed to get concentrated levels of essential nutrients. Avoid refined foods and sugar, alcohol, animal protein, fried foods, artificial sweeteners, nicotine, and caffeine.

Think small: take small meals and small amounts of liquid at any one time. Do not use aluminum cookware, as aluminum gets into food and has been linked to seizures. Improve circulation by getting moderate daily exercise.

The following daily supplement guidelines are for adults; adjust dosages for children.

Most Important

- vitamin B complex (50 mg)—essential to the functioning of the central nervous system, supplemented with vitamin B_3 (50 mg)—improves circulation, vitamin B_6 (100 to 600 mg 3 times daily, under supervision of a doctor), and vitamin B_5 (pantothenic acid) (500 mg)—the anti-stress vitamin

- magnesium (700 mg)

- taurine (500 mg 3 times a day, with water or juice, not with food or milk; for optimal absorption take with 100 mg vitamin C and 50 mg vitamin B_6)—aids brain function

- tyrosine (500 mg 3 times daily)

- folic acid (400 mcg)—promotes nervous system health

Also Recommended

- zinc (25 mg)
- vitamin E (400 IU)
- calcium (1500 mg)
- selenium (100 mcg)

- coenzyme Q10 (30 mg)—improves brain oxygenation

- glycine (500 mg)

- dimethyl glycine (100 mg twice a day)

(Consult your healthcare provider regarding the duration of treatment.)

Aromatherapy

 Some essential oils are said to provoke seizures in sensitive people. Anyone prone to seizures should avoid fennel, hyssop, rosemary, sage, and wormwood essential oils. Research suggests that the more relaxing oils (Roman chamomile, cedarwood, and neroli) can reduce the frequency of seizures.

Ayurvedic Medicine

 An Ayurvedic practitioner may suggest taking an Ayurvedic herbal mixture of *brahmi, punarnava, jatamansi* and *saraswati churna* twice daily. Always consult your doctor before using any new remedy for epilepsy.

Bodywork and Somatic Practices

 CranioSacral Therapy has been helpful with this disorder. Other options may include Feldenkrais, Oriental bodywork, and reflexology.

Herbal Therapy

 The following herbs have a calming effect on the central nervous system and can be quite helpful in treating epilepsy: black cohosh, hyssop, and lobelia. Use these herbs on an alternating basis for optimum effect. For minor, or *petit mal*, seizures, try 1 teaspoon of skullcap tincture 3 times daily.

Herbal products are available in health food stores as well as some pharmacies and supermarkets. Follow package for specific directions. Consult your doctor before starting an herbal regimen to treat epilepsy.

Hydrotherapy

 Under the guidance of a professional, you might want to try constitutional therapy several times weekly. You can also try a relaxing Epsom salts bath several times a week.

Traditional Chinese Medicine

 Acupuncture Acupuncture has been shown to relieve—and, in some cases, prevent—epileptic seizures. Auricular points targeted may include the heart, kidney, stomach, and head.

Acupressure Applying firm pressure to Governing Vessel 26 (located in the indentation between the nose and upper lip), has been shown to revive unconscious seizure victims in less than 30 seconds.

Chinese Herbal Therapy Traditional Chinese Medicine views epilepsy and seizures as "internal damp-wind" diseases, so an herbalist typically begins treatment by advocating herbs used to mollify this imbalance. Formulas that are thought to dispel damp-wind and prevent seizures include Clematis and Stephania, Leonurus and Achyranthes, and Antelope Horn Wind Injury Remedy.

FAINTING

Fainting, known medically as syncope, *occurs when the blood supply to a person's brain is momentarily insufficient. As a result of this sudden shortage of oxygen, the person temporarily loses consciousness. The victim may become pale and lightheaded immediately before fainting. After lying down for a minute or so, blood flow usually returns to the brain, and the victim regains consciousness.*

Despite their dramatic nature, most cases of fainting are not the result of serious medical conditions. For example, some people faint when they see something unpleasant (like a wound or blood), are extremely tired, hungry, or dehydrated, have a severe coughing spell, receive emotionally traumatic news, rise quickly after reclining, or stand too long in a hot room. On the other hand, fainting can be the symptom of a more serious disorder. Several medical conditions, including diabetes, heart disease, and some circulatory problems, can produce fainting spells.

If you see someone faint, it is a good idea to play it safe and assume that the lapse of consciousness is symptomatic of a medical emergency. (If you later discover that the cause of fainting was not serious, your prudence will not have caused any harm.) Lay the victim on her back, then slowly raise her legs above the level of her head—prop her feet up on a chair or a stack of books, if possible. This allows gravity to increase the blood flow to the brain. If the person is wearing a belt, collar, or other forms of constrictive clothing, loosen or remove them. If there is not enough space to lay the victim flat, move her to a seated position with her head between her legs to increase blood flow to the brain.

The victim should regain consciousness within one or two minutes. While her complexion color soon returns to normal, she may continue to feel weak for a short time afterward.

If the victim does not regain consciousness after a minute or two, or if you notice that the victim is not breathing or has a very weak pulse, call for medical assistance immediately. If the victim regains consciousness but complains of chest pain, headache, numbness, extreme muscle weakness, or shortness of breath, the fainting is likely the symptom of an underlying medical disorder—the victim should be examined by a doctor as soon as possible.

FARSIGHTEDNESS

Signs and Symptoms

- Difficulty focusing on objects at close distances
- Eyestrain
- Aching eyes
- Recurring headaches

Description

Farsightedness, or *hyperopia*, is caused by a refraction problem in the eye. When light hits the eye, the cornea and lens refract, or "bend," the light rays so that they converge at the retina, the light-sensitive membrane at the back of the eye. In people with perfect vision, the eye is shaped in such a way that the lens and cornea refract entering light rays so that they converge directly on the retina. In people who are farsighted, the shape of the eye (its length from front to back) is shortened, or compacted, causing the lens and cornea to refract the light rays to a point of convergence behind the retina. As a result, only objects that are some distance away appear in focus, while objects that are too close to the eye appear blurred, out of focus.

Like many vision disorders, farsightedness tends to run in families and, in fact, is usually present to some degree at birth. Yet many children and young adults overcome mild farsightedness because their eye muscles are able to adapt to the condition, changing the shape of the lens to focus the point of convergence on the retina. Thus, many young people do not need treatment for their hyperopia. With age, however, the lens hardens and loses its ability to correct the condition, making vision correction necessary.

Conventional Medical Treatment

If you have difficulty focusing on objects that are close by, see your optometrist or ophthalmologist, who will conduct a series of eye exams to determine if you are farsighted. These tests can also determine the severity of the condition.

Treatment usually includes prescription eyeglass or contact lenses that are customized for your vision. These lenses refract incoming light at an angle that refocuses the point of convergence on your retina, correcting your vision. A new form of eye surgery called *thermokeratoplasty* is available for treating farsightedness, but is not widely used.

For More Information
National Eye Institute (NEI)
National Institutes of Health
2020 Vision Place
Bethesda, MD 20892-3655
301-496-5248
www.nei.nih.gov/publications/lowvis.htm

Health Notes

➤ *When reading, watching TV, performing computer work, or doing crafts or sewing, avoid eyestrain and headaches by giving your eyes a break every 15 minutes. Look away from whatever you have been focusing on for at least five minutes. Closing your eyes for a few minutes can also soothe strained eyes.*

➤ *Do not rely on over-the-counter eye drops to soothe the eyestrain that often accompanies hyperopia. Instead try laying cucumber slices over closed eyelids for five to fifteen minutes.*

➤ *A diet that includes beta-carotene-rich fruits and vegetables, such as carrots and sweet potatoes, is believed to help protect vision. Aim for four servings of fruits and five servings of vegetables each day.*

Complementary and Alternative Treatments

Nutrition and Supplementation

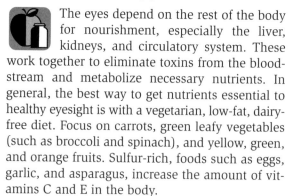

The eyes depend on the rest of the body for nourishment, especially the liver, kidneys, and circulatory system. These work together to eliminate toxins from the bloodstream and metabolize necessary nutrients. In general, the best way to get nutrients essential to healthy eyesight is with a vegetarian, low-fat, dairy-free diet. Focus on carrots, green leafy vegetables (such as broccoli and spinach), and yellow, green, and orange fruits. Sulfur-rich, foods such as eggs, garlic, and asparagus, increase the amount of vitamins C and E in the body.

Supplement your diet with the following daily recommendations:

- vitamin E (400 IU)—assists in healing and building the immune system

- vitamin A (25,000 IU; not to exceed 8000 IU if you are pregnant)—an absolute must to healthy eyesight; also aids liver digestion and metabolism; use emulsion form

- vitamin C (2000 mg 3 times daily)—an antioxidant that cleanses toxins from the bloodstream

- mixed carotenoid formula (15,000 IU)—a precursor of vitamin A

- vitamin B complex (100 mg twice daily)—for intracellular eye metabolism

- zinc (50 mg, not to exceed a total of 100 mg from all supplements)—a deficiency has been linked to retinal detachment; use lozenge form

(Consult your healthcare provider regarding the duration of treatment.)

Traditional Chinese Medicine

 Acupuncture Acupuncture may be used to improve the tone of the liver and balance the flow of energy in the liver meridian. Traditional Chinese Medicine believes imbalances in this organ are responsible for most eye disorders, including farsightedness.

Acupuncture also may be used to actually change the shape of the eye, which can help improve vision.

Chinese Herbal Therapy Herbs that may help rectify blurry vision are *Xiao Yao Wan*, and *Ming Mu Din Wang Wan*.

FATIGUE

Fatigue is a feeling of tiredness that occurs when the body doesn't have enough energy to function comfortably. Fatigue is often caused by non-medical factors, such as having an overly active day, getting less sleep than usual, or enduring emotional turmoil. It also can be the symptom of an underlying medical condition, such as anemia, chronic fatigue syndrome, circulatory problems, diabetes, hyperthyroidism, hypothyroidism, infectious diseases, and malnutrition. Psychological disorders, including clinical depression and anxiety disorders, also may result in fatigue. Even the treatment for medical conditions—such as prescription medication, chemotherapy, or surgery— can cause fatigue.

When non-medical factors are the cause of fatigue, several home care measures can help restore your energy. Regular exercise has been shown to increase energy levels, strengthen the body so that daily tasks are easier, improve quality of sleep, and soothe frazzled nerves. Drinking 8 or more 8-ounce glasses of water daily also helps body systems function efficiently, resulting in adequate levels of energy.

If you wish to explore complementary treatments to alleviate fatigue, you may consider chiropractic. Proper chiropractic spinal manipulation can increase energy levels by removing spinal subluxation and allowing nerves to function freely. Chiropractic care may include invigorating massage to decrease fatigue levels. The chiropractor may also prescribe specific exercises to increase the patient's energy levels. Moderate exercise such as walking or biking may be useful.

If your fatigue is accompanied by other symptoms or lasts more than a few weeks, it may be the sign of an underlying medical condition. In such cases, seek professional medical attention.

SYMPTOM:

FEVER

Fever occurs when a person's body temperature exceeds its normal level, which is usually 98.6° F. Most fevers are not usually noticeable or cause for concern unless body temperature is elevated to 100.5° F or above.

Many everyday occurrences, such as exercise and stress, can cause your body temperature to rise. Fever also can be a symptom of a wide range of medical conditions. Serious medical conditions, such as Hodgkin's disease and leukemia, and less-serious conditions, such as the common cold and flu, include fever among their symptoms. Fever also can occur as a reaction to certain medications. In fact, fever is a symptom of so many conditions that physicians rarely diagnose an illness on the basis of fever alone.

If you have a mild fever, you can usually treat it with home care. Start by increasing your fluid intake—drink large amounts of water and fresh juices. Stay away from solid foods, particularly proteins and fats. Keep the room you are staying in well-ventilated and at a comfortably cool temperature, and keep yourself well-covered. Placing cold compresses on your calves may make you

more comfortable and promote sleep. Aspirin, acetaminophen (Tylenol®, Valadol®), or ibuprofen (Advil®, Motrin®) also can help lower your fever. Children and teenagers should avoid aspirin when they have an infection, since the drug can cause Reye's syndrome, a potentially fatal condition.

If your fever is mild but has continued for three or more days despite home care, or if your fever is moderately high, see your physician as soon as possible. Your doctor needs to know when the fever began, what temperature it reached, and what accompanying symptoms you have, such as chills, muscle aches, vomiting, nausea, and fatigue. Your doctor may also perform a physical examination to determine what illness you have. Medical treatment for fever depends on what is causing the fever as well as other symptoms.

If your fever is above 106° F, or if you are of frail health or elderly, you should see a doctor immediately. Fevers above 108° F are extremely dangerous; if untreated, they can lead to permanent brain damage.

FIBROCYSTIC BREAST DISEASE

Signs and Symptoms

- Breast tenderness and pain, which may subside after menstruation
- Masses under the skin of the breast
- Breast engorgement

Description

Both fibrocystic breast disease and breast cancer are characterized by lumps or growths in the breast tissue. The difference between the two conditions is that while breast cancer is malignant, fibrocystic breast disease is benign. For this reason, the condition is also known as benign breast disease. While the condition may cause discomfort, it will not develop into cancer. However, a woman with fibrocystic breast disease may have difficulty detecting a malignant tumor if one develops. As a result, women with fibrocystic breast disease must be diligent about performing home breast examinations.

The precise cause of fibrocystic breast disease is unknown. It most often strikes women who have a family history of the condition and women of menstruating age. Because fibrocystic breast disease often disappears during menopause, a connection is often made between the condition and ovarian hormones.

Conventional Medical Treatment

Since the symptoms of fibrocystic breast disease are similar to those of breast cancer, see your gynecologist immediately if you feel a lump or experience nipple discharge. Your doctor will conduct a physical examination of the affected area, feeling for lumps and checking for discharge. A mammography or ultrasonography may also be necessary to confirm diagnosis. To determine whether lumps are benign or cancerous, your doctor inserts a needle into the area and takes a tissue core sample for further examination. *Thermography* is a new method of testing that views the heat emitted by targeted regions of the body. While its results are extremely accurate, this diagnostic method is not yet widespread in use.

If you are diagnosed with fibrocystic breast disease, treatment usually includes analgesics or prescription painkillers to ease discomfort. Your doctor also may advise you to wear a supportive bra—even while sleeping—to help reduce pain. If the lumps are extremely painful or increase in size, surgical removal is also an option.

For More Information
American Cancer Society
2420 N. Coliseum Blvd., Suite 200
Fort Wayne, IN 46805
(219) 471-3911
http://www.fwradiology.com/fibrobrst.htm

Complementary and Alternative Treatments

Nutrition and Supplementation

Experts agree that caffeine and dairy products increase breast tenderness and the lumps associated with fibrocystic breasts; so eliminate or limit consumption of these foods.

A diet high in fresh vegetables and low in red meat is believed to be most beneficial for this condition. An iodine deficiency can be corrected by adding iodine-rich seaweeds, such as wakame or kombu, to soups.

Daily recommendations for a supplemental program:

Most Important

- vitamin E (600 to 800 IU)
- mixed carotenoid formula (50,000 IU)
- evening primrose oil (follow directions on package)

Health Notes

➤ *For women with fibrocystic breast disease, weekly breast exams allow them to learn, through touch, which lumps are normal (part of their breast makeup), thus helping them to identify unfamiliar, or irregular, masses immediately.*

➤ *Studies have found that caffeine can cause an increase in lumpy tissue among women with fibrocystic breast disease. If you have the condition, avoid or limit your intake of caffeinated beverages.*

Also Recommended

- zinc (15 to 30 mg)
- vitamin B$_6$ (75 to 100 mg)
- flaxseed oil (2 tbsp)
- vitamin C (1500 mg)
- folic acid (400 mcg)
- iodine (500 mcg)
- choline (500 to 1000 mg)
- methionine (500 to 1000 mg)

(Consult your healthcare provider regarding the duration of treatment; also ask about taking soy isoflavones, especially genestein.)

Ayurvedic Medicine

 Ayurveda considers fibrocystic breasts a kapha condition in which excess kapha builds up, causes congestion, and leads to the development of lumpy, tender tissue. To relieve discomfort and prevent future occurrences, Ayurvedic practitioners often advise gentle massage with warm water and soap and a kapha-reducing diet.

Herbal Therapy

 A blend of herbs may help relieve the tenderness associated with fibrocystic breasts. Herbs for the blend include yellow dock root, dandelion root, burdock root, ginger powder, dong quai, astragalus, licorice root, chaste berry, and pau d'arco. Simmer up to 6 tablespoons of the blend in a quart of water for 20 minutes. Let stand for another 20 minutes. Strain through cheesecloth. Drink 1 cup several times a day for 5 days, take a 2-day break, then repeat. Use for no longer than 3 months.

Alternatively, you might try infusions of any of the following herbs: echinacea, goldenseal, mullein, pau d'arco, or red clover. *Note*: Use goldenseal for no more than a week at a time, and avoid it altogether if you are allergic to ragweed.

Some herbalists also suggest poke root or sage poultices to ease the soreness.

Homeopathy

 Fibrocystic breast disease may respond to homeopathic treatment. However, the selection of a remedy—more than one is available—depends on *your* symptoms and the stage of the condition. Don't try treating this disorder yourself. See a homeopathic professional.

Hydrotherapy

 Contrast therapy (alternate applications of hot and cool moist compresses) can bring welcome relief to tender, sore breasts. Apply for 3 to 5 minutes once a day.

Traditional Chinese Medicine

 Acupuncture Acupuncture can help lessen the pain that often characterizes fibrocystic breast disease. Acupoints commonly used in this treatment include Liver 3, Stomach 18 and 36, Conception Vessel 17, Small Intestine 1, and Gallbladder 41.

Acupressure In addition to massaging the breasts themselves, Conception Vessel 17, Bladder 18, and acupoints located in the armpit also may be involved in the treatment of fibrocystic breast disease.

Chinese Herbal Therapy Chinese herbs are often used to dispel benign cysts and alleviate any discomfort brought on by fibrocystic breast disease. Formulas used to combat fibrocystic breast pain are Bupleurum and Tang Gui, and Bupleurum Sedative Pills.

Yoga and Meditation

 Yoga's ability to help you relax can lessen some of the discomfort associated with tender, lumpy breasts. Try these poses: Locust, Bow, Boast, Spinal Twist, or Shoulder Stand.

FIBROMYALGIA

Signs and Symptoms

- Chronic, widespread pain that lasts three months or more, with no clear cause, combined with tenderness in at least 11 of 18 well-defined tender point sites on the body

- Pains, aches, and stiffness in several muscle groups, joints, and in all four quadrants of the body

- Pain that moves from one part of the body to another, most commonly felt in the neck, chest, arms, legs, hips, and back

- Pain that may be variously characterized as deep aching, radiating, gnawing, shooting, or burning

- Body aches and stiffness upon awakening

- Headaches and jaw pain

- Disturbed sleep patterns

- Fatigue

- Anxiety

- Depression

- Digestive system difficulties, as in swallowing, alternating diarrhea and constipation, or recurring abdominal pain

- Numbness or tingling in parts of the body

- Increased sensitivity to bright lights, noise, odors, and various foods

- Alternating feelings of hot and cold

Description

The word *fibromyalgia* comes from three Latin words, *fibro* ("fibrous tissue"), *my* ("muscle tissue"), and *algia* ("pain"). It is a chronic condition characterized by musculoskeletal pain and many tender points, particularly in the neck, spine, shoulders, and hips. It is called a *syndrome* rather than a *disease*, because not everyone's symptoms are the same.

Fibromyalgia afflicts between three and six million Americans, women more often than men. It often occurs in more than one member of a family, which suggests it may be an inherited disorder. Other possible causes include a virus or an injury that affects the central nervous system. Symptoms may be triggered or exacerbated by stress, anxiety, depression, poor sleep habits, or a change in the weather. For many years, fibromyalgia was thought to be a psychosomatic disorder because no one could find a definitive cause of the pain.

Conventional Medical Treatment

Diagnosis is frustrating, because fibromyalgia mimics the symptoms of other diseases, such as Lyme disease, rheumatoid arthritis, hypothyroidism, or low-back degenerative disease. Diagnosis usually comes after these and other conditions have been investigated and dismissed. There is no known way to prevent fibromyalgia, and the symptoms can come and go, often lasting for months or years. However, the disorder leaves no permanent damage, and in most cases it eventually does subside.

A doctor may prescribe a combination of muscle relaxers, anti-inflammatory, and antidepressant drugs. The antidepressants amitriptyline (Elavil®) or cyclbenzaprine hydrochloride (Flexeril®) are beneficial in relieving some symptoms, but can have side effects, including weight gain, urinary retention, and morning grogginess. Other muscle relaxers and antidepressants are occasionally prescribed.

The treatment for fibromyalgia also includes a combination of healthy diet, exercise, and rest. Stationary biking, low-impact aerobics, swimming, and walking may help alleviate symptoms; slowly work up to 60 minutes of exercise 3 or 4 times per week. Warm up and cool down the muscles gradually before and after exercise, and avoid exercises that can cause joint pain. Proper sleep is also important. Experts recommend eating a wide variety of fruits and vegetables because these foods provide trace elements and minerals that help muscles. High-fiber foods help the digestive system perform its functions. Massage and physical therapy (with heat) may bring some short-term relief.

For More Information

American Fibromyalgia Syndrome Association
6380 E. Tanque Verde, Suite D
Tuscon, AZ 85715
520-733-1570
www.afsafund.org

The Fibromyalgia Network
P.O. Box 31750
Tucson, AZ 85751
800-853-2929
www.fmnetnews.com

When Muscle Pain Won't Go Away:
The Relief Handbook for Fibromyalgia and Chronic
Pain
Gayle Backstrom with B. R. Rubin, D.O., F.A.C.P.
2212 Fort Worth Drive, #64
Denton, TX 76205

Health Notes

➤ *Patient education, stress reduction, and adequate sleep are essential components in any fibromyalgia management strategy.*

➤ *Because fibromyalgia can cause anxiety and depression (a result of chronic pain and fatigue), patients often join one of the numerous fibromyalgia support groups around the country.*

Complementary and Alternative Treatments

Nutrition and Supplementation

When it comes to fibromyalgia, it seems more important to *avoid* certain foods than to *include* particular foods in your diet. Eliminate meat, dairy products, and all other foods high in saturated fats; these fats interfere with circulation and increase pain. Likewise, avoid fried and processed foods, shellfish, white bread, and pasta. Eliminate sugar products from your diet, as sugar in any form disturbs sleep and promotes fatigue. Avoid caffeine and alcohol as well. If you have been consuming these foods on a regular basis, you will go through a short withdrawal period where your symptoms may worsen once you eliminate them from your menu. Before long, however, you will notice improvement.

Center your diet around raw foods and fresh juices. Eat lots of vegetables, fruits, whole grains, nuts and seeds, skinless turkey or chicken, and deep-water fish. These foods provide nutrients that help energize and build immunity. It is important to flush out toxins, so drink steam-distilled water and herbal teas. Eat four or five small meals daily so your body is supplied with a steady intake of proteins and carbohydrates necessary for muscle function.

Malabsorption problems are common in fibromyalgia, so all nutrients are needed in amounts greater than normal. A daily plan would include:

Most Important

- coenzyme Q10 (75 mg)—improves oxygenation of tissues

- lecithin (as directed on label)—energizes and improves circulation

- malic acid and magnesium (as directed on label)—assist in energy production in many cells

- proteolytic enzymes (as directed on label, 6 times daily)—improves the absorption of foods, especially protein

- vitamin A (25,000 IU for 1 month, reduce to 10,000 IU; not to exceed 8000 IU if you are pregnant)—protects the body's cells; use the emulsion form

- vitamin E (800 IU for 1 month, then reduce to 400 IU)—enhances immune function; use the emulsion form

- vitamin C with bioflavonoids (5000 to 10,000 mg)—energizes; use buffered form

- a prodophilus formula (as directed on label)—supports intestinal function

Also Recommended

- vitamin B complex (as prescribed by a doctor)—energizes and increases normal brain function; injections are best

- free-form amino acid complex (as directed on label)—supplies protein necessary for repair and building of muscle tissue

- magnesium glycinate (1000 mg)—a deficiency is common in people with fibromyalgia

- calcium citrate or calcium lactate (2000 mg)—balances with magnesium

- potassium (99 mg)—aids in muscle function

- selenium (200 mcg)—an antioxidant

- zinc (50 mg, not to exceed 100 mg total from all supplements)—helps the immune system function properly

- melatonin (as directed on label, 2 hours or less before bedtime)—promotes sleep

- vanadyl sulfate (as directed on label)—protects muscles and reduces fatigue

- L-glutamine (2 g)—supports immune system functioning

- live cell therapy supplement (as directed on label) (thymus, adrenal, liver, and pancreas)—supports glandular functions

(Consult your healthcare provider regarding the duration of treatment.)

Herbal Therapy

Since fibromyalgia presents a variety of stressing, even incapacitating, symptoms and discomforts, more than one herb is necessary for relief. Try a combination of the following herbal remedies:

- To boost blood circulation, alertness, and the immune system, use astragalus, echinacea, and ginkgo. You might also try these teas: burdock root, dandelion, and red clover. To make the teas, steep 1 to 3 teaspoons dried herb or root in 1 cup boiling water for 5 to 15 minutes; strain. Drink several cups daily. You also can brew a blend of the herbs.

- For relief from muscular pain, use a topical application of 1 part cayenne powder and 3 parts wintergreen oil. You also can try cayenne (in capsule form) and flaxseed oil (as directed on the label, three times daily).

- Sip skullcap or valerian root tea to improve sleep. To make the skullcap tea, steep 2 teaspoons dried leaves in 1 cup boiling water for 10 to 15 minutes; strain. To prepare the valerian tea, steep 2 teaspoons dried, chopped root in 1 cup boiling water for 8 to 12 hours; strain. Both skullcap and valerian are available in tincture form. Be aware that these herbs can cause drowsiness and should not be used to excess.

- Grape seed extract helps to protect muscles from free radical damage. Use as directed on the product label.

Traditional Chinese Medicine

Acupuncture Most of the symptoms and side effects associated with fibromyalgia can be treated with acupuncture. The acupoints to be manipulated will, of course, depend entirely on the symptoms presented by the individual.

Chinese Herbal Therapy There are numerous Chinese herbs that can be used to treat fibromyalgia-related symptoms. Consult the entry for each specific ailment ("Headache," "PMS," etc.) for detailed information or recommended herbs.

Formulas often used for fibromyalgia muscle pain are Corydalis Formula, Ginseng and Tang Gui Ten, Ginseng and Atractylodes, Peony and Licorice, and Tian Qi and Eucommia.

FLATULENCE

Flatulence, or gas (as it is commonly known), is rarely a symptom of a serious condition. Flatulence occurs when natural intestinal gas builds up to uncomfortable levels in your intestines, making your abdomen feel bloated and sore and causing forceful expulsions of gas. Flatulence is usually caused by drinking beverages that contain air (carbonated water or sodas); swallowing excessive air while talking, drinking, or eating; or consuming hard- to-digest fatty or oily foods. Gas also can be caused by eating high-fiber foods, though these foods typically cause flatulence only in individuals who are not used to eating them or do not tolerate them well; once the body is used to consuming fiber regularly, it begins to digest fibrous foods without producing excess gas. Certain medical conditions—such as irritable bowel syndrome, and lactose intolerance—can cause excessive flatulence. Patients re-covering from abdominal surgery also commonly experience flatulence.

In most cases, flatulence can be cleared up by simply avoiding the food or behavior that is causing the gas. If these measures do not work, or if you suspect that your flatulence may have a medical cause, visit your physician. To determine what is causing your flatulence, your doctor asks about the presence of other symptoms, such as belching or snoring (which are other symptoms of excessive air swallowing), and inquires about your stress level, typical daily diet, and elimination habits. The doctor also examines your abdomen for distention, tenderness, and masses. To confirm diagnosis, a blood test, stool analysis, upper gastrointestinal examination, barium enema, or endoscopy may be necessary. Once you receive treatment for the underlying condition, your flatulence will dissipate.

FLU (INFLUENZA)

Signs and Symptoms

- Fever and chills
- Sore throat
- Dry cough
- Nasal congestion and sneezing
- Headache
- General muscle aches
- Fatigue and muscle weakness

Description

Influenza, or flu (as it is commonly known), is an infectious disease caused by one of many strains of influenza virus. Due to its highly contagious nature, influenza is a very common illness, affecting millions of people each year. In fact, few people avoid contracting the flu at least once or twice in their lifetime.

Most people can tell when they are about to "get" the flu (although they are actually infected already)—their neck and shoulder muscles ache, their eyes burn, their throat hurts, and they feel weak or fatigued. Shortly thereafter, the full range of flu symptoms are usually present. Many people have difficulty determining whether they are affected by the flu or a common cold; but influenza symptoms, while similar to those of the common cold, are usually more severe and greater in number.

The influenza virus is transmitted from person to person by hand-to-hand contact or through the air. As a result, influenza spreads quickly in places where large groups of people gather indoors, such as in schools, buses, or offices. To contract the virus, all it takes is one infected person sneezing or coughing on you, near you, or into the air you are breathing. You can also catch the flu by touching a phone, stairway railing, or other surface after it has been touched by an infected person who has recently wiped his nose or eyes, or sneezed or coughed into his hand.

The virus has a one- to four-day incubation period, which means that you will not develop symptoms of the illness for a few days after contracting it. The flu usually lasts for three to five days, though it can last for as little as a day or as long as a week and a half.

Conventional Medical Treatment

In an otherwise healthy person, influenza is generally not dangerous and can be treated with home care measures. While there is no specific treatment for the flu, most doctors recommend bed rest, a nutrient-dense diet, and an increased intake of fluid. Analgesics can temporarily reduce the fever and muscle aches that generally accompany the flu. Antibiotics are ineffective in treating the flu (or any viral infections, for that matter); they are only used to treat bacterial infections.

The elderly, very young children, and people with compromised immune systems should see a doctor immediately for influenza treatment. In these people, influenza can digress into—or be accompanied by—acute sinusitis, bronchitis, or pneumonia. Amantadine, an anti-viral drug, may be prescribed to people in these high-risk groups.

Health Notes

➤ *During flu season, wash your hands frequently to kill any flu germs that you may have come into contact with. Also, avoid touching your face—influenza germs enter the body most quickly through the mucous membranes of the eyes, nose, and mouth.*

➤ *Low humidity weakens the ability of mucous membranes to fight off a viral attack. Use a cold-mist humidifier to add moisture to indoor air and prevent mucous membranes from drying out. Change the water every day to prevent bacteria and mold from growing in the humidifier.*

➤ *To keep your immune system strong, eat a healthy diet, and be sure to get at least 8 hours of sleep a night. A strong immune system is the best way to prevent or fight off a bout of the flu. Also, studies show that stress can weaken the immune system, so keep your stress to a minimum.*

➤ *During a bout of the flu, drink water— more than you usually drink—to flush your body and hydrate cells.*

Although it cannot be administered to someone who currently has the flu, the influenza vaccine is recommended to prevent influenza in people who are at high risk. The immunization is injected into the shoulder in the early fall, just before the traditional fall/winter flu season begins. Yearly vaccination is necessary, as this vaccine does not provide permanent protection. While the vaccine is not 100 percent effective in preventing the influenza virus, it will ensure that the symptoms are mild if you do contract the virus. People who are allergic to eggs and egg products cannot be inoculated for the flu, because they can develop a severe reaction to the vaccine.

Flu (Influenza)

For More Information
Centers for Disease Control and Prevention
1600 Clifton Road
Atlanta, GA 30333
800-311-3435
www.cdc.gov/ncidod/diseases/flu/fluvirus.htm

National Health Information Center
P.O. Box 1133
Washington D.C. 20013-1133
800-336-4797
http://nhic-nt.health.org

Complementary and Alternative Treatments

Nutrition and Supplementation

 Nutritional requirements for the flu are the same as those for the common cold. Garlic has long been used to fight infection, and cilantro has fever-reducing properties. Add 1 clove of chopped raw garlic to each serving of salt-free chicken broth; when the broth is almost hot, add fresh or dried cilantro.

Zinc promotes the proper functioning of the immune system. Vitamin C helps fight infection and liquefy mucus. Practitioners recommend taking zinc and C lozenges at the onset of the flu.

Daily supplements include:

- zinc and vitamin C lozenges (1 lozenge every 2 hours as needed)
- vitamin C (5000 to 20,000 mg in divided doses)—strengthens the immune system
- mixed carotenoid formula (15,000 IU)—a precursor of vitamin A
- vitamin A (15,000 IU; do not exceed 8000 IU if you are pregnant)—a powerful antioxidant
- garlic capsules (as directed on label)
- L-lysine (500 mg, on empty stomach)—combats viral infection and helps prevent outbreak of cold sores. (*Caution*: do not take longer than 6 months at a time.)
- N-acetyl cysteine (2 400 mg dosages at first sign of flu)

(Take supplements until your symptoms subside. If symptoms persist, seek the advice of your healthcare provider.)

Ayurvedic Medicine

 According to Ayurveda, the flu (and its relative in discomfort, the cold) is a vata-kapha disorder in which the body builds up an excess of vata and cool and moist kapha (congestion). To help fight the virus, Ayurvedic practitioners may advise a diet of rice seasoned with ginger powder, ground cumin, and ground turmeric. They also may suggest a combination of *sitopaladi* and *sudarshan* to relieve congestion.

Bodywork and Somatic Practices

 Stay away from massage and try Oriental bodywork, reflexology, polarity therapy, Therapeutic Touch, and Reiki.

Herbal Therapy

 Herbal remedies have long been used to ward off the flu and ease its symptoms. Try any of the following treatments, depending on your needs:

- Before the flu strikes, or at the first sign of illness, take echinacea in tea, tincture, or capsule form to help boost your immune system.

- Once the flu has struck, sip boneset tea several times a day to lessen aches, fever, and congestion. To make the tea, steep 2 to 3 teaspoons dried herb in 1 cup boiling water for 10 to 15 minutes; strain. Drink as hot as comfortable and consume no more than 6 cups in 24 hours. You also might chew a clove of garlic for its anti-viral properties or use elder flowers for their immune-stimulating properties.

- If you're bothered by chills and fever, try yarrow or elder, both of which have anti-inflammatory properties. Either can be taken as a tincture every four hours.

- If you have a cough and congestion, drink peppermint, fenugreek, or slippery elm tea to keep mucus flowing. To make any of the teas, steep 1 to 2 teaspoons of the dried herb in 1 cup boiling water for 5 to 10 minutes; strain. Drink up to 3 times a day. You also might try a pinch or two of cayenne in soups or stews.

Homeopathy

 Homeopathic practitioners recommend at least half a dozen different flu treatments. Which of the following remedies is most helpful depends on your symptoms and the stage of the illness:

- *Oscillococcinum* or "Flu Solution"—for fighting off the flu; must be taken at the first signs of illness; once you come down with the flu, it is not effective

- *Gelsemium*—if you feel tired, chilled, achy, drowsy, and have a headache that starts in the back of your head and settles in your forehead; you may feel as if there's a band around your head

- *Bryonia*—if you feel irritable, hot, achy, and have pain when you move; you may also feel very thirsty and have a headache that becomes worse when you cough

- *Rhus toxicodendron*—if you feel restless and chilled and have stiff, painful muscles; the tip of your tongue might be bright red

- *Nux vomica*—if you feel irritable and have nasal congestion that's worse at night

- *Belladonna*—if you have a very high temperature, sore throat, and flushed face

- *Eupatorium*—if you have severe pain in your limbs and are shivering

Hydrotherapy

 To loosen congestion and improve circulation, you might try a hot bath followed by a cold friction rub. For a cold friction rub, dip a washcloth into 50° to 60°F water and wrap the cloth around your hand. Vigorously rub your arms, legs, feet, chest, and abdomen, dipping the cloth into the cool water as necessary. Dry yourself briskly.

Traditional Chinese Medicine

 Acupuncture Acupuncture can be used to strengthen the immune system, enabling the body to better fight the flu virus. In treating influenza, the acupuncturist is likely to focus on the acupoints related to the organs most affected by the flu, such as the lungs and digestive system. Acupuncture also is helpful in relieving many flu-related symptoms, including chest and nasal congestion, muscle soreness, fatigue, and fever.

Acupuncture points usually used to remedy the flu are Gallbladder 20, Large Intestine 4, 18, and 20, Lung 5, Kidney 7, and Governing Vessel 14. An acupuncturist may manipulate many other points as well, depending on the patient's unique symptoms.

Acupressure This modality can be very helpful in relieving the nausea and sore, stiff muscles brought on by the flu. It can help the immune system work more efficiently and counteract fever and fatigue.

Points that may be manipulated are Governing Vessel 14, Bladder 12, and Large Intestine 4. Other lung, kidney, and stomach points may also be pressed, along with various auricular points.

Chinese Herbal Therapy Chinese herbs, such as akebia, balloon flower, joint fir, and gentian may be used to treat flu-related symptoms, such as sore throat, chest congestion, and stuffy nose.

To reduce a fever, soothe a raw throat, and relieve congestion, take a 1- to 4-gram decoction of licorice twice a day.

Astragalus is a natural immunity booster, as is garlic. Eating a raw clove of garlic can help prevent the flu virus from taking hold (although it shouldn't be taken on an empty stomach). Garlic also can be used as an expectorant to relieve chest congestion.

Two often-prescribed Chinese formulas are Ilex and Evodia (to help relieve fever, sore throat, chills, and stiff muscles), and Lonicera and Forsythia (which herbalists recommend taking at the first sign of illness to lessen the duration and severity of the symptoms).

FOLLICULITIS

Signs And Symptoms

- A rash of small, pus-filled pimples (each pierced by a hair) in a localized area
- When irritated, the pimples develop raised, red borders with yellow or gray centers
- Mild itchiness at the affected site

Description

Folliculitis is characterized by the growth of small, pimple-like bumps on a localized area of skin. Folliculitis can develop on the back of the thighs, on the buttocks, under the arms, or anywhere else on your body. Sometimes the condition is accompanied by mild itching at the affected site, though the symptoms are usually so minor that most people ignore the condition or assume that the bumps are caused by irritation.

Folliculitis is a common skin condition caused by an infection of hair follicles. The infection usually occurs when staphylococci (a type of microorganism), fungi, or bacteria enter hair follicles that have become irritated by clothing friction (such as a tight pair of jeans or a wet bathing suit), follicle blockage (caused when sweat is allowed to dry on the skin), or injury. The condition can occur anywhere on your skin, but folliculitis on the legs, underarms, bikini line, or face is usually caused by shaving. People who suffer from folliculitis often suffer chronically.

Conventional Medical Treatment

Your dermatologist can diagnose folliculitis with a physical examination of the area. If the pustules have become inflamed, your dermatologist will

Health Notes

➤ *A diet rich in fruits and vegetables boosts the immune system, helping the body fight off microorganisms before they can cause folliculitis.*

➤ *Keeping skin well-moisturized and supple reduces the risk of developing small scratches and tears, through which folliculitis-causing microorganisms can enter the skin.*

probably prescribe a topical or oral antibiotic to help clear up the infection.

If you have folliculitis but none of the pustules are inflamed, home care can usually clear the condition. Over-the-counter acne treatments that contain sulfur, salicylic acid, or benzoyl peroxide should clear the condition within three to five days. If your folliculitis is caused by shaving, you may want to consider waxing or a depilatory. Men who develop folliculitis on the face after shaving should use a new razor blade every day to avoid re-infecting the area. Do not shave areas that are affected by folliculitis until after the rash

heals. If your folliculitis is caused by tight clothing, dress in looser fashions—or change out of restrictive clothing (such as bathing suits) as soon as possible.

For More Information
American Academy of Dermatology
930 North Meacham Road
Schaumberg, IL 60173
888-462-DERM
www.aad.org

Complementary and Alternative Treatments

Traditional Chinese Medicine

 Acupuncture This modality can be used to relieve inflammation and improve circulation to the affected follicles. Auricular points that may be targeted include the lung, adrenal gland, back of head, and points that correspond to the affected area.

Chinese Herbal Therapy There are various liniments that can be used. Check with your TCM practitioner.

FOOD POISONING

Signs And Symptoms

Symptoms of food poisoning usually develop within one hour to two days after eating the affected food and vary depending on what substance caused the poisoning. General symptoms include:

- Abdominal cramps and diarrhea
- Nausea and vomiting
- Headache
- Dizziness
- Sweating
- Fever

Description

One in every 10 Americans develops a case of food poisoning each year. Not all cases of food poisoning are the same. In some cases, people develop symptoms within an hour of consuming the

Parasitic Worms

Microorganisms aren't the only outside threat to your digestive system. Small, parasitic worms can also take up residence in the human intestines, causing gastrointestinal distress. The most common species of parasitic worms are *Ascaris,* hookworms, pinworms, and tapeworms.

Ascaris are the most common type of intestinal worm. They thrive in human feces and are especially common in poor countries where overcrowded conditions seriously compromise hygiene. *Ascaris* eggs are found in feces-rich soil; eggs enter the body of humans who eat contaminated food. Symptoms of *Ascaris* infestation include vomiting, stomach pain, and abdominal bloating.

Hookworm larvae live in moist, tropical soil. The larvae enter the body through the skin—usually of the feet—and travel through the bloodstream to the mouth, where they are swallowed. They pass through the stomach and enter the small intestine, where they attach themselves to the intestinal wall and develop into half-inch adult worms. Symptoms of hookworm infestation include a dry cough, low-grade fever, fatigue, loss of appetite, and diarrhea.

Pinworm eggs enter the human body on conta-minated food, in contaminated beverages, or when a contaminated hand is placed in the mouth. The eggs migrate to the lower intestinal tract where they hatch into worms. When the host's body temperature drops—typically at night during sleep—the female worms leave the large intestine. Before dying, the female pinworms lay eggs around the host's anus and in the bed. Symptoms of pinworm infestation include severe anal itching (especially at night) and vague gastrointestinal upset.

Tapeworms can grow up to 75 feet long (though they usually average three feet in length). The worms are introduced into the body via undercooked beef, fish, or pork. Once inside the body, the worms attach themselves to the intestinal wall, where they can live for years. Symptoms of tapeworm infestation include hunger, dizziness, fatigue, and weight loss. However, most people with tapeworm infestations notice no symptoms other than white worm segments found in the stool, bedding, or clothing.

A physician can usually diagnose parasitic worms with a stool sample. Treatment generally consists of a prescription antiparasitic medication to kill the worms.

infected food; in others, symptoms do not manifest themselves until two days after the food is eaten. Duration of symptoms also vary—some bouts last for only 12 hours (in mild cases), while others may remain for five days or more.

Food poisoning is caused by one of more than 10 types of food-borne bacteria, or specific toxins created by the bacteria. Each type of bacteria inhabits a specific type of food—raw or undercooked seafood, egg products, undercooked meat or poultry, dairy products, raw vegetables, or contaminated water. Because such a wide range of bacteria can cause food poisoning, it is often difficult to determine exactly which bacteria contaminated your food.

Conventional Medical Treatment

People who are otherwise healthy, between the ages of 12 and 65, and not pregnant can treat food poisoning with home care. To give your distressed digestive system a rest, do not eat any solid food until your symptoms dissipate. To counteract the loss of fluids caused by diarrhea and vomiting, drink lots of water and electrolyte-rich sports drinks, such as Gatorade. Since continual vomiting usually causes weakness, relaxing indoors—preferably in bed—is wise.

If your symptoms do not go away within 48 hours or you notice blood in your stool or vomit,

Health Notes

➤ Be sure to cook eggs before eating to re-duce the risk of infection by salmonella bacteria, a common cause of food poison-ing.

➤ Be careful when handling raw chicken. At the supermarket, select your chicken after you finish the rest of your shopping and place it in a plastic bag (from the produce department)—this will prevent infected fluids from spilling onto other foods. Once home, store the chicken in the refrigerator until you are ready to cook it. Always wash your hands and any utensils and cutting boards or surfaces used after preparing raw chicken.

➤ Keep meat and fish refrigerated until ready to use. Wash your hands before and after handling meat or fish, and be sure to kill any possible E. coli or other bacteria by thoroughly cooking the meat or fish.

➤ Keep milk, butter, yogurt, cheese, and other dairy products refrigerated.

➤ Fruits and vegetables are often sprayed with pesticides and also have the potential to carry bacteria. Therefore, it is absolutely essential that you wash all fruits and veg-etables before eating them.

➤ To avoid botulism, a potentially fatal form of food poisoning, do not purchase cans of food that have bulges or broken seals.

➤ Drink only bottled water or buy a water fil-ter for your faucet.

see a doctor immediately. Anyone who is over the age of 65 or under the age of 12, is pregnant, or has a compromised immune system should see a doctor at the first signs of food poisoning. A stool culture can help the doctor determine if food poi-soning is cause of your illness. If food poisoning is the diagnosis, a stool sample also can reveal which type of bacteria caused the illness. If the case of food poisoning is severe, your doctor may prescribe antibiotics or recommend intravenous fluid replacement to rehydrate the body.

For More Information
Centers for Disease Control and Prevention
1600 Clifton Road, NE
Atlanta, GA 30333
800-311-3435
www.cdc.gov/ncidod/diseases/foodborn/
foodborn.htm

Complementary and Alternative Treatments

Nutrition and Supplementation

 Avoid solid food, and drink plenty of liq-uids. Take 5 charcoal tablets to absorb toxins; repeat 6 hours later. As you re-cover, experts recommend that you drink several glasses of fresh carrot and beet juice and reduce solid foods in the diet for one to three days. Garlic and citrus help combat any bacterial organisms that may have been ingested.

To replace gut flora after excessive vomiting, follow these daily suggestions:

Most Important

• *Lactobaccillus acidolphilus* and *bifidobacteria* capsules or powders (as directed on label)

• garlic capsules (as directed on package label)

• potassium (99 mg)—restores electrolyte bal-ance

• vitamin C (8000 mg in divided doses)—detox-ifies the system

Also Recommended

• citrus seed extract (as directed on package la-bel)

• glutamine (2 g)—promotes intestinal health

• N-acetyl glucosamine (as directed on label)—promotes intestinal health

Food Poisoning

- gamma orizanol (as directed on label)—promotes intestinal health
- N-acetyl cysteine (200 mg)—detoxifies intestinal tract

(Take supplements until your symptoms subside. If symptoms persist, seek the advice of your healthcare provider.)

Ayurvedic Medicine

To ease the discomfort and symptoms of mild food poisoning, Ayurvedic practitioners may advise first fasting, then drinking cumin-coriander-fennel tea.

Herbal Therapy

Ginger is one of the best remedies for soothing a queasy stomach. Drink a cup of ginger tea every two hours while symptoms last, or take two capsules. To make the tea, boil 1 ounce of the root in 1 cup water for 15 to 20 minutes; strain. Other helpful herbal teas include meadowsweet, catnip, and slippery elm. To make any of these teas, steep 2 teaspoons of the herb in 1 cup boiling water for 15 minutes; strain.

Homeopathy

A homeopathic practitioner may suggest one of the following treatments, depending on your symptoms:

- *Arsenicum album*—for stomach upset from eating bad meat; you may feel extremely weak and anxious
- *Pulsatilla*—for stomach upset from eating overly rich foods

- *Nux vomica*—for stomach upset from overindulgence in food and alcohol
- *Veratrum album*—for stomach upset with diarrhea and vomiting; you may feel extremely cold

Hydrotherapy

To settle your stomach during a bout of food poisoning, sip a mixture of 1/4 cup of activated charcoal mixed into 1 cup of water. Activated charcoal can be found in many health food stores as well as in some pharmacies.

Traditional Chinese Medicine

Acupuncture Acupuncture can be used to improve circulation, thereby speeding toxins out of the body. It can also be used to help relieve an upset stomach (though it should not be used to stop vomiting, as this is the body's way of eliminating the contaminated substance).

Acupressure Applying pressure to Pericardium 6 (on the inner forearm above the wrist) and Stomach 36 (beneath the kneecap) may help relieve food poisoning-induced nausea.

Chinese Herbal Therapy Chinese herbs or herbal formulas should be taken only after you have sought medical attention—and should be used under the guidance of a trained herbalist. Ginger, taken in two 5 to 15 gram decoctions, can help soothe the ravages of food poisoning. The Chinese herbal formula, called Pill Curing, also can help relieve discomfort.

FROSTBITE

Signs And Symptoms

- An area of skin that is hard, white, and cold immediately after prolonged exposure to low temperatures
- After thawing, the affected site becomes red and painful
- Decreased sensitivity at the affected site
- Throbbing pain at the affected site
- Localized swelling or blistering

Description

Frostbite occurs when deep tissue cells freeze and die. In severe cases of frostbite, the underlying blood vessels, muscles, and nerves are damaged. While frostbite can affect any part of the body that is exposed to extremely cold temperatures for a sustained period of time, the nose, ears, feet, and hands are the most commonly affected areas.

Frostbite is typically caused by exposure to temperatures of 0°F or below for two hours or more, though these factors are variable. The process can be accelerated by a very low wind-chill factor, dampness, or returning to the cold environment immediately after thawing from a previous period of exposure.

Although frostbite can affect anyone, people with circulatory problems are at increased risk. Frostbite ultimately destroys tissue by literally freezing the nutrient-rich blood flow to an area of the body. Since people with circulatory problem have sluggish blood flow to begin with, the destruction of tissue by frostbite is accelerated.

Conventional Medical Treatment

If you develop frostbite, the first thing to do is warm the affected tissue. Return to a heated environment, and raise the temperature of the affected area slowly. Do not use heating pads or other direct applications of heat—frostbitten tissue is fragile and burns easily. As soon as you are able, seek medical assistance. A nurse, paramedic, or physician can determine if you have frostbite by conducting a physical examination of the area.

Total recovery from frostbite is not quick—it often takes 6 to 12 months for the site to completely recuperate. During the early stages of recovery, your doctor may place you on antibiotics to ward off the threat of infection. Until you are completely recovered, you should not smoke tobacco products; cigarettes, pipes, and cigars constrict blood circulation, preventing the necessary amount of nutrient-rich blood from reaching the frostbitten site. Unfortunately, you may feel the effects of the episode for the rest of your life:

Health Notes

➤ You can prevent frostbite by wearing multiple layers of clothes, which helps trap heat near the body. Maintain a healthy body temperature by wearing long underwear, pants, a t-shirt, a long-sleeved shirt or sweater, two pairs of socks, two pairs of gloves, a hat, a scarf, and water-resistant outer wear.

➤ If you smoke, quit. Smoking slows blood circulation, putting you at higher risk of developing frostbite.

➤ To maintain healthy blood circulation to your fingers and toes, wiggle them often.

➤ Avoid drinking alcohol before going out in cold weather. Alcohol restricts blood flow, putting you at higher risk for frostbite.

frostbite sometimes causes the affected area to be permanently sensitive to cold temperatures.

In extremely severe cases of frostbite, where large areas of tissue are destroyed, amputation is sometimes necessary. It can take up to three weeks after the initial exposure to cold to verify that the tissue will not recover. In such cases, gangrene may set in and threaten surrounding healthy tissue, making amputation necessary.

For More Information
National Health Information Center
P.O. Box 1133
Washington D.C. 20013-1133
800-336-4797
http://nhic-nt.health.org

Complementary and Alternative Treatments

Nutrition and Supplementation

B vitamins help restore nerve health. Experts recommend a 50- to 75-mg daily dose of vitamin B complex.

Herbal Therapy

Ginger can stimulate the circulatory system. To boost circulation to the affected areas, try drinking hot ginger tea. To make the tea, boil 1 ounce of the root in 1 cup water for 15 to 20 minutes; strain.

Homeopathy

For frostbitten fingers or toes that are red and itchy and tingle, take *Agaricus*.

Hydrotherapy

Frostbitten skin should be warmed slowly. To do so, immerse yourself in a neutral bath (slightly cooler than body temperature), and slowly increase temperature to just above body temperature.

Traditional Chinese Medicine

Acupuncture Following conventional medical treatment, acupuncture can be used to improve circulation, which may help prevent permanent nerve damage.

Acupressure This modality can be used to increase the flow of blood to the affected area, which should speed healing. The acupressure points to be manipulated will depend on the location of the frostbite.

Chinese Herbal Therapy Peony and *Dong Quai* formulas may be helpful in improving circulation to the affected area.

GALLSTONES

Signs and Symptoms

- Intense and very sudden pain in the upper-right portion of the abdomen that may radiate to the right shoulder blade and persist for several hours
- Nausea and vomiting
- Indigestion
- Loss of appetite
- Fever
- Jaundice

Description

The gallbladder is a pear-shaped organ that is located beneath your liver. The gallbladder stores bile, a digestive fluid that the liver produces, until the fluid is required to help digest dietary fats in the small intestine. Normally, the acidic bile prevents cholesterol from becoming too concentrated. However, if too much cholesterol is present in the bile, it crystallizes in the gallbladder, forming gallstones. These crystalline formations may be round or jagged, small as a pea or large as a Ping-Pong ball. Some people with the condition develop only a single gallstone, while others develop several.

Gallstones that remain in the gallbladder typically produce no symptoms. If a gallstone exits the gallbladder, it can cause pain and other symptoms. Gallstones usually begin producing symptoms when they obstruct the duct that leads from the liver to the gallbladder or the duct that leads from the gallbladder to the small intestine. Once lodged in one of these ducts, the stones may produce painful spasms and inflammation at the site of the obstruction.

Gallstones most commonly affect people over the age of 40 and are generally associated with high blood cholesterol levels. Women who have had multiple pregnancies are also at increased risk. In fact, women, in general, have a much higher incidence of gallstones than men do.

Conventional Medical Treatment

While many people who have gallstones never experience any symptoms, some people experience a painful attack that alerts them to visit a doctor. To diagnose the condition, your physician conducts a physical examination (to look for jaundice) and feels your abdomen to determine whether your gallbladder has become obstructed and distended. A blood test and ultrasound examination may be necessary to confirm diagnosis.

Non-surgical treatment is less common now and usually limited to patients who cannot un-

Health Notes

➤ Some studies suggest that moderate alcohol intake of no more than two drinks per day may protect against gallstones.

➤ Studies show that vegetarians who eat a low-fat diet have a lower incidence of gallstones. Fat—especially saturated fat found in animal foods—has been found to be a risk factor for gallstones.

➤ Maintain a healthy body weight. If you are more than ten pounds overweight, you may be at increased risk of developing gallstones.

➤ If you smoke, quit. Cigarette smokers have a higher risk of developing gallstones than people who do not smoke.

dergo surgery. Laparoscopic surgery to remove the gallbladder is the most frequently used treatment. Stones can be broken up by directing high-frequency sound waves at the gallbladder. This is called *lithotripsy*. Alternatively, gallstones may be dissolved with cheno-ursodeoxycholic acid.

While the gallbladder provides a useful service, it isn't necessary in maintaining normal body functions; the liver still can produce bile in the gallbladder's absence.

For More Information

National Institute of Diabetes and
Digestive and Kidney Diseases
2 Information Way
Bethesda, MD 20892-3570
301-654-3810
www.niddk.nih.gov

Complementary and Alternative Treatments

Nutrition and Supplementation

 For gallstones, mix 3 tablespoons of olive oil with lemon or grapefruit juice and drink before breakfast and before bedtime. This treatment often helps eliminate stones in the stool. Your diet should contain 75 percent raw foods and include applesauce, fresh apples, eggs, beets, and plain organic yogurt. Other dairy products, fried and fatty foods, and refined white sugar increase the risk of gallstone formation. Avoid coffee (even decaffeinated), as it contracts the gallbladder and constricts bile flow.

To cleanse the system, drink as much pure apple juice as possible for five days; pear juice may be substituted on occasion.

Obesity is a risk factor. If you are overweight, experts recommend a sensible weight loss program created with the help of a medical expert. *Do not* go on a crash diet, which in itself may be a risk for gallstones.

Supplement your diet with the following on a daily basis:

- vitamin C (3000 mg in divided doses)—a deficiency can result in gallstones

- vitamin E (600 IU)
- lecithin (1200 mg)—aids in the digestion of fats
- choline (1000 mg)—aids in liver and gallbladder function
- L-glycine (500 mg, taken with water or juice)—important for the biosynthesis of bile acids
- taurine (1 g twice daily)—increases bile formation
- vitamin D (400 IU)—may interfere with absorption

(Consult your healthcare provider regarding the duration of treatment.)

Ayurvedic Medicine

 Ayurveda views gallstones as a kapha disorder of slow metabolism (including underactive thyroid). An Ayurvedic practitioner may recommend taking an Ayurvedic formula containing six herbs, including *musta* and *shilajit,* to help prevent gallstones by speeding metabolism. To eliminate gallstones, the practitioner may also suggest a liver flush of olive oil, lemon juice, and spices. *Note*: Use these treatments only with the approval of your doctor and under the supervision of a qualified Ayurvedic practitioner.

Bodywork and Somatic Practices

 Oriental bodywork therapies and reflexology are good first lines of action for these painful conditions. Include Reiki and Therapeutic Touch for extra loving care.

Herbal Therapy

 Numerous herbs are recommended for banishing gallstones, improving the flow of bile, and preventing the formation of new stones. Any of the following treatments are suggested by herbalists: Combine equal amounts of tinctures of wild yam, fringetree bark, milk thistle, and balmony, and take a teaspoonful of the blend several times a day. Drink chamomile or lemon balm tea or a combination tea of balmony and fringetree. To make any of the teas, steep 1 or 2 teaspoons of the herb in 1 cup boiling water for 15 minutes; strain.

Other beneficial herbs for treating gallstones include catnip, cramp bark, dandelion, fennel, ginger root, and horsetail.

Homeopathy

Gallstones may respond to homeopathic treatment. However, the selection of a remedy—more than one is available—depends on *your* symptoms and the stage of the condition. Don't try treating this disorder yourself. See a homeopathic professional.

Hydrotherapy

To help prevent gallstones, drink plenty of water—8 to 12 8-ounce glasses—every day. Water dilutes the bile and helps flush it from the liver.

If you're bothered by gallstones and have frequent attacks, try constitutional hydrotherapy several times a week: apply alternating hot and cold packs to the abdomen and lower back.

Traditional Chinese Medicine

Acupuncture Acupuncture can be used to improve circulation to the gallbladder, thereby helping to prevent the formation of gallstones. It also can be used to relieve gallstone-related pain, inflammation, digestive problems, and fever.

Acupuncture points may include Gallbladder 34, Pericardium 6, Bladder 19, Stomach 36, Large Intestine 11, and related ear points.

Acupressure Acupressure can be useful in improving the flow of bile in the gallbladder and lessening gallstone pain. Points targeted during this treatment include Liver 3; Gallbladder 34; and Bladder 17, 18, and 19.

Chinese Herbal Therapy To improve bile flow and remedy gallstones, a Chinese herbalist may prescribe Corydalis Formula, Liver Strengthening Tablets, Minor Bupleurum Formula, Rhubarb and Scutellaria Formula, and Lidan Tablets. For gallbladder pain, Corydalis Analgesic Tablets are usually recommended.

Yoga and Meditation

Yoga poses that help ward off gallstones by emptying the gallbladder include the Bow, Peacock, and Spinal Twist.

GASTRITIS

Signs and Symptoms

- Upper abdominal discomfort, pain and burning
- Nausea
- Vomiting
- Diarrhea
- Loss of appetite

Description

Gastritis is an inflammation of the stomach lining. It is a very common condition—in fact, most people experience the condition at least once in their lifetime. Fortunately, the symptoms of gastritis are relatively mild, have a short duration, and usually have no lasting effects on the body. The risk of developing a case of gastritis increases with age. The condition also affects more women than men.

Gastritis can result from any of a number of causes, each of which produces slightly different symptoms and intensity. Several types of medications, including aspirin and anti-inflammatory drugs, can bring on a case of gastritis. Severe emotional or physical stress can also induce gastritis. Other causes of the condition include vitamin B_{12} deficiency, excessive smoking or alcohol consumption, and a microorganism called *Helicobacter pylori*.

Conventional Medical Treatment

If you suspect you have a case of gastritis, see your physician, who can diagnose the condition by conducting a physical examination and asking for a history of symptoms. To confirm diagnosis, a barium X-ray or *endoscopy* may be necessary. During an endoscopy, a flexible tube called a fiberoptic endoscope is inserted through your mouth into your esophagus, stomach, and duodenum. This tube is equipped with a lighting and video system that enables a physician to examine your upper digestive tract.

If gastritis is the diagnosis, your physician will first recommend that you discontinue the habit that causes the gastritis. You may need to stop smoking or change your eating or drinking habits. If the gastritis is a side effect of a medication, your doctor may recommend replacing it with another type of drug that should be taken at very specific times of the day. If you have a vitamin B_{12} deficiency, you may need to have monthly vitamin B_{12} shots. If a microorganism is causing the condition, a medication may be prescribed to destroy it.

Antacids are a common—and acceptable—treatment for mild gastritis. If over-the-counter antacids fail to provide relief, your physician may prescribe a medication, such as cimetidine, ranitidine, or famotidine, to decrease the amount of acid produced by your stomach. Medication that protects the lining of the stomach, such as sucralfate or Misoprostol®, also may be prescribed.

Health Notes

➤ *Drink moderately or not at all. Alcohol is a common cause of gastritis.*

➤ *Excess caffeine can cause gastritis. If you are experiencing recurring gastritis, you may want to consider cutting caffeine from your diet.*

➤ *If you experience gastritis, you may want to investigate painkillers that do not contain aspirin or ibuprofen. Studies have found that aspirin and nonsteroidal anti-inflammatory drugs (NSAIDs), such as ibuprofen, can cause gastritis.*

For More Information
National Institute of Diabetes and
Digestive and Kidney Diseases
2 Information Way
Bethesda, MD 20892-3570
301-654-3810
www.niddk.nih.gov

Complementary and Alternative Treatments

Nutrition and Supplementation

 To help aid digestion, eat simple foods in combinations that digest well together. Combine leafy greens with lean proteins, such as non-fat dairy products and lean meats or fish. Get your carbohydrates from sources that do not cause a pronounced blood sugar change; these include rice, fresh fruits, asparagus, broccoli, cauliflower, squash, and green beans.

There are many "don'ts" involved in treating and preventing gastritis. Avoid or severely limit your intake of sugar, alcohol, caffeine, fatty foods, spicy foods, and tomato products. These foods can irritate the stomach lining, increase stomach acid production, and/or weaken the muscular sphincter at the end of the esophagus, almost guaranteeing that all extra acid will find its way into the esophagus. Avoid milk as well; although milk momentarily neutralizes stomach acid, the amount of acid increases almost immediately, leaving you in worse condition.

To relieve symptoms, chew papaya tablets (follow directions on the label). Other daily supplements include:

- L-glutamine (2 g)—heals the stomach lining

- ginger (25 mg)—calms and heals the stomach

- N-acetyl glucosamine (as directed on label)—promotes intestinal health

- gamma orizanol (as directed on label)—promotes intestinal health

- colostrum (as directed on label)—reduces inflammation and aids absorption

(For an *acute* condition, take supplements until your symptoms subside. If symptoms persist, seek the advice of your healthcare provider. For a *chronic* condition, consult your healthcare provider regarding the duration of treatment.)

Herbal Therapy

Meadowsweet is one of the top herbs for digestive upset. It relieves nausea and reduces excess stomach acid. To make meadowsweet tea, steep 2 teaspoons of the dried herb in 1 cup boiling water for 15 minutes; strain.

Following an attack of nausea and vomiting, stomach pain, cramps, and diarrhea, drink a soothing tea made from slippery elm. Simmer 1 part powdered bark in 8 parts water for 15 minutes; strain. Drink 1/2 cup several times a day.

Echinacea and goldenseal can also help heal an irritated stomach lining.

See also "Food Poisoning" and "Indigestion (Dyspepsia)" entries.

Homeopathy

See also "Food Poisoning" and "Indigestion (Dyspepsia)" entries.

Traditional Chinese Medicine

Acupuncture Acupuncture may be used to help alleviate gastritis-induced pain, vomiting, and diarrhea. It also can be helpful in lessening stomach inflammation. Points that may be targeted include Stomach 36, Conception Vessel 12, and Stomach 34 (for acute pain). Additional points may be added as symptoms warrant.

Acupressure To relieve gastritis-related nausea, an acupressure expert probably will focus on Pericardium 6, Stomach 36, Conception Vessel 12 and 17, and Liver 3.

The treatment of diarrhea also may include the manipulation of Stomach 36, along with Stomach 25, Spleen 6 and 9, Conception Vessel 6, and Large Intestine 11.

Chinese Herbal Therapy Aloe vera can be used to calm an upset stomach and relieve inflammation; generally, 0.1 to 1 gram will be given, depending on the severity of symptoms. Other Chinese herbs used to treat gastritis are licorice and various patent formulas as prescribed by a practitioner.

GASTROENTERITIS

Signs and Symptoms

- Diarrhea
- Nausea and vomiting
- Abdominal cramps
- Abdominal pain
- Headaches
- Fever
- Muscle weakness

Description

Gastroenteritis is an infection of the gastrointestinal tract. Sometimes referred to as stomach flu, gastroenteritis can be caused by a number of different factors, including bacteria, virus (usually the rotavirus or Norwalk virus), internal parasites, food poisoning, and tainted drinking water.

Symptoms of gastritis usually come on suddenly, and with the possible exceptions of headache and fever, are limited to the gastrointestinal tract. The severity and duration of symptoms depends solely on what caused the infection. Most cases of gastritis last for no more than 48 hours, though some viral infections and parasites can cause more than a week of discomfort.

Conventional Medical Treatment

If you suspect you have gastritis, see your physician, who conducts a physical examination. A stool sample also may be necessary to confirm the diagnosis and uncover the cause. If the condition is not severe, your doctor may prescribe an anti-diarrheal medication and recommend increased fluid intake to prevent dehydration and replace fluids lost through diarrhea. If you have a severe bacterial infection, your doctor may prescribe an antibiotic.

Health Notes

➤ Only drink bottled water or water that you have boiled or filtered yourself. Some parasites can pass through the filters used by water treatment plants, and others are resistant to the chorine used to purify water supplies.

➤ Microorganisms in human feces—such as E. coli, salmonella, shigella, and giardia—are responsible for a large number of gastroenteritis cases. Always wash your hands thoroughly after changing a baby's diaper or using the restroom.

For More Information
Centers for Disease Control and Prevention (CDC)
1600 Clifton Road
Atlanta, GA 30333
800-311-3435
www.cdc.gov

National Institute of Diabetes and Digestive and Kidney Diseases
2 Information Way
Bethesda, MD 20892-3570
301-654-3810
www.niddk.nih.gov

Complementary and Alternative Treatments

Nutrition and Supplementation

Gastroenteritis often is caused by a viral infection. Follow dietary guidelines for gastritis, and supplement with zinc to stimulate immunity and with vitamin A to help the intestinal lining. Daily supplementation guidelines follow:

- vitamin C (1000 mg)
- zinc (25 to 30 mg; *never* take on an empty stomach)
- vitamin A (5000 IU)
- multivitamin complex

(For an *acute* condition, take supplements until your symptoms subside. If symptoms persist, seek the advice of your healthcare provider. For a *chronic* condition, consult your healthcare provider regarding the duration of treatment.)

Traditional Chinese Medicine

 Acupuncture Gastroenteritis encompasses myriad symptoms, from nausea and vomiting to diarrhea and stomach cramps. Fortunately, acupuncture can be used to remedy most gastroenteritis-related problems, whether viral or parasitic in nature. The areas to be targeted depend on the patient's symptoms, but they will include various stomach, large intestine, kidney, bladder, gallbladder, and related points.

Acupressure To help relieve the discomfort of gastroenteritis, the practitioner may focus on massaging Pericardium 6 (to relieve nausea), along with points on the abdomen and lower back (for other symptoms).

Chinese Herbal Therapy Fresh ginger is a famous nausea remedy; costus and garlic can be used to quell dysentery. Chinese formulas that may be used to help relieve gastroenteritis include Curing Pills, Citrus and Pinellia, Bupleurum and Tang Gui, and Ginseng and Atractylodes.

GENITAL HERPES

Signs and Symptoms

- Pain or itching on the skin of the genital area, anus, or buttocks
- Small, painful blisters or bumps on the affected area
- Swollen lymph nodes in the groin area
- Headaches
- Fever

Description

Herpes is the most common sexually transmitted virus in the United States. In fact, approximately 300,000 new cases of genital herpes are reported each year. The condition is caused by the herpes simplex virus, which is transmitted through vaginal or anal sex.

Within 20 days of exposure to the virus, a herpes victim usually experiences a period of pain and itching in the genital area lasting anywhere from two hours to one week. Immediately after this period, small red bumps begin to appear on the genital area, and urination may become painful. Within four days of developing, the red bumps become fluid-filled blisters that soon rupture and become ulcers. Three or four days after rupturing, the ulcers scab over and heal. During an initial outbreak, the victim may experience flu-like symptoms that disappear once the ulcers have healed. The genital area may be tender until the infection clears.

Unfortunately, the condition is not curable—the virus remains in the victim's bloodstream for the rest of his or her life. The virus may cause recurrent infections over the course of the victim's lifetime. In fact, up to 75 percent of genital herpes victims have a recurrent infection within three

Health Notes

➤ *Celibacy or a mutually monogamous relationship is the only sure way to prevent genital herpes.*

➤ *If you have herpes, consult your physician before starting a family. Genital herpes increases the risk of miscarriage, premature birth, and fetal growth retardation. Caesarean delivery may prevent an infant from contracting herpes during birth.*

➤ *Using a condom decreases your risk of contracting herpes and other STDs.*

➤ *You may be infectious, even when no blisters or sores are visible.*

months of the initial outbreak. While the cause of herpes flare-ups is unknown, there is a higher rate of outbreaks among people with high stress levels or weakened immune systems.

Conventional Medical Treatments

A gynecologist or physician can diagnose genital herpes through a physical examination and culture. Unfortunately, there is no cure or vaccination for genital herpes. Treatment is limited to management of symptoms. Your doctor may prescribe an anti-viral drug, such as acyclovir, to speed the healing of ulcers. Acyclovir, used long-term, can reduce the number of recurrences.

For More Information
Centers for Disease Control and Prevention (CDC)
1600 Clifton Road
Atlanta, GA 30333
800-311-3435
www.cdc.gov

American Social Health Association
P.O. Box 13827
Research Triangle Park, NC 27709
919-361-8488
www.ashastd.org

Managing Outbreaks of Genital Herpes

During the active phases of genital herpes, it is important for partners to take the following precautions:

• Avoid direct skin-to-skin contact with lesions during flare-ups. (*Note*: condoms won't provide complete protection because they don't cover all lesions.)

• Between outbreaks, condoms can help men with herpes protect their partners.

• Avoid sharing items (such as towels) that come in contact with sores.

• If you come into contact with lesions, wash the area immediately with soapy water, which can kill the virus.

Complementary and Alternative Treatments

Nutrition and Supplementation

 During a breakout, eat lightly. Short fruit fasts (not citrus fruits) with lots of pure water and herbal teas can help. Take advantage of the friendly bacteria found in plain organic yogurt, or supplement your diet with acidophilus.

Follow this daily supplement program:

• L-lysine (500 to 1000 mg 3 times daily with water or juice on an empty stomach)—inhibits the growth of the herpes virus

• vitamin A (50,000 IU; do not exceed 8000 IU daily if you are pregnant)—prevents the spreading of infection

- vitamin B complex (50 mg or more 3 times daily)—works with lysine to prevent outbreaks
- vitamin C (5000 to 10,000 mg)—prevents sores and inhibits growth of the virus; use buffered form
- bioflavonoids (30 to 60 mg in divided doses)—works with vitamin C
- zinc (50 to 100 mg, not to exceed 100 mg total from all supplements)—boosts immune function; use a chelate form
- garlic (as directed on label)—stimulates the immune system
- vitamin E (600 IU)—prevents spread of the infection; use emulsion form

(Consult your healthcare provider regarding the duration of treatment.)

Aromatherapy

 The essential oil of tea tree applied to the affected area helps heal the external sore. Use only one drop per application. Bergamot and eucalyptus oils are also helpful.

Ayurvedic Medicine

 An Ayurvedic practitioner may suggest taking an herbal mixture (*shatavari, guwel sattva, kamadudha,* and *neem*) twice daily after meals to pacify genital herpes. Practitioners also suggest taking *tikta ghee* on an empty stomach or *triphala* in warm water every night. *Tikta ghee* also may be applied directly to the affected area.

Herbal Therapy

 To aid healing, wash the area affected by herpes lesions with an infusion of lemon balm, which has anti-viral properties. To make the infusion, steep 2 to 3 teaspoons finely cut fresh or dried leaves in 1/2 cup boiling water for 20 to 30 minutes; strain the mixture. Saturate a clean cloth with the solution and apply to the herpes lesions several times a day.

St. John's wort and echinacea are also beneficial for their anti-herpes activity and immune-stimulating properties. (*Caution:* Do not use St. John's wort in conjunction with antidepressants. St. John's wort may act as a mild monoamine oxidase inhibitor (MAOI); consult your healthcare provider regarding potential dietary and medication restrictions.) Other herbs that may soothe symptoms and assist healing include cayenne (take in capsule form or apply oil), goldenseal, and licorice root. (*Cautions:* Don't take goldenseal or licorice for more than a week at a time. Avoid goldenseal if you are allergic to ragweed; avoid licorice if you have high blood pressure.)

Homeopathy

 Genital herpes may respond to homeopathic treatment. However, the selection of a remedy—more than one is available—depends on *your* symptoms and the stage of the condition. Don't try treating this disorder yourself. See a homeopathic professional.

Hydrotherapy

 Sitz baths in warm saline (salt) water can lessen the itching and burning that accompanies an outbreak of herpes. If heat aggravates the condition, use a neutral (slightly lower than body temperature) or a brief cool bath. You also can apply a cool compress to the inflamed area.

Traditional Chinese Medicine

 Acupuncture Acupuncture can be used to promote relaxation and lessen anxiety, which can reduce recurrent herpes outbreaks (stress is the main factor in recurrent eruptions). It also can be used to strengthen the immune system, which can lessen the frequency and severity of outbreaks.

Acupressure As with acupuncture, this modality can be very effective in reducing stress and promoting feelings of well-being, which can deter herpes outbreaks.

Chinese Herbal Therapy This condition is treated as a damp-heat syndrome with formulas such as Gentiana Formula.

ⓖ GERMAN MEASLES (RUBELLA)

Signs and Symptoms

German measles may not produce symptoms. If any symptoms are present, they may include:

- A pink, fine rash that typically appears first on the face then spreads to the rest of the body
- Enlarged glands behind the ears and on the neck
- Low-grade fever
- Loss of appetite
- Irritability

Description

German measles is a mild viral infection—so mild, in fact, that symptoms are sometimes unnoticeable—caused by the rubella virus. It is a condition that primarily affects children. The rubella virus is transmitted via droplets of body fluid expelled when someone sneezes, coughs, or exhales.

After contracting the virus, a child may incubate the illness (have no discernable symptoms) for two or three weeks. Thereafter, the child may develop a slight rash for two or three days—though approximately half of all victims do not develop a rash. The condition is contagious for the week prior to the rash developing. Like chickenpox, once you have German measles, you are usually immune to the virus for life.

If a pregnant woman contracts the rubella virus, her child is at high risk of developing one or more serious birth defects, including growth retardation, cataracts, chronic rashes, deafness, and congenital heart and organ defects.

Conventional Medical Treatment

If you suspect that you or your child has German measles, see your physician, who can diagnose the virus with a blood sample. If diagnosed, the infection is usually allowed to run its course. Your doctor may recommend bed rest and acetaminophen to help ease any symptoms.

Fortunately, the disease is easily prevented with an immunization. Ask your doctor about the measles/mumps/rubella (MMR) vaccination, if your child has not already had one.

Health Notes

➤ *Do not use aspirin to reduce a child's fever. When used to reduce the fever of a virus, aspirin can increase a child's risk of contracting Reye's syndrome, a potentially fatal condition.*

➤ *If you are considering becoming pregnant, see your doctor to determine whether you need to be immunized against rubella. To avoid possible birth defects, you must wait at least three months after a rubella vaccination before conceiving.*

For More Information
Centers for Disease Control and Prevention (CDC)
1600 Clifton Road
Atlanta, GA 30333
800-311-3435
www.cdc.gov

National Institute of Allergies and Infectious Diseases
Building 31, Room 7A50
31 Center Drive, MSC 2520
Bethesda, MD 20892-2520
301-496-5717
www.niaid.nih.gov

Complementary and Alternative Treatments

Nutrition and Supplementation

Diet can't do much to treat Rubella. Avoid processed foods and drink plenty of fluids, including water, herbal teas, vegetable juices, and vegetable broths.

The following daily supplemental guidelines are for adults. For a child between 12 and 17, use three-quarters the dose. For a child between 6 and 12, use one-half the dose. Use one-quarter the dose for a child under six.

- proteolytic enzymes (as directed on label, on an empty stomach)—reduces infection (Do not give this supplement to a child)

- vitamin C with bioflavonoids (5000 to 20,000 mg in divided doses)—important for immune function; controls fever and infection

- zinc lozenges (1 15-mg lozenge 3 times for 4 days, then reduce to 1 lozenge daily)—repairs tissue (For adults and children over 5 only)

(Consult your healthcare provider regarding the duration of treatment.)

Herbal Therapy

Some herbalists suggest the following herbs for boosting immune response and lessening the symptoms of German measles: catnip, peppermint, or yarrow tea. To make the teas, steep 1 teaspoon of the dried herb for 10 minutes; strain. Drink several times a day. Echinacea and goldenseal extracts can also be beneficial.

Homeopathy

Homeopathic practitioners might advise one of the following treatments for German measles, depending on your symptoms:

- *Aconite*—if the onset of the illness is sudden

- *Belladonna*—if your face is red, you have a throbbing headache, and you feel drowsy noise or a jarring motion makes you feel worse, and your limbs twitch slightly

- *Gelsemium*—if the onset of the illness is slow; you feel heavy, tired, and apathetic and have a headache with pain at the nape of your neck

- *Euphrasia*—if you have bitter tears, a noticeable nasal discharge, and your eyes are sensitive to light

Hydrotherapy

If a high fever accompanies German measles or the rash is itchy, a cool sponge bath can lessen discomfort. Wash with a mild salt solution.

Traditional Chinese Medicine

Acupuncture If the patient is an adult, the illness is treated as a damp-heat syndrome; if a child, then the illness is allowed to run its course.

Chinese Herbal Therapy Burdock can relieve swollen glands and other rubella symptoms. Lonicera and Forsythia and *Hui Chun Tan* are two commonly-used German measles formulas. Bupleurum and peppermint can be used to force the rash to a head, which speeds healing. Powdered cicada is often used locally to treat German measles as well, but may be difficult for a parent or caregiver to put on a child who is suffering from weeping sores.

GINGIVITIS

Signs and Symptoms

- Soft, swollen, red gums
- Tender gums that bleed easily, especially when brushing or flossing
- Bad breath
- Change in the contours of gums

Description

Gingivitis is an inflammation of the gums. The condition is caused by deposits of plaque—a sticky, gum-irritating film that forms on the exposed portion of teeth. If enough plaque develops, the gums become red and swollen, and have a tendency to bleed, especially when brushing. Although gingivitis is seldom painful, it can lead to *periodontitis*—a more serious gum condition that can lead to gum and tooth loss if left unchecked.

Poor dental hygiene is the primary cause of gingivitis. Most people can prevent gingivitis by brushing their teeth after meals, flossing daily, and getting routine professional cleanings at the dentist's office. Gingivitis can also be caused by poor-fitting orthodontia or dentures. People with a severe overbite or underbite are also at increased risk of developing the condition.

Conventional Medical Treatment

If your gums are swollen and red or bleed easily, visit your dentist, who will examine your gums carefully, looking for inflamed tissue and excess deposits of plaque at the base of your teeth. If your dentist or dental hygienist discovers gingivitis, he or she will thoroughly clean all the plaque and tartar off your teeth.

Hormones vs. Gingivitis

Hormonal fluctuations during menopause and pregnancy may affect a woman's oral health. Experts believe that the presence of estrogen may encourage bacteria growth. In women, gingivitis often develops during menstruation, pregnancy (60 to 75% of all pregnant women develop gingivitis), and menopause, and while taking birth control pills. Dental hygiene professionals recommend that women in these high risk groups take extra care to brush and floss their teeth.

Once you are diagnosed with gingivitis and receive a cleaning, you must maintain a strict program of oral hygiene to keep the condition in remission. This includes brushing your teeth after all meals and flossing at least once a day. Your dentist or dental hygienist can show you exactly

Health Notes

➤ If you use any tobacco products, quit. Tobacco use of any type has been shown to promote gingivitis.

➤ Reduce your stress levels. When the immune system is under stress it releases chemicals that can lead to uncontrolled inflammation, including gingivitis.

➤ Anti-depressants, antihistamines, chemotherapy, steroids, and calcium channel blockers can all make the gums more susceptible to gingivitis.

how—and how long—to brush and floss to prevent the condition from returning. You also will need to return to your dentist twice a year for professional cleanings.

For More Information
American Dental Association (ADA)
211 East Chicago Avenue
Chicago, IL 60611
312-440-2500
www.ada.org

Complementary and Alternative Treatments

Nutrition and Supplementation

 It's no surprise that there is such a high rate of gingivitis and other dental disorders. Today's diet of refined foods fuels bacteria, and our resistance to those bacteria is lowered by the high intake of sugar. So the bacteria are able to flourish and spread throughout the mouth. Avoiding refined foods and those high in sugar is a good starting point.

Your diet should consist of fresh fruits, green leafy vegetables, lean meat, and whole grains. These foods require chewing, a form of exercise for the teeth and gums. High-fiber foods, such as whole grains, legumes, and vegetables, are also important.

Vitamin C is essential for the prevention of gingivitis, while vitamin A aids in general health of the gums. Recent research found that the same compounds in cranberries that prevent urinary tract infections may also reduce your risk of gum disease by inhibiting plaque from forming. More research needs to be done, but it can't hurt to add cranberry juice to your diet. Follow the daily supplement guidelines below to help prevent and/or treat gingivitis.

- vitamin C (4000 to 10,000 mg in divided doses throughout the day)—retards plaque growth and promotes healing

- coenzyme Q10 (chewable form; 100 mg)—increases tissue oxygenation

- calcium (1500 mg)—helps prevent bone loss

- magnesium (750 mg)—works with calcium

- vitamin A (25,000 IU for 1 month, then reduce to 10,000 IU, do not exceed 8000 IU daily if you are pregnant)—heals gum tissue (Use emulsion form for best assimilation)

- mixed carotenoid formula (as directed on label)—manufactures vitamin A on an as-needed basis

- vitamin E (400 IU, increase slowly to 1000 IU)—heals gum tissue. (Open a capsule and rub the oil on the gums 2-3 times daily)

- zinc (2 15-mg lozenges)—prevents infection and promotes healing

- oral glutathione spray (as directed on label)—promotes healing of gums

(For an *acute* condition, take supplements until your symptoms subside. If symptoms persist, seek the advice of your healthcare provider. For a *chronic* condition, consult your healthcare provider regarding the duration of treatment.)

Aromatherapy

 For a soothing rub to maintain gum health, combine 1 ounce canola, sunflower, or sesame oil; 10 drops tea tree oil; 6 drops myrrh oil; 3 drops lemon oil; and 1 drop peppermint oil. Blend well. Massage mixture into your gums after brushing your teeth and using a mouthwash. Take care not to swallow.

For a refreshing mouthwash, try adding either of these combinations to 1 cup cooled boiled water: 1 drop myrrh oil and 1 drop peppermint oil, or 2 drops clove oil and 1 drop thyme (linalol) oil.

Ayurvedic Medicine

 Ayurveda views excess pitta and vata doshas as responsible for the receding, bleeding, and swollen gums associated with gingivitis. For general gum care, practitioners may advise brushing your teeth with a toothpaste containing *neem* or another bitter, astringent herb.

Rinsing with *neem* tea also may be beneficial. Such products and herbs are available in health food stores.

For bleeding and receding gums, practitioners may suggest rubbing your gums with sesame or coconut oil; drinking diluted lemon juice; and eating raw apples, pears, and melons.

Herbal Therapy

A number of herbal mouthwashes, toothpastes, and teas can be effective in treating and preventing gingivitis. Bloodroot and stinging nettle, which are available in toothpastes and mouthwashes, can help prevent plaque buildup.

Chamomile can reduce inflammation and bacteria. Look for it in toothpaste form or prepare a strong chamomile tea and drink it between meals or use as a mouthwash. To make the tea, place 2 to 3 teaspoons of the herb in 1 cup boiling water, steep for 10 minutes, and strain. (If you notice an allergic reaction, such as itching, discontinue use.)

Echinacea and peppermint also have antibacterial properties. To use echinacea, add a dropper or two of tincture to a tea or mouthwash. For peppermint tea or mouthwash, add 2 teaspoons crushed peppermint leaves to 1 cup boiling water and steep for 10 minutes; strain.

Homeopathy

Gingivitis may respond to homeopathic treatment. However, the selection of a remedy—more than one is available—depends on *your* symptoms and the stage of the condition. Don't try treating this disorder yourself. See a homeopathic professional.

Hydrotherapy

Apply alternating hot and cold compresses to your face several times a day to increase blood flow and lessen inflammation.

You can also rinse your mouth with a mixture of ½ teaspoon sea salt in 1 cup warm water. Follow this rinse with a mouthwash of 1 dropperful each of myrrh and goldenseal in 1 cup warm water. Salt, myrrh, and goldenseal all have antimicrobial effects.

Traditional Chinese Medicine

Acupuncture Oral acupuncture, in which saline or local anesthetics are injected in various acupuncture points within the mouth, has been successful at remedying gingivitis.

Acupressure This modality is thought to quell bleeding gums and prevent teeth from loosening. In most cases, the acupressure points to be massaged include Large Intestine 14 (on the hand), and Stomach 6 and 7 (on the face).

Chinese Herbal Therapy Some Chinese herbalists recommend pseudoginseng and achyranthes, which can be used to heal bleeding gums. Stomach herb formulas also may be prescribed.

GLAUCOMA

Signs and Symptoms

- Blurred vision
- Headaches
- Loss of peripheral vision
- Seeing halos around lights
- Pain and sensitivity in the affected eye
- Redness in the affected eye
- Teary eyes

Description

Glaucoma is one of the leading causes of blindness. It occurs when increased fluid pressure within the eyeball causes progressive damage to the optic nerve. As the optic nerve deteriorates, the result is often blind spots, blurred vision, lack of peripheral vision, and even headaches. If the condition is not treated, the victim may eventually be left with reduced or complete lack of sight.

The area of the eye between the iris and the lens is bathed in a fluid called aqueous humor. In a healthy eye, the aqueous humor is continually produced and then drained out of the eye through the canal of Schlemm. In an eye affected by glaucoma, the aqueous humor does not exit the eye as it should. In some cases, the canal of Schlemm is blocked, preventing the fluid from leaving the eye. In other cases, too much aqueous humor is produced, causing the eye to fill with more fluid than it can release. The consequence in either case is that pressure within the eye increases, damaging the optic nerve and retina.

Glaucoma often develops so slowly that most victims do not realize they have the condition until their peripheral vision is completely gone. Also, the condition has few early warning signs. While peripheral vision gradually declines, cen-

tral vision usually remains intact until the final stages of the disease.

Acute glaucoma, on the other hand, is a form of the condition that appears suddenly and requires immediate medical attention. If any early warning signs develop, they come in the form of fuzzy vision, halos around lights, and tenderness in the eye in the weeks before the acute attack. The attack itself is usually so severe that it can cause nausea and vomiting.

Age is the primary risk factor for developing glaucoma—the risk of developing the condition increases after the age of 40. People with diabetes are also at increased risk; in fact, they are three times as likely to develop chronic glaucoma than those without diabetes. People of African descent are more likely to have glaucoma than those from other ethnic groups. Heredity is also believed to play a role in developing the disease.

Conventional Medical Treatment

Since glaucoma has few warning signs, regular eye exams—especially once you reach age 40—are essential in detecting and treating glaucoma before it severely affects your vision. Your ophthalmologist will most likely perform a tonometry test, which reveals fluid buildup by testing the tension on the surface of the eye. Your physician also may use an *ophthalmoscope* to get an unobstructed view of the eye's interior, allowing him or her to locate any optic nerve damage.

If glaucoma is diagnosed, your doctor may prescribe special eye drops (usually epinephrine, pilocarpine, or beta-adrenergic blockers) to help decrease the pressure in the eye by increasing the rate at which fluid drains from the eye. Oral medication, such as acetazolamide, may be prescribed to lower pressure in the eye by decreasing the formation of aqueous humor.

Glaucoma

In severe cases of glaucoma, surgery may be required to open blocked drainage canals. Laser surgery is a simple out-patient procedure that is usually performed in the doctor's office. A filtration procedure is another surgical option. This operation creates a drainage passage between the interior of the eye and the conjunctiva to relieve interior pressure.

If you suspect you are having an attack of acute glaucoma, immediately contact your ophthalmologist or go to the nearest emergency room. Acute glaucoma is treated with *laser iridotomy*, an emergency operation that uses a laser to create a drainage hole in the iris. While laser iridotomy is an emergency operation, many people are able to resume normal activities hours after receiving the treatment.

For More Information
Glaucoma Research Foundation
200 Pine Street, Suite 200
San Francisco, CA 94104
800-826-6693
www.glaucoma.org

Prevent Blindness America
500 East Remington Road
Schaumberg, IL 60173
800-331-2020
www.preventblindness.org

Health Notes

➤ *If you have a family history of glaucoma, be sure to get an annual eye exam. And everyone between the ages of 40 and 65 should receive an eye examination every two to four years, while those over the age of 65 should have one every one to two years.*

➤ *If you drink large amounts of caffeinated beverages, you should reduce your intake. Experts believe that heavy caffeine intake (two or more cups of coffee a day) can lead to glaucoma.*

The Marijuana Prescription

Many experts believe that marijuana is the perfect medication for treating glaucoma. While marijuana can't cure glaucoma, it has been shown to help slow the disease's progression. Currently, legislation in 26 states has established clinical research programs to study the effects of marijuana on different medical conditions. In addition to helping glaucoma patients, proponents claim that medical marijuana can help forestall AIDS-related muscle wasting, ease the nausea brought on by cancer chemotherapy, and counter the symptoms of epilepsy and multiple sclerosis. While prescription medications are available that offer relief similar to marijuana, these drugs often have unpleasant side effects and can be toxic to the liver and kidneys.

Complementary and Alternative Treatments

Nutrition and Supplementation

 A dairy-free, low-fat vegetarian diet gives you all the nutrients essential for eye health. The nutrients associated with the eyes are vitamins E and D as well as A (liver metabolism) and C (rids bloodstream of toxins). Also important are glutathione, B vitamins, omega-3 and -6 fatty acids, and calcium (along with magnesium). Carrots; green leafy vegetables such as broccoli and spinach; and yellow, red, and orange fruits are great sources of vitamin A. Fish oils supply fatty acids, and sulfur-rich foods, such as garlic and asparagus, increase the amount of vitamins C and E in your body. Finally, drink 8 to 10 glasses of water every day. Avoid caffeine, alcohol, and carbonated beverages.

These daily supplements are recommended by nutritionists:

- lecithin (1000 to 2000 mg)
- glutathione (500 mg 2 times daily, on empty stomach)

- vitamin B complex (50 mg 3 times daily)—essential for eye health

- vitamin A (50,000 IU; do not exceed 8000 IU if you are pregnant)—essential for night vision

- vitamin C (2000 to 4000 mg)—lowers eye pressure

- vitamin E (400 IU)—protects eye lens; reduces eye pressure

- zinc (30 mg, not to exceed 100 mg total from all supplements)—essential in activating vitamin A from the liver

- taurine (as directed on label)—protective supplement

(Consult your healthcare provider regarding the duration of treatment.)

Ayurvedic Medicine

 According to Ayurvedic theory, glaucoma is a kapha dosha disorder. An Ayurvedic practitioner may suggest drinking *punarnava* tea to slowly decrease the pressure or tension in the eye during the early stages of the disorder. Consult your doctor before starting a new eye-care regimen. Glaucoma that's not properly treated can lead to blindness.

Bodywork and Somatic Practices

 The eye as a sensory organ is deeply connected with the mind/body experience and its function is constantly influenced by the emotions. Therefore, movement re-education options are ideal to help the mind/body evolve and change. Other modalities to consider include CranioSacral Therapy, massage, Trager, reflexology, and Oriental bodywork.

Traditional Chinese Medicine

 Acupuncture Chinese medical practitioners use acupuncture to help relieve the pressure caused by glaucoma, which can eliminate the need for prescription medications, and in some cases, surgery. Acu-

puncture points typically utilized are Stomach 1, Bladder 1, Large Intestine 4, and Liver 2 and 3. Additional points may be added as symptoms warrant.

Acupuncture also may be used to improve circulation and rid the body of toxins and waste, which can sometimes cause glaucoma.

Acupressure To relieve the pressure caused by glaucoma, a practitioner may focus on the various acupressure points that ring the eye socket.

Chinese Herbal Therapy Rehmannia and Dogwood Fruit Formula is often prescribed in cases of glaucoma. Also commonly prescribed is a liver formula, such as *Xiao Yao Wan.*

SYMPTOM:

GOITER

Goiter is an enlargement of the thyroid gland, which is located at the base of the neck. It is most commonly associated with a deficiency of iodine, which is necessary to manufacture thyroid hormones. Fortunately, iodine deficiency is an extremely rare condition in the United States, because of the widespread use of iodized salt. Goiter is also associated with other conditions, including Hashimoto's disease, an inflammation of the gland that leads to hypothyroidism, thyroid cancer, and subacute thyroiditis.

An enlarged thyroid may appear as a small lump on the neck or a generalized enlargement of the neck. In some cases, the swelling causes a slight pressure on the throat, but in most cases there is no discomfort. In rare instances, the gland becomes so enlarged that it makes breathing and swallowing uncomfortable.

Medical treatment for goiter usually involves treating the condition that is causing the swelling. If the goiter becomes so enlarged that it causes discomfort, a rarity, surgical removal of part of the thyroid may be necessary.

GONORRHEA

Signs and Symptoms

- Thick, pus-like discharge from the penis or vagina
- Burning sensation during urination
- Increased frequency of urination
- Pelvic and lower abdominal pain
- Pain during intercourse
- Nausea and vomiting
- Fever and chills

Description

Gonorrhea is a sexually transmitted disease (STD) caused by the bacterium *Neisseria gonorrhoeae*. Men usually experience symptoms in two to fourteen days after exposure to the bacteria. Symptoms begin with a tingling sensation in the urethra during urination; in two to four hours urination becomes very painful and is accompanied by a pus-like discharge. As the condition progresses, the pain worsens, and the discharge becomes thick and is produced in greater amounts.

Women, on the other hand, may experience no symptoms at all until the condition is quite advanced. In the early stages, a gynecologist may be able to detect slight cervical inflammation or light vaginal discharge during a pelvic examination. If the condition is not detected and treated, it can progress to the point that urination becomes painful, urgent, and frequent. Even at this advanced stage, gonorrhea is often mistaken for a bladder infection unless a thick, pus-like discharge is present.

If it is not treated promptly, gonorrhea can develop into prostitis or urethritis in men. In women, it can spread to the fallopian tubes and uterus, causing pelvic inflammatory disease (PID) which, in turn, can lead to infertility. The bacteria also can travel through the bloodstream to other parts of the body, potentially causing heart problems or arthritis.

Conventional Medical Treatment

Because gonorrhea is so difficult to self-diagnose, sexually active adults who are not in a monogamous relationship should be tested for gonorrhea annually. To diagnose the condition, your physician or gynecologist conducts a pelvic examination, checking for inflammation or discharge; if either is present, the doctor will collect a specimen of the discharge or infected tissue for further testing.

Gonorrhea is a highly contagious disease. If you are diagnosed with gonorrhea, your doctor will ask that you contact all present (and, if necessary, past) sexual partners. Antibiotics, such as the Ceftriaxone® (which is taken in a single dose) plus doxycyline may be prescribed. Doxycyline is prescribed for 7 days to treat chlamydia, which often occurs simultaneously with gonorrhea.

For More Information

Centers for Disease Control and Prevention (CDC)
1600 Clifton Road
Atlanta, GA 30333
800-311-3435
www.cdc.gov

Planned Parenthood Federation of America
810 Seventh Avenue
New York, NY 10019
800-230-PLAN
www.plannedparenthood.org

Health Notes

➤ *The spermicide nonoxynol-9 weakens the bacteria that causes gonorrhea, reducing a woman's risk of becoming infected. However, the spermicide can cause rashes in some women and is not 100 percent protective.*

➤ *Celibacy or a mutually monogamous physical relationship are the only sure ways to prevent sexually transmitted diseases. Consistent use of condoms is a good way to reduce your risk of contracting an STD.*

➤ *If you are thinking about starting a family, visit your physician to be screened for gonorrhea and other sexually transmitted diseases before conceiving. Exposure to the bacteria that causes gonorrhea can cause blindness in newborns.*

Complementary and Alternative Treatments

Nutrition and Supplementation

 Although diet doesn't have a direct role in treating or preventing sexually transmitted diseases, supplementation can help. Follow the daily guidelines below:

- a prodophilus formula (as directed on label, 3 times daily, on empty stomach)—restores friendly bacteria often killed by antibiotics

- garlic (as directed on label)—an immune stimulant and natural antibiotic
- free-form amino acid complex (as directed on label)— needed for tissue repair
- vitamin C (750 to 2500 4 times daily)—an antiviral agent
- zinc (not to exceed 100 mg)—essential for the health of reproductive organs
- colloidal silver (as directed on label)—reduces inflammation and promotes healing
- vitamin B complex (50 mg 3 times daily)—aids in cellular reproduction
- raw glandular complex (as directed on label)—promotes immune function
- vitamin K (100 mcg)—destroyed by antibiotics, but necessary for blood clotting

(Consult your healthcare provider regarding the duration of treatment.)

Traditional Chinese Medicine

 Acupuncture Although acupuncture cannot prevent or cure gonorrhea, it can be used to help fortify the immune system so that the body is better able to fight this bacterial intruder. This modality also can offer pain relief, reduce a fever, and lessen inflammation.

Chinese Herbal Therapy See your practitioner for a full diagnosis; strong herb formulas may be prescribed.

GOUT

Signs and Symptoms

- Acute, severe pain in a joint, usually in the big toe or ankle
- Swelling and redness in the affected joint
- Chills and fever

Description

Gout usually strikes without warning. One moment the victim is feeling fine; then, within a matter of hours, a particular joint becomes acutely painful, red, and swollen. The most commonly affected joint is the one at the base of the big toe, but joints elsewhere in the feet, ankles, knees, hands, and wrists may be affected. While the affected joint will ache for anywhere from 3 to 10 days, the pain will gradually fade over the course of the next week. Sixty percent of gout sufferers have a more severe and prolonged recurrence of the condition within a year of the initial attack.

Gout, also known as crystal-induced arthritis, occurs when uric acid crystals accumulate in a joint. Uric acid is produced by the body (and a small amount is derived from a substance in some foods called purine) to help with the digestive process. When the amount of uric acid in your body blood stream increases, the acid accumulates in the synovial fluid around your joints and forms crystals. The accumulation of a significant amount of crystal in a joint results in gout. (Sometimes uric acid crystal deposits form in the kidneys, resulting in kidney stones.) If left untreated, the high uric acid levels associated with gout can cause permanent joint damage or kidney problems.

Ninety percent of all gout victims are men over the age of 40. One out of every four sufferers has a family history of the ailment. Other suspected risk factors include: a diet high in purine-rich foods (such as sardines, anchovies, sweetbreads, liver, and kidney), obesity, hypertension, and use of thiazide diuretics (for treating high blood pressure). An attack of gout also can be caused by the stress of an injury, such as a bone fracture or a surgical procedure.

Conventional Medical Treatment

If you are suffering from an attack of gout, visit your physician. To diagnose the condition, your physician withdraws a small amount of fluid from

Health Notes

➤ People who are at risk for gout should avoid foods that contain large amounts of uric-acid producing compounds, such as anchovies, shellfish, goose, duck, kidneys, liver, sardines, roe, and sweetbreads.

➤ Drinking two or more quarts of water daily can help the body flush out accumulated uric acid.

➤ People with gout should avoid products that contain salicylate derivatives, which can worsen symptoms. Two products that contain salicylate derivatives are aspirin and Pepto-Bismol®.

➤ Menopausal and postmenopausal women who are at risk for gout should talk to their doctors about hormone replacement therapy. Estrogen protects against high uric acid levels, which usually rise after menopause.

the affected joint, and examines the white blood cells for uric acid crystals.

Medication can be helpful in treating acute attacks of gout, and also can prevent future attacks. Anti-inflammatory drugs are first used to treat inflammation. Then medications are prescribed to reduce the amount of uric acid in the body—four of the most widely used medications are colchicine, indomethacin, probenecid, and allopurinol. With treatment, an attack of gout typically runs its course in four days to four weeks; after treatment, the affected joint usually returns to normal.

Although physicians are divided about whether certain foods can cause gout, it is always wise to avoid excessive alcohol consumption, keep weight within healthy limits, and avoid foods that contain high levels of purine.

Complementary and Alternative Treatments

Nutrition and Supplementation

Since gout is the result of too much uric acid in the blood, tissues, and urine, it makes sense to limit foods that contribute to that surplus. Avoid anchovies, asparagus, herring, meat gravies and broths, mushrooms, mussels, and sardines. Meat also contains extremely high levels of uric acid, so do not eat meat (including organ meats) of any kind. Eliminate alcohol from your diet, as it contributes to the production of uric acid. Likewise, limit your intake of caffeine, cauliflower, lentils, fish, eggs, oatmeal, peas, poultry, spinach, and yeast products. White flour and sugar products are not healthy foods, so avoid cakes and pies.

Do eat only raw fruits and vegetables for two weeks when an attack of gout strikes. If you are susceptible to gout, always include an abundance of strawberries and cherries, which neutralize uric acid. Focus on grains, nuts, and seeds.

If you're overweight, lose those excess pounds. Do so sensibly, however, avoiding any sort of crash diet. Sudden elimination of foods sometimes results in an increase in uric acid.

Follow these recommended daily supplement guidelines:

essential fatty acids (as directed on label, with meals)—repairs tissue and aids in healing. This disorder is often caused in part by an excess of saturated fats.

Most Important

- omega 3 fatty acids (fish or flaxseed oil; 2 tbsp)—acts as an anti-inflammatory
- vitamin B complex (100 mg)—aids proper digestion
- vitamin C with bioflavonoids (3000 to 5000 mg in divided doses)—lowers serum uric acid levels
- folic acid (200 mcg)—assists with nucleoprotein metabolism

Also Recommended

- kelp (1000 to 15,000 mg)—reduces serum uric acid
- potassium (99 mg)—necessary for proper mineral balance
- zinc (30 mg, not to exceed a total of 100 mg from all supplements)—repairs tissues and aids in protein metabolism
- calcium (1500 mg)—reduces the stress caused by gout; Take before bedtime with magnesium (750 mg)

(For an *acute* condition, take supplements until your symptoms subside. If symptoms persist, seek the advice of your healthcare provider. For a *chronic* condition, consult your healthcare provider regarding the duration of treatment.)

Bodywork and Somatic Practices

CranioSacral Therapy, Reiki, Therapeutic Touch, and polarity therapy are good starting points. As inflammation lessens, reflexology and Oriental bodywork can be effective. As healing ensues and the pain subsides, Feldenkrais can begin to bring gentle integrated activity back to the body.

Chiropractic

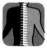

In many cases, gout affects the ankles and lower extremities, as uric acid crystals are deposited in the joints. After appropriate medical and nutritional consultation, patients with gout may seek chiropractic care, which can be effective in decreasing the swelling and pain associated with the condition.

Herbal Therapy

To help eliminate uric acid from your system, drink an infusion of celery seed or gravelroot up to three times a day. Infuse 2 teaspoons of either herb in 1 cup boiling water; strain.

To relieve pain and inflammation, try willow tea. Since willow contains salicylates, avoid using it if you're allergic to aspirin.

Homeopathy

Your homeopathic practitioner may recommend one of the following treatments for gout, depending on your symptoms: *Colchicum* (an extract of autumn crocus) if your big toe is painful, especially when touched or moved; *Ledum* if your foot feels better when placed in ice water.

Hydrotherapy

To ease discomfort, apply a cold compress or ice pack to the affected joint for 20 minutes several times a day. Don't exceed 20 minutes, as prolonged exposure to cold can damage the skin. A full-body steam bath excluding the head (a Russian bath) can also bring relief.

Traditional Chinese Medicine

Acupuncture Acupuncture can be instrumental in relieving the pain and swelling caused by gout. It also can be used to help reduce a gout-induced fever. The acupuncturist works on points related to (but not near) the swollen joint, to avoid causing additional pain.

Acupressure Acupressure points that correspond to the kidneys may be massaged to regulate the flow of uric acid. In addition, points and meridians that relate to the affected joint(s) may be targeted, to allay pain and reduce swelling.

Chinese Herbal Therapy Herbs that may be given to treat gout and control uric acid production are Clematis and Stephania Formula (a common Chinese gout medicine) and Polygonum Tablets to relieve pain.

Hair Loss (Alopecia)

Signs and Symptoms

- Noticeably thinning hair on the scalp
- Receding hairline
- Bald spot on the crown of the head

Description

Hair loss is usually associated with aging men: thinning scalp hair, receding hairline, a shiny spot of scalp at the crown, or total baldness. Male pattern baldness, as it is known, is the most common type of balding, affecting 50 percent of Caucasian men over the age of 50. Yet this is not the only type of hair loss. Some women suffer from a similar thinning of hair, called female pattern baldness. Women's hair loss differs in appearance from men's: female pattern baldness involves an all-over thinning of scalp hair, but rarely progresses to total baldness. Female pattern baldness is most common in postmenopausal women, though it can affect women of any age. This type of hair loss is usually permanent, for men or for women.

There are other types of hair loss, as well; among them are thinning hair due to hormonal changes (caused by pregnancy or some types of birth control pills) or nutritional deficiencies, and partial or total hair loss due to chemotherapy or overly tight hairstyles. In these instances, the hair loss is usually temporary. The hair should grow back after the cause is discontinued.

Alopecia areata is another type of temporary hair loss that causes patches of hair—usually the size of silver dollars—to fall out. In some instances, these patches overlap, causing large tracts of bare scalp. Body and facial hair also may fall out, although this is less common. In approximately 90 percent of all alopecia areata cases, the lost hair grows back within six months to two years.

Female and male pattern balding are hereditary; those with a family history of the condition are at increased risk. Alopecia areata, on the other hand, is caused by an immune disorder wherein the body's immune system rejects its own hair. While the exact cause of the condition is unknown, experts believe that extreme stress, surgery with anesthesia, a weakened immune system, or a reaction to a medication may contribute.

Conventional Medical Treatment

Most cases of hair loss are not threatening to general health. If you choose to seek conventional treatment, your physician will find the cause of your condition in order to determine the proper treatment. If the problem is due to nutritional deficiencies, you will have to change your diet and

---

Male Baldness and Heart Disease

Researchers have noticed a correlation between male baldness and the risk of heart attack. Men under 55 with bald spots on the top of their heads have been found to have a slightly increased risk of heart attack. The more extensive the baldness on top (called vertex baldness), the higher the risk. Mild to moderate vertex baldness indicated a risk of heart attack about 40 percent greater than that for men with a full head of hair; severe vertex baldness indicated up to a 340 percent greater risk. Researchers believe that there is a relationship between this phenomenon and the male sex hormone *dihydrotestosterone*.

perhaps take dietary supplements. If the balding is caused by a tight hairstyle, you will obviously need to try a new way of wearing your hair. If the hair loss is caused by hormonal changes, your doctor may prescribe estrogen therapy or a new type of birth control pill.

Minoxidil—a topical, over-the-counter preparation that was once available only by prescription—is often recommended for people who suffer from hereditary or alopecia-induced hair loss. Unfortunately, the hair growth produced by minoxidil is often very fine, not thick like the original strands.

Some dermatologists treat alopecia with cortisone—either via tablets, ointment, or injecting the substance into the bald areas. However, because alopecia often is temporary, many experts resist the use of cortisone therapy due to its side effects.

Another option for treating hair loss is hair transplant surgery. While transplant surgery is not a cure, it can help cosmetically enhance bald spots for those suffering from male or female pattern baldness. Tiny plugs of hair—usually about ten strands per plug, with their root systems intact—are removed from dense areas of hair and transplanted to sparse areas. The results of this surgery are permanent. Unfortunately, most people need multiple surgeries (usually two to four) to achieve the desired result, the treatment is expensive, and hair can continue to fall out in non-transplanted areas.

Health Notes

➤ If you experience sudden hair loss, consult your physician. Hair loss can be a sign of extreme stress or an indication of lowered immunity.

➤ Prevent hair breakage that can cause thinning hair by always treating your hair gently. Avoid using harsh styling products, repeated blow drying, or hairstyles that pull the hair too tight.

For More Information
American Hair Loss Council
401 N. Michigan Ave.
Chicago, IL 60611
888-873-9719
www.ahlc.org

Complementary and Alternative Treatments

Nutrition and Supplementation

Biotin is necessary for healthy hair. Good natural sources include brewer's yeast, brown rice, green peas, lentils, soybeans, sunflower seeds, and walnuts. Avoid raw eggs, which contain avidin, a protein that prevents biotin from being absorbed. If you suspect a hormonal reason for your hair loss, consult your healthcare professional about taking soy isoflavones.

In addition, the following daily supplement recommendations help keep the hair and scalp healthy:

Most Important

- essential fatty acids (1000 mg)—improves hair texture and prevents dryness

- raw thymus glandular (500 mg)—stimulates immune function (Do not give to children.)

- vitamin B complex with vitamin B_3 (50 mg), plus additional vitamin B_5 (100 mg 3 times daily), vitamin B_6 (50 mg 3 times daily), and biotin (50 mg 3 times daily)—deficiencies have been linked to hair loss

- inositol (100 mg 2 times daily)—essential for hair growth

- vitamin C (3000 to 10,000 mg)—improves scalp circulation

- vitamin E (start with 400 IU and slowly increase to 800 to 1000 IU)—improves health and growth of hair

- zinc (50 to 100 mg, not to exceed this amount)—stimulates hair growth

Also Recommended

- coenzyme Q10 (60 mg)—improves scalp circulation
- dimethylglycine (100 mg)—improves scalp circulation
- kelp (500 mg)—provides minerals necessary for proper hair growth
- copper (3 mg)—works with zinc; use a chelate form

(Consult your healthcare provider about the duration of treatment.)

Ayurvedic Medicine

 An Ayurvedic practitioner may suggest *Ashwagandha* and *amla*, which are Indian herbs, or *bhringaraj* or *brahmi* oil to stimulate hair growth.

Bodywork and Somatic Practices

 Massage may help bring better blood circulation to the head, but therapies that vitalize the systems of the body may be more useful. Try Oriental bodywork therapies and CranioSacral Therapy.

Traditional Chinese Medicine

 Acupuncture Chinese medicine views alopecia as a condition related to the kidneys, so acupuncture may be used to help tone and strengthen this organ and related meridians. The practitioner may focus on the kidney, lung, head, and ear points. If the hair loss is sudden (alopecia areata) and caused by an underlying medical condition, additional points may be targeted.

Acupressure An acupressurist may work on the Governing Vessel 14 and Gallbladder 20 points, in addition to performing a vigorous scalp acupressure to stimulate hair follicles.

Chinese Herbal Therapy Biota leaves may be steeped in a 60 percent alcohol solution for 1 week and then rubbed on bald spots 3 times a day to promote hair growth. Aloe vera juice is another Chinese alopecia remedy, as is *Gotu Kola*, which can be taken as a decoction or mixed with water or oil and used as an external ointment. Six Flavor Tea is a kidney tonic that may also be recommended to counteract hair loss. *No Shou Wu* is used and there are a number of Chinese herbal topical formulas that may be useful for balding. Few are useful for male pattern balding, however.

HEADACHE, CLUSTER

Signs and Symptoms

- Extreme, sometimes throbbing, pain in and around one eye
- Redness and watering in the affected eye
- Nasal congestion on the affected side of the head
- Flushing of the face

Description

Cluster headaches are extremely painful occurrences that are focused right around one of eyes. This type of headache usually causes the affected eye to become red and watery, and causes nasal congestion in that side of the face. Cluster headaches typically occur within a few hours of sleep onset, reaching their peak within 15 minutes of appearing and lasting less than two hours.

Unfortunately, cluster headaches are a chronic condition. Sufferers may have one headache or more each day for multiple days, weeks, or months before a remission period that can last from weeks to years. While cluster headaches are a cause of recurring discomfort, they do not cause any permanent harm.

Cluster headaches are a relatively rare condition, and their exact cause is unknown. The leading theory is that the headaches are caused when a brain chemical provokes blood vessels to enlarge, putting pressure on facial nerves. Men are more susceptible to cluster headaches than women. Heavy smokers are at the highest risk for developing the condition. Alcohol consumption also can trigger attacks in people who suffer from cluster headaches.

Conventional Medical Treatment

Cluster headaches do not respond well to treatment used for other types of headaches, namely over-the-counter analgesics. Many sufferers do not seek medical treatment, instead opting to manage the pain themselves. While this is certainly an option that will not cause you any permanent harm, you may want to visit your physician for a pro-

gram of pain management. Because this type of headache is notoriously unresponsive to any one medication, conventional treatment typically involves a combination of two or three medications, such as oxygen inhalation, ergotamine tartrate, prednisone, methysergide maleate, lithium carbonate, and calcium channel blocking agents.

Although cluster headaches are easy to diagnose, your physician may want to conduct a urinalysis, sinus X-ray, skull X-ray, or CAT scan to rule out other ailments that have similar symptoms, such as brain tumors, aneurysms, or sinusitis.

For More Information
National Headache Foundation
428 West St. James, 2nd Floor
Chicago, IL 60614-2750
800-843-2256
www.headaches.org

National Institute of Neurological Disorders and Stroke
P.O. Box 5801
Bethesda, MD 20824
800-352-9424
www.ninds.nih.gov

Complementary and Alternative Treatments

Nutrition and Supplementation

 In addition to the information given under the "Tension Headache" entry, take the following daily supplements to relieve cluster headaches.

- L-tyrosine (as directed on label) (Do not take if you are currently using a monoamine oxidase (MAO) inhibitor.)

- L-glutamine (500 mg twice daily)

- quercetin (500 mg twice daily)

(For an *acute* condition, take supplements until your symptoms subside. If symptoms persist, seek the advice of your healthcare provider. For a

---

Health Notes

➤ *Reduce stress levels. Stress can trigger an acute cluster headache in people susceptible to the condition.*

➤ *If you smoke, quit. Smokers have considerably higher rates of cluster headaches than people who do not smoke.*

➤ *If you are prone to cluster headaches, avoid alcoholic beverages, which can trigger cluster headaches.*

chronic condition, consult your healthcare provider regarding the duration of treatment.)

Ayurvedic Medicine

Ayurveda has three classifications for headaches: vata type, pitta type, and kapha type.

For vata headaches—which are associated with tension in the neck and shoulders and start as throbbing pain in the back of the head—an Ayurvedic practitioner may suggest trying an enema or a sesame-oil massage.

For pitta headaches—which are associated with nausea and dizziness and start as shooting pains in the temples—a practitioner may advise drinking a cooling cumin-coriander tea.

For kapha headaches—which are associated with sinus congestion and usually start in the sinus area—a practitioner may recommend sipping spicy ginger-cinnamon tea and using a saline solution to wash the nasal passages.

Chiropractic

To understand how chiropractic can help those who suffer from cluster headaches, it is important to know a little bit of anatomy: a nerve, an artery, and a vein flow out of every hole in the spine. In cluster headaches, the first and second cervical vertebrae may be involved. When a chiropractor relieves the pressure of a vertebral subluxation through specific chiropractic adjustment (SCA) to the cervical (upper neck) portion of the spine, blood flow, and nerve flow are restored. Therapy also may involve electromuscle stimulation and moist-heat application.

Homeopathy

Homeopathic practitioners may suggest one of the following treatments for a tension headache, depending on your symptoms:

- *Glonoine*—for an acute, or sudden, headache from sun exposure; there is pounding pain, and your head feels as if it were bursting; you feel confused
- *Belladonna*—for a headache from sun exposure; your face is bright red, and you have throbbing pain
- *Nux vomica*—for a headache that results from overindulging in alcohol; the pain is severe and worsens when you move—even just your eyes—ever so slightly
- *Gelsemium*—for a headache from fright or anxiety; your head feels heavy and hard to lift

Traditional Chinese Medicine

Acupuncture Because cluster headaches are thought to be sinus-related, acupuncture may be helpful in opening blocked nasal passages and alleviating sinus pressure, which, in turn, may reduce the frequency and severity of this type of headache. The acupuncturist's targets points may include Large Intestine 14; Gallbladder 20 and 41; Triple Warmer 3, 5, and 23; and related points in the ear.

Cluster headaches are usually related to a liver imbalance, and treating the liver with acupuncture can be useful in preventing future episodes.

Acupuncture also can be used to promote relaxation, as cluster headaches are believed to be stress-induced.

Acupressure Acupressure can encourage feelings of tranquility, which may help alleviate cluster headaches. Relevant acupressure points include: Gall bladder 20 and 34, Stomach 3 and 36, Large Intestine 4 and 14, Liver 3, Bladder 1 and 2, Triple Warmer 5, and related auricular points.

Chinese Herbal Therapy Chinese medical practitioners believe that headaches are a yang condition, caused by excessive heat and dysfunctions in hollow yang-related organs, such as the large and small intestine, liver, bladder, gallbladder, stomach, and triple warmer. To counteract chronic cluster headaches, an herbalist would recommend therapies that balance the energy within these organs and their corresponding meridians.

Herb formulas commonly used to treat cluster headaches include Bupleurum and Tang Gui Formula, Bupleurum and Dragon Bone Formula, and Leonurus and Achyranthes Formula. Further diagnosis may be required to achieve desired results.

HEADACHE, MIGRAINE

Signs and Symptoms

In some cases, migraine headaches are preceded by an aura—blank spots, streaks of colors, flickering lights, or floating shapes in the field of vision. During the migraine attack, symptoms may include:

- Intense, throbbing pain
- Nausea and vomiting
- Dizziness
- Numbness on one side of the body
- Sensitivity to lights, sounds, and odors

Description

Migraines are often-debilitating headaches that feature intense, throbbing pain that begins on one side of the head and may slowly spread. The pain becomes most extreme in ten minutes to two hours after onset and can last anywhere from three hours to two days. In many cases, migraine sufferers are unable to work, talk, or conduct normal daily activities.

Migraines are a chronic condition, but the frequency of attacks varies from person to person. One person may get a migraine almost daily, while another person may experience one every seven or eight months. Most sufferers begin experiencing migraines in adolescence or early adulthood, and the frequency of attacks tends to lessen with age.

Although the exact cause of migraine headaches is unknown, there is a correlation between the condition and the constricting of blood vessels in the head; for this reason, migraines are also referred to as vascular headaches. Any of a number of factors can cause this vascular constriction. Eating certain foods—such as chocolate, aged cheese, red wine, dried fruit, milk, chicken livers, smoked meats, and foods containing monosodium glutamate (MSG)—can bring on a migraine headache. Use of birth control pills and alcohol consumption also can result in a migraine headache, as can stress, menstruation, pregnancy, sunlight, vigorous exercise, or a period of hard work followed directly by a period of relaxation. Hereditary plays a major role in whether an individual develops reccurring migraines.

Conventional Medical Treatment

If you are experiencing symptoms of a migraine headache, see your physician immediately. Your doctor can make a more certain diagnosis if he or she can see you while you are still suffering from the headache—though an immediate appointment is not mandatory. Your physician may give you a thorough examination to rule out other neurologic illnesses that have symptoms similar to those of migraines. Your physician also may ask you detailed questions about your activities and diet, medical history, and family's medical history.

There is no cure for migraine headaches. Instead, your physician advises you to avoid the triggers that prompted your attack. In addition, he or she may prescribe nonsteroidal anti-inflammatory drugs (NSAIDs) to lessen the pain, or recommend that you use over-the-counter analgesics, such as aspirin, acetaminophen, and ibuprofen. If you have frequently reccurring migraines, your doctor may prescribe a daily oral dose of a beta-adrenergic or calcium-entry blocker, sumatriptan (Imitrex®) or an ergotamine to reduce blood pressure in the head, and thus, prevent future attacks.

For More Information
National Headache Foundation
428 West St. James, 2nd Floor
Chicago, IL 60614-2750
800-843-2256
www.headaches.org

National Institute of Neurological Disorders and Stroke
P.O. Box 5801
Bethesda, MD 20824
800-352-9424
www.ninds.nih.gov

Health Notes

➤ Talk to your physician about taking aspirin to prevent migraine headaches. According to a recent study, people who take one aspirin every other day have 20 percent fewer migraines than people who do not take aspirin.

➤ Getting proper sleep is integral in preventing migraine headaches. Irregular sleeping habits trigger migraine attacks in some people.

➤ Moderate aerobic exercise performed three to seven times a week can lessen the frequency and severity of migraine headaches.

Complementary and Alternative Treatments

Nutrition and Supplementation

Migraines are frequently triggered by allergic reactions to foods, additives, or food combinations. To determine if any of these trigger your migraines, eliminate suspect foods and then reintroduce them one at a time, keeping track of your reaction to them. People are often allergic to red wine or beer as well as the amino acid tyramine (cheese, yogurt, smoked fish) and MSG (an additive found in salad dressings, commercial Chinese food, soups, and frozen foods). Sodium nitrate (hot dogs and cold cuts) has also been implicated. Similarly, chocolate, coffee, and soda have been known to trigger these headaches. Flaxseed oil (1 tblsp daily) is extremely helpful to migraine sufferers. Ask your healthcare provider about L-arginine. This amino acid is able to dilate blood vessels and is most effective when taken at the first sign of a migraine.

Chiropractic

Specific chiropractic adjustment (SCA) can be effective in relieving the pain, intensity, and frequency of migraine headaches in some sufferers, by removing vertebral subluxation in the upper cervical spine (typically, the first and second cervical vertebrae). The chiropractor may also apply moist heat, electromuscular stimulation, or ultrasound to the posterior cervical musculature to decrease spasms and pain in those muscles. Some patients find relief with chiropractic care alone, while others utilize a combination of medical intervention and chiropractic care.

Traditional Chinese Medicine

Acupuncture Acupuncture can be very effective in relieving migraine pain, migraine-induced nausea and vomiting, and in reducing recurrences. Points that may be targeted are Governing Vessel 4 and 19, Gallbladder 5 and 6, Large Intestine 4 and 10, Stomach 36 and 44, and Spleen 6. Points in the ear may be added to the session, if necessary. Liver points may be targeted to build up the system, if the migraine headaches are caused by a liver deficiency.

Because migraines are thought to be caused by improperly dilated blood vessels in the head, acupuncture also can be used to help improve circulation and energy flow within these vessels.

Acupressure Acupressure is very helpful in encouraging relaxation, which is usually in short

supply during a migraine episode. The particular acupressure points depends on the location of the pain. In most cases, the practitioner works on points along the bladder, gallbladder, lung, and stomach meridians.

Acupressure also can help improve the flow of energy in the blood vessels of the head, which may have preventive benefits.

Chinese Herbal Therapy Bupleurum Sedative Pills, Corydalis Analgesic Tablets, and Cnidium and Tea Formula also can help reduce migraine pain.

HEADACHE, TENSION

Signs and Symptoms

- Dull, gripping pain in the scalp, temples, and/or back of the neck
- Inability to concentrate
- Muscle stiffness in the neck and front of the head

Description

Tension headaches are believed to be the most common type of headache. The primary symptom of this type of headache is a tight, gripping pain on the top of the head that sometimes spreads to the back of the neck. In addition to the feeling of constriction, sufferers may also feel a stinging, tingling, or burning sensation on the skin of the head and neck. Tension headaches come on slowly and may last for hours if untreated. The pain accompanying the condition typically varies in severity over the course of one to six hours.

Tension headaches are caused by a tight contraction of the cranial and cervical muscles outside the skull. Although these headaches are sometimes caused by poor posture, which can

strain the neck muscles, they are most commonly caused by stress, illness, and fever.

Conventional Medical Treatment

Tension headaches respond well to over-the-counter analgesics, such as aspirin, acetaminophen, and ibuprofen. As a result, most tension headaches can be treated at home without having to see a doctor.

Easy On the Aspirin

Over-the-counter analgesics, such as aspirin, acetaminophen, and ibuprofen, are popular and effective ways to treat tension headaches. However, overuse of these drugs has been linked to a "drug rebound headache," wherein the body becomes resistant to previously effective drugs, and a headache results. When taking these painkillers, limit yourself to no more than five pills a day, every other day.

Health Notes

➤ *Be sure to maintain proper posture. In some instances, tension headaches can be triggered by spinal misalignment or poor posture.*

➤ *If you are trying to reduce your caffeine intake, do so slowly over a two- or three-week period. Abrupt caffeine withdrawal can cause tension headaches.*

➤ *Studies have shown that eating smaller, more frequent meals may lessen the frequency of tension headaches.*

➤ *If you are suffering from tension headaches, be sure to get a good night's sleep (or at least take a nap). Sleep helps to ease and even prevent tension headaches.*

If, on the other hand, you experience more than two tension headaches a week for an extended period of time, visit your physician. To rule out other disorders that also cause headaches—such as brain tumors, vision impairment, or sinus conditions—your doctor may want to perform a urinalysis, vision test, sinus X-ray, skull X-ray, or CAT scan. If over-the-counter medications do not offer relief, your doctor may prescribe nonsteroidal anti-inflammatory drugs (NSAIDs) to reduce the pain.

For More Information
National Headache Foundation
428 West St. James, 2nd Floor
Chicago, IL 60614-2750
800-843-2256
www.headaches.org

National Institute of Neurological Disorders and Stroke
P.O. Box 5801
Bethesda, MD 20824
800-352-9424
www.ninds.nih.gov

Complementary and Alternative Treatments

Nutrition and Supplementation

 Eat a well-balanced diet in small meals, and feel free to eat between meals. This helps stabilize your blood sugar levels. Be sure to include pineapple, cherries, almonds, garlic, parsley, and fennel in your diet. All are rich in nutrients—such as bromelain, vitamin E, vitamin C, and anti-inflammatories—that minimize pain. Get a daily supply of fiber.

Foods to avoid include sugar, caffeine, alcohol, chewing gum, ice cream, and salt. Eliminate foods containing tyramine and the amino acid phenylalanine; reintroduce them one at a time to determine which foods cause your headaches. Tyramine is found in chicken, alcoholic beverages, bananas, cheese, chocolate, citrus, cold cuts, onions, peanut butter, pork, smoked fish, sour cream, vinegar, wine, and fresh-baked yeast products. Tyramine raises blood pressure, which can cause a dull headache. Phenylalanine is found in aspartame, monosodium glutamate (MSG), and the preservatives used in hot dogs and lunch meats. Check for other food sensitivities, such as dairy or wheat.

Try to get a daily dose of exercise, which improves blood circulation to the brain. In addition, the following recommended daily supplements should help treat those nasty headaches.

- D-L-phenylalanine (DLPA) (500 mg 3 times before meals)
- bromelain (500 mg as needed)—regulates inflammation
- calcium (lactate or citrate form, not carbonate) (1500 mg)—alleviates muscular tension
- magnesium (glycinate form) (1000 mg)
- coenzyme Q10 (30 mg twice daily)—improves tissue oxygenation
- glucosamine sulfate (as directed on label)—a natural alternative to aspirin
- potassium (99 mg)—helps provide the proper sodium and potassium balance, which helps prevent water retention

- vitamin B₃ and niacinamide (up to 300 mg, not to be exceeded; stop and maintain the dosage that provides relief)—aids in the functioning of the nervous system (Do not take niacin if you have a liver disorder, gout, or high blood pressure.)

- vitamin C with bioflavonoids (2000 to 8000 mg in divided doses)—assists with the production of anti-stress hormones

- vitamin E (start with 400 IU and slowly increase to 1200 IU)—improves circulation

(For an *acute* condition, take supplements until your symptoms subside. If symptoms persist, seek the advice of your healthcare provider. For a *chronic* condition, consult your healthcare provider regarding the duration of treatment.)

Aromatherapy

All of the following remedies can help relax the muscles of your face, neck, upper back, and shoulders, thereby keeping headaches at bay.

- Combine 1 teaspoon sunflower oil and 1 drop peppermint oil. Apply to your forehead, neck, and shoulders the moment you feel a tension headache coming on.

- Combine 3 drops Roman chamomile oil, 3 drops lavender oil, 2 drops marjoram oil, 2 drops thyme oil, and 1 drop coriander oil. Add to warm bath water. Soak for 20 to 30 minutes.

- Blend together 1 teaspoon canola or sunflower oil and 1 drop each of marjoram oil, Roman chamomile oil, lavender oil, coriander oil, helichrysum oil, basil oil, and ginger oil. Use to massage your neck and shoulders.

- Massage a few drops of lavender oil into your temples. You can also blend lavender oil and peppermint oil, and massage a few drops of the blend into your temples. If the essential oils themselves feel too harsh on your skin, blend them with 1 teaspoon of canola or sunflower oil.

Chiropractic

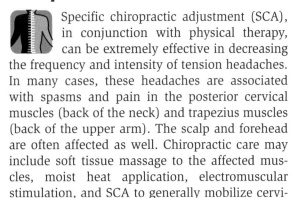

Specific chiropractic adjustment (SCA), in conjunction with physical therapy, can be extremely effective in decreasing the frequency and intensity of tension headaches. In many cases, these headaches are associated with spasms and pain in the posterior cervical muscles (back of the neck) and trapezius muscles (back of the upper arm). The scalp and forehead are often affected as well. Chiropractic care may include soft tissue massage to the affected muscles, moist heat application, electromuscular stimulation, and SCA to generally mobilize cervical vertebrae.

Herbal Therapy

Tension headaches respond quite nicely to infusions of valerian, skullcap, willow bark, or thyme. Drink 1 cup of valerian tea before bedtime. To prepare skullcap tea, brew 2 teaspoons dried leaves in 1 cup boiling water for 10 to 15 minutes; strain. Drink up to 3 times a day. For thyme tea, stir 1 teaspoon dried herb into 1 cup boiling water; steep for 10 minutes; strain.

Another soothing brew contains equal parts dried wintergreen, willow bark, and meadowsweet. Steep 1 teaspoon of the blend in 1 cup boiling water for 10 minutes; strain. Drink once a day.

Evening primrose oil is believed to promote healthy circulation and relieve pain. Experts recommend taking 500 mg 3-4 times daily.

Herbal products are available in health food stores and in some pharmacies and supermarkets. Follow package for specific directions.

Hydrotherapy

Some sufferers of tension headaches find relief by applying heat and cold. Soak your feet in hot water and at the same time apply a cold cloth or ice pack to your forehead. Remember to limit use of the ice pack to 20 minutes; extended exposure to cold can damage your skin.

Traditional Chinese Medicine

 Acupuncture To treat pain in the neck and back of the head, an acupuncturist may focus on the following points: Bladder 10, 60, and 65; Gallbladder 20; Governing Vessel 15; Small Intestine 3; and Large Intestine 4.

If the pain is concentrated on the top of the head, Bladder 60, Governing Vessel 20, and Liver 2 and 3 may be added to the session. Additional points may be incorporated as symptoms warrant.

Acupressure Applying firm pressure to Large Intestine 4 (located in the webbing of the hand between the thumb and forefinger) and Gallbladder 20 (on either side of the spine at the base of the head) should help relieve the discomfort associated with a tension headache. Additional acupressure points (including those mentioned in the acupuncture section, above) also may be included.

Chinese Herbal Therapy Bupleurum and Tang Gui Formula may provide some relief of tension headache pain, and Pueraria Combination can be used if the patient has a stiff neck and a tendency to coldness.

Yoga and Meditation

 Several yoga positions can bring welcome relief from headache pain. They include the Neck Roll, Moon Salutation, Boat Pose, Hidden Lotus, Bow Pose, Spinal Twist, Half Moon I, and Standing on the Toes. Do these exercises up to three times a day for maximum benefit. *Cautions*: Avoid the Neck Roll if you have neck problems or neck pain. Avoid inverted poses (such as the Headstand, Shoulder Stands, and the Plow pose) when you have a headache.

SYMPTOM:

HEARING LOSS

Hearing is a complex process, requiring many different parts of the ear to function properly. When sound waves strike the eardrum, the membrane vibrates. These vibrations are transmitted through the tiny bones of the middle ear and into the inner ear through the oval window. The vibrations are then directed into the cochlea, where they are converted into electrical impulses that are transmitted to the brain via the auditory nerve. If any parts of the ear are damaged— through injury or illness—hearing loss may occur.

Hearing loss (either partial or complete) is a symptom that accompanies a wide variety of ear problems. An infection of the inner or middle ear can cause temporary hearing loss in the infected ear. An eardrum that has been damaged—for example, punctured by a cotton swab or ruptured by the pressure of a sharp blow to the outer ear—cannot vibrate properly, thus affecting hearing in one ear. A buildup of excess ear wax also can cause temporary hearing loss. Prolonged exposure to noise over 85 decibels also can diminish hearing. With age, the shape of the cochlea and surrounding nerves changes, thus affecting hearing.

If you notice a loss of hearing, visit your physician or otorhinolaryngologist, who will examine your ears. If your doctor discovers an injury or underlying medical condition, you will receive treatment, hopefully regaining your hearing capacity. If your hearing loss is found to be permanent, you may be fitted with a hearing aid, an electronic device that is placed in the bowl of the ear to amplify the sounds around you.

For a complementary treatment, you may consider Ayurvedic medicine, which uses a combination of herbs and oils to strengthen nerves associated with hearing. Practitioners may suggest taking yogaraj guggulu, *an herbal compound, several times daily. Or they may advise placing garlic oil in the affected ear. Note: Before using the oil, be certain the ear is not infected. Ayurvedic products are available at many health food stores and Indian pharmacies.*

HEARTBURN

Signs and Symptoms

- A burning sensation usually felt behind the breastbone of the chest

Description

Heartburn is experienced on occasion by about one in three American adults. It is the result of acidic gastric juices from the stomach washing upward into the esophagus, or food pipe. Because gastric acids are required for food digestion, they occur naturally in the stomach, where the stomach lining is tough enough to resist them without harm. However, if the same strong digestive acids wash back up into the esophagus, they may irritate the lining of the esophagus, and the resulting burning sensation is commonly called heartburn, acid indigestion, or sour stomach.

Heartburn usually follows a rich meal or vigorous exercise and may be exacerbated by stress, bending over, or the strain of lifting heavy objects. The symptoms often are felt at night, upon lying down for sleep. Pregnant women also experience frequent heartburn. The burning sensation can last from a few minutes to several hours and range from mild discomfort to intense, heart-attack-like pain.

Conventional Medical Treatment

Generally, the condition is easily treated with over-the-counter antacids that neutralize the gastric acids; liquid antacids are more effective than tablets.

Long-term antacid use, however, may disguise other diseases, cause acid rebound, or contribute to hypertension or congestive heart failure if their sodium content is high.

Health Notes

Heartburn and gastroesophageal reflux disease (GERD) can be chronic disorders. In addition to antacids, you also may want to try these strategies for relief:

➤ *Elevate the head of your bed by six to eight inches to help prevent reflux by counteracting it with gravity.*

➤ *Eat several small meals each day, rather than one or two large meals. Make breakfast or lunch your main meal, not dinner.*

➤ *Avoid eating or drinking up to three hours before bedtime.*

➤ *Reduce your intake of caffeine, alcohol, chocolate, acidic foods (such as fruit juices and tomato products), mints, onions, garlic, pepper, carbonated drinks or other foods that cause burping, and very hot beverages.*

➤ *Lose weight, avoid fatty foods and overeating.*

➤ *Drink lots of water, especially with meals.*

➤ *Avoid heavy lifting or strenuous bending after meals.*

➤ *Avoid tight garments.*

➤ *Quit smoking.*

➤ *Avoid aspirin.*

➤ *Ask your doctor if any medication you are taking, such as aspirin or ibuprofen, asthma medications, certain antibiotics, hormone therapies, tranquilizers, or narcotics, could affect your lower esophagus.*

Is It Heartburn, GERD, or a Heart Attack?

Those who suffer from GERD (as many as one in ten Americans) experience more intense and more frequent episodes of heartburn, generally because an abnormality in the lower esophagus sphincter muscle prevents it from completely closing off from the stomach. GERD sufferers may also have a hiatal hernia, which may increase the incidence of heartburn. Another symptom of GERD is regurgitation of bitter fluid from the stomach. Less common symptoms include constant hoarseness, a frequent need to clear the throat, an unexplained cough, and chest pain. Wheezing, asthma, and frequent respiratory infections may accompany the disorder.

If your symptoms persist, your physician may recommend drugs such as cimetidine (Tagamet®), ranitidine (Zantac®), famotidine (Pepcid®), and nizatidine (Axid®). Once available only by prescription, most are now available over-the-counter and do not interfere with food digestion. Called histamine$_2$ receptor antagonists (H$_2$RAs), they reduce the production of acid in the stomach and can help eliminate symptoms in up to 60 percent of those with GERD.

You also may be advised to try proton-pump inhibitors, such as omeprazole (Prilosec®), lansoprazole (Prevacid®), and pantoprazole, which reduce acid production. Also available are the promotility (prokinetic) drugs, which speed the clearance of fluids from the esophagus, such as cisapride (Propulsid®) and metoclopramide (Reglan®).

In severe cases, your physician may recommend an operation called *fundoplication surgery*, which strengthens the lower esophageal sphincter muscle that connects to the stomach.

If left untreated, GERD can lead to esophagitis (a serious inflammation of the esophagus lining that can cause sores or bleeding and eventually may lead to anemia). If you spit up black or bloody material or pass black tarry stools, see your doctor immediately to be evaluated for a possible esophageal ulcer. A rare condition called Barrett's esophagus is one of the most serious results of GERD. The condition is characterized by a change in the esophagus lining, which may indicate a slightly increased risk of cancer of the esophagus.

Since the symptoms of heartburn or GERD may be mistaken for a heart attack, seek emergency treatment if:

- your pain increases with exertion and decreases with rest (physical activity does not generally affect heartburn)

- you do not receive prompt relief from your heartburn pain by taking antacids

- you feel pain in the jaw or arm (heartburn pain is not felt in these areas)

- your pain is accompanied by shortness of breath, an irregular pulse, sweating or dizziness

Heartburn also may indicate the existence of more serious medical problems, such as gastroesophageal reflux disease (GERD) or peptic ulcer disease. Such severe conditions often do not respond to antacid treatment, so consult a physician if pain is persistent.

HEART DISEASE (CARDIOVASCULAR DISEASE)

Signs and Symptoms

- Chest pain—either sharp and stabbing or tight and suffocating; the pain may radiate up to the jaw or through the shoulder down the arms
- Pounding, fluttering, or racing heartbeat
- Shortness of breath
- Lightheadedness
- Dizziness
- Fatigue and muscle weakness
- Fainting
- Visible fluid retention in the ankles, legs, or abdomen

Description

Heart disease and *cardiovascular disease* are general terms referring to several conditions that affect the heart. *Atherosclerosis* is an inflammation of the coronary arteries, resulting in hardening of the arteries. *Arrhythmia* is a disturbance in your heart's normal beating pattern, and includes *tachycardia* (when the heart beats too quickly) and *bradycardia* (when the heart beats too slowly). *Cardiomyopathy* is a thickening or stretching of the heart muscle. Problems with the heart valves, including *mitral valve prolapse*, can cause leakage or obstruction of blood flow in the heart. *Pericardial diseases* cause inflammation of the membrane that surrounds the heart. All of these conditions affect the heart's ability to efficiently pump oxygen-rich blood through the body; and all of these conditions can lead to a heart attack.

While heart conditions most commonly affect men over the age of 45, they are of increasing concern to women as well. In fact, heart disease is the number-one cause of death in both men and women. Heart disease is often a hereditary condition. Other risk factors include: obesity, high blood pressure, smoking, high blood cholesterol, sedentary lifestyle, and diet high in animal products.

Conventional Medical Treatment

If you experience severe constriction in the chest, shortness of breath, and pain that radiates out from your heart, immediately call an ambulance—you may be experiencing a heart attack. If, instead, you experience mild, chronic symptoms of heart disease, visit your physician, who may perform one or more tests to diagnose the condition. Heart disease diagnostic tests include: serum cholesterol test, blood pressure reading, echocardiogram, electrocardiogram, exercise tolerance test (also known as a treadmill test), and angiogram.

Treatment for heart disease usually consists of a combination of lifestyle modifications and medication to regulate the heartbeat, lower blood pressure, lower blood cholesterol levels, treat heart swelling, or thin the blood for travel through the arteries to the body. In more serious cases, surgery may be required. During bypass surgery, an artery is removed from the leg and implanted in another area of the body to bypass blocked arteries. Valve surgery is used to replace or repair faulty valves. A balloon catheter can be inserted into arteries to dislodge mild blockages. This is called *angioplasty*. If the heart is not beating regularly, an electronic device called a pacemaker can be implanted in the heart to regulate heartbeat.

For Further Information
American Heart Association
7272 Greenville Avenue
Dallas, TX 75231
888-AHA-USA1
Women's Health Line: 888-MY-HEART
www.americanheart.org

Do You Need a Stress Test?

A stress test is one of several techniques for determining cardiac problems. It is used to help diagnose the extent of coronary artery disease (CAD) in people suffering with chest pain, to monitor those being treated for heart conditions, and to identify risks for those beginning vigorous exercise programs. You may need a stress test if:

- You are a man over 40 or a woman over 50.

- You have two or more risk factors for CAD. These include high blood pressure, cholesterol, tobacco use, obesity, or a family history of premature CAD.

- You have cardiovascular or lung disease or a metabolic disorder such as diabetes.

How The Test Works

A stress test shows how your heart and blood vessels respond to physical activity. Here is what you expect during the test:

- Prior to the test, electrodes are placed on your chest and back to transmit signals from your heart to the machine.

- During the test, your heart's activity is monitored on an electrocardiograph while you work out on a treadmill or stationary bicycle for 10 to 15 minutes.

- As your pace gradually increases, the ECG monitor changes in response to the rate, rhythm, and electrical activity of your heart; your blood pressure is also monitored throughout the procedure.

- During a "maximal" test, you exercise until fatigue causes you to stop or until warning signs occur, such as chest pain, dizziness, or abnormalities in ECG, heart rate, rhythm, or blood pressure.

- During a "submaximal" tests, you stop exercising once you reach a predetermined heart rate.

- A cardiologist will evaluate the results of your stress test and make a determination based on your age, sex, and medical history.

Health Notes

➤ Many psychological disorders—such as depression, generalized anxiety disorder, panic disorder, and phobias—are associated with an increased risk of having a heart attack. If you believe you might suffer from one of these disorders, consider getting psychological counseling as a preventive measure.

➤ If you smoke, quit. Experts claim that the simple act of quitting smoking may reduce your risk of a fatal heart attack by at least 50 percent.

➤ If you drink, do so in moderation. While drinking one or two glasses of red wine each day has been shown to lower your risk of developing heart disease, heavy alcohol intake—more than two drinks daily—can raise blood pressure and increase your risk for developing heart disease.

➤ Stress plays a significant role in the development of heart disease. Learn to manage your stress, through the use of various stress-reduction techniques (for example, meditation or biofeedback) or regular exercise. A social support network or counseling can also be effective.

➤ Regular exercise can significantly lower your risk of heart disease by increasing heart efficiency and burning excess body fat. Try to get a minimum of 30 minutes of moderate exercise each day. The more you exercise, the greater the benefit in terms of cardiovascular health.

➤ A woman's risk of developing heart disease increases greatly after menopause, due to decreased estrogen levels. Hormone replacement therapy can counter this estrogen loss, reducing a postmenopausal woman's risk of heart disease by half.

(h)

Heart Disease (Cardiovascular Disease)

National Heart, Lung, and Blood Institute
P.O. Box 30105
Bethesda, MD 20824-0105
301-592-8573
www.nhlbi.nih.gov

Complementary and Alternative Treatments

Nutrition and Supplementation

 Nutrition plays a vital role in preventing and treating heart disease. Numerous studies show that diet and exercise directly affect cardiovascular health.

Complex carbohydrates—found in fruits, vegetables, beans, and whole grains—are at the core of this diet. Bioflavonoids, which are plant pigments found in vegetables, fruits (oranges, grapefruits, grapes, plums, cherries, and blackberries), and some grains and beans, provide protection against heart disease that can't be obtained from any other source. Research shows that an increased intake of fish combats heart disease. Use soy protein in place of animal protein when possible. Tofu is a good high-fiber, high-protein source, low in saturated fat.

Water is also important. Pure water, and lots of it, keeps your cells hydrated and helps balance blood pressure. A good guideline to follow is to drink half your body weight in ounces daily.

Protein is important, but Americans consume far too much of the stuff. To get your protein, eat broiled fish and skinless turkey and chicken. With these, you get the protein without the fat. Reduce your cholesterol level by eating garlic, onions, and lecithin-rich grains, legumes and fish. Raw nuts (except peanuts), olive oil, trout, salmon, and mackerel contain essential fatty acids. Eliminate all sources of sodium from your diet, and avoid stimulants such as coffee and tea. Stay away from tobacco, alcohol, chocolate, sugar, butter, margarine, red meat, fats, fried foods, soft drinks, white flour products, and refined or processed foods.

Nutritionists recommend the following daily supplements:

Most Important

- Coenzyme Q10 (50 to 200 mg for less severe cases, up to 400 mg for those more severe)—increases oxygenation of the heart tissue; has been shown to prevent recurrences in those who have had a heart attack
- calcium (1500 to 2000 mg in divided doses)—helps cardiac muscle function
- magnesium (750 to 1000 mg in divided doses)
- garlic (as directed on label)—lowers blood pressure and thins the blood
- lecithin (2400 mg 3 times daily, with meals)—emulsifies fat
- L-carnitine (500 mg two times daily, on empty stomach)

Also Recommended

- B vitamin complex (50 mg)—with at least 400 mcg of folic acid to prevent homocysteine buildup, supplemented with vitamin B_3 (consult a healthcare provider for dosage; can hamper liver function if incorrect dosage is given)—helps prevent heart attack
- Omega-3 fatty acids (fish or flax, as directed on label)—protects against heart disease
- vitamin E (start with 100 to 200 IU and increase slowly, adding 100 IU weekly until daily dosage is 800 to 1000 IU; do not exceed 400 IU daily if you are taking an anticoagulant drug)—strengthens the heart muscle and improves circulation (Use this supplement only under the direction of a healthcare provider.)
- vitamin C (500 to 1000 mg in divided doses)—prevents heart disease
- bioflavonoids (100 to 300 mg)—protect against cardiovascular disease and heart attacks
- taurine (500 mg 2 times daily)—an antioxidant that enhances the flow of blood from the heart
- selenium (200 mcg)—deficiencies found in people with heart disease
- melatonin (2 to 3 mg, taken near bedtime)—an antioxidant that helps prevent stroke and aids sleep

- potassium (99 mg)
- L-carnitine (500 mg 2 times daily, on empty stomach)
- Omega-3 fatty acids (fish or flaxseed oils) (as directed on label)—protects against heart disease

(Consult your healthcare provider regarding the duration of treatment.)

Ayurvedic Medicine

 Ayurvedic practitioners use a variety of treatments to strengthen the heart muscle and rid the body of free radicals—the heart-damaging by-products of eating meat, smoking, and drinking alcohol. For healing the heart and encouraging circulation, an Ayurvedic practitioner may advise taking *arjuna,* an herb that acts as a vasodilator, twice a day.

In addition, a practitioner may recommend *pancha karma* techniques to detoxify and purify the body and heart. A complete *pancha karma* program, however, should be carried out only under the guidance of a qualified practitioner.

Consult your doctor before embarking on any new regimen; proper heart care is critical.

Bodywork and Somatic Practices

 Bodywork can enhance a total medical and complementary treatment program. Direct manual approaches would be Oriental bodywork, reflexology, and CranioSacral Therapy or SomatoEmotional Release. Consider trying Reiki, polarity therapy, and Therapeutic Touch.

Herbal Therapy

 If you're suffering from angina pain, both foxglove and hawthorn berry have powerful effects on the heart and can relieve discomfort and improve heart function by dilating blood vessels. Use these herbs only under the supervision of a qualified medical herbalist and with your healthcare provider's approval.

Garlic and ginger may be helpful in managing high cholesterol and high blood pressure, both of which are associated with clogged arteries. Garlic is available as fresh cloves and in tablet form. Fresh ginger (often called ginger root) is available in most supermarkets and also can be found in tablet, capsule, and tea form.

Traditional Chinese Medicine

 Acupuncture To combat the hardened arteries associated with atherosclerosis (the main cause of heart disease), acupuncture may improve circulation to the area, thus reducing the risk of an angina episode. It also can be used to lessen atherosclerosis symptoms, such as chest pain, dizziness, irregular heartbeat, leg cramps, confusion, and forgetfulness.

In addition, acupuncture can be used as anesthesia during open heart surgery. In this case, the Lung 7 and Circulation 6 points on the wrist may be manipulated, along with related points in the left ear.

Acupressure This modality may help lessen the symptoms of heart disease. In the case of angina, for instance, the practitioner may apply pressure to Conception Vessel 17, Pericardium 6, and Heart 7 to help relieve pain. Palpitations also are treated by manipulating Pericardium 6 and Heart 7, along with related ear points. Various bladder, spleen, and stomach points may be added.

Chinese Herbal Therapy Ginseng, which has been shown to prevent myocardial infarction, may be used as a preventive treatment to strengthen the heart, regulate blood pressure, and lower cholesterol levels. Take a 5- to 10-gram decoction once a day. Pseudoginseng is a related herb that is also very effective, although it should not be used during pregnancy.

Garlic has anti-clotting properties.

Dan Shen Tablets (whose main ingredient is salvia), and Ginseng Restorative Pills are Chinese patent medicines that may be recommended to counteract heart disease.

Because Chinese medicine views heart disease as a condition related to digestive problems, herbs may be given to cleanse and strengthen the gastrointestinal system.

Yoga and Meditation

Several yoga positions help increase blood flow, improve circulation, and make the veins more elastic—all of which will help protect the heart. Try these poses several times a day: Sun Salutation, Locust, Lotus, Bridge, Dog and Cat, Camel, Bow, Cobra, Forward Bend, and Knee Squeeze. Also try the Supported Shoulder Stand; build up slowly to holding it for five minutes. Remember to consult your doctor before embarking on any new exercise program; proper heart care is extremely important.

HEAT EXHAUSTION

Signs and Symptoms

- Fatigue and muscle weakness
- Dizziness
- Extreme thirst
- Heavy sweating
- Hyperventilation
- Headache
- Rapid heartbeat
- Elevated temperature of up to 103°F
- Nausea and vomiting
- Pale, moist skin

Description

Heat exhaustion occurs when the body is unable to acclimate to an extremely warm environment, and it begins to overheat. The symptoms of heat exhaustion, or heat collapse, as it is sometimes called, usually come on very quickly after prolonged exposure to high temperatures—whether working in a room that is very hot or exercising outdoors in the summer heat.

Many conditions can increase a person's risk

Health Notes

➤ Avoid heat exhaustion on a hot day by wearing non-restricting, cool, light-colored cotton clothing and a broad-brimmed hat. Also, avoid being outdoors between 11 a.m. and 3 p.m., when the sun is at its hottest.

➤ Be aware that humidity makes you especially vulnerable to heat exhaustion. High humidity prevents sweat from evaporating.

➤ Avoid drinking alcoholic or caffeinated beverages in a hot environment. Both alcohol and caffeine act as diuretics and increase the body's need for liquid.

➤ Be aware that certain medications put you at higher risk for heat exhaustion. Laxatives, appetite suppressants, diuretics, sedatives, antihistamines, some thyroid hormones, and medications for treating Parkinson's disease all make the body more sensitive to warm temperatures.

The Elderly and Heat

The elderly are at a increased risk of heat exhaustion, because they are unable to efficiently regulate body temperature. The hypothalamus is a gland located in the brain that functions as the body's temperature regulator. When the body temperature changes, the hypothalamus stimulates temperature-regulating mechanisms—such as sweat production and blood vessel dilation in the skin—to lower the body's temperature. With age, the hypothalamus is less efficient at regulating temperature. Illnesses, such as lung and heart disease, also can increase an older person's vulnerability to heat exhaustion. To prevent heat exhaustion, elderly individuals should stay in a climate-controlled environment—such as an air-conditioned building—during the hottest part of the day. Frequent bathing, keeping physical exertion at a minimum, and drinking lots of water also may help prevent the condition.

of experiencing heat exhaustion. People who are obese and of advanced age are at increased risk, because their bodies are unable to regulate temperature efficiently. Physical activity also puts people at greater risk, because such exercise raises the body's core temperature to begin with.

Conventional Medical Treatment

Most cases of heat exhaustion can be treated with homecare measures. If you suspect you are experiencing heat exhaustion, get yourself into a cooler environment immediately. An air-conditioned room is ideal, but any cooler area—such as a shady area or a room in the house where a breeze is blowing—will suffice if it is all that's available.

After moving to a cooler location, lie down and elevate your feet to help increase blood flow to the heart. Loosen or remove any restrictive clothing. If you are wearing multiple layers of clothing, remove as much of it as possible to help the body cool down. It is also necessary to replenish your body's fluid supply to prevent dehydration; drink as much cold water as you can. (Do not drink ice water, because it can cause shock by dropping the temperature of certain tissues too rapidly.)

If you are with someone who is experiencing heat exhaustion, take measures to help him or her cool down. If the person's skin is hot and dry, or if he or she has lost consciousness, call an ambulance immediately or go to the nearest emergency medical center.

Complementary and Alternative Treatments

Traditional Chinese Medicine

Acupuncture Acupuncture may help alleviate the dizziness, rapid pulse, and headache associated with heat exhaustion or heatstroke.

Acupressure Pressure may be applied to Governing Vessel 26 (in the crescent above the upper lip) and Kidney 11 (below the ball of the foot) to relieve symptoms of heat stroke.

Chinese Herbal Therapy Ilex Compound Pills, as well as many herbal formulas made with animal products, are used in cases of heat exhaustion, but generally the most important course of action is to get the person to the hospital.

Hemorrhoids (Piles)

Signs and Symptoms

- Tenderness or pain in the anal region, especially during bowel movements
- Anal itching
- Straining during bowel movements
- Blood on the stool
- Soft tissue protruding from the anus

Description

Hemorrhoids occur when the blood vessels in the lower rectum and anus swell due to straining during bowel movements. These swollen blood vessels cause a stretching and irritation of the membrane that lines the rectum and anus. Often, the swollen blood vessels cause small, visible protrusions in the wall of the anus.

Hemorrhoids can occur either internally or externally. Internal hemorrhoids develop in the rectum, and are rarely noticeable. Often, the only sign of internal hemorrhoids is blood in the stool, caused when the swollen blood vessels rupture. External hemorrhoids, on the other hand, develop on the anus itself and can be extremely uncomfortable. This type of hemorrhoid is often visible, turning red or purple as the vessels fill with blood. Fortunately, both types of hemorrhoids are usually not serious.

Conventional Medical Treatment

If your hemorrhoids do not cause much discomfort, you may safely choose to ignore them. If, on the other hand, you experience severe symptoms of hemorrhoids, visit your physician, who can conduct a physical examination of the area to arrive at a diagnosis. In order to rule out more serious conditions, such as polyps or colon cancer, your doctor also may perform a sigmoidoscopy or colonoscopy (where a fiber optic tube is used to view the inside of the rectum and colon).

If hemorrhoids are diagnosed, your physician may recommend over-the-counter analgesics to reduce the pain or prescribe a topical preparation containing a general anesthetic. You also may be advised to take warm baths whenever your hemorrhoids bother you. Since hemorrhoids are caused by straining during bowel movements, your doctor may recommend a high-fiber diet with increased water intake to keep the stool soft.

Hemorrhoid removal is another medical option. One removal method involves tying a rubberband-like thread around the base of the hemorrhoid. Within a few days, the hemorrhoid atrophies to the point where it painlessly falls off. Other procedures include injecting a fluid into the hemorrhoid to close it off, or a *hemorrhoidectomy*, which involves surgically removing the hemorrhoid.

Health Notes

➤ Constipation is a primary cause of hemorrhoids. Avoid constipation by eating fiber-rich foods, such as whole grains and raw fruits and vegetables, and drinking at least 8 8-ounce glasses of water each day.

➤ Daily aerobic exercise helps prevent hemorrhoids by improving the digestive process, which ensures that food is moved quickly and efficiently through the intestines.

Complementary and Alternative Treatments

Nutrition and Supplementation

 This condition is due to a systemic imbalance, and therefore, can be improved through diet. Eat a high-fiber diet. Foods high in fiber include whole grains, wheat bran, fresh fruits, and almost all vegetables. Apples, broccoli, carrots, green beans, pears, and peas are especially good. Adequate water (8 to 10 glasses each day) is the best stool softener and helps prevent constipation.

Try to stay away from fats and animal products. High-protein diets are more difficult to digest.

Bleeding hemorrhoids can be helped by eating foods high in vitamin K, such as alfalfa and dark-green, leafy vegetables.

Nutritionists recommend the following daily supplements for help in treating hemorrhoids:

- calcium (1500 mg)—essential for blood clotting
- magnesium (750 mg)—balances calcium
- vitamin C (3000 to 5000 mg)—encourages normal blood clotting; promotes healing
- bioflavonoids (100 mg)
- vitamin E (600 IU)—promotes healing and blood clotting
- vitamin B complex (50 to 100 mg 3 times daily, with meals)—aids in proper digestion, which puts less strain on the rectum
- potassium (99 mg)—commonly deficient in those with constipation
- vitamin D (600 IU)—heals mucous membranes and tissues; needed for calcium absorption

Aromatherapy

 A warm sitz bath with one of the following combinations can bring welcome relief from itching: 10 drops cypress oil, 20 drops juniper oil or 10 drops lavender oil. Before getting into the tub, stir up the water to distribute the oils throughout the water.

Ayurvedic Medicine

 Any of the doshas (vata, pitta, and kapha) can have imbalances leading to hemorrhoids, but most are associated with vata and pitta disturbances. Your Ayuredic practitioner may recommend applying an anti-itch, gentle-healing mixture of turmeric and ghee (clarified butter) to tender tissues at bedtime. (*Note:* Turmeric will permanently stain whatever fabric it touches; use a soft disposable cloth to apply the mixture.) Alternatively, your practitioner may suggest applying castor oil or *tikta ghee*, or taking *triphala guggulu* tablets.

Ayurvedic products are available at many health food stores and Indian pharmacies.

Bodywork and Somatic Practices

 Hemorrhoids respond well to classic massage, reflexology, Oriental bodywork, CranioSacral Therapy, and Therapeutic Touch.

Herbal Therapy

To soothe the itching and burning of external hemorrhoids, dab them with a chilled salve containing pilewort or St. John's wort. To make a pilewort salve, simmer 2 tablespoons of fresh or dried herb in 7 ounces of petroleum jelly for 10 minutes. Strain and allow to cool. Apply once or twice a day. Prepared St. John's wort salves can be found in many health food stores. Follow package directions.

Compresses soaked with witch hazel can offer additional relief.

Herbal products are available in health food stores and in some pharmacies and supermarkets. Follow package for specific directions.

Homeopathy

 A homeopathic practitioner may suggest *Aesculus, Collinsonia*, or *Hamamelis* for the throbbing and swelling of hemorrhoids. For additional pain relief, you also might apply *Hamamelis* or *Aesculus* ointment twice a day following a sitz bath.

Hydrotherapy

 As mentioned earlier, a sitz bath can provide very welcome relief from the discomfort, swelling, and itching of hemorrhoids. Soak in warm (100°F to 105°F) water that is hip deep for 10 to 15 minutes, one to three times a day. This is particularly effective following a bowel movement.

To obtain additional relief from itching and swelling, apply a cold cloth moistened with witch hazel. Hold the compress on the swollen tissue for 15 minutes several times a day.

Traditional Chinese Medicine

 Acupuncture Acupuncture can be used to both relieve hemorrhoid pain and tone the area in order to prevent recurrences. Governing Vessel 20 is the most oft-targeted point. Stomach 25 and 36; Large Intestine 11; Bladder 25, 30, 32, and 57; and Governing Vessel 1 and 14 also may be used to treat this condition. In addition, acupuncture may also be used in place of traditional anesthesia during surgery to correct hemorrhoids.

Acupressure Strangely enough, Governing Vessel 20, located on the top of the head, has been shown to relieve hemorrhoids. Other points that may be used to remedy the condition are Governing Vessel 1 and 9, as well as Bladder 18, 23, 25, 26, and 40, along with various ear points.

Chinese Herbal Therapy Aloe vera juice can be applied topically to relieve hemorrhoid pain. Japanese honeysuckle can be used as a decoction or an external wash.

Depending on the root cause of an individual's hemorrhoids, various herbal formulas may be suggested, including Ginseng and Tang Gui, Apricot Seed and Linum, Cimicifuga, Ginseng and Longan, or Fargelin High Strength (also called Fargelin for Piles).

If the condition is accompanied by bleeding, the first-aid pills *Yunnan Pai Yao* may be prescribed (they should *not* be used during pregnancy).

Yoga and Meditation

 When executed properly, several yoga postures help blood flow away from hemorrhoids, and therefore, ease pain. Try one or more of the following poses daily: Bridge, Half Shoulder Stand, Plow, Shoulder Stand, and Downward Facing Dog.

HEPATITIS

Signs and Symptoms

- Loss of appetite
- Low-grade fever
- Fatigue

- Muscle or joint pain
- Nausea and vomiting
- Abdominal pain
- Headache

- Dark urine
- Jaundice (yellowing of the eyes and skin)

Description

Hepatitis, an inflammation of the liver, is a very serious disease. The liver is responsible for processing most of the nutrients that are absorbed from the intestine. Besides converting many of these nutrients into forms that can be used by the body, the liver also stores nutrients, manufactures cholesterol and blood-clotting substances, and detoxifies the blood. Hepatitis interferes with these vital liver functions.

Hepatitis is caused by one of a number of viruses. The three most common types are hepatitis A, hepatitis B, and hepatitis C—all of which have similar symptoms. Hepatitis A is the least dangerous form of hepatitis, and is usually contracted through contaminated food or water. Hepatitis B is the most common form of hepatitis, and can be spread through sexual contact, blood transfusions, infected needles, or from mother to child. Hepatitis C is a rare but dangerous form of the disease, and is transmitted primarily through tainted blood.

While many people who develop hepatitis recover after a few weeks, the condition can be quite dangerous. Hepatitis can cause cirrhosis of the liver, a potentially fatal condition. Even in people who do recover from the virus, it may take months for the liver to return to normal.

Conventional Medical Treatment

If you experience symptoms of hepatitis, see your doctor as soon as possible. Your physician needs to conduct a physical examination and a blood test, as well as take a detailed medical history, to diagnose the condition.

There is no specific medical treatment for hepatitis A. Most physicians require their patients to abstain from alcohol and medications to rest the liver. A nutritious diet with adequate caloric intake is also important in recovering from hepatitis. For three or four months after your diagnosis,

Health Notes

➤ *A vaccine is available for preventing Hepatitis B; vaccination is advisable for adults at risk of exposure to the virus. If you are a healthcare style worker or your sex partner has hepatitis B, you should consider yourself "at risk."*

➤ *Avoid high-risk behaviors that can lead to hepatitis, including unprotected sex and intravenous drug use.*

➤ *If you are exposed to hepatitis A, you should notify your doctor, who may advise an injection of immune serum globulin (protective antibodies) to prevent the disease.*

your physician may take an occasional blood test to determine whether your liver has regained its function.

Hepatitis B and C also may resolve spontaneously, but in many patients, B and C infections develop into chronic hepatitis. The drug interferon is used to treat chronic hepatitis B and hepatitis C. Approximately 30 percent of patients have an initial response to the medication, but only half or fewer of these individuals maintain a sustained response. Since interferon eradicates or cures infection in only a small number of patients, the common goal of the treatment is to suppress infection enough to minimize its effects on the liver.

For More Information
American Liver Foundation
1425 Pomptom Avenue
Cedar Grove, NJ 07009
800-GO-LIVER
http://sadieo.ucsf.edu/alf/alffinal

Centers for Disease Control and Prevention (CDC)
1600 Clifton Road
Atlanta, GA 30333
800-311-3435
www.cdc.gov

Complementary and Alternative Treatments

Nutrition and Supplementation

 Drink steam-distilled water and fresh juices, such as apple, carrot, or cranberry juice. "Green" drinks (those high in chlorophyll) purify the system. Avoid chemicals, food additives, alcohol, fats, sugars, and highly processed foods.

Follow this daily supplement guideline:

Most Important

- free-form amino acid complex (as directed on label)—supplies vital proteins; takes the strain off the liver

- glutathione (500 mg twice daily, on empty stomach)—protects the liver

- raw liver extract (as directed on label)—promotes liver function

- coenzyme Q10 (60 mg)—enhances tissue oxygenation

- lecithin (1200 mg 3 times daily, before meals)—protects cells of the liver; mobilizes fat

- vitamin B complex (50 to 100 mg 3 times, with meals)—essential for normal liver function

- vitamin C with bioflavonoids (5000 to 10,000 mg)—improves hepatitis quickly with high doses

- vitamin E (start with 400 IU and increase to 1200 IU over the course of a month)—a powerful antioxidant

Also Recommended

- calcium (1500 mg)—essential for blood clotting

- magnesium (1000 mg)

- essential fatty acids (as directed on label)—fights inflammation of the liver

- raw pancreas glandular (as directed on label)—aids in digestion and function of the pancreas

(Consult your healthcare provider regarding the duration of treatment.)

Ayurvedic Medicine

 Several Ayurvedic herbal preparations may have the power to cleanse and heal the digestive system, including the liver. An Ayurvedic practitioner may advise taking *shatavari* or *Chyavan prash* or an herbal mixture of *kutki*, *guduchi*, and *shanka pushpi*. Other remedies include yogurt with a pinch of baking soda, and basmati rice with spices, such as coriander and turmeric, which are said to clean the liver.

Remember to consult your doctor before embarking on any new regimen; hepatitis can do serious and permanent damage to your liver if not treated properly.

Traditional Chinese Medicine

 Acupuncture An acupuncturist tries to improve the individual's overall immunity while fortifying the liver and improving the flow of *chi* along the liver meridian. Points usually targeted include Bladder 18 and 19, Stomach 36, and Kidney 3.

If there is muscle pain, Gallbladder 40 may be added to the regimen. Jaundice requires the inclusion of Gallbladder 34. Additional points may be added as warranted by symptoms.

Chinese Herbal Therapy There are many Chinese herbal formulas to cleanse and build the liver; consult a professional. Astragalus may be given to combat the symptoms of jaundice and boost immunity. Licorice is a time-honored Chinese remedy for liver toxicity. Capillaris, mishmi bitter, dandelion, prunella, and gentian can be used to treat hepatitis-related jaundice.

HERNIA, GENERAL

Signs and Symptoms

- Tender lump or swelling in the groin area, especially after heavy lifting or straining
- In men, pain in area of scrotum

Description

A hernia occurs when internal tissue bulges out through a weakened area of the abdominal muscles. Although there are many types of hernias, most people associate the term with an inguinal hernia. This type of hernia generally affects men and is located where the spermatic cord that suspends the testis passes out of the abdomen and into the scrotum. It occurs when the inguinal ring—the ring of muscular tissue surrounding this opening—becomes weakened, allowing part of the intestine to push through. This portion of intestine often produces a noticeable bulge.

There are other types of hernias. An umbilical hernia occurs when a portion of the small intestine pushes through the abdominal wall near the navel. This type of hernia is most common among pregnant and obese women. Another type of hernia, known as an incisional hernia, is caused when intestines pass through the site of a previous surgery.

Conventional Medical Treatment

If you suspect that you have a hernia, see your physician, who can usually diagnose the condition by physically examining and pressing on the tender area. While some mild hernias heal on their own, others can result in the intestinal tissue becoming tightly pinched by the abdominal muscle. This can cause the affected portion of intestine to die, which results in a life-threatening situation. For this reason, your physician may suggest surgery to repair the hernia.

Health Notes

➤ *It is important to maintain a healthy body weight. Overweight people have an increased risk of developing hernias.*

➤ *If you have a chronic cough, consider being examined for a hernia. An ongoing cough can weaken groin muscles and contribute to a hernia.*

➤ *Improper lifting of heavy objects is a primary cause of hernias. Always use a proper lifting technique when lifting heavy objects: stand close to the object, bend at the knee, and use your legs to help you lift.*

Surgery for hernias usually entails physically pushing the intestine back into the abdomen (while the patient is anaesthetized) and sewing together any weakened muscles. Recovery after surgery usually takes six to eight weeks, during which time you must abstain from strenuous physical activity.

Complementary and Alternative Treatments

Bodywork and Somatic Practices

 Some initial therapy could include Oriental bodywork, reflexology, Cranio-Sacral Therapy, Trager, Aston-Patterning, or Therapeutic Touch.

Traditional Chinese Medicine

 Acupuncture Acupuncture may be used to strengthen the spleen.

HERNIA, HIATAL

Signs and Symptoms

In many cases, hiatal hernias produce no symptoms. If symptoms are present, they usually include:

- Heartburn
- Pain in the upper abdomen that may radiate into the neck; especially after large meals or when lying down

Description

In between the mouth and the stomach, the esophagus passes through an opening in the diaphragm called the hiatus. If the tissue around the hiatus weakens, part of the stomach or esophagus may push through the opening into the chest cavity—a condition known as a hiatal hernia.

While many people with hiatal hernias do not even know that they have the condition, it can be problematic if left untreated. Because the valve that separates the esophagus and stomach is weakened, stomach acid can move backward into the esophagus and cause pain and inflammation. This is known as *reflux esophogitis*, and is the cause of most symptoms related to hiatal hernia.

The cause of this weakening of the hiatus is unknown. Researchers believe that increased pressure in the abdomen—caused by obesity or other factors—stresses the tissue, causing it to weaken or tear.

Conventional Medical Treatment

Because the majority of hiatal hernias are asymptomatic, a great number go undetected. Fortunately, a small hiatal hernia is unlikely to cause any health problems and is not considered dangerous. If you are experiencing discomfort that may be associated with a hiatal hernia, see your physician, who can take a barium X-ray of the area to locate the hernia. A physician may first recommend sleeping with your head propped up to keep food down in the stomach, eating smaller meals late in the evening, and avoiding snacking—all of which can worsen irritation of the esophagus and stomach.

A number of medications can improve symptoms. These include antacids, H_2 receptor blockers (Zantac®, Pepcid®, Tagamet®), omeprazole (Prilosec®) and asapride (Propulsid®). Surgery is required to repair the condition only in situations where the pain is very severe and all other conservative methods have failed.

For More Information
National Institute of Diabetes and
Digestive and Kidney Diseases
2 Information Way
Bethesda, MD 20892-3570
301-654-3810
www.niddk.nih.gov

Health Notes

➤ *The abdominal burning that often accompanies a hiatal hernia can usually be avoided by eating smaller meals. Try to break up eating into four or five smaller meals over the course of the day.*

➤ *To keep from aggravating the symptoms of a hiatal hernia, avoid reclining after eating.*

Complementary and Alternative Treatments

Nutrition and Supplementation

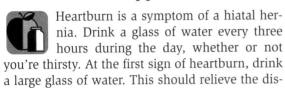 Heartburn is a symptom of a hiatal hernia. Drink a glass of water every three hours during the day, whether or not you're thirsty. At the first sign of heartburn, drink a large glass of water. This should relieve the discomfort.

Rather than eating three large meals, eat smaller meals throughout the day. Avoid spicy, fatty, and fried foods, and stay away from coffee, alcohol, tea, and cola. A high-fiber diet prevents constipation and the resulting straining. Nutritionists recommend the following daily supplements:

- proteolytic enzymes plus pancreatin (as directed on label)—improves digestion (*Do not* give to children.)

- papaya enzyme (2 tablets 3 or more times daily)—aids digestion and healing; use chewable tablet form

- zinc (50 mg, not to exceed a total of 100 mg from all supplements)—repairs tissue; use lozenge form

- vitamin A (50,000 IU for 1 month, then 30,000 IU for 2 weeks, then reduce to 20,000 IU; do not exceed 8000 IU daily if you are pregnant)—combats excess acid; use emulsion form

- vitamin B complex (100 mg twice daily, with meals)—aids in proper absorption of nutrients

- vitamin C (up to 1500 mg)—builds immunity and heals tissues

(Consult your healthcare provider regarding the duration of treatment.)

Traditional Chinese Medicine

 Acupuncture Acupuncture may be used to strengthen the spleen to aid digestion.

Hiccups

Hiccups are a harmless condition that affects almost everyone at some point in their life. Hiccups occur when an irritation in the chest or abdomen prompts a series of contractions in the diaphragm. During these contractions, the glottis (the part of the larynx that contains the vocal cords) claps shut, cutting off the intake of air. The strange noise that accompanies a hiccup is the result of air rushing past the closed vocal cords into the lungs.

The cause of hiccups varies from person to person. People can get them from eating spicy foods, drinking carbonated beverages, or accidentally swallowing air. In many cases, there is no explainable reason why someone starts hiccuping.

While everyone can (and generally does) get hiccups, there are people who are prone to frequent bouts. People with brain stem lesions, chronic renal failure, gastritis, pancreatitis, and lung conditions are all at increased risk.

Common home remedies for hiccups include holding one's breath, breathing into a paper bag, and drinking water quickly. The theory behind these methods is that raising CO_2 levels in the blood will stop hiccups. Usually hiccups go away without treatment, but if they don't, see your doctor, who may recommend medications such as sedatives or muscle relaxants.

For a complementary treatment, try one of these modalities. Ayurvedic practitioners believe hiccups are caused by a low blood supply to the diaphragm. To alleviate the spasms, practitioners may suggest taking a blend of honey and castor oil. They also may suggest alternate nostril breathing. Simply inhale deeply through one nostril (start with the right) while holding the other one shut. Hold your breath. Exhale through the left. Repeat, but reverse the nostrils. Continue alternate breathing until the hiccups have stopped.

(h)

HIGH BLOOD PRESSURE (HYPERTENSION)

Signs and Symptoms

In most cases, high blood pressure does not produce any symptoms. When symptoms do occur, they typically include:

- Headaches
- Dizziness
- Nosebleeds
- Ringing in the ears
- Tingling sensation in the hands and feet
- Blurred vision
- Heart palpitations
- Depression

Description

High blood pressure, also known as hypertension, is a condition wherein the blood is pumped through the body under abnormally high pressure—a pressure that is dangerous to your health. A normal blood pressure reading is 120/80. This means that the heart is exerting a maximum pressure that measures 120 during its pumping phase and 80 when the heart is at rest. Blood pressure is generally considered to be high when it measures 140/90 or higher.

High blood pressure is thought to affect between 50 and 60 million Americans, or roughly 20 percent of the U.S. population. Yet, only half of those affected are aware they have the condition. In fact, hypertension is frequently called "the silent killer" because it is often asymptomatic—a large percentage of people who suffer from it have no symptoms at all. However, hypertension is very dangerous. It overworks your cardiovascular system, causing damage to your heart, blood vessels, and kidneys—all of which can lead to a premature death. It also puts you at increased risk for stroke.

Fewer than 1 in 10 cases of hypertension can be pinpointed to a specific cause. In other words, more than 90 percent of all cases have no identified cause. When a cause cannot be determined, high blood pressure is known as essential hypertension.

When a cause can be identified, high blood pressure is called secondary hypertension, because the increased pressure is the result of some other ailment. Conditions that can result in hypertension include: endocrine disorders (such as Cushing's syndrome), tumors of the adrenal gland, kidney disease (such as pyelonephritis), and vascular disorders (such as coarctation). Sometimes a medication—such as oral contraceptives, antidepressants, corticosteroids, lithium, and decongestants—can cause high blood pressure.

Other risk factors for hypertension include a family history of the condition, pregnancy, high

Temporary Hypertension?

Millions of Americans are diagnosed as having hypertension, but in some of these people, their blood pressure returns to normal once they leave the doctor's office. For some people with normal blood pressure, even the most simple medical examination puts them under enough stress to temporarily raise their blood pressure to high levels. Called "white coat hypertension," the condition was discovered more than 250 years ago when a German physician noticed changes in a patient's pulse "on the appearance of the doctor." Unfortunately, it is difficult for a physician to distinguish true hypertension from white coat hypertension. To get an accurate blood pressure reading, some physicians ask their patients to take their blood pressure at home several times and record the results to share with the doctor.

alcohol intake, high dietary sodium intake, stress, obesity, and physical inactivity.

Conventional Medical Treatment

The most effective and easiest way to diagnose hypertension is with a blood pressure reading. If you are diagnosed with essential hypertension, your doctor may recommend a low-fat/low-sodium diet, moderate exercise, stress reduction, smoking cessation, and reduction of alcohol consumption. For some people, these lifestyle changes are enough to lower blood pressure.

Other people, however, require medication to reduce blood pressure. Among the most commonly prescribed medications are: diuretics (to decrease the amount of fluid in the blood vessel walls which, in turn, decreases the resistance to blood flow), beta-adrenergic blockers (to block the heart stimulating effects of adrenaline in your body), calcium channel blockers (to block the entry of calcium into the cells, thus decreasing the tendency of the small arteries to become narrow), and angiotensin-convert enzyme inhibitors (to keep arteries dilated).

If you are diagnosed with secondary hypertension, your doctor will conduct the tests and recommend treatment for the underlying condition.

For More Information
American Heart Association
7272 Greenville Avenue
Dallas, TX 75231
800-AHA-USA1
Women's Health Line: 888-MY-HEART
www.americanheart.org

National Heart, Lung, and Blood Institute
P.O. Box 30105
Bethesda, MD 20824-0105
301-592-8573
www.nhlbi.nih.gov

Health Notes

➤ *Increase your calcium intake to three or four servings per day. According to a recent study, individuals with high calcium levels have lower incidences of hypertension. Some studies also have shown that magnesium and potassium can play an important role in controlling high blood pressure.*

➤ *If you suffer from a mood disorder, seek counseling. A recent study found that patients with symptoms of anxiety or depression were more likely to develop hypertension.*

➤ *Exercise to prevent or lessen the effects of hypertension. A recent study showed that regular aerobic exercise (three to five times per week) reduced the amount of medication required to treat severe hypertension and improved heart strength.*

➤ *According to one study, a low-fat diet rich in fruits and vegetables (8 to 10 servings per day) significantly lowered blood pressure within two weeks.*

➤ *Lose weight. Every 10 pounds you drop may reduce your blood pressure as much as 2 to 3 points.*

Complementary and Alternative Treatments

Nutrition and Supplementation

 Formerly, if you suffered from high blood pressure, you were told to eliminate salt from your diet. This meant no foods with ingredients that include "salt," "soda," "sodium," or the symbol "Na." You were told to avoid the additive monosodium glutamate (MSG), baking soda, commercially prepared foods, canned vegetables, toothpastes that contain saccharin or baking soda, ibuprofen, diet soda, preservatives, sugar substitutes, meat tenderizers, and soy sauce.

These days we know that not everyone is so sensitive to salt, and it may be enough to simply stay away from all processed foods, as they tend to be heavy in salt.

Eat lots of fruits and vegetables and get plenty of fiber from whole grains. Drink nutrient-rich fresh juices, such as carrot, watermelon, cranberry, citrus fruit, and celery. Shiitake mushrooms can help reduce high blood pressure. Drink plenty of water as well.

Avoid all animal fats. Skinless turkey and chicken are acceptable, but only in moderation. Get your protein from vegetables sources and grains and legumes. Stay away from aged cheese, meats, chocolate, sour cream, alcohol, caffeine, and tobacco.

Nutritionists recommend the following daily supplements:

Most Important

- calcium (1500 to 3000 mg)—deficiencies have been linked to high blood pressure

- magnesium (750 to 1000 mg)

- L-carnitine (500 mg twice daily)—transports fatty acid chains

- L-glutamine (500 mg, on empty stomach)—detoxifies ammonia

- selenium (200 mcg)—deficiencies have been linked to heart disease

Also Recommended

- coenzyme Q10 (100 mg)—lowers blood pressure and improves heart function

- vitamin C (3000 to 6000 mg in divided doses)—reduces blood-clotting tendencies

- lecithin (1 tblsp 3 times daily)—emulsifies fat

- vitamin E (400 IU)—improves heart function; use emulsion form

- bromelain (as directed on label)—aids in the digestion of fat

- kelp (1000 to 1500 mg)—provides minerals and iodine

- shiitake (as directed on label)—reduces high blood pressure

- proteolytic enzymes (as directed on label)—completes protein digestion

- raw heart glandular (as directed on label)—strengthens the heart

- vitamin B_6 (50 mg 3 times daily)—reduces water content in tissues, thereby relieving pressure on the cardiovascular system; keeps homocysteine at bay

- potassium (99 mg)

(Consult your healthcare provider regarding the duration of treatment.)

Ayurvedic Medicine

Any of the doshas—vata, pitta, and kapha—are subject to high blood pressure, but the condition is most often seen in pitta and kapha types. To help control hypertension, Ayurvedic practitioners encourage a low-salt, low-cholesterol diet. They also suggest alternate-nostril breathing to help relax the body and invigorate the cardiovascular system. Simply inhale deeply through one nostril (start with the right) while holding the other one shut. Hold your breath. Exhale through the left. Repeat, but reverse the nostrils. Do this exercise several times daily.

In addition, the following Ayurvedic-approved herbs may be beneficial: *convolvulus pluricaulis, ashwaganda,* and *musta.* All have a calming effect. Ayurvedic products are available at many health food stores and Indian pharmacies.

Remember to consult your doctor before embarking on any new regimen; maintaining normal blood pressure is critical to good health.

Bodywork and Somatic Practices

Persons with high blood pressure should exercise caution when it comes to massage, so check with your healthcare provider. Some gentle therapies would include reflexology, polarity therapy, Reiki, Therapeutic Touch, and CranioSacral Therapy.

Herbal Therapy

 Many herbalists recommend taking garlic capsules daily to help lower blood pressure. Look for the capsules in health food stores and follow package directions. Consult your healthcare provider before using this herbal regimen as a complementary treatment.

Flaxseed oil is also recommended to improve circulation and lower blood pressure. Try taking 1 tablespoon daily.

Other herbs that may be helpful in controlling high blood pressure are mistletoe, American snakeroot, prickly ash bark, valerian, dandelion leaf, motherwort, yarrow, and *coleus forskohlii*. Consult your doctor before using these herbs as complementary treatments.

Traditional Chinese Medicine

 Acupuncture Chinese medicine believes that deficient flow of energy or *chi*—brought on by anything from stress to depression to anger—is responsible for high blood pressure. Consequently, acupuncture is used to help improve the flow of *chi* throughout the body. Points that may be focused on are Liver 3, Stomach 9 and 36, Large Intestine 11, and Gallbladder 20.

This modality may also help improve general immunity and fortify kidney yin, believed to be a contributing factor in hypertension.

Acupressure Acupoints usually targeted in the treatment of hypertension include Stomach 9 (on the throat), Pericardium 6 (above the wrist), Stomach 36 (below the kneecap), Kidney 3 (behind the ankle bone), and related auricular points.

Chinese Herbal Therapy Patent medicines that may be used to treat hypertension include Compound Cortex Eucommia Tablets, Hypertension Repressing Tablets, Gentiana, Rehmannia Six, Ginseng and Longan, and Eight Immortal Long Life Pills.

Yoga and Meditation

 If you're bothered by stress, yoga can ease body tension, improve circulation, and help lower blood pressure. Try the following poses every day: Mudra, Moon Salutation, Knee Squeeze, and Corpse. Avoid the Shoulder Stand.

Yoga practitioners also recommend 10 to 20 minutes of meditation twice daily for relaxing.

HIVES

Signs and Symptoms

- A batch of raised, red or white bumps on a localized area of skin

- Bumps may appear and disappear suddenly

- The affected area may be mildly or severely itchy

Description

Hives are a sudden eruption of red and white bumps on the skin. While hives are usually itchy, and therefore bothersome, they are generally not dangerous—except in cases of bee or insect stings, when hives indicate a true medical emergency. A case of hives may last for less than 30 minutes or as long as a week.

Hives

When the body comes into contact with a substance it considers dangerous, it floods the skin with histamine to combat the problematic substance. Hives result when there is excess buildup of histamine on a particular area of skin. Substances that cause this histamine release differ from person to person, though common irritants include animal dander, pollen, aspirin, penicillin, insect bites, and foods to which the person is allergic.

Conventional Medical Treatment

Hives often do not usually require medical treatment, but if the hives remain for an extended period of time, see your doctor. After taking your medical history, your physician may ask about your exposure within the last two weeks to any possible irritants. Unfortunately, hives can be caused by such a wide range of irritants that your physician may not be able to identify the exact cause. If the cause is identified, you will be urged to avoid the substance that caused the outbreak. In severe cases, your doctor may prescribe a medication, usually an antihistamine, to treat the condition.

If the hives are accompanied by shortness of breath, fever, nausea, or abdominal cramps, immediately seek medical help. You could be suffering from anaphylactic shock.

For More Information
American Academy of Allergy, Asthma, and Immunology
611 Wells Street
Milwaukee, WI 53202
800-822-2762
www.aaaai.org

American Academy of Dermatology
930 North Meacham Road
Schaumburg, IL 60173
888-462-DERM
www.aad.org

Complementary and Alternative Treatments

Nutrition and Supplementation

 Your hives may be caused by any number of things, including food additives and preservatives. Try to pinpoint what causes your outbreak and avoid that substance.

Alcohol and processed foods deplete nutrients, so avoid them when possible. Also stay away from foods high in saturated fat, cholesterol, and sugar, and from dairy products, eggs, chicken, and nuts.

The following daily supplements should help your hives:

Most Important

- a prodophilus formula (as directed on label)—reduces allergic reactions and replaces friendly bacteria

- garlic (10 drops in water 3 times daily)—destroys bacteria

- quercetin (as directed on label)—reduces inflammation and reactions

- vitamin C (1000 mg 3 times)—acts as an anti-inflammatory

- vitamin D (400 IU)—reduces outbreaks

- vitamin E (600 IU)—improves circulation to the skin tissues

- zinc (50 mg, not to exceed a total of 100 mg from all supplements)—heals skin tissue

Also Recommended

- calcium lactate (1000 mg)
- pantothenic acid (500 mg)
- vitamin B complex (50 mg)—maintains healthy skin, supplemented with vitamin B_{12} (2000 mcg)—prevents nerve damage, and B_6 (100 mg)

(For an *acute* condition, take supplements until your symptoms subside. If symptoms persist, seek the advice of your healthcare provider. For a *chronic* condition, consult your healthcare provider regarding the duration of treatment.)

Aromatherapy

 German chamomile oil can help bring relief from itching. Simply place a drop directly on the itchy skin and massage in.

Ayurvedic Medicine

 Hives come from excessive heat in the body, say Ayurvedic practitioners. To cool the heat and soothe the maddening itch, they favor eating watermelon as well as drinking coriander milk or cilantro.

Herbal Therapy

 Parsley and amaranth have antihistamine compounds that can control itching. To benefit from parsley's anti-itch properties, steep 1 teaspoon dried parsley (or 3 teaspoons fresh) in 1 cup boiling water for 5 to 10 minutes; strain. Drink up to 3 cups a day. Or brew 2 teaspoons crushed amaranth seeds in 3 cups of boiling water for 15 minutes; strain. Dab over the itchy area with a cotton cloth.

You also can calm intense itching by applying aloe vera gel to the affected area. Look for a commercial product in health food stores or in drug stores, and follow the directions on the label.

Homeopathy

 A homeopathic practitioner may suggest one of the following treatments for hives, depending on your symptoms: *Apis* if the hives are red, produce a burning sensation, and improve after a cold compress has been applied; *Urtica urens* if the hives are caused by an allergic reaction—especially from eating shellfish.

Note: if the allergic reaction is severe, and you experience swelling and difficulty breathing, immediately seek medical help.

Hydrotherapy

 Soothe the itch of hives with a relaxing 20- to 30-minute bath. Experiment to see which of the following soaks works best for you:

- Add 5 tablespoons of oatmeal to warm bath water; swish to distribute well. (Use regular or quick oats, or grind regular oats in a food processor until powdered. You also can purchase a powdered oat solution in almost any drugstore.) When done bathing, gently pat yourself dry; do not rub.

- Add 3 to 8 tablespoons of baking soda (sodium bicarbonate) to a tepid bath; stir to distribute. When done bathing, gently pat yourself dry; do not rub.

- Stir 1 cup of cider vinegar into warm bath water; mix well. When done bathing, gently pat yourself dry; do not rub.

To restore the skin's natural pH balance and blunt the itching, apply cool, diluted vinegar compresses to irritated skin. Use cider vinegar or white distilled vinegar. Flush toxins from the system by drinking large amounts of water.

Hypoglycemia

Signs and Symptoms

- Headaches
- Nervousness
- Weakness
- Sweating
- Dizziness
- Blurred vision
- Tingling sensation in hands and feet
- Heart palpitations
- Severe hunger
- Nausea
- Pale skin
- Trembling

Description

Hypoglycemia is condition that results when blood sugar levels are low. The body's cells, especially those in the brain, must receive a steady, consistent supply of sugar from the blood in order to function correctly. After eating, blood sugar levels normally rise as food is digested. The pancreas releases insulin, which transports the sugar from the bloodstream to the body's cells. As blood sugar levels drop, insulin levels subside, and stored sugar is released from the liver into the bloodstream.

Even when they do not eat, most people maintain a relatively constant blood sugar level, somewhere between 60 to 100 milligrams per deciliter of blood. In a small number of people, however, this mechanism of transporting blood sugar does not work properly and blood sugar levels fall too low. To compensate, the body releases adrenaline, which in turn releases sugar from the liver, but also causes rapid heartbeat, sweating, trembling and other symptoms.

Hypoglycemia is a very rare condition—less than 1 percent of the general population experiences it. While hypoglycemia sometimes occurs in pregnant women who skip a meal, it is most common among people with diabetes. In people with diabetes, hypoglycemia often occurs if they take a large dose of insulin, miss a meal, or engage in vigorous physical activity. In people without diabetes, hypoglycemia can occur when a large amount of alcohol is consumed on an empty stomach or after eating a meal full of carbohydrates.

Conventional Medical Treatment

If you suspect you have hypoglycemia, visit your physician. To diagnose hypoglycemia, your doctor needs to test your blood sugar levels.

Treatment for hypoglycemia is simple: for people with and without diabetes, eating a simple carbohydrate—such as a glass of fruit juice, or a piece of candy will correct the situation within 10 to 15 minutes. You may need to consume more carbohydrates if you see little or no improvement after 15 minutes. After the symptoms have resided, you may want to consume a bit more of the carbohydrate to prevent recurrence. Immediate treatment for a bout of hypoglycemia is essential for anyone with diabetes, who can slip into unconsciousness or experience convulsions, and require emergency medical assistance.

For More Information
American Diabetes Association
1660 Duke Street
Alexandria, VA 22314
800-DIABETES
www.diabetes.org

Health Notes

➤ *If you suffer from hypoglycemia, carry a concentrated simple carbohydrate—such as a candy bar or a sugar packet—in case of emergency.*

➤ *Maintain even blood sugar by eating five to six small meals a day rather than three large ones.*

➤ *Avoid simple carbohydrates found in foods such as cookies and candies. Simple carbohydrates cause a faster drop in blood sugar than complex carbohydrates, found in fruits, vegetables, bread, pasta, and cereals.*

➤ *Restrict or eliminate intake of caffeinated and alcoholic beverages. Both can cause a rapid drop in blood sugar one to three hours after consumption.*

National Institute of Diabetes and
Digestive and Kidney Diseases
1 Information Way
Bethesda, MD 20892-3560
301-654-3810
www.niddk.nih.gov

Complementary and Alternative Treatments

Nutrition and Supplementation

Naturopaths target diet and supplements to treat hypoglycemia. Although each patient needs an individualized treatment plan, there are some basic "dos and don'ts" that pertain to all hypoglycemics.

Eat adequate amounts of protein, either from animal sources such as fish, eggs, lean meats or vegetable sources, such as nuts, seeds, legumes, and soy products. Avoid all refined grains, choosing only complex carbohydrates. Fiber slows down the absorption of glucose, which allows for a more gradual release of insulin; eat fiber-rich plant foods. Carry plain raw almonds with you in case your blood sugar drops.

Avoid caffeine, nicotine, or alcohol; these rob your body of essential nutrients. Simple sugars are another no-no. They cause your pancreas to overproduce insulin. Simple sugars are found in sugar, fructose, glucose, corn sweeteners, corn syrup, table sugar, and brown sugar. Check food labels; avoid anything ending in -ose (sucrose, maltose, dextrose, etc.).

Never skip meals; eat frequent small meals throughout the day. Some people find that a snack before bedtime helps. The following daily supplements are useful.

Most Important

- brewer's yeast (as directed on label)—stabilizes blood sugar levels

- chromium picolinate (300 to 600 mcg)—is essential for optimal insulin activity

- pancreatin (as directed on label)—aids in protein digestion

- proteolytic enzymes (as directed on label)—aids in protein digestion (Do not give to children.)

- vitamin B complex (50 to 150 mg in divided doses)—counteracts the effects of malabsorption disorders; aids in carbohydrate and protein metabolism

- zinc (50 mg, not to exceed 100 mg total from all supplements)—essential for proper release of insulin

Also Recommended

- manganese (as directed on label)—maintains blood glucose levels; deficient in most people with hypoglycemia

- vitamin C with bioflavonoids (3000 to 8000 mg in divided doses)—for adrenal insufficiency, common in this disorder

- L-glutamine (1000 mg on an empty stomach)—reduces craving for sugar

- N-acetyl cysteine (600 mg)
- L-carnitine (as directed on label)—converts body fat into energy
- liver and adrenal extracts (as directed on label)
- phosphatidyl serine (500 mg 3 times daily, with food)—stabilizes glandular function

(Consult your healthcare provider regarding the duration of treatment.)

Ayurvedic Medicine

Hypoglycemia, or low blood sugar, is common in people with a pitta imbalance, according to Ayurveda. To stabilize blood sugar levels, Ayurvedic practitioners may advise drinking *brahmi*-licorice tea or taking a combination remedy containing *guduchi* and other Indian herbs.

Bodywork and Somatic Practices

Practitioners of reflexology, Oriental bodywork, massage, and CranioSacral Therapy can help regulate the relevant body systems.

Herbal Therapy

When combined with small, light snacks several times a day, herbal teas made from burdock, dandelion, or licorice can help stabilize blood sugar levels.

Herbal products are available in health food stores and in some pharmacies and supermarkets. Follow package for specific directions.

Traditional Chinese Medicine

Acupuncture Hypoglycemia is a very complicated condition with many contributing factors. Acupuncture can help alleviate certain symptoms of hypoglycemia by reducing stress and regulating digestion, which may improve the body's ability to absorb essential nutrients.

Chinese Herbal Therapy Ophiopogon can be used as a tonic to strengthen the lungs and heart, believed by Chinese herbalists to be associated with low blood sugar. Take a 3- to 6-gram decoction twice a day. Codonopsis fortifies the blood; take in a 5- to 7-gram decoction twice a day.

Ginseng is a famous blood sugar regulator; daily dosages vary from 6 grams of the powdered herb to 10 grams if taken in decoction form.

Yoga and Meditation

At least four yoga positions help strengthen the pancreas and maintain even blood sugar levels: the Peacock, Camel, Locust, and Elevated Lotus.

HYPOTHERMIA

Signs and Symptoms

- Body temperature below 94°F
- Pale skin that is cold to the touch
- Lethargy
- Muscle stiffness
- Loss of motor coordination
- Confusion or delirium

- Shivering
- Body swelling
- Unconsciousness or coma (in severe cases)
- Fixed pupils (in severe cases)
- Very slow pulse (in severe cases)

Description

Prolonged exposure to cold temperatures causes your body to lose more heat than it can generate, resulting in a condition called hypothermia. Symptoms of the condition do not usually appear immediately; often signs of hypothermia come on so gradually that the person suffering from it has no idea anything is wrong. Hypothermia may occur in any number of cold environmental situations, including being underdressed in the middle of winter, falling into cold water, and wearing damp clothing in a cool environment.

Hypothermia can strike anyone who is exposed to extremely cold temperatures over a prolonged period of time. People who are at increased risk include very thin people (who have little natural fat insulation), elderly people, and infants. Alcoholics and people with hypothyroidism, diabetes, malnutrition, or heart disease also stand a greater chance of developing hypothermia.

Conventional Medical Treatment

Hypothermia is an emergency situation. If someone you know has the condition, get the person out of the cold environment and remove any damp clothing. If you are unable to get the victim indoors, move him or her to an area that is sheltered from the wind, remove all damp clothing, and layer blankets, jackets, and any other dry clothing over the victim to create insulation.

Next, call an ambulance. While waiting for the medical assistance to arrive, check the victim's pulse and breathing. Once at the hospital, the victim's body temperature will be gradually increased with a combination of intravenous fluid and lukewarm water therapy.

Complementary and Alternative Treatments

Nutrition and Supplementation

Drink plenty of warm, quality beverages and take a supplement with vitamin B complex (50 mg 3 times daily).

Traditional Chinese Medicine

Acupuncture Acupuncture can be used to improve circulation, which may help prevent permanent nerve damage in the affected area.

Hypothermia

Acupressure Acupressure can help increase the flow of blood to the affected area, which hastens healing. The specific acupressure points vary, depending on the location of the hypothermia.

Chinese Herbal Therapy Peony and *Dong Quai* formulas may be helpful in improving circulation, which can prevent permanent nerve damage.

IMPETIGO

Signs and Symptoms

- Patch of itchy, red blisters on the face, arms, or legs
- When blisters break they become oozing sores that eventually scab

Description

Impetigo is a skin infection caused by either the stapphococci or streptococci bacterium. The condition occurs when bacteria enter a wound—such as a scratch, cut, abrasion, or insect bite—and cause a rash of red blisters that ooze a highly contagious fluid. Any physical contact with this fluid, including scratching or even touching, can spread blisters to other parts of the body or transmit the infection to other people. Two or three days after developing, the blisters scab, developing yellow or brown crusts. These sores heal slowly—taking up to five weeks to fully heal.

While impetigo can strike anyone, it is most prevalent among children. It is also common among people who have poor hygiene, are malnourished, or live in unhygienic conditions.

Conventional Medical Treatment

Most cases of impetigo do not require a visit to the doctor and clear up within a few days. To prevent the condition from spreading, everyone in the household, including the infected person, should practice good hygiene, including frequent hand washings.

If the infection lasts for more than a few days or infects a very young child, visit a physician or dermatologist, who can diagnose impetigo with a tissue sample biopsy. Conventional treatment includes topical antibiotic creams or oral antibiotic therapy.

Animal Kingdom Antibiotics

Some frogs secrete a class of antibiotics called *magainins* (Hebrew for "shield"). Most conventional antibiotics act by destroying an enzyme within a bacterium; once the organism learns to alter that enzyme, the antibiotics are no longer effective. However, magainins attack the bacterium's cell membrane, causing a fatal wound. Researchers believe this different mechanism prevents bacteria from developing resistance to magainins. Magainin has not yet been approved for use on humans, although a magainin-based treatment for impetigo and diabetic foot ulcers has passed laboratory tests and is currently being tested in clinical trials on humans.

Health Notes

➤ *Think twice before asking your doctor for oral antibiotics. A bacterial skin infection, such as impetigo, does not always warrant systemic antibiotic therapy and usually can be treated with topical antibiotic preparations.*

➤ *Washing the infected area of skin with an antibacterial cleanser three times a day can soften the crusts of the sores, so they can be removed gently.*

➤ *To avoid spreading impetigo, do not share your clothing or razors, and avoid touching other people.*

Impetigo

For More Information
American Academy of Dermatology
930 North Meacham Road
Schaumburg, IL 60173
888-462-DERM
www.aad.org

Complementary and Alternative Treatments

Nutrition and Supplementation

Nutritionists recommend the following daily supplements:

- vitamin A (10,000 IU for 5 days, then stop for 2 days; do not exceed 8000 IU daily if you are pregnant)—adult dose; reduce for child

- vitamin D (400 IU)—for 5 days then stop for 2 days—adult dose; reduce for child

- vitamin E (100 to 400 IU)

- vitamin C (500 mg twice daily)

- zinc (30 mg)

- selenium (200 mcg)

Aromatherapy

For this infectious disease, apply a compress using 2 drops each of myrrh, German chamomile, and tea tree oil. Apply to the infected areas often.

Herbal Therapy

Marigold, with its antibacterial properties, can help fight infection and aid healing. Mix 5 drops marigold tincture in 1 cup cooled, boiled water and apply directly to the infected skin. Repeat several times a day, as long as necessary.

Herbal products are available in health food stores and in some pharmacies and supermarkets. Follow package for specific directions.

Homeopathy

Impetigo may respond to homeopathic treatment. However, the selection of a remedy—more than one is available—depends on *your* symptoms and the stage of the condition. Don't try treating this disorder yourself. See a homeopathic professional.

Hydrotherapy

Bathe red, blistered areas with a solution of *Hypericum* and *Calendua*. Add 5 drops of each tincture to 1 cup of cooled boiled water; use several times a day. These remedies can be purchased at health food stores.

Traditional Chinese Medicine

Acupuncture While acupuncture cannot cure impetigo, it can be used to help make the patient more comfortable by lessening the pain associated with impetigo blisters. Many times it can help correct an balance, especially when used in combination with diet modification and herbs.

Chinese Herbal Therapy Although antibiotics are almost always recommended in the treatment of a highly contagious bacterial infection, such as impetigo, herbs can be helpful in alleviating symptoms until the condition is cured.

The Chinese herbal formula known as *Lien Chiao Pai Tu Pien* may be used to help stave off secondary infections and heal skin ulcers.

IMPOTENCE (ERECTILE DYSFUNCTION)

Signs and Symptoms

- Inability in males to achieve or sustain an erection for sexual intercourse more than 25 percent of the time or a tendency to sustain only brief erections

Description

Impotence, also called erectile dysfunction, is estimated to affect between 10 and 30 million men in the United States. Previously thought to be mainly a psychological problem or caused by the aging process, physicians now believe that more than 80 percent of cases stem from physical causes, including disease, injury (especially spinal cord injury), substance abuse, or the side effects of prescription medications. And while incidence increases with aging, it is not an inevitable result. Because the term *impotence* has developed a negative connotation, it is now rarely used in technical literature.

Among the most common causes are diseases that affect blood flow, such as heart disease, arteriosclerosis, and high blood pressure. Other common causes are diabetes, kidney disease, chronic alcoholism, liver failure, elevated cholesterol level, hormonal abnormalities, and neurological disorders, such as multiple sclerosis or spinal cord damage. Smoking also restricts blood flow. Drugs, such as cocaine, marijuana, anti-depressants, narcotics, blood pressure medications, anti-fungals, and beta-blockers may also cause impotence.

Psychological factors—such as stress, anxiety, guilt, depression, or low self-esteem—are estimated to cause between 10 and 20 percent of cases.

Conventional Medical Treatment

Since achieving and sustaining an erection involves the man's mental state—as well as the nerves, muscles, and circulatory system—physicians often take a team approach to treatment. Your doctor generally begins by taking a medical and sexual history and giving you a complete physical examination. Typical tests ordered include a blood count, urinalysis, lipid profile, measurements of creatinine and liver enzymes, and a blood testosterone analysis. Since healthy men have involuntary erections during sleep, you may also be asked to monitor your erections during the night, to help evaluate the possibility of psychological problems.

Though today about 95 percent of cases of erectile dysfunction are treatable, only 5 to 10 percent of men seek treatment. Among the most successful and least invasive treatments is the prescription medicine sildenafil, sold as Viagra®, originally used to treat high blood pressure disorders. Viagra® works by inhibiting a particular enzyme in the body, therefore allowing blood to flow into the penis. It is not recommended for men with certain types of heart disease, but is effective for about 65 to 70 percent of men, including those with physical and psychological problems.

Before Viagra® became available, other medications recommended included testosterone and yohimbine hydrochloride, but both are controversial. Testosterone is effective in only a small percentage of men with hormonal imbalances. Yohimbine, which is derived from tree bark and has been used for centuries as an aphrodisiac, has not been proven effective in clinical trials.

Several mechanical devices also have been used with varying degrees of success. One of these, a vacuum constriction device, pulls blood into the penis by means of a vacuum created when the penis is inserted into a plastic tube and air is then pumped out of the tube. The result mimics an erection, which can be maintained for about a half an hour by placing an elastic band around the penis.

With penile injection therapy, medication is in-

Impotence (Erectile Dysfunction)

jected into the side of the penis to create an erection. The drawbacks, however, include the pain of the injection and the possibility of a prolonged erection of two hours or more. In the treatment known as *intra-urethral* therapy, a soft pellet of medication, about the size of a grain of rice, is inserted into the urethra with an applicator. The medication is absorbed directly into the erection chambers of the penis, resulting in an erection in between 30 to 80 percent of men that can last 30 minutes to an hour.

In some cases, especially in young men with vascular injuries, physicians may recommend surgery. Surgery may be used to implant a prosthesis to cause the penis to be erect, reconstruct arteries to increase blood flow to the penis, or repair veins that may allow a too-rapid exit of blood from the penis. Two types of implants are used: one consists of two semi-rigid but malleable rods; the other is an inflatable implant that can be expanded with a pressurized saline fluid. Men and their partners using prosthesis report a 93 percent satisfaction rate.

For More Information:
American Foundation for Urologic Diseases
1128 North Charles Street
Baltimore, MD 21201
410-468-1800
www.afud.org

National Institute of Diabetes and Digestive and Kidney Diseases
31 Center Drive, MSC 2560
Bethesda, MD 20892-2560
301-654-3810
http://www.niddk.nih.gov/health/urolog/pubs/impotnce/impotnce.htm

Complementary and Alternative Treatments

Nutrition and Supplementation

 The Association for Male Sexual Dysfunction recognizes over 200 drugs that may cause impotence, including alcohol, narcotics, nicotine, sedatives, and antihistamines. Avoid use of these drugs, and stay away from animal fats, sugar, and fried or junk foods. The same plaques that clog arteries leading to the heart also clog arteries leading to the genitals, contributing to dysfunction. Make sure the problem is not psychological or relational.

Eat a well-balanced diet that includes pumpkin seeds, which nourish the prostate gland. Follow the recommended daily supplement program outlined below:

- vitamin E (start with 200 IU and increase to 400 to 1000 IU)—increases circulation

- zinc (80 mg, not to be exceeded)—important in prostate gland function and reproductive organ growth

- dimethylglycine (as directed on label)—increases oxygen supply in the blood

- raw orchic glandular supplement (as directed on label)—promotes function of male reproductive organs

- L-arginine (500 mg 3 times daily)

- human growth hormone co-factors (as directed on label)

(Consult your healthcare provider regarding the duration of treatment.)

Aromatherapy

Use jasmine, an essential oil known for its aphrodisiac properties, in a candle diffuser. Inhale it from a handkerchief or tissue, or apply it to your body. Clary sage, sandalwood, and ylang-ylang essential oils also can aid romance; add these to a massage oil or to a warm bath.

Traditional Chinese Medicine

Acupuncture Acupuncture has proven quite successful in the treatment of impotence. Typically, the Conception Vessel meridian is utilized, along with various bladder and spleen points, to improve the flow of *chi* to sexual organs. Stomach 36, Bladder 23, and Triple Warmer 4 may also be included.

Acupressure Acupressure can help stimulate the sex drive and strengthen the kidneys which, in turn, may prevent impotence. Relevant acupoints include Conception Vessel 1, 2, 4 and 8; Governing Vessel 3 and 4, Spleen 6, Stomach 36, and Bladder 23.

Chinese Herbal Therapy Because impotence is viewed as being caused by a kidney deficiency, herbs may be prescribed to strengthen that organ and improve the flow of energy along the kidney meridian.

The aptly named herb horny goat weed has been shown in studies to increase semen secretion and stimulate the male sex drive; it is most potent if steeped in spirits for three months and then taken as a tonic liquor.

Lycium Combination and Golden Book Tea are commonly prescribed Chinese patent medicines that also claim to boost libido.

INCONTINENCE, URINARY

Signs and Symptoms

- Inability to control urination
- Urine leakage during physical activity, laughing, coughing, or sneezing

Description

Incontinence is the inability to fully control urination. For someone suffering from the condition, simple actions, such as sneezing, laughing, physical activity, and hugging, can cause urine leakage. In some cases, the sufferer may lose bladder control despite the lack of a definite physical cause. Women are twice as likely as men to be affected by urinary incontinence.

Elderly women are the segment of the population most commonly affected by the condition, because their urinary muscles and ligaments become less efficient with age. Declining estrogen levels after menopause also contribute to bladder control problems. While incontinence is a medical condition that usually develops late in life, it is also a symptom of several illnesses and physical conditions that can affect men and women of any age. The muscular and neural systems that control the retention and release of urine can be affected by medications, urinary tract infections, diabetes, prostate gland problems, weakened pelvic floor muscles, operations on the urinary tract, stroke, Alzheimer's disease, and even psychological factors, such as depression, anger, or confusion.

Middle-aged women who have given birth are at increased risk of developing incontinence because the muscles at the pelvic floor (which support the bladder and close off the top of the urethra) can become stretched during pregnancy. With any subsequent pregnancy, it becomes even more difficult for the pelvic muscles to resume their original tautness. Episiotomies and deliveries involving forceps may cause further damage. The pelvic floor can also deteriorate as a result of obesity and hysterectomies.

Men often experience incontinence as a symptom of a prostate condition, wherein an inflamed, enlarged prostate pushes against the bladder, interfering with its opening and closing mechanism. In children, incontinence most often takes the form of bed-wetting.

Conventional Medical Treatment

If you are suffering from incontinence, see your family doctor or primary care physician, who may refer you to a urologist or urogynecologist (a specialist who focuses on treating women's urological problems). The specialist takes a detailed medical history, including any medications, operations, or infections that you may have had. The doctor also may conduct a physical examination of your genitals, rectum, and abdominal area, and take a urine specimen for analysis. In some cases, an ultrasound, pelvic X-ray, or cystoscopy (a microscopic examination of cells) may be necessary to confirm diagnosis.

Treatment for incontinence depends on what is causing the condition. For example, if a prostate gland problem is the cause, treatment for that condition can cure incontinence. In severe cases, an artificial sphincter, which allows you to control its open and closed settings, can be surgically implanted. Collagen injection therapy—wherein collagen is injected into the external bladder to add bulk to the urethra—is effective in some cases for women with sphincter deficiency and for men who experience urinary stress incontinence after prostate surgery. Medication also may be prescribed to treat incontinence; commonly prescribed drugs are anticholinergic agents (Pro Banthene®), alpha-adrenergic agonist drugs, tri-

cyclic antidepressant drugs, and antispasmodics (Bentyl®, Ditropan®, and Urispas®). Postmeonpausal women with stress incontinence may benefit from estrogen either orally or by applying a cream to the vagina.

For More Information

National Association for Continence
P.O. Box 8310
Spartanburg, SC 29305-8310
800-BLADDER
www.nafc.org

Simon Foundation for Continence
Box 835-F
Wilmette, IL 60091
800-22-SIMON
www.simonfoundation.org

Exercises to Prevent and Treat Incontinence

Women can help reduce their chances of developing incontinence from pregnancy or aging by strengthening their pelvic floor with Kegel exercises, preformed daily. Kegel exercises strengthen the pubococcygeal muscles, which surround the anus and vagina and are responsible for controlling bladder function. To perform the exercise, begin by squeezing, or contracting, your vaginal muscles as you would to start or stop the flow of urine. (Do not contract your abdominal, thigh, or buttocks muscles.) Hold for a count of 10. Relax the muscle, then repeat the contraction 10 times. To produce benefits, the exercise must be repeated several times per day. To learn how to isolate the correct muscle, perform the exercise while urinating. Halt the flow of urine and hold for 10 seconds, then release. Repeat the exercise several times. If Kegel exercises do not work for you, talk to your physician about muscle training with weighted vaginal cones to increase the strength of the pelvic floor muscles.

Health Notes

➤ *Maintain a healthy weight. People who are overweight have a higher incidence of incontinence.*

➤ *If you smoke, quit. Smokers have higher rates of incontinence than non-smokers.*

➤ *If you are incontinent, avoid diuretic pills or diuretic substances, such as caffeine. Diuretics cause your body to produce an increased amount of urine in a short period of time—too much for an incontinent bladder to comfortably process.*

Complementary and Alternative Treatments

Ayurvedic Medicine

Ayurveda views incontinence as a vata disorder that's caused by a weak bladder sphincter. Your Ayurvedic practitioner may recommend taking an Indian herbal blend containing *ashwagandha* and also may suggest eliminating or reducing your intake of alcohol and coffee and other caffeine-containing foods, which intensify the urge to urinate as well.

If symptoms persist, see your doctor for evaluation and assistance.

Bodywork and Somatic Practices

Oriental bodywork, reflexology, massage, Therapeutic Touch, Reiki, polarity therapy, and CranioSacral Therapy are helpful first options.

Traditional Chinese Medicine

Acupuncture Chinese medical experts believe that incontinence is caused by a lack of energy in the kidney and spleen and their related meridians. To combat this imbalance, they work on the points that correspond to these areas and to the bladder.

Acupressure Points that may be focused on during an acupressure session to treat incontinence are Conception Vessel 2, Spleen 6, and related auricular points.

Chinese Herbal Therapy Herbs may be given to help tone the kidney and spleen and to strengthen bladder functions.

Yoga and Meditation

Exercise is always beneficial for strengthening muscles, including those of the bladder and surrounding areas. Try these easy yoga exercises several times daily to combat incontinence: Ashwini Mudra and Stomach Lock. Consult a trained practitioner for proper technique. Avoid these poses if you're pregnant.

INDIGESTION (DYSPEPSIA)

Signs and Symptoms

- Abdominal tenderness and distention
- Feeling of fullness and discomfort in the upper abdomen
- Burning sensation in the chest, often originating in the upper abdomen and radiating to the neck
- Regurgitation of bitter liquid into the throat or mouth, commonly when lying down
- Nausea and vomiting

Description

Indigestion is a symptom that is caused by a number of stomach conditions, including hiatal hernia, gastroesophageal reflux disease (GERD), *Helicobacter pylori*, heartburn, and dyspepsia. Because many of these conditions can pose serious health risks, it is important to visit your healthcare provider in order to properly diagnose the reason for your indigestion. The condition usually occurs after eating. People experience indigestion for a variety of reasons—after eating a specific food, after eating too much food, after drinking alcohol or carbonated beverages, or after smoking cigarettes. The frequency of occurrence also varies from person to person. Approximately one in ten adults experiences indigestion weekly, while approximately one in three experiences it monthly.

Heartburn, a problem affecting the esophagus, is perhaps the most common type of indigestion. Your esophagus is a 10-inch-long tube leading from the back of your mouth to your stomach. Food travels down the esophagus to the lower esophageal sphincter, a muscle that opens to allow food to pass into the stomach and closes to prevent food and acids from escaping from the stomach into the esophagus. Heartburn occurs when this lower esophageal sphincter is weak or dysfunctional, allowing stomach acid to escape.

People who are overweight are at increased risk for developing indigestion because excess weight can increase pressure on the abdomen which, in turn, can make it difficult for the lower esophageal sphincter to stay tightly shut. Pregnant women also experience a higher incidence of the condition because they, too, experience increased pressure on the abdomen. In addition, people who smoke are at increased risk because cigarettes relax the lower esophageal sphincter.

Heartburn or Heart Attack?

Prodromes is the term used for the subtle warning signs that sometimes occur several days or weeks before a heart attack. These may include:

- Aching, burning, or feeling of pressure in the chest and upper abdomen
- Nausea
- Discomfort or tingling in the left or right arm, the jaw, or the teeth
- Sweating
- Shortness of breath
- Dizziness

Unfortunately, these symptoms are easily mistaken for symptoms of heartburn; as a result, many people ignore them. One way to tell the difference between indigestion and prodromes is that prodromes usually follow a predictable pattern not related to eating—worsening with activity and dissipating with rest. If you have the slightest suspicion that your symptoms are indicative of a heart attack, immediately visit a hospital emergency room.

Health Notes

➤ *In some people, heartburn can be triggered by eating rich or spicy foods. To offset the acid produced by these foods, eat a small amount of bread, rice, or pasta, which neutralizes stomach acid.*

➤ *Chocolate, fatty foods, peppermint, alcohol, antihistamines, aspirin, ibuprofen, birth control pills, anti-spasmodic drugs, and asthma medications all relax the lower esophageal sphincter, increasing the risk of developing heartburn.*

➤ *Do not recline after eating. Lying down on a full stomach can cause gastric acid to leak into the esophagus, causing heartburn. Instead, try taking a walk after a heavy meal to stimulate digestion and move food into the intestines.*

➤ *Over-the-counter antacids that contain magnesium may be hazardous to elderly people. With age, the kidneys slowly lose their ability to eliminate magnesium, putting the elderly at risk for a condition called* hypermagnesemia, *an overabundance of magnesium that can lead to paralysis and death. If you are an elderly person seeking relief from indigestion, ask your doctor for alternate treatments.*

➤ *Avoid eating late at night.*

➤ *If you smoke, quit.*

Conventional Medical Treatment

If you suffer from indigestion only occasionally, you may experience relief by taking over-the-counter antacids, which neutralize gastric acids. You also can prevent future cases of indigestion by avoiding any food or drink that irritate your stomach.

If you experience indigestion frequently, see your doctor, who will try to determine when your indigestion occurs, what foods and drinks seem to trigger it, in what part of the abdomen the discomfort is strongest, and how long it typically last. Your physician also may want to run a series of tests to make sure that your indigestion is not being caused by a more serious condition, such as gastroesophageal reflux disease, colon cancer, stomach ulcer, gastritis, pancreatic disease, or irritable bowel syndrome. A barium X-ray, endoscopic examination of the digestive tract, or stool sample may be necessary. In order to rule out disorders of the pancreas, liver, or gallbladder, your doctor also may recommend an ultrasound examination of those organs.

If over-the-counter products do not offer relief, your physician may prescribe cimetidine (Tagamet®), ranitidine (Zantac®), famotidine (Pepcid®), or omeprazole (Prilosec®) to block acid production in the stomach. A medication that increases the strength of the lower esophageal sphincter, such as metocopramide or bethanechol, also may be prescribed.

Complementary and Alternative Treatments

Nutrition and Supplementation

 Adding papaya and fresh pineapple to your diet may help, as both contain enzymes beneficial to digestion. Limit your intake of lentils, peanuts, and soybeans; they contain an enzyme inhibitor. Check with a health practitioner to make sure you don't have food sensitivities or serious illnesses, such as gastroesophageal reflux disease. A well-balanced diet high in fiber (fresh fruits, vegetables, and whole grains) is ideal.

The following daily supplement program helps prevent and/or treat digestive disorders:

Most Important

• proteolytic enzymes (as directed on label)— break down protein for absorption

Indigestion (Dyspepsia)

- a prodophilus formula (as directed on label)—important for normal digestion; replaces friendly bacteria
- vitamin B complex (50 mg 3 times daily, with meals)—necessary for normal digestion

Also Recommended

- L-methionine (as directed on label)—detoxifies liver
- multi-enzyme complex (as directed on label)—improves digestion
- gamma orizanol (as directed on label)—protects and heals the stomach mucosa
- bovine colostrum (as directed on label)—heals damaged stomach tissue
- curcumin (as directed on label)—anti-inflammatory agent
- N-acetyl glucosamine (as directed on label)—heals the stomach wall

(For an *acute* condition, take supplements until your symptoms subside. If symptoms persist, seek the advice of your healthcare provider. For a *chronic* condition, consult your healthcare provider regarding the duration of treatment.)

Aromatherapy

 Prepare a comforting essential oil by combining 1 teaspoon canola or safflower oil and 4 drops of any of the following essential oils: ginger, Roman chamomile, coriander, fennel, lavender, peppermint, or rosemary. Lie down and massage this preparation into your stomach using a gentle circular motion. Alternately, you can apply a hot compress spiked with essential oil to your abdomen. Repeat as often as necessary.

Ayurvedic Medicine

 Good digestion, according to Ayurveda, depends on a strong *agni*, or digestive fire. To kindle the fire and speed digestion, Ayurvedic practitioners may advise trying one or more of the following treatments: Take *shatavari*, Ayurveda bitters, *Gasex* (2 to 3 tablets after meals), or *Bonnisan*. Snack on ginger root, drink bay leaf tea, or munch on a small handful of fennel or cumin seeds daily.

Ayurvedic products are available at many health food stores and Indian pharmacies.

Bodywork and Somatic Practices

 Try reflexology, polarity therapy, Oriental bodywork, CranioSacral Therapy, and massage. Reiki and Therapeutic Touch can enhance treatment.

Homeopathy

 Homeopathic practitioners may recommend one of the following treatments for indigestion, depending on your symptoms:

- *Nux vomica*—for heartburn and sour burps brought on by overeating and drinking too much coffee or alcohol
- *Pulsatilla*—for discomfort from heartburn accompanied by queasiness, a bad taste in the mouth, and a heavy, bloated feeling that often comes from eating rich foods
- *Carbo vegetabilis*—to help settle gas and eliminate rancid belching from overeating
- *Lycopodium*—to relieve the painful gas produced by intolerance to beans, cabbage, onions, and garlic
- *Arsenicum album*—to help relieve indigestion accompanied by a burning pain in the middle of the night

Hydrotherapy

 For heartburn, try sipping a mixture of 2 to 3 tablespoons activated charcoal mixed with 10 ounces of water. Activated charcoal is available in most health food stores and in some drugstores.

Traditional Chinese Medicine

Acupuncture This modality may be used to help control the symptoms of indigestion (heartburn, gas, abdominal pain, nausea), though it won't necessarily cure any underlying causes, especially if used only short-term.

In most cases of indigestion, the practitioner begins by focusing on points related to the large and small intestine, stomach, pancreas, gallbladder, and spleen.

Acupressure To alleviate symptoms of indigestion, the practitioner may apply firm pressure to Stomach 25 and 36, and Large Intestine 4. Add Spleen 6 and Bladder 60 to counteract gas. Heartburn may be treated by manipulating Conception Vessel 6 and 12, Stomach 36, and Pericardium 6.

Chinese Herbal Therapy Codonopsis and fennel are two other commonly prescribed herbs for this condition and are thought to boost the body's ability to absorb nutrients from food and speed digestion; take a 5- to 7-gram codonopsis decoction twice a day, or a 1- to 3-gram fennel decoction three times a day.

Cardamom seed, nutmeg, and mint all have a soothing effect on digestive upset, while licorice and trifoliate orange act as stomach tonics.

Yoga and Meditation

Try a yoga position that massages the large colon which improves digestion by easing constipation. Yoga specialists favor the Wind Removal, Half Spinal Twist, Peacock, and Half Locust poses.

INFERTILITY

Signs and Symptoms

- The inability to conceive after one year of regular, unprotected sexual intercourse

Description

Infertility is a condition that currently affects some five million Americans. The condition is defined by the inability to conceive a child after having healthy sexual relations for one year without using birth control. The condition can be caused by a problem with either the male or the female reproductive system. In fact, in approximately 40 percent of infertility cases, the problems are attributed to the man; and 40 percent are related to the woman. In approximately 20 percent of infertility cases, no cause is determined.

There are a multitude of physical factors, in both men and women, that can lead to infertility. In men, infertility can be caused by impotence, low sperm count, absence of sperm in the semen, or production of malformed sperm. In women, the condition can result from irregular ovulation, obstruction or dysfunction of the fallopian tubes, or abnormalities of the cervix or uterus, such as polyps. One major risk factor for infertility in women is age. Many women today are waiting until their thirties or forties to conceive a child, which increases their risk of becoming infertile.

Conventional Medical Treatment

If you (or your partner) are unable to conceive after a year of trying, visit your physician or fertility specialist for a fertility evaluation. This evaluation involves ruling out underlying conditions in both partners that can impair fertility, such as sexually transmitted diseases, an overactive or underactive thyroid, substance abuse, pelvic conditions, and prostate conditions.

A man should visit his urologist for an examination and tests, many of which are non-invasive and painless. Usually, ejaculated semen is collected or is examined for quality and quantity.

A woman should visit her gynecologist for examination and testing. These tests include any of the following:

- Hormonal tests to confirm that ovulation is occurring monthly

- Endometrial biopsy—a small portion of endometrial tissue is tested to determine whether and when ovulation is occurring and whether the uterine lining is hormonally prepared

- Hysteroscopy—a flexible fiberoptic device used to examine the interior of the cervix and uterus for irregularities

- Hysterosalpingography—radiography (often performed under general anesthesia) to evaluate the condition of the uterus and fallopian tubes

- Laparoscopy—an incision is made beneath the navel, and a needle inserted into the abdominal cavity to test whether there are any blockages in the fallopian tubes and uterus

If any of these tests reveal an underlying condition that is affecting fertility, the condition is treated and fertility may be restored.

For example, if a man has a low sperm count, artificial insemination—implanting healthy donor sperm into a woman's uterus—is one option. Women who do not produce eggs regularly may be prescribed a medication—such as clomipene citrate (Clomid®) or human menopausal gonadotropin (Pergonal®)—to induce ovulation or encourage the body to produce more than one egg at a time.

For those in whom no precise cause for infertil-

Fertility Treatments and Multiple Births

Although most fertility specialists do not intend to produce multiple births, they are more likely to occur when fertility medications are used. "Superovulation," an advanced reproductive technique in which drugs spur ovulation, results in a 20 percent chance of multiple conception. This is because several eggs are extracted, fertilized, and reimplanted. The more embryos reimplanted, the greater the chance of successful—and possibly multiple—conception.

Pollutants and Infertility

Exposure to pollution and other environmental chemicals can lead to infertility in men and women. Chronic exposure to metal particles released into the air by incinerators and certain manufacturing plants appear to inhibit the sperm's ability to penetrate the ovum. Results of laboratory tests showed that non-toxic concentrations of cadmium, nickel, manganese, or zinc could all be involved in male infertility. Lead, toluene, cadmium, and carbon disulfide are potential reproductive hazards in the workplace that can affect female fertility. While anyone who has lived in a city plagued by air pollution for a long time is at risk, metal workers—such as smelters, welders, and people who manufacture alkaline batteries—are at greatest risk. Metal workers and urban residents should consider using protective measures, such as breathing units or air filters.

Health Notes

➤ Drink alcohol only in moderation. Men and women who drink three or more alcoholic drinks daily have higher infertility rates than moderate drinkers and non-drinkers.

➤ Douching, which is not necessary for cleanliness, has been associated with an increased risk of pelvic inflammatory disease, a leading cause of infertility.

➤ Obesity is a risk factor for infertility. In women, obesity can interfere with conception by stopping ovulation. In men, obesity has been linked with reduced sperm counts.

➤ Sexually transmitted diseases can cause infertility. Be sure to use safe-sex practices, and always use a condom (unless you are trying to conceive).

➤ Stress can lead to irregular ovulation or loss of menstrual function in women and reduced sperm counts in men.

➤ Researchers have discovered that the motility of a man's sperm (its ability to move to the egg) decreases by approximately 10 percent after the loss of a partner, whether by death, divorce, or separation.

Counseling is often essential for the couple experiencing infertility.

For More Information

American Society for Reproductive Medicine
1209 Montgomery Highway
Birmingham, AL 35216-2809
205-978-5000
www.asrm.org

Fertility Foundation
P.O. Box 18627
Charlotte, NC 28205
704-531-8345
www.fertilityfoundation.org

RESOLVE, Inc.
The National Infertility Association
1310 Broadway
Somerville, MA 02144
617-623-0744
www.resolve.org

Complementary and Alternative Treatments

Nutrition and Supplementation

A well-balanced diet is important to fertility, but don't rule out psychological issues. Stress often plays a major role in infertility. Avoid fats and food additives. The following substances inhibit fertility in both sexes: nicotine products, caffeine, alcohol, heavy metals (hair analysis can detect poisoning), and drugs (such as marijuana and cocaine). In some cases, a gluten-free diet has helped both men and women overcome their infertility. Also, ask your healthcare provider about deoxyhydroepiandosterone (DHEA) supplementation.

Intense exercise, hot tubs, and saunas have been known to impact ovulation and reduce sperm count. Although each person needs an individualized program, the following recommended daily

ity is found, or for whom other treatments have failed, there are still available options. In vitro fertilization, a form of assisted fertility, is one possibility. During this procedure, the man's sperm and an egg extracted from the woman are combined in a petri dish; the fertilized egg is then implanted into the woman's uterus. It is important to remember that many of these tests and therapies are stressful, expensive, and time-consuming.

nutritional supplement plan is a good place to begin:

- selenium (200 to 400 mcg)—deficiency has been linked to infertility in men and women

- vitamin C (2000 to 6000 mg in divided doses)—keeps sperm from clumping; increases motility

- vitamin E (start with 200 IU and increase to 400 to 1000 IU)—balances hormone production; carries oxygen to the sex organs

- zinc (80 mg, not to exceed a total of 100 mg from all supplements)—important for normal functioning of reproductive organs

- liver extract (as prescribed by a healthcare provider)—promotes proper functioning of the sex organs

- essential fatty acids (as directed on label)—vital for normal glandular activity, especially for the reproductive system

- L-carnitine (for men, 3000 mg for four months)—increases sperm motility

- soy isoflavones, including genestein (as directed on label)

- uva ursi (as directed on label)—cleanses urinary tract

- DHEA supplementation, as administered by your healthcare provider

(Consult your healthcare provider regarding the duration of treatment.)

Traditional Chinese Medicine

 Acupuncture In infertile men, acupuncture can be used to improve general circulation which can, in turn, enhance the mobility of sperm. Female infertility is sometimes caused by a hormonal disorder, and acupuncture can be used to increase the body's production of fertility-boosting hormones and to regulate the fertility cycle.

Points targeted to treat infertility in either gender are Spleen 6 and Liver 3. Kidney 7 is added to the male's routine, and Spleen 9 is added to the female's routine.

Chinese Herbal Therapy Herbs often prescribed in the treatment of female infertility include cnidium (a 3-gram capsule or decoction, 3 times a day) and leonurus (5- to 7.5-gram decoction 2 times a day).

Additional herbs used to treat male and female infertility are horny goat weed, cordyceps, schisandra, and Chinese raspberry. The patent medicine Dang Gui Four Combination is another common remedy. Once again, if desired results are not achieved, a better diagnosis of the individual's true imbalance is necessary.

INSOMNIA

Signs and Symptoms

- Difficulty falling asleep
- Inability to fall asleep after waking up in the middle of the night
- Waking up earlier than usual
- Anxiety over whether or not you will be able to fall—and remain—asleep
- Daytime sleepiness

Description

Insomnia is an extremely frustrating condition, during which normal sleep patterns are consistently interrupted—either when falling asleep, in the middle of the night, or very early in the morning. One, two, or three consecutive sleep-deprived nights can make you less alert, easily confused, and unusually fatigued. Four or more consecutive nights without adequate sleep can interfere with motor skills, physical coordination, and problem-solving abilities. It also can make you moody, prone to depression, and susceptible to infectious illnesses, such as the common cold and flu. In some people, prolonged sleeplessness can even cause hallucinations, psychosis, and delusions.

Insomnia is a very personalized condition; it can be caused by a multitude of factors, including job stress, money concerns, depression, alcohol or drug use, hyperthyroidism, sleep apnea, jet lag, caffeine, sleep deprivation due to having a newborn infant, and trying to sleep in a noisy environment.

Conventional Medical Treatment

If you have not had a good night's sleep for four or more days in a row, visit your physician, who will examine you to ensure that a physical ailment, such as hyperthyroidism or sleep apnea, is not the cause of your insomnia. Insomnia is also a symptom of depression, which your doctor also may explore. If a medical or psychological cause of your insomnia is determined, it must be ad-

Insomnia and the Elderly

It is estimated that half of all people over the age of 65 suffers from chronic sleep disturbance. Among elderly people—even those who are healthy—the frequency of sleep disorders is associated with an impairment of melatonin production. Melatonin, produced by the pineal gland at night, plays a role in regulation of the sleep-wake cycle. A recent study investigated the effect of melatonin on sleep quality in 12 elderly subjects who complained of insomnia. In all 12 subjects, the amount of melatonin excreted during the night was lower than in non-insomniac elderly people. After the subjects were treated with 2 mg of controlled-release melatonin each night for three weeks, it was determined that melatonin replacement therapy effectively improved sleep quality in the study population.

Health Notes

➤ Try using a white-noise machine as an alternative to ear plugs if you are a light sleeper, or if street noise is keeping you awake. These gadgets cover up loud noises with a steady hum or dull roar, which is less noticeable than sudden sounds. Studies indicate that they can improve sleep for many people, including infants.

➤ Recent Swiss research indicates that warming your feet with a pair of socks or a hot water bottle may help you to fall asleep. The body typically prepares for sleep by dilating blood vessels in the hands and feet to radiate heat away from the body. Warming the feet may help to speed up this process.

➤ Save your bed for sleeping and sex. Refrain from paying bills, reading, or watching television in bed. If you spend more than 30 minutes trying to fall asleep, or wake up in the middle of the night, go to a quiet, dimly lit area of your house and engage in a non-stimulating activity (such as needlework or reading a dull book) until you feel sleepy again. This will keep you from subconsciously associating your bed with wakefulness.

➤ Birth control pills and other drugs can interfere with caffeine removal, prolonging caffeine's stimulating effects.

➤ Regular aerobic activity—performed five or six hours before bedtime—is an effective way to prevent insomnia. Studies have shown that fit individuals typically fall asleep faster, and sleep more soundly and deeply, than people who do not exercise. Typically, metabolism and core body temperature rise in the day and fall at night. But for many insomniacs, their core body temperature does not decrease adequately at night. Exercise forces the body temperature to rise. Five to six hours later it will drop, facilitating the onset of sleep.

dressed in order for your usual sleep patterns to resume.

Often, there is no underlying medical factor behind a person's sleep difficulties. Instead, the problem may be rooted in poor "sleep hygiene." Sleep hygiene means following a fixed routine of activities that the body associates with sleep onset, including adhering to set sleep and waking times (even on weekends), avoiding stimulating activities (such as exercising, watching an emotional movie, or reading an upsetting book) within three hours of bedtime, avoiding all stimulants (such as caffeine) within six hours of retiring, creating a noise-free environment for sleep, and ensuring that the bedroom is a comfortable temperature. Other sleep hygiene measures include eliminating daytime naps and setting aside time during the day to attend to (or simply keep a journal of) the worries that keep you awake at night.

Complementary and Alternative Treatments

Nutrition and Supplementation

To treat insomnia, avoiding certain substances is more important than consuming particular foods. Alcohol can help induce sleep initially, but will disrupt those deeper sleep cycles later in the night. Contrary to popular belief, nicotine does not calm one's system. It is a neurostimulant and can cause sleep problems. Stay away from caffeine in any form; some people are even sensitive to decaf, which still contains some caffeine. Avoid bacon, cheese, chocolate, ham, potatoes, sugar, sausage, spinach, tomatoes, and wine as bedtime grows near. These foods contain tyramine, a brain stimulant.

Do eat turkey, bananas, figs, dates, yogurt, milk, tuna, and whole grain crackers in the evening. These foods contain tryptophan, which promotes sleep.

There are a handful of supplements that can assist you in establishing regular sleep patterns. Follow this daily guideline:

- calcium (1500 to 2000 mg in divided doses, after meals and especially at bedtime)—has a calming effect

- magnesium (half as much as your calcium dose)—balances with calcium; relaxes muscles; if bowels become loose take less

- melatonin (start with 1.5 mg, taken 2 hours or less before bedtime; if this doesn't help, gradually increase the dosage until an effective level has been reached; do not exceed 5 mg)—promotes sleep

- vitamin B complex (50 mg), supplemented with vitamin B_5 (50 mg)—relieves stress

- inositol (100 mg at bedtime)—enhances rapid eye movement (REM) sleep

- St. John's wort (300 mg 3 times daily with each meal; must include .3 percent hypericum)—promotes restful sleep (Do not use in conjunction with antidepressants. St. John's Wort may act as a mild monoamine oxidase inhibitor (MAOI); consult your healthcare provider regarding potential dietary and medication restrictions.)

- kava kava (as directed on label)—reduces anxiety

(For an *acute* condition, take supplements until your symptoms subside. If symptoms persist, seek the advice of your healthcare provider. For a *chronic* condition, consult your healthcare provider regarding the duration of treatment.)

Aromatherapy

For occasional restlessness, essential oils of Roman chamomile and lavender can provide relaxing effects. Add 5 to 15 drops to a tub of warm (not hot) water. Soak in the bath for 20 to 30 minutes before bedtime. Aromatherapists also suggest putting a drop or two of lavender and marjoram on a tissue or handkerchief and inhaling a few times. Alternatively, you can place the drops of oil on your pillow case.

Ayurvedic Medicine

According to Ayurveda, insomnia is a vata problem or imbalance, and to bring on sound, peaceful sleep, the overactive vata must be calmed. If you suffer from restless, sleepless nights, Ayurvedic practitioners may suggest trying one or more of the following remedies:

- Drink warm milk before retiring.

- Apply coconut oil, sesame oil, or mustard oil to your head and feet to calm your nervous system.

- Take a warm (not hot) bath or shower to help you relax.

Bodywork and Somatic Practices

Massage is always a great relaxing therapy. CranioSacral Therapy/Somato-Emotional Release, reflexology, Trager, polarity therapy and Oriental bodywork, can also induce sleep.

Herbal Therapy

Of all the herbal remedies for insomnia, valerian (a central nervous system depressant) is probably the best known and most effective. To make a cup of valerian tea, steep 2 teaspoons chopped root in 1 cup boiling water for 15 minutes; strain. Drink half an hour before bedtime. You can also take 20 drops valerian tincture in water at bedtime. Use occasionally, not nightly.

St. John's wort tea has also been used to treat insomnia. An infusion of 1 teaspoon of dried St. John's wort (3 teaspoons fresh) to each 8 ounce cup of boiling water is used. The tea should be steeped for 15 minutes before drinking.

Chamomile tea is another highly effective sleep aid. Steep 2 teaspoons chopped flowers in 1 cup boiling water for 10 minutes; strain. Drink half an hour before bedtime. Do not drink chamomile tea if you're allergic to ragweed.

Other teas that have a calming effect include lime blossom, passion flower, hops, and skullcap.

To make one of these teas, steep 1 teaspoon dried herb in 1 cup boiling water for 10 minutes; strain. You also can find blends of these herbs in teas, tinctures, and capsules in most health food stores. Follow the directions on the package label.

Herbal products are available in health food stores and in some pharmacies and supermarkets. Follow package for specific directions.

Homeopathy

Persistent sleeplessness should be treated by a professional homeopath. For a sudden bout of insomnia, one of several remedies may be recommended by practitioners:

- *Nux vomica*—for sleeplessness after mental strain or overindulgence; you get to sleep early in the morning and wake up feeling tired and unrefreshed

- *Ignatia*—for sleeplessness caused by grief

- *Coffea*—for sleeplessness from mental activity brought about by exciting or distressful news

- *Arnica*—for sleeplessness from physical or mental overexertion

- *Aconite*—for sleeplessness brought on by fear or panic following a fright or shock

Hydrotherapy

A leisurely soak in an Epsom salts bath can help you relax and feel sleepy. Add 2 cups Epsom salts to a tub of warm (not hot) water. Soak for 20 to 30 minutes. Repeat nightly as needed.

Traditional Chinese Medicine

Acupuncture Traditional Chinese Medicine believes that insomnia is caused by kidney disorders or imbalances, so acupuncture is used to improve the flow of *chi* and restore harmony within this organ and the related meridians. Acupuncture points relating to the kidney, brain, and heart are involved.

Acupressure To relieve insomnia, an acupressure expert may apply pressure to the following points: Heart 7, Spleen 6, Kidney 3, and the extra point known as Yin Tang, which lies between the eyebrows.

Chinese Herbal Therapy There are many Chinese herbal formulas used to counteract insomnia. If sleeplessness is accompanied by irritability and restlessness, Gentiana Formula may be recommended. Insomnia accompanied by nightmares, night sweats, and heart palpitations, or brought about by constant worrying, may call for Ginseng and Ziziphus or Concha Marguerita and Ligustrum. Sleep disorders marked by fatigue and lack of appetite may respond best to Ginseng and Longan or Ginseng and Tang Gui Ten. Emperor's Tea is another popular insomnia remedy.

Yoga and Meditation

 Meditating in the Corpse position can help you unwind and fall asleep. First, concentrate on vanquishing tension from one muscle at a time from the bottoms of your feet to the top of your head; then, focus on slow, deep breathing. Finally, repeat a mantra, such as "ohm" or "hum," for 10 to 15 minutes. Don't fret if you fall asleep before you finish meditating.

IRRITABLE BOWEL SYNDROME (IBS)

Signs and Symptoms

Symptoms of irritable bowel syndrome usually occur shortly after meals and include:

- Abdominal or intestinal cramps
- Abdominal bloating
- Diarrhea
- Constipation
- Abnormal bowel habits

Description

Irritable bowel syndrome—also known as IBS or spastic colon—is a condition that affects at least 10 to 15 percent of all American adults. In fact, IBS is second only to the common cold as a cause of missed workdays. Most people with IBS typically develop the condition in their 20s and have it, either periodically or frequently, for life.

Each IBS sufferer has a slightly different mix of symptoms as well as different triggers, which set off an "attack" or episode. The severity of symptoms also varies among IBS sufferers. Yet there is one thing that all sufferers have in common: during an attack of IBS, their colons do not contract properly. Some people's colons may contract too vigorously, producing cramps and diarrhea. Others may not contract enough, causing constipation. And in some sufferers, the bowels alternate between the two extremes, causing the sufferer to vacillate between periods of diarrhea and constipation.

While the exact cause of IBS is unknown, some experts believe that certain people have hypersensitive colons, which react adversely to different foods. Since many female IBS sufferers experience more severe symptoms during menstruation, hormonal changes are thought to play a role as well. Stress also appears to worsen symptoms, probably because the colon is partially controlled by the nervous system.

Conventional Medical Treatment

If you notice recurring changes in your bowel movements, visit your doctor. To rule out other bowel conditions—such as colon cancer, colitis, or Crohn's disease—your physician may perform a digestive stool analysis and rectal examination, and might administer a barium enema.

If you are diagnosed with IBS, your doctor may recommend that you try to limit stress and change your diet. You may need to increase your fiber intake by adding bran, oatmeal, whole grains, beans, fruits, and vegetables to your diet or by using an over-the-counter fiber preparation, such as methylcellulose (Citrucel®) to help ease constipation, promote regular bowel movements, and normalize watery stools. However, fiber alone will not prevent or cure a case of IBS. You also need to avoid foods that trigger episodes. For some people, this means staying away from acidic foods, such as tomato-based dishes. Other people experience IBS symptoms after eating any type of sugar, including fructose and corn syrup. Caffeine and carbonated beverages can cause problems for many IBS sufferers. Other common triggers include lactose-based foods (such as milk and ice cream), fatty foods (such as packaged snack foods, chocolate, pastries, and red meat), and certain vegetables, such as brussel sprouts, beans, carrots, celery, and onions. If your symptoms are severe, you may require medication. The medications your doctor prescribes will depend on your symptoms. For example, if chronic diarrhea is the main problem or if frequent stools occur, cholestyramine or loperamide may be useful.

In some cases, medications, such as antianxiolytics and antidepressants, are prescribed to improve symptoms associated with stress, but their use poses the risk of dependency. New medications that act on serotonin receptors in the digestive tract are being tested for use in IBS.

For More Information
National Institute of Diabetes and
Digestive and Kidney Diseases
2 Information Way
Bethesda MD 20892-3570
301-654-3810
www.niddk.nih.gov

Health Notes

➤ If you have been told to add more fiber to your diet, increase your fiber consumption very gradually over a period of two weeks. At the same time, don't forget to drink 8 or more 8-ounce glasses of water each day to help keep fiber soft and passable.

➤ Switch to a low-fat, plant-based diet. High-fat foods—especially animal products that contain saturated fat—have been shown to aggravate IBS.

➤ A major trigger of IBS is stress. Try to identify and address relationships and situations in your life that increase your stress level.

Complementary and Alternative Treatments

Nutrition and Supplementation

To help keep the bowel clean and clear, eat a high-fiber diet that includes lots of fruits and vegetables as well as whole grains and legumes. Supplement with fiber; psyllium powder works well because it regulates bowel movements. Drink 6 to 8 glasses of pure water daily.

Alcohol and tobacco irritate the lining of the stomach and colon; limit your intake—or better yet, eliminate them from your diet. Other foods prevent the absorption of nutrients and are mucus-forming. These include: animal fats, carbonated beverages, caffeine in any form, candy, chocolate, dairy products, fried foods, ice cream, junk food, margarine, processed foods, sugar, wheat products, and sugar-free gum. Be sure to check for your own particular food sensitivities.

During an attack, eat a bland diet. Organic baby food can help at a time like this. At all times, avoid eating directly before bed; wait at least 2 hours before lying down.

The following recommended daily supplements will help the IBS sufferer lead a healthy, active life.

Most Important

- vitamin B complex (50 to 100 mg 3 times daily)—promotes proper muscle tone in the gastrointestinal tract

- a prodophilus formula (as directed on label)—replaces friendly bacteria; important for digestion and for the production of B vitamins

- garlic (as directed on label)—aids in digestion; destroys toxins in the colon; use liquid form

- psyllium fiber (as directed on label)—heals and cleanses

- free-form amino acid complex (as directed on label)—repairs mucous membranes of the intestines

- N-acetyl glucosamine (as directed on label)—protects the intestinal lining from digestive enzymes

Also Recommended

- flaxseed oil (as directed on label)—supplies essential fatty acids that protect the intestinal lining

- calcium (1000 mg in divided doses)—helps the central nervous system

- magnesium (1000 mg in divided doses)—prevents colon cancer; cut back if bowels become loose

- calcium carbonate (500 mg)—to absorb intestinal toxins

- ginger (25 mg)

- gamma orizanol (as directed on label)—protects and heals the stomach mucosa

- bovine colostrum (as directed on label)—heals damaged stomach tissue

- curcumin (as directed on label)—anti-inflammatory agent

(For an *acute* condition, take supplements until your symptoms subside. If symptoms persist, seek the advice of your healthcare provider. For a *chronic* condition, consult your healthcare provider regarding the duration of treatment.)

Aromatherapy

If you're prone to cramping, some aromatherapists recommend massaging and kneading the abdomen with anti-spasmodic essential oils. Combine 3 drops of peppermint oil and 1 teaspoon of carrier oil (canola or safflower). You can also add 3 drops of Roman chamomile to 2 teaspoons of the blend, and you can substitute lotion for the carrier oil. Apply to your stomach and massage very gently in a circular pattern.

Ayurvedic Medicine

An Ayurvedic practitioner may advise taking *triphala*, a mild Indian laxative, twice a day to ease the alternating constipation and diarrhea associated with irritable bowel syndrome. Triphala is made from three Indian fruits and may help restore a healthy tone to the intestinal tract.

Ayurvedic products are available at many health food stores and Indian pharmacies. Remember to consult your doctor if symptoms persist.

Herbal Therapy

Peppermint has anti-spasmodic properties and is a good choice for relieving the intestinal cramps that accompany irritable bowel syndrome. There are two ways to take peppermint: Mix 2 or 3 drops peppermint oil in 1/4 cup warm water. Drink 3 or 4 times a day. Or infuse 1 teaspoon dried peppermint leaves in 1 cup boiling water for 10 minutes; strain. Drink several times a day, as needed.

Chamomile, marshmallow root, and slippery

elm teas are also calming to the intestinal tract. Steep 1 teaspoon of one of those dried herbs in 1 cup boiling water for 10 minutes; strain. Drink 3 to 4 times a day.

Herbal products are available in health food stores and in some pharmacies and supermarkets. Follow package for specific directions.

Homeopathy

 Irritable bowel syndrome may respond to homeopathic treatment. However, the selection of a remedy—more than one is available—depends on *your* symptoms and the stage of the condition. Don't try treating this disorder yourself. See a homeopathic professional.

Hydrotherapy

 Constitutional therapy (alternating applications of hot and cold towels to the front and back of the body) may provide some relief. Apply several times a week.

Traditional Chinese Medicine

 Acupuncture Acupuncture can be helpful in reducing stress, which can exacerbate irritable bowel syndrome. It can also be used to lessen inflammation and relieve gas, diarrhea, nausea, pain, or constipation.

The acupuncture points targeted will vary, depending upon the patient's complaints, although treatment probably will include points along the spleen, liver, kidney, and large intestine meridians.

Acupressure The practitioner may concentrate on Liver 3 and 13, Stomach 25 and 36, Pericardium 6, and Spleen 6. Additional points may be added, as warranted by the patient's specific symptoms.

Acupressure can also help reduce stress and enhance relaxation, which can have a positive impact on this condition.

Chinese Herbal Therapy Fennel is a time-honored nausea remedy. Some TCM practitioners believe that anxiety or sadness also may be a contributing factor in the development of irritable bowel syndrome and may recommend herbs that address these conditions as well. Ginseng and Astragalus Formula can be used to build the system.

Yoga and Meditation

 If stress is the cause of your irritable bowl syndrome, try a daily routine of deep breathing exercises, three or four yoga poses, and meditation to help you relax. Vary the poses from day to day, but be sure to include the Corpse, Baby, Wind Removal, and Root Lock.

ITCHING

Itching can affect the eyes, nasal membranes, throat, ear canal, anus, and skin. An itch can be fleeting and occur for no apparent reason, or it can be a chronic symptom of an underlying medical condition. Body-wide itching is sometimes the symptom of a systemic illness, such as liver disease, leukemia, Hodgkin's disease, or kidney failure; it can also be the side effect of a drug, such as aspirin or codeine-related pain relievers. Localized itching often accompanies localized conditions, including hemorrhoids, conjunctivitis, and many sexually transmitted diseases. Skin itching is a common side effect of many skin conditions, including hives, dermatitis, insect bites or stings, athlete's foot, psoriasis, or dehydrated skin.

As tempting as it is to scratch an itch, it is not advisable. Too much scratching can tear the epidermis (the outer layer of skin), cause irritation and inflammation, and possibly lead to an infection. Itchiness can often be controlled with topical preparations, including cortisone ointment, caspium cream (available at health stores), and calamine lotion. Oatmeal preparations—such as homemade oatmeal rubbed on the itchy area or an oatmeal bath made by holding a handful of oatmeal tied in cheesecloth under running lukewarm water—can also alleviate itching. A starch- and-soda bath also can be used to treat itching—add 8 ounces of baking soda and 16 ounces of laundry starch to a tub of lukewarm water and soak in it for a half hour. Other itch-fighting strategies include keeping itchy skin well-moisturized with a non-perfumed body lotion, avoiding the drying effects of soap and hot water, and using a humidifier to add moisture to your environment.

If none of the above homecare measures ease the itching, contact your healthcare provider.

JAUNDICE

Jaundice is a yellowish cast to the skin or whites of the eyes. In the vast majority of cases, jaundice is symptomatic of a liver condition, such as hepatitis, cirrhosis, liver cancer, liver abscess, or Gilbert's syndrome. In other people, jaundice is caused by a blockage of bile, from gallstones, for example. Jaundice generally disappears when the condition that is causing it is successfully treated. Jaundice sometimes appears in newborns and young children, but in these cases it is usually not dangerous.

The liver regulates the composition of the blood, controlling the amounts of glucose, protein and fat that enter the bloodstream. The liver also is responsible for removing bilirubin—a yellow pigmentation that is created during the breakdown of red blood cells—from the blood. In the liver, bilirubin is chemically altered so that it becomes water-soluble; it is then added to the bile, which enters the intestinal tract and is eliminated. Jaundice is an indication that the liver is not adequately removing and processing bilirubin. Bilirubin levels in the body elevate and the substance is deposited in the skin and membranes of the eye, creating a yellow cast.

JET LAG

Signs and Symptoms

- Fatigue
- Drowsiness
- Loss of mental acuity
- Irritability
- Headaches
- Mild physical coordination problems

Description

Jet lag occurs when the body is thrust abruptly into a new time zone, requiring a whole new pattern of sleeping, waking, and eating. The sudden time readjustment to these activities brings about jet lag—feeling out of sorts, tired, uncoordinated, testy, irritable. Fortunately, the symptoms are temporary. Most people adjust to a new time schedule at a rate of about one hour a day. For example, after changing four time zones, the body requires about four days to reset its usual rhythms.

Conventional Medical Treatment

Most cases of jet lag can be treated without medical assistance. Some people have success trying to ignore their fatigue entirely and just eat and sleep on the schedule of their new time zone, until their symptoms subside. Others go straight to bed at the first opportunity—no matter what time of day they arrive in the new time zone. Others take short naps throughout the first few days of their stay to keep them well rested. Experts believe that exposure to sunlight immediately upon arrival in a new time zone helps the body adjust more quickly.

Health Notes

➤ *Prevention is one of the best ways to lessen the effects of jet lag. Two or three days before a trip, try adopting a sleep-wake-eat pattern similar to what you will experience at your destination.*

➤ *You may want to try arriving at your destination at the hour you usually start your day—having slept during the flight—so that your body immediately begins to orient itself to the new time schedule.*

➤ *Drink lots of liquid when traveling, but avoid beverages that contain alcohol and caffeine, both of which can upset your body's sleep-wake patterns.*

Complementary and Alternative Treatments

Nutrition and Supplementation

Though it may sound surprising, you can control jet lag by resetting your body clock through diet. The rule is *feast, fast, feast, fast*. Three days before departure, feast on foods high in protein and carbohydrates. Eat foods such as steak, eggs, green beans, pasta potatoes, starchy vegetables, and even sweet desserts. High-protein foods stimulate your active cycle, while foods high in carbohydrates stimulate sleep. Do not consume caffeine except between 3 and 5 p.m.

The next day, fast on light meals such as salads, clear soups, fruits, and juice. Again, no caffeine except between 3 and 5 p.m. Fasting depletes the liver's store of carbohydrates and allows you to re-set your body's clock.

On the day before you leave, feast again. The day you leave, follow this guideline: if you're traveling west, drink caffeine in the morning if you drink caffeine regularly and fast for only half the day. If traveling east, consume your optional caffeine between 6 and 11 p.m., and fast the whole day.

Another helpful tip is to take melatonin one hour before going to sleep in the new location. Doing this for one or two nights sends your brain the message that you need to do some adjusting. Drink plenty of fluids as well; you cannot combat fatigue if you are dehydrated.

St. John's wort is sometimes helpful; take 300 mg 3 times daily before meals. (Do not use in conjunction with antidepressants. St. John's wort may act as a mild monoamine oxidase inhibitor (MAOI); consult your healthcare provider regarding potential dietary and medication restrictions.)

Aromatherapy

Many airlines now provide moist face cloths enhanced with essential oils of lavender, geranium, lemon, or rosemary for combating fatigue and in-flight jitters. To prepare your own jet-lag kit, pack a moist cloth in a self-sealing plastic bag. Just before using, place a drop or two of lavender, geranium, lemon, or rosemary oil on the cloth. Gently wipe your forehead. Once at your destination, boost your energy by taking a warm bath to which you've added about a dozen drops of geranium oil. Aromatherapists also recommend placing a drop or two of rosemary oil on a tissue or handkerchief and inhaling whenever you feel drowsy.

Ayurvedic Medicine

Because of the speed of jet travel, too much vata is produced in the body, according to Ayurvedic theory. To prevent fatigue and lethargy, Ayurvedic practitioners may suggest taking ginger before your flight and drinking lots of water (no alcohol, coffee, or tea) during the flight.

Homeopathy

Homeopathic practitioners may suggest one of the following treatments for jet lag, depending on your symptoms: *Ar-*

nica if you feel restless and overtired while still on the plane; *Cocculus*, if after arriving, you feel disoriented, as if you're still flying.

Hydrotherapy

To prevent dehydration and much of the resulting jet lag, drink at least 1 8-ounce glass of water each hour during the flight.

Traditional Chinese Medicine

Acupuncture This modality can help regulate the body's energy level, which may prevent or remedy jet lag.

Chinese Herbal Therapy *Gotu Kola* may be effective in reducing jet-lag-induced disorientation, while astragalus, eucommia, and codonopsis can be helpful in relieving fatigue. Ginseng Tonic Pills and Eight Treasure Tea are commonly used Chinese energy tonics.

Yoga and Meditation

Deep-breathing exercises and meditation can help relieve the grogginess that accompanies jet travel. Perform these exercises while on the plane and after you reach your destination: Sun Salutations, Warrior, and Triangle.

JOCK ITCH

Signs and Symptoms

- Itching in the anal and groin area; the rash may spread to the inner thighs and buttocks
- Burning in the affected area
- Fine, red rash covering the affected area

Description

Jock itch, or groin ringworm, is a fungal infection of the skin that causes an intense itching and burning sensation in the groin area and inner thigh that may extend to anus and abdomen. The condition is caused by a variety of fungi, which also cause athlete's foot. While jock itch is much more common in men, women can suffer from it as well. (In women, the condition is usually caused by a yeast infection.)

The fungus that causes jock itch thrives on moist, sweaty skin; for this reason, people who sweat a lot, such as athletes and obese people, are at increased risk for developing the condition. People with diabetes are also at increased risk.

Conventional Medical Treatment

Jock itch can be treated—and prevented—with homecare. Wash the affected area two or three times per day, and after drying the skin thoroughly, apply an anti-fungal drying powder to the area. (Do not overuse anti-fungal powder—if you use it on an area more than three times a day,

Health Notes

➤ To avoid developing jock itch, change your undergarments at least once a day—particularly if you have been sweating.

➤ Some health experts believe that fungi thrive on sugar, so they recommend cutting refined sugar out of your diet if you are prone to fungal infections, such as jock itch.

your skin can become dry and irritated.) You also may want to smooth on an over-the-counter antifungal cream before going to bed at night. If your jock itch persists despite continued homecare, contact your healthcare provider.

For More Information
American Academy of Dermatology
930 North Meacham Road
Schaumberg, IL 60173
888-462-DERM
www.aad.org

Complementary and Alternative Treatments

Nutrition and Supplementation

 Fungi thrive on sugar, so avoid all sugars and refined carbohydrates. Equally important to avoid are colas, grains, processed foods, and fried or greasy foods. Dairy and meat produce mucus, so steer clear of those. Nutritionists recommend the following daily supplements:

Most Important

- a prodophilus formula (as directed on label)—replaces friendly bacteria usually deficient in people with fungal infections

- garlic (as directed on label)—neutralizes most fungi

- vitamin B complex (50 mg 3 times daily)—correctly balances friendly bacteria

- vitamin C with bioflavonoids (5000 to 20,000 mg)—aids in proper immune function

- vitamin E (400 to 800 IU)—necessary for proper immune function

- zinc (50 mg, not to exceed a total of 100 mg from all supplements)—necessary for proper immune function

Also Recommended

- vitamin A (25,000 IU; do not exceed 8000 if you are pregnant)—heals skin and mucous membranes

- olive leaf extract supplement (as directed on label)

- caprylic acid formula (taken internally as directed on label)

(For an *acute* condition, take supplements until your symptoms subside. If symptoms persist, seek the advice of your healthcare provider. For a *chronic* condition, consult your healthcare provider regarding the duration of treatment.)

Traditional Chinese Medicine

 Chinese Herbal Therapy Cnidium monnieri, eucommia, and licorice may be made into an external wash and used to treat jock itch. The patent medicines Margarite Acne Pills and *Lien Chiao Pai Tu Pien* also may help alleviate any itchiness.

KELOIDS

Signs and Symptoms

- Firm, smooth, elevated scar that extends past the borders of the initial wound and may continue to grow over a period of years, often with claw-like projections
- Itchiness, tenderness, or pain at the affected site
- Irregular pigmentation of the scar, either lighter or darker than normal

Description

A keloid is a type of scar characterized by an overgrowth of fibrous scar tissue. It looks raised—sometimes even puffy—and often continues to grow long after the original wound has healed.

A keloid can be caused by a cut or wound, an acne scar, or even a patch of itchy skin that was scratched too vigorously. Though the condition can strike anyone, people with dark complexions tend to be at higher risk, possibly because of an abnormality in melanocytic-stimulating hormones. In fact, keloids are up to 20 times more common in people of African and Asian descent than they are in people of Caucasian ancestry; Hispanics also have a higher incidence of keloids. The condition tends to run in families.

Conventional Medical Treatment

If you develop what appears to be a keloid scar, see your dermatologist, who can diagnose the condition by physically examining the scar. Treatment usually consists of getting monthly corticosteroid injections in the site for six months to a year. This treatment causes the scar to atrophy into a patch of flat, shiny skin. If a keloid is detected as a wound heals, further growth can be prohibited with a pressure bandage, which is usu-

ally worn constantly for six months to a year. Surgery to repair a keloid is generally ineffective, since an incision is likely to prompt the formation of new keloid tissue. On the other hand, in instances where the keloid is very large, skin can be grafted from another part of the body to replace the scarred tissue.

For More Information
American Academy of Dermatology
930 North Meacham Road
Schaumberg, IL 60173
888-462-DERM
www.aad.org

Complementary and Alternative Treatments

Traditional Chinese Medicine

 Acupuncture Acupuncture is effective at improving blood flow and circulation, which may enhance the skin's ability to heal and prevent the formation of an unsightly keloid scar.

Chinese Herbal Therapy Blood-moving formulas may help; check with your practitioner.

KIDNEY DISEASE (CHRONIC)

Signs and Symptoms

- Increased need to urinate at night
- Decrease in urine output
- Bloating and fluid retention
- Appetite and weight loss
- Fatigue
- Headaches
- Impaired mental ability
- Hypertension
- Muscle cramps and twitches
- Dry and itchy skin
- Pale skin
- Blood in the urine
- Nausea and vomiting

Description

The kidneys are two small organs located at the back of the abdominal wall—one on each side of the lower spine. Their job is to remove toxins from the blood and filter the waste into the urine, where it can be carried out of the body. They also produce hormones that help produce red blood cells, regulate blood pressure, and form bones. Chronic kidney failure, or renal disease, is a life-threatening condition that results when the kidneys deteriorate to the point that they are unable to perform their necessary functions. Kidney disease often develops slowly, usually over the space of many years. In fact, it comes on so slowly that by the time symptoms appear, the organs' function has often decreased to 25 percent of their normal capacity.

As the kidneys lose function, waste builds up in the blood, which in turn can affect a wide range of metabolic and endocrine functions. In fact, virtually all the body systems are affected by the buildup of fluid toxins: bones weaken and become susceptible to fractures, the heart is prone to congestive failure, ulcers may form in the stomach, anemia occurs, the central nervous system can be damaged (making thinking and concentrating difficult), muscles twitch in the arms and legs, and sensitive nerve endings cause skin itching.

The most common causes of chronic kidney disease or kidney failure are diabetes mellitus and hypertension. Autoimmune diseases, such as systemic lupus erythematosis and obstruction of the urinary tract by an enlarged prostate, also can lead to kidney failure.

Conventional Medical Treatment

If you notice any of the symptoms of kidney disease, see your doctor—kidney disease is a very serious condition that requires immediate medical attention. Your doctor may take X-rays, blood tests, and urine analysis to determine whether you have kidney disease. A needle biopsy, where the doctor takes a sample of kidney tissue for examination, may be necessary to confirm diagnosis.

Treatment for kidney disease begins with measures to control elevated blood pressure; the aim is to keep blood pressure around 130/80 mm Hg. Diuretics are one way to lower blood pressure and regulate extra water retained by the body. Angiotensin-converting enzyme (ACE) inhibitors are also prescribed to slow the progress of the disease. Unfortunately, unless it is treated early, kidney disease usually continues to worsen until *dialysis* (use of an artificial device to clean the blood) and eventually kidney transplant are necessary.

Health Notes

➤ *If you are at increased risk for developing kidney disease, avoid using aspirin, ibuprofen, and acetaminophen. Also avoid over-the-counter products that contain any of these medications. After reviewing 750 studies on analgesics and kidney disease, the National Kidney Foundation has concluded that long-term use of these drugs is damaging to the kidneys.*

➤ *A low-protein diet has been shown to reduce the risk of kidney disease and slow the progression of the disease in people who have the condition.*

For More Information
National Kidney Foundation
30 East 33rd Street, Suite 1100
New York, NY 10016
800-622-9010
www.kidney.org

National Institute of Diabetes and
Digestive and Kidney Diseases
31 Center Drive, MSC 2560
Bethesda, MD 20892-2560
301-654-3810
www.niddk.nih.gov

Complementary and Alternative Treatments

Nutrition and Supplementation

Include garlic, potatoes, asparagus, celery, cucumbers, papaya, and bananas in your diet. Sprouts and most green vegetables are also beneficial, as is watermelon. Eat the melon by itself so it can pass quickly through the body; otherwise, toxins begin to form. Foods containing arginine are helpful for kidney function: these include seeds, legumes, and especially soybeans.

Limit your intake of animal protein and dairy products (except those that are soured, such as yogurt, buttermilk, and cottage cheese). Obtain protein from peas, beans, lentils, soybeans, and whole grains. Soy protein powders are an excellent source of protein for kidney patients—take as directed by your healthcare provider. Stay away from chocolate, cocoa, eggs, fish, spinach, tea, and rhubarb.

Pure water is especially important for urinary tract health. Drink 6 to 8 ounces of pure water every waking hour. Unsweetened or fruit-juice-sweetened cranberry juice is helpful because it destroys bacteria buildup and promotes healing of the bladder. Drink 8 ounces 3 times daily, and follow this daily supplement program:

Most Important

- a prodophilus formula (as directed on label)—replaces friendly bacteria; especially important if you're taking antibiotics

- vitamin B complex (50 mg), supplemented with vitamin B_6 (50 mg 3 times daily)—reduces fluid retention, and vitamin B_2 (25 mg 3 times daily)—necessary for nephritis

- vitamin C with bioflavonoids (2000 to 4000 mg)—acidifies the urine and promotes healing

Also Recommended

- glutathione (400 mg)

- calcium (1500 mg)—helps attain proper mineral balance

- magnesium (750 mg)—balances with calcium

- L-arginine (500 mg 4 times daily)—for kidney disease

- L-methionine (as directed on label)—improves kidney circulation

- lecithin (1200 mg 3 times daily)— needed for nephritis

- multi-mineral complex (as directed on label)—corrects mineral depletion, common in kidney disease

- potassium (99 mg)—stimulates kidney; necessary for nephritis

- vitamin A (25,000 IU; do not exceed 8000 IU daily if you are pregnant)—heals urinary tract lining; use emulsion form, not pill

- vitamin E (800 IU daily)—destroys free radicals

- zinc (50 to 80 mg, not to exceed 100 mg)—promotes healing and inhibits crystal growth; use in lozenge form

(Consult your healthcare provider regarding the duration of treatment.)

Ayurvedic Medicine

General discomfort in the area of the kidneys is often a pitta problem. To combat the discomfort and strengthen the kidneys, Ayurvedic practitioners advise drinking a coriander-cumin-fennel tea or taking an herbal blend of *punarnava*, *gokshura*, *kamadudha*, and *jatamansi*. Ayurvedic products, including herbs, are available at many health food stores and Indian pharmacies.

Remember to consult your doctor before embarking on any new regimen for kidney disease.

See also "Kidney Stones" entry.

Traditional Chinese Medicine

Acupuncture Acupuncture can be used to help fortify weak kidneys and improve the flow of energy to the organ itself and within the kidney meridian. This can enhance the body's ability to process and eliminate toxins. Acupuncture also can help relieve edema and shortness of breath, both symptoms of kidney disease. The points most likely targeted are those that lie along the kidney and bladder meridians.

Chinese Herbal Therapy Patent formulas that may help with edema are Rehmannia Eight and Poria Five Herb Combination.

Yoga and Meditation

Yoga poses that stretch the kidney area can be very helpful in relieving discomfort. Try the Cobra, Pyramid, and Locust poses.

KIDNEY INFECTION

Signs and Symptoms

- Pain in the lower back that may spread to the groin area

- Frequent and urgent urination

- High fever

- Severe nausea and vomiting

Description

Kidney infections, or renal infections, are caused when a bacteria—usually *E. coli*—enters the kidneys through some other part of the body. The most common type of kidney infection occurs when bacteria from a bladder infection travels up the ureters and into the kidneys. The result is swelling and inflammation in one or both of the kidneys.

In the early stages, the symptoms of a kidney infection usually resemble the symptoms of a bladder infection, such as increased frequency and urgency of urination. If left untreated, a kidney infection may cause flu-like symptoms—such as fever, chills, nausea, and perhaps vomiting—as it progresses. These symptoms are accompanied by aches on both sides of the abdomen or upper back.

People with kidney stones, diabetes mellitus (which can impair the kidney's filtering system), or scar tissue from a previous kidney infection are at increased risk of developing a kidney infection. Pregnancy is also a time of increased risk. Use of a catheter (used to empty the bladder after surgery) also increases a person's risk of developing a kidney infection.

Conventional Medical Treatment

If you suspect you have a kidney infection, see your doctor immediately. Prompt medical attention is crucial to prevent complications, such as a kidney abscess, bloodstream infection, or shock or permanent scarring of the kidneys. To diagnose a kidney infection, your physician may take a urine specimen and urine culture to test for bacteria. An X-ray of the kidney and bladder or a kidney ultrasound may be necessary to look for the underlying cause of the kidney infection, such as a kidney stone. Treatment for a kidney infection generally consists of one to two weeks of antibiotic therapy.

For More Information

National Kidney Foundation
30 East 33rd Street, Suite 1100
New York, NY 10016
800-622-9010
www.kidney.org

National Institute of Diabetes and Digestive and Kidney Diseases
31 Center Drive, MSC 2560
Bethesda, MD 20892-2560
301-654-3810
www.niddk.nih.gov

Complementary and Alternative Treatments

Traditional Chinese Medicine

 Acupuncture Acupuncture may be used to help lessen the inflammation and pain associated with a kidney infection.

Acupressure A frequent urge to urinate may be diminished by applying firm pressure to Conception Vessel 3, Bladder 23, Spleen 6, and Liver 3.

Chinese Herbal Therapy The Chinese herbal formulas Energetics Yin and Energetics Yang may be taken simultaneously to help strengthen kidneys that have been weakened by infection. Achryanthes also may be given as a kidney tonic. Dianthus Combination may be taken to help strengthen kidneys that have been weakened by infection.

KIDNEY STONES

Signs and Symptoms

- Persistent urge to urinate
- Blood in the urine
- Pain in the side that moves toward the groin
- Sweating
- Nausea and vomiting
- Fever and chills

Description

When urine becomes too concentrated, mineral deposits—usually calcium salts or uric acid—form in the kidneys, causing a condition known as kidney stones. Most kidney stones are small enough that they easily pass through the ureter and out of the body with the urine. Larger stones, on the other hand, may irritate the ureter as they are passed from the body, resulting in extreme pain. In other cases, kidney stones grow so large that they become lodged in the ureter, blocking the flow of urine.

An estimated 5 percent of American women and 10 percent of American men develop kidney stones by the time they reach age 70. While most people have only one episode of kidney stones, it is not at all uncommon to have the condition several times—and there are even people who pass stones annually. The condition tends to run in families.

Conventional Medical Treatment

If you suspect you have kidney stones, see your physician, who can perform a blood analysis to look for an underlying cause, such as elevated calcium. A 24-hour collection of urine and urine culture also may be necessary. Obtaining the stone for analysis is the most important study. This test is needed to determine the chemical makeup of your kidney stones, which, in turn, influences the type of treatment you receive.

To treat kidney stones, your physician may prescribe a thiazide diuretic, which inhibits the growth of calcium salt stones, or allopurinol, which are helpful in treating uric acid stones. Without medication, up to 90 percent of all kidney stones pass on their own, usually within 72 hours. In the meantime, your doctor may prescribe painkillers to help you manage the pain of passing a stone.

If an X-ray reveals a kidney stone that is too large to pass, the stone may be crushed using a procedure called *lithotripsy*, where shock waves are used to break up a stone so it can pass more easily in the urine. For stones that are too large to be crushed, a tube can be inserted into the kidney to remove the stones.

New Thinking on Calcium

For years, doctors told patients suffering from kidney stones to avoid dairy products and reduce calcium intake because most kidney stones are made primarily of calcium. However, several recent studies have doctors recommending the opposite. One study revealed that men who consume diets high in calcium cut their risk of developing kidney stones by 50 percent. Another study found that women who consume fewer than 500 milligrams of calcium daily were at relatively high risk of suffering stones. *Caution*: People who rely on calcium pills to meet their daily allowance of calcium are more likely to suffer kidney stones than those who get their calcium from food. The best food sources of calcium are dairy products, leafy, green vegetables, and canned fish with bones.

Health Notes

➤ *To help prevent kidney stone formation, keep your salt intake to a minimum.*

➤ *Consume a low-protein diet. High-protein intake disrupts metabolism and causes the system to throw off calcium. A low-protein diet helps the body utilize calcium more efficiently, and thus, prevent kidney stones.*

➤ *To prevent kidney stones, drink at least 8 to 12 glasses of water a day. This keeps urine diluted, reducing the likelihood that kidney stone crystals will form.*

➤ *Excess intake of oxalate-rich foods (such as spinach, rhubarb, parsley, and cocoa) may contribute to the incidence of stones by interfering with calcium absorption.*

For More Information
National Kidney Foundation
30 East 33rd Street, Suite 1100
New York, NY 10016
800-622-9010
www.kidney.org

National Institute of Diabetes and
Digestive and Kidney Diseases
31 Center Drive, MSC 2560
Bethesda, MD 20892-2560
301-654-3810
www.niddk.nih.gov

Complementary and Alternative Treatments

Nutrition and Supplementation

Water is essential for healthy kidneys. Drink at least 3 quarts of pure water daily. Mix the juice of a fresh lemon in a glass of warm water and drink that each morning to help prevent stones from forming. Unsweetened cranberry juice controls bacterial growth. To relieve pain, drink the juice of half a fresh lemon in 8 ounces of water every half hour until the pain subsides. You can alternate apple juice with lemon juice.

Because vitamin A is beneficial to the urinary tract and discourages the formation of stones, eat foods such as alfalfa, apricots, cantaloupes, carrots, pumpkin, sweet potatoes, and squash.

Eliminate foods that contain or lead to the production of oxalic acid. This includes asparagus, beets, eggs, fish, parsley, rhubarb, spinach, and vegetables belonging to the cabbage family. Other foods to avoid include chocolate, dried figs, nuts, pepper, poppy seeds, black tea, alcohol, and caffeine. Dairy products and animal protein are not recommended. Diets high in animal protein cause the body to excrete calcium, and this results in excessive amounts of calcium, phosphorus, and uric acid in the kidneys. This, in turn, leads to kidney stones.

Nutritionists recommend a daily supplement program such as the following:

Most Important

- L-methionine (500 mg, on empty stomach)— destroys free radicals and reduces kidney stones

- magnesium (500 mg)—reduces calcium absorption

- zinc (50 to 80 mg, not to exceed 100 mg)—inhibits crystallization, which can lead to stone formation

- vitamin B complex (including 50 mg each of folate, B_6, and B_{12})—promotes healing

Also Recommended

- L-arginine (500 mg)—improves kidney disorders

- raw kidney glandular (500 mg)—strengthens the kidneys

- vitamin A (25,000 IU; do not exceed 8000 IU if you are pregnant)—heals urinary tract lining

- vitamin C (3000 to 6000 mg)—discourages stone formation

- glutathione (200 mg)

Kidney Stones

(Consult your healthcare provider regarding the duration of treatment.)

Ayurvedic Medicine

 According to Ayurveda, kidney stones can be a vata, pitta, or kapha disorder, and may be composed of calcium, phosphate, or oxalate. Ayurvedic practitioners may recommend eating barley soup with *dugdapachan bhasma, gokshura,* and *mutral churna* or *punarnava* three times daily to promote passing of stones. They also may suggest applying alternating hot and ice compresses to the kidney area until the pain lessens or disappears.

Ayurvedic products are available at many health food stores and Indian pharmacies.

Bodywork and Somatic Practices

 Oriental bodywork therapies and reflexology are good first lines of action for these painful conditions. Include Reiki and Therapeutic Touch for extra loving care.

Traditional Chinese Medicine

 Acupuncture Acupuncture can reduce the pain of kidney stones and help prevent infection. The practitioner focuses on points along the kidney and bladder meridians, along with related points in the ear.

Chinese Herbal Therapy Long-term use of *Te Xiao Pai Shi Wan* pills is helpful.

LACTOSE INTOLERANCE

Signs and Symptoms

Symptoms of lactose intolerance appear after consuming dairy products and include:

- Abdominal cramps
- Abdominal bloating
- Diarrhea
- Vomiting
- Flatulence

Description

Lactose is the primary sugar found in cow's milk. To digest lactose, the human body manufactures an enzyme called lactase, which is produced by the lining of the small intestine. However, not everyone's small intestine produces enough lactase to properly digest milk, cheese, ice cream, and other dairy products, resulting in a condition known as lactose intolerance. For those who suffer from lactose intolerance, consumption of dairy products may result in an array of abdominal symptoms, including cramps, gas, bloating, and diarrhea. These signs usually occur within an hour after ingestion and are the result of bacterial fermentation of undigested lactose in the colon, which disrupts fluid reabsorption and produces watery diarrhea.

It is unknown why some people are lactose intolerant while others can enjoy dairy products without problems. Ethnicity seems to play the largest role in determining whether a person can or cannot tolerate milk products. It is estimated that nearly 100 percent of indigenous North Americans (Native Americans) do not produce enough lactase; approximately 80 to 90 percent of people of African, Asian, Mediterranean, and Middle Eastern descent are lactose intolerant. On the other hand, only 3 to 5 percent of all Northern and Western European descendants have the problem.

In a small number of instances, a person's lactose production may be hampered by illness, such as an infection of the small intestine, cystic fibrosis, inflammatory bowel disease, or AIDS.

Conventional Medical Treatment

If you have digestive distress after consuming dairy products, see your physician, who can diagnose lactose intolerance by taking a detailed history of incidences, including what was eaten prior to the onset of symptoms. Your doctor also may wish to conduct a lactose absorption test, hydrogen breath test, digestive stool analysis, or stool acidity test to confirm diagnosis. Treatment for lactose intolerance consists of taking over-the-counter lactase tablets before ingesting dairy products and drinking low-lactose milk, available in the refrigerated section of most supermarkets.

Are You Really Lactose Intolerant?

A recent study tested individuals who described themselves as lactose intolerant but who had not been tested for the condition. The study found no difference in the amount of gastrointestinal distress after a week of drinking a cup of regular whole milk each day and a week of drinking a daily cup of treated milk (in which the lactose had been pre-digested). The researchers concluded that lactose intolerance has become a popular scapegoat for individuals facing gastric distress brought on by other sources.

➤ *Yogurt with active cultures is generally a good dairy option for people with lactose intolerance. The bacteria in yogurt actually contain lactose, which successfully passes through the acidic environment of the stomach and is released into the intestine, where it aids in the digestion of lactose.*

➤ *Aged cheese often causes no problems for individuals who are lactose intolerant. Most of the lactose is removed from the milk during cheesemaking. In addition, the remaining lactose is converted into lactic acid during the aging process.*

Complementary and Alternative Treatments

Nutrition and Supplementation

The most important rule is to avoid milk and all dairy products, although yogurt is often tolerated because it contains cultures that digest the lactose contained in the product. Foods high in calcium are important: broccoli, collards, calcium-fortified orange juice, rhubarb, kale, tofu, and yogurt. Consider taking calcium supplements.

Do not eat solid foods during an attack. Instead, drink plenty of pure water. The following recommended daily supplements help treat lactose intolerance:

Most Important

- charcoal tablets (4 tablets hourly during an attack; take until symptoms subside)—absorb toxins and relieve diarrhea
- a prodophilus formula (1 tsp in distilled water, 2 times daily)—replaces friendly bacteria; use a non-dairy formula like *Lactobacillus sporogenes*
- a digestive enzyme supplement (as directed on label)—assures normal digestion and absorption

Also Recommended

- calcium carbonate (1000 mg)—absorbs intestinal toxins
- magnesium (500 mg)—necessary for calcium absorption
- vitamin D (400 IU)—necessary for calcium absorption
- vitamin E (400 to 1000 IU)—protects cells that line the colon wall
- zinc (30 mg)—maintains immune system

(Consult your healthcare provider regarding the duration of treatment.)

LARYNGITIS

Signs and Symptoms

- Hoarse or whispery voice, or loss of voice
- Itching, tickling, or rawness of the throat
- Constant urge to clear the throat
- Pain when speaking
- Fever
- Coughing

Description

The larynx is a part of the windpipe that contains the vocal cords. Laryngitis occurs when the mucous membranes of the larynx become irritated or infected, causing the vocal chords to become inflamed and swollen. As a result, the enlarged vocal chords are unable to open and close properly, producing a hoarse, soft whisper—or complete loss of voice.

Laryngitis can be caused by a number of factors. Excessive smoking, alcohol consumption, or recreational drug use can irritate the larynx. Laryngitis also can be caused by inhaling airborne chemicals or by talking or singing more than usual. Laryngitis is often the result of a viral or bacterial infection that originated with a cold, flu, bronchitis, or pneumonia.

Conventional Medical Treatment

Whether irritation or infection is to blame, laryngitis is usually treated with voice rest, over-the-counter analgesics (painkillers), and avoidance of all irritating substances (including alcohol, smoke, and household chemicals). If the condition does not improve after taking these measures, see your doctor, who may analyze throat tissue for signs of bacterial infection. In cases of severe bacterial infection, antibiotics also may be prescribed.

Health Notes

➤ *You can ease a case of laryngitis by drinking increased amounts of water, juice, herbal tea, or other non-alcoholic, non-caffeinated beverages. Liquids help soothe the throat by keeping mucus secretions liquefied and throat tissue moist.*

➤ *Another way to soothe irritated vocal cords is to directly inhale steam, either from a steaming tea kettle or humidifier.*

Complementary and Alternative Treatments

Nutrition and Supplementation

 Avoid refined carbohydrates and focus on whole foods with plenty of raw fruits and vegetables. Drink plenty of pure water and herbal teas, and follow these suggested daily guidelines for supplements:

- vitamin A (50,000 IU for 3 days; do not exceed 8000 IU daily if you are pregnant)
- vitamin C (2000 mg)
- garlic capsules (as directed on label)
- zinc (15 mg lozenge twice daily)
- a prodophilus formula (as directed on label)—is especially important if you are taking antibiotics
- glutathione (oral spray form) (as directed on label)

(For an *acute* condition, take supplements until your symptoms subside. If symptoms persist, seek the advice of your healthcare provider. For a *chronic* condition, consult your healthcare provider regarding the duration of treatment.)

Aromatherapy

 The essential oils of lavender, frankincense, sandalwood, and red thyme can relieve the hoarseness and discomfort associated with laryngitis. You can add several drops to a steam inhalation or place a drop or two on a tissue or handkerchief and inhale. Alternately, you can add 3 drops of lavender, sandalwood, or lemon oil to half a glass of water and gargle with the mixture.

Ayurvedic Medicine

 To ease the discomfort of laryngitis and recover your voice, Ayurvedic practitioners often favor an infusion of cloves, ginger, or mint.

Bodywork and Somatic Practices

Polarity therapy, reflexology, and Oriental bodywork techniques can be helpful.

Herbal Therapy

Gargle with cooled goldenseal or sage tea to ease the sore, inflamed, raspy throat that usually accompanies laryngitis. To make goldenseal tea, stir 1 teaspoon dried leaves into 1 cup boiling water; steep for 10 minutes; strain. For sage tea, chop 2 teaspoons fresh leaves and add to 1 cup boiling water. Steep for 10 to 15 minutes and strain. Both teas can be used for 2 to 3 days.

You also can try gargling with bayberry, red sage, yarrow, or chamomile teas. Make standard infusions of 1 teaspoon dried herb in 1 cup boiling water and let cool before using.

Echinacea, taken internally as a tea or tincture, can blunt the discomfort of laryngitis.

Homeopathy

Your homeopathic practitioner may recommend one of the following treatments for laryngitis, depending on your symptoms: *Argentum nitricum* if you've overused your voice, and your throat feels raw and sore; *Arum triphylum* if your voice is hoarse and cracks.

Hydrotherapy

Apply alternating hot and cold compresses once or twice daily to the neck and throat to soothe general discomfort and aching in the area.

You also can try steam inhalation for 10 minutes or so every hour throughout the day. For directions, see "Hydrotherapy" in the "Introduction to Complementary Therapies" section.

Traditional Chinese Medicine

Acupuncture This modality can lessen the pain and inflammation of laryngitis, and also can help quiet a cough. Acupuncture points include those related to the pharynx and larynx, heart, and lungs.

Acupressure To alleviate the symptoms of laryngitis, the practitioner may focus on Liver 4, Lung 7, and Conception Vessel 22.

Chinese Herbal Therapy Mint is a very soothing herb often prescribed in cases of laryngitis. It can be taken in infusion, powder, or decoction form (up to 4 grams a day). Chinese herbalists also suggest brewing mint leaves into a tea and taking with honey, as needed. The Chinese over-the-counter medicine known as Laryngitis Pills are also useful for treating this condition.

LEAD POISONING

Signs and Symptoms

In early stages of exposure, lead poisoning often produces no symptoms. If symptoms are present, they usually include:

- Headaches
- Sluggishness
- Inability to concentrate
- Irritability

- Personality changes
- Poor appetite
- Unexplained weight loss
- Vomiting
- Constipation
- Severe abdominal pain
- Metallic taste in mouth
- Confusion
- Seizures

Description

Lead is a poisonous substance that, if ingested or inhaled, can accumulate in the kidneys, nerves, and bone marrow. Unfortunately, lead poisoning often produces no symptoms in its early stages. In other cases, its signs are so subtle that the victim does not recognize the illness. Symptoms generally appear gradually, becoming more obvious after many years of continuous exposure.

Ongoing accumulation of lead in the body can result in serious health problems. Brain damage is rare in adults, but even mild elevations of blood levels in children can lead to impaired intellectual ability. Long-term exposure can lead to permanent brain damage.

While lead is no longer used in most consumer products, many Americans still come into contact with it in the form of lead-based paint and pipes (typically found in buildings built prior to 1980) and in auto emissions. People who engage in hobbies in which lead is present—including pottery (some glazes still contain lead), target shooting, car or boat repair, and old home restoration and remodeling—are also at increased risk. Individuals who are exposed to lead at work are in danger of developing lead poisoning. Jobs in bridge abatement (which involves sandblasting lead paint), radiator repair, painting, plumbing, auto body repair, building and bridge construction, glass and electronic component manufacturing, ship building, steel working, ammunition manufacturing, and lead mining and smelting put workers at increased risk. (The Occupational

Standards and Health Administration [OSHA] has standards and rules in place for the protection of workers, but studies have found that many companies do not meet the regulations, and guidelines are often ignored.)

Conventional Medical Treatment

If you suspect that you have lead poisoning, visit your physician, who may take a blood test to detect traces of the metal in the bloodstream. Blood levels of 10 micrograms per deciliter in children and 30 micrograms in adults are unhealthy.

Health Notes

➤ *Homes built before 1980 should be checked for lead pipes, lead soldering, lead paint, and lead particles in soil around the home. For more information, including where to turn for help in checking for lead, contact your local Environmental Protection Agency (EPA) office.*

➤ *If older paint surfaces are to be sanded or scraped, pregnant women, young children, people with high blood pressure, and pets should be kept away from the area.*

➤ *If you have an infant or young child, keep his or her crib and playpen away from radiators, exposed pipes, and painted walls and windowsills.*

➤ *Always have children wash their hands after playing outdoors, since you never know what surfaces they touched. This is particularly true before meals and nap or bedtime, when they may be using their hands or sucking their thumbs.*

➤ *Frequent home cleaning with a phosphate solution may help protect you and your family against lead poisoning.*

Lead Poisoning

Most cases of childhood lead poisoning are detected during a routine screening. If you are diagnosed with lead poisoning, your doctor may prescribe a chelation drug, which binds to the lead in your blood and ushers it out of your body through the urine. This type of therapy is most effective during the condition's early stages. If it is allowed to progress, lead poisoning can cause kidney damage, which often leads to kidney disease. In such cases, chelation therapy is used in combination with kidney disease treatments, such as angiotensin-converting enzyme (ACE) inhibitors. Medication to keep blood pressure at around 130/80 mm Hg also may be prescribed, in order to ease the kidney's workload.

For More Information
Environmental Health Center-Division of
National Safety Council
1025 Connecticut Avenue NW, Suite 1200
Washington, DC 20036
(202) 293-2270
National Lead Information Hotline:
800-424-LEAD
www.nsc.org/ehc/lead.htm

Complementary and Alternative Treatments

Nutrition and Supplementation

 If you suspect lead poisoning, have a hair analysis done. This will confirm long-term accumulation, whereas blood tests identify only the most recent exposure. Foods that rid the body of lead include legumes, beans, eggs, onions, and garlic. Your diet should be high in fiber and contain pectin, which is found in apples. Drink only pure water and do not smoke, or expose yourself to secondhand smoke.

Nutritionists recommend the following daily supplements:

Most Important

- apple pectin (as directed on the label)—removes toxins and metals from the body

- calcium (2000 mg)—prevents lead from being deposited in the body tissues. Use chelate form, and *do not* obtain it from bone meal or cow's milk, which also can contain lead

- magnesium (1000 mg)—balances with calcium

- garlic (as directed on label)—binds with and excretes lead

- kelp (as directed on label)—removes unwanted metal deposits

- L-lysine (500 mg, on empty stomach)—improves calcium absorption

- vitamin C with bioflavonoids (5000 to 20,000 mg)—neutralizes the effects of lead

- zinc (80 mg, not to exceed a total of 100 mg from all supplements)—displaces lead

Also Recommended

- glutathione (250 mg)

- N-acetyl cysteine (250 mg)

- Inositol hexaphosphate (IP_6, as directed on label)—removes heavy metals from body

(Consult your healthcare provider regarding the duration of treatment.)

Traditional Chinese Medicine

 Acupuncture Acupuncture can be used to enhance overall immunity and improve the flow of *chi* throughout the body, which can help speed the elimination of toxins such as lead. It also can be used to help remedy various symptoms of lead poisoning, such as fatigue, mental confusion, anxiety, high blood pressure, tinnitus, headaches, muscle pain, and gastrointestinal ailments.

Acupressure While acupressure cannot cure lead poisoning, it can be used to relieve the symptoms brought about by the condition.

Chinese Herbal Therapy Generally, almost any liver formulas will help to some extent.

LICE

Signs and Symptoms

- Intense itching at the infested site (usually in the hair of the head or pubic area)
- Tiny eggs on shafts of hair
- Lice bodies or eggs on the clothing or in bedding
- Tiny bite marks or rash at the infested site
- Tiny pinprick-sized spots of blood in underwear (in women, not related to menstruation)

Description

Lice are tiny parasites that feed on the blood of their hosts. Although they do not represent a serious medical threat, lice can cause uncomfortable itching and are highly contagious. They usually infest areas of the body that are covered by hair—the head or pubic region.

Head lice are tiny parasites that are very difficult to locate; often the only signs of infestation are intense itching and tiny red bumps on the scalp, caused when the lice burrow into the skin to feed. Sometimes their tiny white eggs, called nits, are visible where they are attached to hair

Health Notes

➤ If someone in your family has lice, everyone he or she has come in contact with—whether or not they have visible parasites—should also undergo treatment.

➤ If you have lice, do not scratch the area to relieve itching. Scratching the small bites can lead to bleeding or infection.

➤ To prevent your children from getting lice, teach them not to share combs, brushes, hair ornaments, or hats with other children.

shafts. Head lice are easily spread from person to person, especially among young children, who often share combs, brushes, and hats and have frequent physical contact with one another.

Pubic lice are also known as crab lice because they resemble crabs in appearance and use their crab-like claws to affix themselves to the host. Tiny and gray, pubic lice are as difficult to locate and cause the same intense itching as head lice. And like head lice, pubic lice lay eggs on the shafts of hair—eggs that are not easily washed off during bathing. They are usually transmitted during sex, though they also can spread via infested bedding, clothing, or toilet seats.

Conventional Medical Treatment

Unless they are extremely severe, lice can be treated without medical intervention. Apply an over-the-counter anti-lice lotion or shampoo to the affected area according to the package directions. Most treatments require several applications over a two-week period—the amount of time it takes for louse eggs to hatch. Any remaining eggs or dead lice should be removed with tweezers or special, thin-pronged lice combs. In addition, all bedding, towels, grooming items, clothes, and rugs should be washed in hot, soapy water. To treat pubic lice, you may wish to shave the pubic area. In severe cases, your physician can prescribe a stronger anti-lice product to apply.

Complementary and Alternative Treatments

Traditional Chinese Medicine

 Chinese Herbal Therapy Several Chinese herbs can be made into a wash or ointment and used to treat head lice. These include Chinaberry bark, cnidium monnieri, alum, camphor, and acorus.

LOW BLOOD PRESSURE (HYPOTENSION)

Signs and Symptoms

- Dizziness
- Lightheadedness
- Headaches
- Fatigue

Description

Low blood pressure, or hypotension, does not get as much attention as high blood pressure, probably because it does not affect as many people. The primary symptom of low blood pressure is lightheadedness, caused by decreased blood flow to the brain. This lightheadedness most commonly occurs when someone with hypotension stands up from a seated or reclining position. In fact, some sufferers even faint when rising. This condition is referred to as orthostatic hypotension. It is not an uncommon symptom, but if it occurs frequently, it may be caused by medications, hormone deficiencies, heart problems, or neurologic disorders. Orthostatic hypotension can also occur after an illness, such as gastrointestinal infection, which causes dehydration.

Blood pressure is described in terms of systolic pressure, measured when the heart contracts to send blood through the veins, and diastolic pressure, measured when the heart relaxes and draws blood into its chambers. A normal blood pressure reading has a systolic pressure of 140 and a diastolic pressure of 85—or 140/85. When blood pressure falls below 90/60, it is considered unusually low.

Conventional Medical Treatment

If you know you have low blood pressure—or frequently feel dizzy upon standing—visit your physician, who can diagnose low blood pressure

Health Notes

➤ If you have low blood pressure, make a conscious effort to rise slowly, even holding onto a piece of furniture as you go. If, at any time, you stand and feel faint, slowly sit back down again until the feeling passes.

➤ If you have hypotension, and are unnaturally tired after performing physical tasks or suffer from daily fatigue, consider being tested for chronic fatigue syndrome. New research has uncovered a link between chronic fatigue syndrome and blood pressure lower than 90/60.

➤ Regular, moderate exercise increases blood circulation throughout the body, making it especially useful in combating symptoms of low blood pressure.

➤ If you have hypotension, avoid becoming overheated, which can worsen symptoms of the condition.

by taking a blood pressure reading. You also may want to ask your physician to determine your sodium/potassium ratio. If there is an underlying cause, your doctor will treat that, but in most cases, medication is not used to treat low blood pressure.

Complementary and Alternative Treatments

Nutrition and Supplementation

 Ask your healthcare provider to check your sodium/potassium ratio for possible imbalance. Nutritionists recommend the following daily supplements:

- Kelp (1 to 3 tablets daily)—if you are taking thyroid medication, kelp may decrease the need for the amount you are taking; consult your healthcare provider

- multivitamin and amino acid-chelated mineral complex (1 tablet or capsule 2 times daily)

- an antioxidant formula containing alpha- and beta-carotene, lutein, lycopene, vitamins C and E, selenium, ginkgo biloba, coenzyme Q10, soy isoflavones, bilberry, L-glutathione, grape seed extract, and green tea extract (1 tablet or capsule 2 times daily)

(Consult your healthcare provider regarding the duration of treatment.)

Traditional Chinese Medicine

Acupuncture Acupuncture can be used to help regulate blood pressure and remedy dizziness, headaches, and poor circulation. The points most likely involved are Liver 3, Triple Warmer 25, and auricular points relating to the heart and adrenal gland.

Acupressure Pressing the Yin Tang spot between the eyebrows and Liver 3 (in the webbing between the big and middle toe) may help prevent dizziness. Headaches can be relieved by pressing Large Intestine 4 (which lies between the thumb and forefinger) and Gallbladder 20 (at the base of the skull on either side of the spine).

Chinese Herbal Therapy Aloe vera and ginseng may be useful in regulating low blood pressure. The practitioner's goal is to bring about a balance and to build the patient's strength.

LUPUS

Signs and Symptoms

- Severe joint pains and joint swelling
- Rash across the nose and cheeks
- Sensitivity to sunlight
- Weakness and fatigue
- Weight loss
- Ulcers of the mouth or throat
- Mental confusion
- Anemia
- Kidney dysfunction

Basic Description

Lupus is a chronic disease in which the immune system attacks the connective tissue of joints, muscles, and skin as well as the membranes surrounding other body organs. People with lupus are often constantly tired and especially sensitive to sunlight. On the other hand, the rashes and joint pain that also characterize the disorder are episodic—one day symptoms are present, the next day they are not.

The exact causes of lupus are unknown, though heredity is believed to play a role in determining risk. African Americans are three times as likely as Caucasian Americans to develop the condition. The vast majority of lupus victims are women, and the condition most often strikes between the ages of 15 and 35.

Conventional Medical Treatment

If you have symptoms of lupus, see your physician, who can diagnose the condition with a blood test. For many lupus victims, the only treat-

In a Different Light

Ultraviolet light can trigger painful flare-ups in lupus sufferers, prompting many to head indoors when the sun shines. On the other hand, recent research has found that one type of ultraviolet light actually improves lupus. Although UVB light can trigger lupus, patients who were administered pure UVA-1 light experienced decreased fatigue, joint pain, headaches, and other problems, which allowed them to reduce their medication intake. This light may help repair the internal skin damage that accounts for many of the symptoms of lupus. Unfortunately, sunlight contains both UVB and UVA light, so simply spending time in the sun is not a safe way to get UVA rays, and pure UVA treatment is still in experimental stages. Also, equipment needed to deliver pure UVA-1 light costs thousands of dollars, meaning funding is needed to study the therapy and earn FDA approval.

Health Notes

➤ *If you suffer from lupus, talk to your healthcare provider about dehydroepiandrosterone (DHEA) supplements. Several studies have found that lupus patients have abnormally low levels of the hormone. Oral DHEA supplements have been shown to relieve rashes, joint pain, headaches, and fatigue in some patients.*

➤ *If you are a woman, talk to your healthcare provider about the estrogen in oral contraceptives and hormone replacement therapy. Some estrogen studies have found the hormone to lessen symptoms as well as the frequency of bouts in women with lupus; other studies have found that estrogen puts women at a greater risk for developing lupus.*

➤ *Silicone breast implants may put women at increased risk for developing lupus and other autommimune disorders.*

ment necessary is avoidance of excessive sunlight and constant use of a strong sunscreen lotion. In most cases the disease is not considered serious, and approximately 40 percent of victims experience a spontaneous—and total—remission.

Mild cases of lupus may only require the use of aspirin to relieve symptoms. In serious cases, lupus can lead to inflammation around the heart and lungs, kidney disease, or serious joint damage. If you suffer from a severe case of lupus, your physician may place you on corticosteroids to limit joint inflammation. You also must undergo checkups on a monthly basis so that you can treat any of the above complications as they arise.

For More Information
Lupus Foundation of America, Inc.
1300 Piccard Drive, Suite 200
Rockville, MD 20850-4303
800-558-0121
www.lupus.org

Complementary and Alternative Treatments

Nutrition and Supplementation

Lupus is often triggered by an allergic reaction to food. People with lupus commonly have trouble with foods such as peanuts, soy, wheat, corn, meat, dairy, and oranges. A diet that is easy on the kidneys is low in fat, salt, and animal protein. Get plenty of sardines (a good source of essential fatty acids), brown rice, fish, green leafy vegetables, oatmeal, whole grains, and non-acidic fresh fruits. Asparagus, eggs, garlic, and onions contain sulfur, which you need to repair bone, cartilage, and connective tissue. It also enhances the uptake of calcium. Consume fiber daily.

It is important to get your iron from food sources rather than supplements. Iron supplements can cause pain and swelling. Eat fresh pineapple often, as it contains bromelain, which is great for reducing inflammation. However, avoid peppers, eggplant, tomatoes, and white potatoes, as these foods contain solanine, which contributes to inflammation and pain. Also avoid alfalfa, caffeine, tobacco, and any foods that contain sugar.

Follow these daily recommendations:

Most Important

- calcium (1500 mg)—balances pH and protects against bone loss
- magnesium (750 mg 2 times daily)—balances with calcium
- N-acetyl cysteine and L-methionine (500 to 1000 mg each, on empty stomach)—vital to skin formation and in white blood cell activity
- L-lysine (500 to 1000 mg)—prevents mouth sores

Also Recommended

- flaxseed oil (as directed on label)—protects skin cells; aids in the reproduction of all body cells
- glucosamine sulfate (as directed on label)—important for healthy skin, bones, and connective tissue
- N-acetyl glucosamine (as directed on label)—may help to prevent lupus erythematosus

- garlic (as directed on label)—protects enzyme systems
- zinc (50 to 100 mg; do not exceed this amount)—promotes healing; protects organs
- vitamin B complex (including 50 mg each of folate, B_6, and B_{12})

(Consult your healthcare provider regarding the duration of treatment; also ask about DHEA supplementation.)

Traditional Chinese Medicine

 Acupuncture Acupuncture may be helpful in reducing the pain and inflammation associated with lupus. It also can be used to strengthen the patient's immune system.

Chinese Herbal Therapy Many of the same herbs used to treat arthritis can be helpful in cases of lupus joint pain as well. See "Traditional Chinese Medicine" in the "Arthritis" entry for more information on specific Chinese herbs and dosages. Likewise, see the "Kidney Disease" and "Kidney Infection" entries for herbs that may be used to treat lupus-induced kidney problems.

LYME DISEASE

Signs and Symptoms

- Circular "bulls eye" rash, often with a red border and clear center, at the site of a tick bite
- Headache
- Fever and chills

- Body aches
- Sore throat
- Joint pain and inflammation
- Fatigue
- Loss of mental acuity
- Irregular heartbeat or chest pain

Lyme Disease

Description

Lyme disease was named after Lyme, Connecticut, where the disease was discovered. The disease is spread by ticks, though only a few species of ticks carry the bacterial organism that causes Lyme disease. One species is the deer tick, or black-legged tick, which lives in the Northeastern, Southern, and Midwestern United States. Another is the Western black-legged tick, which inhabits the Pacific coastal states. Victims rarely feel the insect's bite because it injects an anesthetic (which numbs the area of skin) both when it punctures the skin and when it withdraws. Many experts believe that the tick must be attached to the body for at least 24 hours for infection to occur.

The first symptoms of Lyme disease appear anywhere from 3 to 32 days after infection. One of the most recognizable early signs is a circular, red "bull's-eye" rash at the site of the bite (though the rash does not appear in many cases). In its initial stages, other symptoms of the illness resemble those of the flu—intermittent fatigue, fever, nausea, headache, and chills. If the condition is not treated in its early stages, serious secondary symptoms can occur weeks or months later. These include arthritis, joint disability, muscle problems, and heart, nervous system, and even brain disorders.

Health Notes

➤ When walking in wooded or grassy areas, always wear long sleeves, a hat, and long pants tucked into shoes or boots. Always perform a full body check for ticks after returning.

➤ May through August are prime months for Lyme disease, mainly because the infected ticks are in their infancy stage and easily escape detection due to their small size.

➤ If you need to remove a tick, do so with with thin-tipped tweezers. Do not twist the tick right out; instead, cover the area with petroleum jelly or clear nail polish (to cause it to release) and exert a slow steady pull. If you are worried that the tick could carry Lyme disease, place it in a small jar of alcohol, and take it to the doctor for identification. Disinfect the site of the bite with alcohol after removal.

Conventional Medical Treatment

If you suspect you may have Lyme disease, visit your doctor immediately. If it is detected and treated early, the disease often causes no lasting harm; if, on the other hand, it is left to worsen, it can cause permanent complications involving the joints, heart, and brain. Your doctor can diagnose the condition with a blood test. Treatment for Lyme disease includes antibiotics to fight the bacteria and aspirin to help relieve any joint inflammation.

For More Information
Lyme Disease Foundation
One Financial Plaza, 18th Floor
Hartford, CT 06103
800-886-LYME
www.lyme.org

Complementary and Alternative Treatments

Nutrition and Supplementation

 Garlic is a natural immune booster, so you would benefit from eating it in its natural state or taking it in supplement form. "Green drinks" provide chlorophyll, which detoxifies, along with vital nutrients and enzymes. These can be found in your natural foods store.

To improve your condition, follow these recommended daily guidelines:

Most Important

- essential fatty acids (as directed on label)—reduce joint stiffness and inflammation
- pancreatin and bromelain (as directed on label)—aid digestion
- evening primrose oil (1000 mg 2 to 3 times daily)—combats pain and inflammation

Also Recommended

- garlic (as directed on label)
- kelp (1000 to 1500 mg)—detoxifies the body
- selenium (200 mcg)—a free radical scavenger
- multivitamin and mineral complex (as directed on label)—use a high-potency formula for necessary nutrients

- glutathione (600 mg)
- thymic extract (as directed on label)
- maitake D fraction (as directed on label)—boosts immunity

(Consult your healthcare provider regarding the duration of treatment.)

Traditional Chinese Medicine

 Acupuncture Acupuncture treatment can be used to help relieve the fatigue, joint pain, and related side effects of Lyme disease.

MACULAR DEGENERATION

Signs and Symptoms

- Blurred vision in one or both eyes that grows increasingly worse
- Straight vertical or horizontal lines appear crooked or broken
- Blank spots in central vision

Description

Macular degeneration is a loss of central vision in the eye; usually, the peripheral vision remains intact. It is the most common form of vision loss in the United States. The condition usually occurs when abnormal small blood vessels grow in the eye's macular region, which is located between the retina and its supporting layer of tissue. These new vessels often leak blood onto the retina, killing retinal cells. When this occurs, central vision is affected.

The exact cause of macular degeneration is unknown, though heredity is thought to play a role. The condition most commonly strikes people over the age of 65. Other risk factors include: light eye color, cardiovascular disease, short height, lung infections, a history of excessive sunlight exposure, and cigarette smoking.

Conventional Medical Treatment

If you notice changes in your vision, visit an ophthalmologist, who can evaluate the blood vessel pattern in the eye and look for abnormal blood vessels. If you are diagnosed with macular degeneration, your doctor may recommend laser therapy to seal abnormal blood vessels, to slow or prevent further vision loss. To help your eyes heal—or prevent untreated eyes from growing worse—your ophthalmologist also may suggest wearing sunglasses with UV protection whenever you are exposed to sunlight.

Health Notes

➤ Wear sunglasses in all weather and avoid the sun when it is at its brightest, from 11 a.m. to 3 p.m. Damage from lifetime sun exposure is one of the most common causes of macular degeneration in the United States.

➤ According to two studies, smoking at least a pack of cigarettes a day more than doubles your risk of developing age-related macular degeneration. Smoking can lead to diseases of the blood vessels, slower blood flow, and impaired circulation, which may lead to retinal damage.

For More Information

Macular Degeneration Foundation
P.O. Box 9752
San Jose, CA 95157
888-MDF-EYES
www.eyesight.org

National Eye Institute (NEI)
2020 Vision Place
Bethesda, MD 20892-3655
301-496-5248
www.nei.nih.gov

Complementary and Alternative Treatments

Nutrition and Supplementation

 Increase your intake of legumes, yellow vegetables, berries (blueberries, blackberries, and cherries), and foods rich in vitamins E and C, such as raw fruits and vegetables. Avoid all sugars, saturated fats, cigarette smoke, and alcohol, plus drink lots of water.

Follow this daily supplement program to prevent and treat macular degeneration.

Most Important

- mixed carotenoid formula (2000 IU)—improves all eye disorders
- grape seed extract (as directed on label)—is a powerful antioxidant
- selenium (400 mcg)—is an antioxidant
- vitamin A (50,000 to 100,000 IU; do not exceed 8000 IU if you are pregnant)—is a powerful antioxidant important to eye function
- vitamin C with bioflavonoids (1000 to 2500 mg 4 times daily)—prevents eye damage
- vitamin E (600 to 800 IU)—destroys free radicals
- zinc (45 to 80 mg, not to exceed a total of 100 mg from all supplements)—a deficiency has been linked to macular degeneration; use zinc picolinate form

Also Recommended

- glutathione (600 mg)
- riboflavin (B$_2$, 50 mg)

(Consult your healthcare provider regarding the duration of treatment.)

Traditional Chinese Medicine

 Acupuncture TCM attributes most eye and vision problems to liver dysfunction. A TCM practitioner, therefore, treats macular degeneration by using acupuncture to tone the liver and improve circulation to the eyes, which may enhance the eyes' ability to function properly. Also, due to the degenerative nature of the disease, the practitioner works on the kidney as well, as it is pinpointed to be the basis of all other organ function.

Chinese Herbal Therapy Patent medicines that may be used to combat macular degeneration are *Ming Mu Dihuang Wan*, Rehmannia and Magnetitum Formula, and Dendrobium Moniliforme Night Sight Pills.

MASTITIS

Signs and Symptoms

- Red, tender, painful lump or swollen area in the breast
- Swelling of the nearby gland in the armpit
- Fever
- Pus discharge from the nipple of the affected breast

Description

Mastitis is a common breast infection among lactating women. It is caused when bacteria enters a breast through a cracked or abraded nipple. The bacteria causes a localized infection and an abscess of pus develops.

Conventional Medical Treatment

If you suspect you have mastitis, visit your physician, who will physically examine the breast. A needle biopsy of the lump may be necessary to confirm diagnosis. Most cases of mastitis can be treated with oral antibiotics and analgesics (pain-killers). If the abscess is severe, it may need to be drained. Talk to your physician about alternative

Health Notes

➤ If you have mastitis, continue to massage the infected breast gently to expel milk and prevent painful engorgement.

➤ If you are breastfeeding, keep your nipples clean and dry between feedings and avoid clothing that irritates them.

➤ Do not allow your baby to bite or chew on your nipple. Small cuts can allow bacteria to enter the breast, causing mastitis.

feeding options for your baby while you are being treated for mastitis.

For More Information
American College of Obstetricians and Gynecologists
409 12th Street, SW
P.O. Box 96920
Washington, DC 20090-6920
800-673-8444
www.acog.org

Complementary and Alternative Treatments

Nutrition and Supplementation

 Other than drinking plenty of fluids, there isn't much in the way of diet that can be done to treat mastitis. *Do not* stop nursing or the ducts will remain full. Over-filled ducts can exacerbate the problem.

These daily supplements help the nursing mother and baby:

- free-form amino acid complex (as directed on label)—supplies necessary protein
- calcium (1000 to 1500 mg)—needed by both mother and baby

- magnesium (500 to 750 mg)—balances with calcium
- vitamin B complex (50 mg 2 times daily)—necessary for milk production; relieves stress
- prenatal vitamins (continue prescribed regimen)

(Consult your healthcare provider regarding the duration of treatment.)

Herbal Therapy

 Echinacea, with its antibiotic compounds, is very helpful in treating mastitis and healing nipple fissures. Add a dropperful of tincture and 1 or 2 cloves of garlic to ½ cup carrot juice. Blend well in a blender. Drink several times a day.

To aid healing and ease pain, gently massage aloe vera gel into cracked nipples.

Homeopathy

 A homeopathic practitioner may advise one of the following treatments for mastitis, depending on your symptoms:

- *Belladonna*—for breasts that are inflamed, red, hot, tender; throb; and have red streaks radiating from the nipples
- *Bryonia*—for breasts that are hot, hard, and painful, especially when you move
- *Silicea*—if your nipples are cracked and infected
- *Phytolacca*—for breasts that are very firm, sensitive, and have a purple hue; this remedy is also helpful if you feel pain throughout your body when you breastfeed your baby

Hydrotherapy

 Apply warm, moist compresses to the affected breast before feedings to ease discomfort and help ensure that ducts drain.

Traditional Chinese Medicine

 Acupuncture To lessen the inflammation caused by mastitis, the practitioner uses acupuncture to target the following points: Stomach 18 and 44, Gallbladder 41, Large Intestine 4, Small Intestine 1, and Conception Vessel 17. In addition, ear points that correspond to the mammary gland, internal secretion, back of head, and adrenal gland also may be included.

Acupressure To treat mastitis, the practitioner may focus on Stomach 18, Conception Vessel 17, and Bladder 18, 20, and 21.

Chinese Herbal Therapy Leonurus may be used to quell the swelling associated with mastitis. Dandelion also may reduce breast pain and inflammation. The dosage varies, depending upon the severity of the condition and the form in which the herb is taken—check with your TCM practitioner.

MEASLES (RUBEOLA)

Signs and Symptoms

- Body-wide rash
- Fever
- Sore throat
- Runny nose
- Sneezing
- Persistent cough
- Swollen eyelids
- Tiny white spots on the inside of the cheek

Description

Measles, a severe illness that usually strikes children, is caused by a virus that is transmitted via infected droplets—usually the droplets are inhaled from an infected person's sneeze or cough. In healthy people, measles usually poses little health threat. Infants, the elderly, and people with poor health, on the other hand, can develop serious complications, such as pneumonia or encephalitis (inflammation of the brain). Fortunately, people who have had measles become permanently immune, preventing them from getting the disease again.

A few days after being infected with the virus, the measles victim will develop flu-like symptoms, such as a fever, coughing, sneezing, and sore throat. After three to five days, white spots begin to develop on the inside of the cheek, followed by the characteristic red blotchy rash, which appears on the face and slowly spreads to the neck, torso, arms, and legs. This rash may last up to 10 days before slowly fading. Unfortunately, measles is most infectious during the 10 to 14 days after infection, particularly before the rash appears.

Conventional Medical Treatment

If you suspect you have measles, call your physician (rather than making an office visit, since the virus is highly contagious) to see if you need an appointment. Measles usually does not require medical attention and is cared for in isolation until the rash disappears. Acetaminophen and

Measles (Rubeola)

over-the-counter cough medicine can be used to treat individual symptoms.

If, however, you are unsure that you have measles, or are particularly uncomfortable with the illness, your physician may ask to see you. A physical exam is usually all that is necessary to diagnose the condition, although your doctor may take a blood sample. Call your physician immediately if you begin to vomit, since this can be a sign of encephalitis, a dangerous inflammation of the brain.

For More Information
Centers for Disease Control and Prevention
1600 Clifton Road
Atlanta, GA 30333
800-311-3435
www.cdc.gov

Complementary and Alternative Treatments

Nutrition and Supplementation

Drink plenty of fluids, including water, juices, and vegetable broth. Boost your immune system with these daily supplements:

- vitamin A (10,000 IU twice for 1 week, then reduce to 10,000 IU once; do not exceed this dosage; do not exceed 8000 if you are pregnant)

- cod liver oil (as directed on label)—for children who can't swallow capsules

- proteolytic enzymes (as directed on label)—reduces infection

- raw thymus glandular (500 mg twice daily)—stimulates the immune system

- vitamin C (300 to 1000 mg in divided doses for children; 1000 to 3000 mg in divided doses for adults)—vital to immune function; controls fever and infection

- vitamin B complex (50 mg 3 times daily)—promotes healing; for a child under eight, use a formula specifically designed for children

- zinc (1 15-mg lozenge 3 times daily for 4 days, then reduce to 1 lozenge daily)—speeds healing; relieves itchy throat and cough

(Consult your healthcare provider regarding the duration of treatment.)

Traditional Chinese Medicine

Acupuncture Rubeola, also known as hard measles, cannot be cured with acupuncture (as is true of any viral infection), but this treatment can be helpful in lessening associated symptoms, such as fever and rash. Acupuncture also can be used to bolster the immune system, which may help lessen the risk of additional complications, such as bronchitis and ear infections.

Chinese Herbal Therapy A TCM practitioner may recommend that burdock be taken internally, or mixed with water and used as an external wash to combat a measles rash. Red, irritated eyes may be remedied with Chinese black cohosh. A child's dose of Ilex and Evodia (*Gan Mao Ling*) may be used to speed recovery.

m

SYMPTOM:

MEMORY LOSS

Memory loss is frightening—both for the person whose memory is faltering and for those around him or her. In some cases, memory loss is caused by the onset of senility or Alzheimer's disease or recurrent strokes. Fortunately, though, many cases of memory loss can be traced to certain behavioral factors, and thus, are reversible. Memory loss can be caused by such everyday occurrences as stress, overwork, fatigue, depression, preoccupation, or even the use of prescription drugs, such as those used to treat heartburn or diabetes.

If you are experiencing memory loss, speak to your doctor. Disorders such as Alzheimer's disease need immediate medical attention. If, on the other hand, your memory loss is caused by behavioral factors, your doctor may suggest changes in lifestyle or medication to help you regain your memory. For example, recent studies have shown that a high-fiber, plant-based diet, combined with moderate exercise and stress reduction, can help improve memory. Other research shows that intellectual disuse can cause memory decline: older adults improved their memories after five one-hour training sessions.

MÉNIÈRE'S DISEASE

Signs and Symptoms

- Episodes of severe vertigo (dizziness), often accompanied by nausea and vomiting
- Muffled or distorted hearing in the ear
- Ringing in the ears (tinnitus)
- Hearing loss
- Feeling of pressure in the ear
- Headache

Basic Description

Named after Prosper Ménière, who first described the condition over a century ago, Ménière's disease is marked by problems in the inner ear, which is responsible for hearing and balance. Most attacks are accompanied by severe vertigo, or dizziness, and various hearing problems, including hearing loss, ringing in the ear, or a sensitivity to loud noises. An attack can last anywhere from an hour to days or months—there was even an instance of an attack lasting over two years. In one-quarter to one-half of all cases, it will move to the other ear.

While the exact cause of Ménière's disease is not known, there seems to be a connection to an increase of fluid in the labyrinth, a part of the inner ear that helps to control balance. The excess fluid creates pressure within the labyrinth, distorting and sometimes even rupturing the tissue in that area.

Conventional Medical Treatments

If you think you may have Ménière's disease, see your physician, who can perform a variety of

Health Notes

➤ *Although it is not know exactly why, a low-sodium diet has been shown to lessen the frequency and severity of Ménière's symptoms.*

➤ *If you have Ménière's disease, avoid caffeine, alcohol and nicotine—all of which affect the central nervous system and can worsen symptoms of dizziness and vertigo.*

tests. One test measures how well you hear sounds of various frequencies. Another involves flooding the ear with water and monitoring the eyes' response—when performed on a healthy inner ear, the eyes should flicker.

There is no cure for Ménière's disease. Instead, treatment is limited to treating symptoms, not the condition itself. Treatment may include medication to combat the vertigo, dizziness, and nausea, or diuretics to decrease the fluids in the body. However, most Ménière's disease attacks come and go on their own. If you feel an attack coming on, lie down until the symptoms have passed, then call your physician.

In severe cases, or in cases that slip in and out of remission, surgery may be required to relieve the pressure within the inner ear. In some severe cases, parts of the inner ear can be removed in a procedure called *labyrinthectomy*.

Complementary and Alternative Treatments

Nutrition and Supplementation

The exact cause of this disorder is not known, although some doctors recommend a high-protein, low-refined-carbohydrate diet because they have found that people with this disorder have high blood insulin levels. Other factors that may contribute to this disorder

include obesity, alcohol use, smoking, high cholesterol, allergies, stress, and excessive salt intake. Some doctors recommend a hypoglycemic diet (see "Hypoglycemia" entry). Avoid fats, fried foods, salt, and sugar in any form, as well as caffeine.

Nutritionists recommend the following daily supplements:

- manganese (5 mg, taken separately from calcium)—a deficiency may cause this disorder
- chromium picolinate (200 mcg)—controls blood sugar levels
- coenzyme Q10 (100 mg)—improves circulation
- vitamin B_3 (50 mg twice; do not exceed this amount without consulting your doctor)—improves circulation. Do not take if you have a liver disorder, gout, or high blood pressure.
- vitamin B complex (50 mg)—stabilizes the nervous system
- vitamin B_6 (100 mg twice)—reduces fluid retention
- calcium (1500 mg)—stabilizes the nervous system and aids in muscle contraction
- magnesium (1000 mg)—balances calcium; reduce amount if bowels become loose

(Consult your healthcare provider regarding the duration of treatment.)

Aromatherapy

To help relieve the stress brought on by this disorder, try soaking in a warm bath to which you've added no more than 15 drops of the essential oils of lavender, geranium, and sandalwood.

Bodywork and Somatic Practices

CranioSacral Therapy is usually a first therapy for ear and inner ear problems. Other modalities that may help include reflexology, polarity therapy, Oriental bodywork, Therapeutic Touch, and Reiki.

Chiropractic

As a complement to standard medical care, chiropractic may be extremely helpful in reducing the frequency and intensity of the symptoms of this disorder. The chiropractor will typically concentrate on adjusting the upper cervical vertebrae (C1 and C2), which are related to one's center of balance. In conjunction with specific chiropractic adjustment (SCA), heat or ice may be used on a case-by-case basis, depending on the duration and intensity of the patient's symptoms.

Homeopathy

Ménière's disease may respond to homeopathic treatment. However, the selection of a remedy—more than one is available—depends on *your* symptoms and the stage of the condition. Don't try treating this disorder yourself. See a homeopathic professional.

Traditional Chinese Medicine

Acupuncture Acupuncture can be extremely effective in alleviating the dizziness and tinnitus associated with this condition by improving the flow of energy and stimulating circulation to the ears. Auricular therapy may focus on the kidney, heart, internal ear, bladder, and head acupuncture points. The practitioner's focus is on balancing liver function.

Acupressure To relieve the symptoms of Ménière's disease, a practitioner may focus on the "extra points" known as Tai Yang (at the temples) and Yin Tang (between the eyebrows), along with Gallbladder 20, Liver 3, and Triple Warmer 20.

Chinese Herbal Therapy Anemarrhena, Phellodendron, and Rehmannia Formula may be recommended to treat Ménière's disease, but as is always the case in chronic disorders, it is best to work with an herb-trained acupuncturist.

Meningitis

Signs and Symptoms

- Fever
- Severe headache
- Vomiting
- Confusion
- Drowsiness
- Stiff neck
- Shooting pain in the neck and back
- Dark red or purple rash anywhere on the body
- Seizures

Description

Bacterial meningitis is a rare, but serious, condition caused by one of several strains of bacteria that spread from another infected part of the body to the brain or spine. The bacteria attacks the membranes, or meninges, surrounding your brain and spinal cord. While it is not generally considered contagious, meningitis can be spread in confined environments (such as college campuses, boarding schools, and military bases) via infected, exhaled droplets.

Although bacterial meningitis is a medical emergency, it does not always get the emergency medical care it requires because its symptoms resemble a severe flu. The longer an infected person goes without treatment, the greater the risk of permanent neurological damage, hearing loss, blindness, or even death.

There is also a form of meningitis that is caused by a viral infection. The symptoms of viral meningitis are usually very mild—just a headache and malaise. The condition usually improves on its own within one or two weeks.

Conventional Medical Treatment

If you suspect you have bacterial meningitis, immediately seek emergency medical treatment. If you are unable to reach your physician, go to the nearest emergency clinic or hospital. To diagnose the condition, the physician examines your head, ears, skin, and spine for possible infected areas. Inspection of fluid extracted from the spinal area and X-rays of the head and chest also may be necessary to confirm diagnosis.

Treatment for bacterial meningitis always in-

cludes antibiotic therapy, either intravenous or oral. If fluid has accumulated in the sinuses, mastoids, or between your brain membrane layers, surgery may be necessary to drain the excess fluid.

For More Information

Centers for Disease Control and Prevention
1600 Clifton Road
Atlanta, GA 30333
800-311-3435
www.cdc.gov

National Institute of Allergies and Infectious Diseases
31 Center Drive, MSC 2520, Building 31, Room 7A-50
Bethesda, MD 20892-2520
301-496-5171
www.niaid.nih.org

Complementary and Alternative Treatments

Nutrition and Supplementation

Avoid animal protein and its by-products, caffeine, dairy products (except yogurt), processed foods, salt, sugar, and white flour products—all of which encourage the formation of mucus. Once recovery has begun, eat a well-balanced diet that includes fresh fruits and vegetables, grains, nuts, seeds, yogurt and other soured products. Add fresh papaya and pineapple to your diet. Papaya aids digestion and pineapple reduces inflammation.

Drink plenty of quality fluids and take the following daily supplements:

- acidophilus (as directed on label)—replaces friendly bacteria

- dimethylglycine (125 mg twice daily)—relieves many symptoms

- free-form amino acid complex (as directed on label)—repairs tissues and protects membranes

- garlic (2 capsules 3 times daily)—a natural antibiotic that stimulates the immune system

Health Notes

➤ A vaccine is currently available that protects against one of the bacteria strains that causes meningitis. The Hib vaccine protects against the bacterium Haemophilus influenza B which is the most common cause of childhood meningitis. The vaccine is given in a series of 3 to 4 shots, usually at ages 2 months, 4 months, and 6 months. Vaccines to protect against other meningitis-causing bacteria are currently being developed.

➤ Studies have shown that alcoholics, smokers, and obese people are at increased risk of developing meningitis. If you are in one of these high-risk groups, talk to your doctor about ways to decrease your risk.

- shiitake (as directed on label)—fights viral infection
- vitamin A emulsion (50,000 IU; do not exceed 8000 IU if you are pregnant)—boosts the immune system

- vitamin C with bioflavonoids (3000 to 10,000 mg)—cleanses the bloodstream

(Consult your healthcare provider regarding the duration of treatment.)

MENOPAUSE

Signs and Symptoms

Not all women experience menopausal symptoms. Among those who do, symptoms may include:

- Hot flashes
- Dry skin
- Headaches
- Sleep disturbances
- Vaginal dryness, which may result in pain during intercourse
- Vaginal inflammation
- Night sweats
- Insomnia
- Breast tenderness
- Increased need to urinate
- Psychological changes (fatigue, irritability, nervousness, mood swings)

Description

Menopause is not an illness. For women, it is a natural and unavoidable stage of life. While the term *menopause* literally means "the cessation of menstrual periods," it also is used to describe the period of life following a woman's final period. Menopause typically occurs between the ages of 50 and 52, though some women experience menopause as early as their late 30s or as late as their late 50s.

Approximately 25 percent of women experience few or no symptoms during menopause. Some 50 percent experience mild symptoms, and another 25 percent experience moderate to severe symptoms. Of these symptoms, perhaps the best known is the hot flash—a sudden feeling of heat, usually accompanied by a reddening of the face and sweating. Other reported symptoms include vaginal dryness, difficulty sleeping, and psychological changes that range in intensity and duration and may take the form of mood swings or increased irritability or anxiety. Due to the decreased levels of estrogen in the body, osteoporosis and cardiovascular disease become major health risks after menopause. Bone loss progresses most rapidly during the first five years of menopause and then slows to about 1 to 2 percent each year.

Not all the effects of menopause are negative. Among the benefits are the ability to have conception-free sex without birth control. In addition, women who suffer from endometriosis or fibrocystic breast disease often report diminished symptoms or complete remission of symptoms upon reaching menopause.

Conventional Medical Treatment

Menopause does not usually require medical treatment. If you experience any bothersome menopausal symptoms—such as hot flashes—see your gynecologist, who can recommend therapies

389

Health Notes

➤ *Women who start smoking before the age of 17, or those who've smoked a pack of cigarettes a day for 20 years or more, may be three to four times more likely to go through menopause before age 40 than nonsmokers.*

➤ *Women who follow a vegetarian, high-soy diet report fewer menopausal symptoms than other women. Foods made from soy contain high levels of naturally occurring plant estrogens (phytoestrogens), which may provide estrogenic benefits without the attendant risks sometimes associated with hormone replacement therapy.*

➤ *While a low-fat diet can benefit anyone, it is especially important for postmenopausal women who are not on HRT, to lower their risk of developing cardiovascular disease.*

➤ *Menopausal women with diabetes may need HRT even more than those without diabetes, because they have a markedly increased risk of developing cardiovascular conditions such as heart attack and stroke.*

➤ *A combination of aerobic exercise (20 minutes or more) and strength training (light weightlifting) performed three times a week has been shown to help alleviate common menopausal problems, such as hot flashes, bone loss, cardiovascular disease, and sleep disturbances.*

tailored to treat individual symptoms. Hormone replacement therapy (HRT)—a prescription drug therapy that replenishes estrogen or more commonly delivers a combination of estrogen and progesterone—is often prescribed to elevate a woman's hormones to the premenopausal level. This generally lessens all symptoms of menopause. HRT has the added benefit of protecting

against osteoporosis and reducing the risk of cardiovascular disease. These long-term benefits usually require long-term HRT, and for some women this brings with it an increased risk of breast cancer. The decision whether or not to go on hormone replacement therapy is medically complex and should be made by each woman in consultation with her doctor.

For More Information

Office on Women's Health
Department of Health & Human Services
200 Independence Avenue SW, Room 730 B
Washington, DC 20201
202-690-7650
www.4women.org/owh

Power Surge (Web Resource)
www.power-surge.com/intro.htm

Complementary and Alternative Treatments

Nutrition and Supplementation

 Take a protein supplement to stabilize your blood sugar level, and aim to get 40 percent of your calories from high quality proteins, including soy proteins. Your diet should include broccoli and other leafy greens, kelp, salmon with bones, sardines, and white fish. Limit your intake of dairy products and meat. These are high in protein, which works against calcium absorption. It's best to get calcium from plant sources or supplements. Avoid caffeine, sugar, alcohol, spicy foods, and hot soups or drinks, which can trigger hot flashes and make mood swings worse.

Drink 2 quarts of water daily to prevent drying of the skin and mucous membranes. Studies have shown that plant estrogens found in soy products are helpful in fighting off symptoms of menopause. Soy products include tofu, tempeh, miso, soy milk, and soybeans. Cashews, almonds, alfalfa, and apples also contain this natural estrogen, but in more modest amounts. Ask your healthcare provider about taking soy isoflavones, including genestein.

Try the following daily supplements to help ease menopause:

Most Important

- lecithin (1200 mg 3 times daily, before meals)—emulsifies vitamin E, which reduces hot flashes
- hydrochloric acid (as directed on label)—production declines with age; do not take if you have ulcers
- evening primrose or flaxseed oil (as directed on label)—good for hot flashes
- vitamin B complex (50 mg), supplemented with vitamin B_5 (100 mg 3 times daily)—a potent anti-stress vitamin, and vitamin B_6 (50 mg 3 times daily)—minimizes water retention; eases symptoms
- vitamin E (start with 400 IU and slowly increase until hot flashes are relieved, up to 1600 IU)—reduces hot flashes and other symptoms; use emulsion form for easier assimilation

Also Recommended

- boron (3 mg; do not exceed this amount)—enhances calcium absorption
- calcium (1500 to 2000 mg individual doses)—relieves nervousness and irritability; protects against bone loss
- magnesium (750 to 1000 mg)—balances with calcium; cut back if bowels become loose
- silica (as directed on label)—enhances calcium absorption
- zinc (50 mg; not to exceed a total of 100 mg from all supplements)—protects against bone loss; reduces symptoms
- vitamin C (3000 to 10,000 mg)—for hot flashes
- potassium (99 mg)

(Consult your healthcare provider regarding the duration of treatment; also ask about supplementation with soy isoflavones, including genestein and glycitein.)

Aromatherapy

When you feel a hot flash coming on, use the essential oil of clary sage or geranium in a home diffuser for speedy relief. Alternately place a drop of clary sage oil on a tissue or handkerchief and inhale whenever you feel a flash is coming on. Sage oil can help lessen the sweating that accompanies hot flashes.

Ayurvedic Medicine

Ayurveda views menopause as a natural occurrence, not a disease or harmful condition. To help you move comfortably through this stage of life, Ayurvedic practitioners may suggest taking aloe vera gel 3 times daily. Be sure to buy the aloe gel intended for internal use, and get one that doesn't have a laxative effect. Alternatively, practitioners may advise using the Ayurvedic formula *Geriforte* according to your needs.

Ayurvedic products are available at many health food stores and Indian pharmacies.

Bodywork and Somatic Practices

Many therapies could be helpful, but it is important to find the combination that is right for you. Initial therapies could include polarity therapy, CranioSacral Therapy, reflexology, and Oriental bodywork.

Herbal Therapy

Black cohosh, with its phytoestrogens (plant estrogens), is the most effective herbal remedy for calming hot flashes, vaginal dryness, and other discomforts of menopause. It's most convenient to buy the herb in a standardized preparation (under the trade name Remifemin®), which is available in health food stores. Follow package directions, and use this potent herb under medical supervision.

Other herbs useful in reducing the severity of menopausal symptoms include dong quai, chasteberry, and wild yam.

Homeopathy

Menopausal symptoms may respond to homeopathic treatment. However, the selection of a remedy—more than one is available—depends on *your* symptoms and the stage of the condition. Avoid self-treatment. See a homeopathic professional.

Hydrotherapy

Apply cold compresses to the neck and chest to diminish hot flashes. Keep the cloth in place for 3 minutes. Rewet as necessary. You can also take a cool bath for 20 minutes every morning.

For vaginal dryness, try a perineal wash with plain water once a day.

Traditional Chinese Medicine

Acupuncture Acupuncture may be used to control a host of menopause-related symptoms, including hot flashes, mood swings, back pain, depression, and anxiety. The various points targeted depend upon the patient's individual symptoms, so a full diagnosis is needed.

Chinese Herbal Therapy Angelica and ginseng may be prescribed to alleviate hot flashes. Patent formulas to relieve menopausal symptoms include Rehmannia Eight, Rehmannia Six, or Bupleurum and Dragon Bone, among others. If these therapies do not help you achieve desired results, see an herb-trained acupuncturist.

Yoga and Meditation

Exercise and stretching to strengthen the lower abdominal area is very helpful for soothing vexing menopausal symptoms. Beneficial yoga poses include the Sun Salutation, Lotus, Locust, Bow, Boat, Spinal Twist, Leg Lifts, Chest-Knee, Reclined Lunges, and Reclined Cobblers.

MENSTRUATION, ABSENCE OF (AMENORRHEA)

Signs and Symptoms

- Absence of menstruation for six months or longer in a non-pregnant adult woman

- Not having had a menstrual period by the age of 16

Description

It is normal to not have a period while pregnant, while breastfeeding, and after menopause. The menstrual cycle is closely linked to levels of body fat. Women who lose a great deal of weight very quickly may stop getting their menstrual periods, a condition known as amenorrhea. This condition occurs most often in women who have a very low body-fat percentage, such as high-performance athletes (for example, long-distance runners), dancers, and women suffering from anorexia (see "Anorexia" entry). Women who stop taking oral contraceptives may also experience a cessation of periods due to the body's hormonal fluctuations. Other causes include hormonal abnormalities, such as thyroid disease. Young women who have reached the age of 16 without starting to menstruate may be too thin and usually will begin menstruating once they gain adequate body weight.

While the absence of menstrual periods may seem convenient, it can contribute to certain health conditions, including loss of bone density, which increases a woman's risk of developing osteoporosis later in life.

Conventional Medical Treatment

If you are 16 or older and have not yet had your first period, or if you are an adult whose periods have stopped, visit your gynecologist or primary care physician. The doctor can perform a physical and a pelvic examination to look for any irregularities that could be causing the condition. To confirm diagnosis, the physician takes a blood test and/or X-rays.

If rapid weight loss caused your amenorrhea, you will be advised on how to lose weight at a more gradual pace—usually one or two pounds per week. In underweight women, a weight gain of as few as five pounds can often reinitiate menstruation. Athletes may be directed to reduce their weekly workout schedules by a few hours and add more calories to their daily diet. Women who have ceased ovulating after going off the pill may be given an oral dose of hormones to prompt the body to ovulate.

For More Information

American College of Obstetricians and Gynecologists
409 12th Street, SW
P.O. Box 96920
Washington, DC 20090-6920
800-673-8444
www.acog.org

Association of Reproductive Health Professionals
2401 Pennsylvania Avenue, NW, Suite 350
Washington, DC 20037
202-466-3825
www.arhp.org

Health Notes

➤ If you need to lose weight, concentrate on slimming slowly. Weight loss of more than five pounds a week can bring on amenorrhea in some women.

➤ If you experience amenorrhea, be aware that you are at risk for bone loss. Eat three to five servings of calcium-rich foods daily. You also may want to speak to your physician about calcium supplements.

Complementary and Alternative Treatments

Nutrition and Supplementation

 If you're underweight, eat at least 500 calories more than you are currently getting on a daily basis. Be sure these are healthy foods, not junk, processed, or highly refined. Also be sure you're getting enough healthy fats in your diet. Hormones cannot be produced without dietary fat. Over-exercising is another cause of amenorrhea. Supplement your diet with vitamin A (10,000 IU daily) to help regulate hormone production.

Traditional Chinese Medicine

 Acupuncture Acupuncture may be very useful for treating amenorrhea, but requires a full diagnosis. The practitioner typically focuses on the uterus, adrenal gland, ovary, kidney, and internal secretion points in the ear, by stimulating circulation and regulating the body's production of estrogen.

Acupressure Acupressure targeting Conception Vessel 4, 6, and 12; Bladder 18, 20, 23, 31, and 34; Governing Vessel 3 and 4; Stomach 36; and

Spleen 6 and 10 may help remedy amenorrhea by improving the flow of *chi* and blood through the pelvic area and uterus.

Chinese Herbal Therapy The practitioner may recommend over-the-counter preparations, including Tang Gui Four, White Phoenix Pills, Rehmannia Six, or Ginseng and Tang Gui Ten. Usually, this condition is due to weakness, so be sure to eat a variety of grains and vegetables; organic calves liver also is recommended. A practitioner may also recommend using a hot water bottle (not a heating pad) on the abdomen twice a day for half an hour.

MENSTRUATION, HEAVY (MENORRHAGIA)

Signs and Symptoms

- Menstrual periods that last for more than seven days
- Having menstrual periods more often than once every 28 to 32 days
- Unusually heavy bleeding during menstrual periods

Description

Menorrhagia is the medical term for heavy periods. Some women naturally have heavy periods—especially during adolescence or early adulthood. Others develop the condition suddenly, often for no identifiable reason. Most cases of menorrhagia are a result of a hormonal disorder that affects the normal menstrual cycle. Factors known to contribute to heavy periods include uterine fibroids; obesity; some types of blood disorders; IUD use; ectopic pregnancy; heavy aspirin use; or an ovarian, uterine, or endometrial condition.

Although heavy periods are inconvenient and uncomfortable, in most cases the only health risk associated with the condition is anemia.

Conventional Medical Treatment

If you suddenly experience heavy periods, make an appointment with your gynecologist. Even women who have consistently heavy periods can benefit from a doctor's advice. To uncover any possible abnormalities or conditions that could be causing menorrhagia, your gynecologist asks about your medical and health history and performs a thorough physical, a pelvic examination, a Pap smear, and possibly, a biopsy of the uterine lining and an ultrasound of the uterus and ovaries. A blood test may be necessary to determine whether the condition is causing anemia.

If menorrhagia is caused by an underlying medical condition, addressing the health problem usually causes the periods to lighten on their own. If no underlying health condition is present, your physician may suggest that you begin taking birth control pills or change your current pill; the estrogen and progesterone contained in birth control pills can sometimes cause periods to lighten.

For More Information

American College of Obstetricians and Gynecologists
409 12th Street, SW
P.O. Box 96920
Washington, D.C. 20090-6920
800-673-8444
www.acog.org

Association of Reproductive Health Professionals
2401 Pennsylvania Avenue NW, Suite 350
Washington, DC 20037
202-466-3825
www.arhp.org

Health Notes

➤ *Prolonged heavy bleeding can cause anemia. To avoid developing anemia, increase your intake of iron-rich foods, such as dark leafy greens, whole grains, nuts, dried fruits, and meats. Iron supplements also may be an option; discuss this course with your doctor.*

➤ *Ask your gynecologist about oral contraceptives. For many women with menorrhagia, the estrogen and progesterone in the Pill lightens menstrual flow considerably.*

Complementary and Alternative Treatments

Nutrition and Supplementation

 Bioflavonoids, found in the white pulpy part of citrus fruits, maintain the strength of your blood vessels. Supplement your diet daily with the following:

- iron (3 mg)
- vitamin C with flavonoids (1000 mg)
- vitamin A (10,000 IU)—controls hormone production

- zinc (30 mg)—a deficiency can contribute to this disorder

(For an *acute* condition, take supplements until your symptoms subside. If symptoms persist, seek the advice of your healthcare provider. For a *chronic* condition, consult your healthcare provider regarding the duration of treatment.)

Ayurvedic Medicine

 Raspberries are especially helpful in decreasing a heavy menstrual flow, according to Ayurveda. Your practitioner may suggest drinking raspberry tea or eating raspberries several times daily.

Traditional Chinese Medicine

 Acupuncture Acupuncture can be used to regulate hormone production and balance energy levels, which may help lessen heavy menstrual flow. The acupuncturist may focus on body or auricular points relating to the uterus, internal secretion, liver, kidney, spleen, and brain.

Chinese Herbal Therapy *Yunnan Pai Yao* pills may also be effective in cases of menorrhagia. Also used is *Erjiao,* or donkey gelatin, which helps restore blood integrity.

MENSTRUATION, INFREQUENT (OLIGOMENORRHEA)

Signs and Symptoms

- Fewer than 11 menstrual periods per year

Description

Most women menstruate 11 to 13 times a year. If a woman misses many menstrual periods a year, the condition is known as oligomenorrhea. Infrequent periods can be caused by a number of factors, including frequent dieting, excessive exercise, high levels of androgens (male hormones) in the body, an ovarian tumor, low estrogen levels, or oncoming menopause. In some cases, the condition has no discernible cause.

If you are not ovulating every month, it can be

very difficult to conceive a child—something to keep in mind if you are planning to become pregnant. Another potential concern is the development of endometrial hyperplasia—an overgrowth of the uterine lining that can lead to uterine cancer. This occurs because the lining of the uterus is not shedding regularly. Alternatively, if low estrogen levels are causing infrequent menstruation, you are at risk for bone loss and osteoporosis.

Conventional Medical Treatment

If you are experiencing infrequent menstruation, visit your gynecologist, who can conduct a physical and pelvic examination, and blood and urine tests to determine hormone levels. Treatment for the condition depends on its cause. For example, if over-dieting is to blame, your physician may recommend nutritional or psychiatric counseling. An excess of androgen may be treated with steroid drugs or oral contraceptives, and estrogen deficiency may be treated with oral estrogen. Treatment of the underlying condition usually restores regular menstrual activity. If the approach

Health Notes

➤ Consult your gynecologist before increasing your level of exercise, whether it is for weight loss or athletic training. A sudden increase in exercise levels can cause irregular menstruation. Opt instead for an exercise regimen that gradually increases the frequency and intensity of your workouts.

➤ Establish a regular sleep schedule. Erratic sleep can lead to erratic periods in some women.

➤ A recent study showed that oligomenorrhea was less common among vegetarians than among women who eat meat, poultry, and fish.

of menopause is causing oligomenorrhea there are several options for treatment, such as low-dose estrogen oral contraceptives or progesterone. Discuss these options with your doctor.

For More Information
American College of Obstetricians and Gynecologists
409 12th Street, SW
P.O. Box 96920
Washington, DC 20090-6920
800-673-8444
www.acog.org

Association of Reproductive Health Professionals
2401 Pennsylvania Avenue, NW, Suite 350
Washington, DC 20037
202-466-3825
www.arhp.org

Complementary and Alternative Treatments

Traditional Chinese Medicine

 Acupuncture Chinese medicine views infrequent or irregular menstruation as being caused by one of two factors: either an organ in the body is malfunctioning with regard to the menstrual cycle, or the body's energy level is excessive in one direction over another, towards either too little or too much energy, causing erratic periods. Acupuncture may be used to regulate this imbalance and promote regular menses. Acupuncture points in the treatment of oligomenorrhea typically include: Spleen 9 and 10, Stomach 36, and Bladder 20.

Acupressure A practitioner may help regulate infrequent menstruation by focusing on points related to the conception vessel, bladder, stomach, and spleen meridians. Pericardium 6 also may be used to treat this condition.

Chinese Herbal Therapy Certain patent medicines also may be prescribed to remedy irregular menstruation, including Rehmannia Eight, Ginseng and Longan, or Bupleurum and Tang Gui.

MENSTRUATION, PAINFUL (DYSMENORRHEA)

Signs and Symptoms

- Intense pain or cramps in the lower abdomen during menstruation (the pain may extend to the hips, lower back, and thighs)
- Nausea and vomiting during menstruation

Description

Some women experience periods that are so painful they cause nausea and vomiting. This condition, known as dysmenorrhea, is usually not related to an underlying health or gynecological disorder. Experts believe that painful menstruation is caused when the hormone prostaglandin—which causes the uterus to contract to shed its old lining—is present in very high levels in the body. An excess of this hormone can cause strong, painful contractions within the uterus. Severe menstrual pain can also be caused by endometriosis and uterine fibroids.

Adolescents and young adults—particularly those who have not had a child—are at the highest risk of developing dysmenorrhea. The condition usually disappears when the woman reaches her mid-twenties or gives birth to a child.

Conventional Medical Treatment

If you are experiencing painful menstruation, visit your gynecologist. The visit includes an informational interview, during which the physician may ask questions about your diet, lifestyle, and sexual history as well as the history of your menstrual pain. A full physical and pelvic examination also may be necessary.

Fortunately, there are effective drug treatments for dysmenorrhea. These include nonsteroidal anti-inflammatory drugs, such as ibuprofen, naproxen, mefenamic acid, and Anaprox®. These relax the uterine muscle, greatly lessening the painful contractions. Oral birth control pills can also make periods less painful.

For More Information

American College of Obstetricians and Gynecologists
409 12th Street, SW
P.O. Box 96920
Washington, DC 20090-6920
800-673-8444
www.acog.org

Association of Reproductive Health Professionals
2401 Pennsylvania Avenue, NW, Suite 350
Washington, DC 20037
202-466-3825
www.arhp.org

Health Notes

➤ Studies have shown that meat, caffeine, and salty foods contribute to painful cramps by increasing levels of prostaglandin, the substance responsible for uterine contractions.

➤ Vitamin C, vitamin E, vitamin B_6, and magnesium help lessen cramps by lowering the body's prostaglandin levels.

➤ If you have dysmenorrhea, exercise regularly. Moderate physical activity performed daily before and during your periods can lessen the pain of cramps by releasing endorphins (natural painkillers).

Complementary and Alternative Treatments

Nutrition and Supplementation

 Eat a diet plentiful in whole grains, legumes, fruits and vegetables, and seeds and nuts. Avoid dairy products, saturated fats, salt, sugars, and caffeine. (See "Hypoglycemia.")

Supplement with the following daily dosages:

- vitamin B complex (should include 50 mg each of vitamin B_3 and vitamin B_6)
- vitamin C (1000 mg)
- calcium (500 mg, citrate form)
- magnesium (500 mg, glycinate form)
- potassium (99 mg)
- zinc (30 mg)
- essential fatty acids (as directed on label)

(Consult your healthcare provider regarding the duration of treatment.)

Aromatherapy

 To lessen cramping and discomfort, try massaging your abdomen with an antispasmodic essential oil. Combine 5 drops (total) of the essential oils of marjoram, Roman chamomile, clary sage, or jasmine with 1 teaspoon of vegetable oil. Apply to your abdomen and massage gently in a circular pattern.

Ayurvedic Medicine

 According to Ayurveda, painful menstruation can be classified as vata, pitta, and kapha, according to your symptoms. Ayurvedic practitioners may advise taking a mixture of aloe vera (look for a non-laxative type) and black pepper until the symptoms subside. They also may suggest a *guggulu* herbal compound, such as *triphala guggulu,* which is available in tablet form.

Ayurvedic products are available at many health food stores and Indian pharmacies.

Chiropractic

 Painful cramping associated with menstruation can be relieved with applications of dry heat and specific chiropractic adjustment (SCA). The chiropractor may utilize soft tissue massage to the paraspinal lumbar muscles (along the spine) to facilitate relaxation of skeletal and visceral (internal) muscles. The practitioner works to adjust the lumbar and sacral vertebral segments to induce proper nerve flow and relax these muscles.

Herbal Therapy

 A number of herbal teas can tame cramping uterine muscles and soothe discomfort. Experiment to see which of the following works best for you.

The most effective of the teas is made from cramp bark. Simmer 2 teaspoons in 1 cup water for 15 minutes. Drink 3 times a day while needed. Other teas worth trying include feverfew, skullcap, black cohosh, and valerian. Consult a medical herbalist for directions.

Herbal products are available in health food stores and in some pharmacies and supermarkets. Follow package for specific directions.

Homeopathy

 Your homeopathic practitioner might advise one of the following treatments for painful menstruation, depending on your symptoms:

- *Colocynthis*—if the pain eases when you lie down, draw up your legs, or put pressure firmly on your abdomen
- *Chamomilla*—if you feel irritable and have intense, labor-like pains
- *Belladonna*—if the onset is sudden and you have throbbing pains which are worse on the

right side; you feel a sensation similar to bearing down

- *Magnesia phosphorica*—if the pain eases when you draw up your knees and place a hot water bottle on your abdomen

Hydrotherapy

Place a hot pack over the abdomen for 5 to 30 minutes to relax the muscles, diminish cramping, and lessen discomfort. For relief from cramps, apply cold compresses to the belly. Here are some additional useful remedies:

- drink 2 glasses of cold water on arising to help flush area
- sit in a cool shallow bath with feet in a hot bath

Traditional Chinese Medicine

Acupuncture Menstrual pain may be greatly relieved by acupuncture. Typically, the points targeted include Conception Vessel 4 and Spleen 6, and uterine- and ovarian-related auricular points. Abdominal cramps or bloating may be relieved by targeting Stomach 30, Spleen 4, and Liver 5. Other points may be included, as symptoms warrant. A hot water bottle (not a heating pad) also can be very helpful.

Acupressure Acupressure can be very effective in lessening menstrual pain. Acupressure points that may be targeted include: Conception Vessel 3, 4, and 6; Spleen 6, 9, 10, 12 and 13; Liver 3; Large Intestine 4; Stomach 36; and Bladder 23, 31, 32, and 60.

The practitioner often may recommend that the patient receive treatment the week before the onset of menstruation to help prevent dysmenorrhea from recurring.

Chinese Herbal Therapy Chinese combination medicines are often used to combat dysmenorrhea, including Bupleurum and Tang Gui, Corydalis Formula (or Corydalis Analgesic Tablets), and Ginseng and Atractylodes.

Yoga and Meditation

Spend a few minutes every day doing yoga to keep your body strong and relaxed. Gentle Spinal Twists can be helpful. Take a break from yoga during your menstrual period.

MONONUCLEOSIS (EPSTEIN-BARR VIRUS)

Signs and Symptoms

- Fever
- Sore throat
- Swollen lymph nodes
- Pain on the upper left side of the abdomen
- Lack of appetite
- Fatigue, weakness, and lethargy
- Sore muscles and/or muscle stiffness
- Rapid heartbeat
- Nausea
- Headaches

Description

The Epstein-Barr virus is a strain of the herpes virus that causes infectious mononucleosis, also known as "mono." Although mononucleosis is seldom serious (it is only dangerous in rare cases when the spleen becomes enlarged and ruptures, or when a vital organ, such as the heart or brain becomes affected), it can be extremely inconvenient. The illness can last anywhere from a couple of weeks to two or three months or even longer, during which time sufferers experience extreme fatigue and weakness and must limit their daily activities.

The Epstein-Barr virus can affect anyone, but it most commonly affects individuals between the ages of 10 and 35. The condition is also known as the "kissing disease," because the virus that causes it is spread through infected saliva. Since mononucleosis is highly contagious, it often occurs as an epidemic within a closed population, such as a college or boarding school. In children and adolescents, the disease incubation period is usually 7 to 14 days, while adults may harbor the illness for 30 to 50 days before developing symptoms.

Conventional Medical Treatment

Due to its broad range of symptoms, mononucleosis can be difficult to diagnose by symptoms alone. In most cases, a monospot blood test is performed to confirm the presence of the Epstein-Barr virus in the bloodstream.

Unfortunately, there is no specific anti-viral medication to treat the disease. Drinking large amounts of fluid, getting plenty of bed rest, and taking aspirin or acetaminophen are common treatments. (*Caution*: Children should not take aspirin because of the small risk of Reye's syndrome, which can be fatal.) Be prepared to take it easy for the full duration of your illness—however long that may be.

If you have mononucleosis and experience sudden jabs of pain in the upper left side of your abdomen, call your physician immediately or go to a hospital emergency room. The cause could be a ruptured spleen, a rare complication, but one that requires immediate surgical attention.

Health Notes

➤ If you have mononucleosis, take it easy. Exercise may lead to a ruptured spleen, a potentially fatal complication of infectious mononucleosis.

➤ If you've been diagnosed with mononucleosis, ask your physician whether you are still contagious. If you are, stay home until you get the doctor's okay to return.

➤ To boost your body's immune system, increase your intake of nutrient-rich fresh vegetables and fruits.

➤ Studies show that after a bout of mononucleosis, the Epstein-Barr virus remains in the body and slightly suppresses the immune system, putting you at greater risk for contracting other infectious illnesses.

➤ Moderate, daily exercise boosts immunity, helping you fight attacks of viruses, such as the Epstein-Barr virus.

Epstein-Barr Strikes Again

The Epstein-Barr virus is best known as the cause of mononucleosis, but numerous studies have shown that the virus is also associated with Hodgkin's disease. In one study of 80 people with Hodgkin's disease—none of whom had ever had mononucleosis—60 were found to be carrying the virus. In another study of people with Hodgkin's disease, 25 individuals out of 77 were carrying the Epstein-Barr virus. The exact relationship between the virus and Hodgkin's disease is still unclear.

Centers for Disease Control and Prevention
1600 Clifton Road
Atlanta, GA 30333
800-311-3435
www.cdc.gov

National Institute of Allergies and Infectious Diseases
31 Center Drive, MSC 2520, Building 31, Room 7A50
Bethesda, MD 20892-2520
301-496-5171
www.niaid.nih.org

Complementary and Alternative Treatments

Nutrition and Supplementation

Drink 8 8-ounce glasses of pure water as well as fresh juice daily. "Green drinks" made from leafy green vegetables are also beneficial. Eat a diet that emphasizes wholesome soups, root vegetables, and whole grains, including brown rice. Avoid coffee, fried foods, processed foods, soft drinks, stimulants, sugar, tea, and white flour. These depress immune function. Consume as much raw food as possible.

Nutritionists recommend these daily supplements:

- a prodophilus formula (as directed on label)—replaces friendly bacteria

- vitamin A (25,000 IU for 2 weeks, then slowly reduce to 15,000 IU; do not exceed 8000 IU if you are pregnant)—is essential for the immune system; use emulsion form

- vitamin E (400 IU)

- vitamin C with bioflavonoids (5000 to 10,000 IU in divided doses)—destroys the virus; boosts the immune system

- free-form amino acid complex (1/4 tsp 2 to 3 times daily, on empty stomach)—provides the protein necessary for healing and rebuilding tissue

- vitamin B complex (100 mg 3 times daily, with meals)—increases energy, supplemented with vitamin B_{12} (15 mg 2 times daily)—prevents anemia

- omega-3 fatty acids (as directed on label)

- thymus and liver live cell therapy (as directed)

(Take supplements until your symptoms subside. If symptoms persist, seek the advice of your healthcare provider.)

Herbal Therapy

To fight a mononucleosis infection and regain pep, take tincture of myrrh or of echinacea. For myrrh, drink 1/4 to 3/4 teaspoon in 1 cup warm water, 3 times a day. For echinacea, use 15 drops in a glycerin form, twice a day. To reduce a fever, try drinking a tea made from elder flowers or yarrow. Infuse 1 to 2 teaspoons of either dried herb in 1 cup boiling water for 10 minutes; strain. Take up to 3 times a day. In addition, garlic is a natural antibiotic. Take garlic supplements as directed on the product label.

Herbal products are available in health food stores and in some pharmacies and supermarkets. Follow package for specific directions.

Traditional Chinese Medicine

Acupuncture This treatment can help boost immunity and tone organs that may be affected by the disease, including the liver, spleen, heart, and (always) the kidneys.

Chinese Herbal Therapy Formulas that are helpful for immune disorders very often include herbs such as Chinese wolfberry, but in a weakened form. It is always best to seek an herb-trained acupuncturist.

Yoga and Meditation

Use yoga, which is an extremely gentle form of exercise, to reduce fatigue; select non-strenuous poses, such as the Cobra, Locust, and Bow.

SYMPTOM:

MORNING SICKNESS

Morning sickness has nothing to do with the time of day. This combination of nausea, dizziness, vomiting, headaches, and diarrhea can strike a pregnant woman at any time. In fact, it can plague a pregnant woman around the clock. Fortunately, most expectant mothers who experience this unpleasant side effect find that it disappears after the first three or four months of pregnancy. Because symptoms are worse when the stomach is empty, many obstetricians recommend eating several small meals and drinking water throughout the day.

There are numerous theories as to what causes morning sickness. The most common explanations include hormonal changes, low blood sugar, low blood sodium, and slow digestion.

Morning sickness can be dangerous—55,000 pregnant women are hospitalized each year for morning-sickness complications, including dehydration, anemia, and disrupted metabolism caused by excessive vomiting. Unfortunately, there is no medication available for morning sickness.

m

MOTION SICKNESS

Signs and Symptoms

- Nausea
- Vomiting
- Pallor
- Sweating
- Weakness, fatigue, and/or malaise
- Feeling of panic
- Hyperventilation

Description

Motion sickness is not really an illness, but the body's response to unusual motion, such as turning, twisting, winding, or rocking. This type of motion may be caused by a riding in a boat, car, plane, or amusement park ride. The condition occurs because there is a discrepancy between what the eyes see (a series of seemingly speeding objects in the window, or no motion at all if you are reading or looking down at your lap) and what the inner ear feels (rocking or swaying movement, for instance). The nervous system responds to this discordant perception by triggering a feeling of nausea.

Conventional Medical Treatment

Motion sickness can be treated without medical intervention. The easiest solution is to get off the vehicle that is causing the problem. If that is not a possibility, move to another area of the vehicle. If you are in the back seat of a car, sit in front so you can look forward out the window at the horizon instead of having to see scenery rushing by through the side windows. If you are in a boat or plane, move to the middle of the craft, where there is less of a rocking sensation.

Health Notes

➤ If you are in a car or train and experience motion sickness, open the windows; if you are in a plane, direct the air vent to blow air on you. Circulating air can help alleviate symptoms of motion sickness.

➤ If you are reading when motion sickness strikes, stop reading. For many people, nothing sparks a bout of motion sickness like reading while on a moving vehicle.

➤ If you are experiencing motion sickness symptoms, try to sleep. Sleeping is one of the most effective ways to alleviate symptoms.

If you regularly suffer from motion sickness, ask your doctor for a prescription for a scopolamine patch. Applied eight hours before travel, the patch releases a medication that prevents motion sickness. Antihistamines, such as diphenhydramine (Benedryl®) and dimenhydrinate (Dramamine®), are also commonly used to prevent motion sickness. These are available over the counter or by prescription, and are most effective if taken 30 to 60 minutes before traveling. If you will be operating a vehicle, do not take motion sickness medication, because the drugs have sedative qualities. Also, these drugs should not be taken with alcohol or tranquilizers.

Complementary and Alternative Treatments

Nutrition and Supplementation

 Melatonin, the same nutrient that treats jet lag, is also helpful in treating motion sickness. Take 1 to 3 mg during your trip. Avoid foods that contribute to nausea, such as fried, junk, processed, spicy, heavy, or fatty foods. Stay away from alcohol, since it disrupts

communication between the eyes, the brain, and the inner ears.

These supplements may help prevent motion sickness:

- charcoal tablets (5 tablets 1 hour before travel)—detoxifies
- magnesium (500 mg 1 hour before trip)—acts as a nerve tonic
- vitamin B_6 (100 mg 1 hour before trip, then 100 mg 2 hours later)—relieves nausea

(Take supplements until your symptoms subside. If symptoms persist, seek the advice of your healthcare provider.)

Aromatherapy

 Many aromatherapists recommend peppermint essential oil for easing nausea. Mix 1 drop with 1 teaspoon honey or vegetable oil and take internally, or place 1 drop on your tongue. You also can place a few drops on a tissue or handkerchief and inhale whenever you feel queasy. Alternately, combine 4 drops with 4 drops ginger essential oil and mix with 1 teaspoon vegetable oil or lotion. Massage this blend into your chest just before traveling.

Ayurvedic Medicine

Ayurvedic practitioners might suggest taking ginger capsules before your trip, chewing candied ginger during your trip, or taking the Ayurvedic formula *Gasex* (two or three tablets chewed after meals) or *Bonnisan* before and during your trip. Ayurvedic products are available at many health food stores and Indian pharmacies. See package directions for details.

Herbal Therapy

 Ginger is extremely effective for preventing motion sickness. Take it on an empty stomach in one of the following forms: chew on fresh peeled ginger root, eat candied ginger, drink ginger tea, or take 2 capsules (500 mg each) of dried ginger root every 4 hours, starting the day before traveling.

Homeopathy

Homeopathic practitioners often recommend one of the following treatments for motion sickness, depending on your symptoms:

- *Tabacum*—for extreme seasickness if you have a death-like pallor, are vomiting, feel icy cold, and must lie with your eyes closed

- *Chocculus*—for motion sickness that comes from side-to-side motion; this remedy is most useful after a sea voyage when the ground feels as if it's moving

- *Nux vomica*—for a queasy feeling that's accompanied by a splitting headache and a loathing for food; you may gag, vomit without bringing anything up, and feel chilly

- *Petroleum*—for persistent nausea that's accompanied by the pooling of water in your mouth; this remedy is helpful if your stomach feels empty and the nausea eases when you eat something

Hydrotherapy

Place a cool compress at the base of your skull to lessen nausea. Rewet as necessary.

Traditional Chinese Medicine

Acupuncture Acupuncture may be useful in alleviating the nausea, dizziness, and anxiety brought on by motion sickness. Points that may be targeted to treat nausea include Pericardium 6, Stomach 36, and related ear points. To lessen dizziness, the practitioner may focus on Liver 3, Stomach 40, Triple Warmer 17 and 21, and Conception Vessel 6 and 12.

Acupressure As with acupuncture, the points that are typically targeted are Pericardium 5 and 6, Stomach 36, and Small Intestine 17 (the latter helps regulate inner ear balance). Over-the-counter seasickness bands use the point P6.

Chinese Herbal Therapy Dried ginger and angelica are time-honored Chinese herbal remedies to treat motion sickness. Curing Pills, an over-the-counter herbal preparation, may also be used to quell motion sickness.

MULTIPLE SCLEROSIS (MS)

Signs and Symptoms

- Blurred vision, double vision, loss of central vision

- Dizziness or vertigo

- General fatigue

- Brief shooting pain or tingling sensations anywhere in the body

- Numbness, weakness, or paralysis in one or more limbs

- Occasional tremors

- Lack of coordination

- Unsteady gait

- Lack of bladder or bowel control

Description

Multiple sclerosis is a disease of the central nervous system characterized by bouts of symptoms that may last from two weeks to four months. Experts believe that during a bout the body's own white blood cells mistakenly attack the myelin, a sheath that insulates nerve fibers. This attack causes inflammation and eventual scarring of the myelin, which, in turn, affects muscle coordination, visual sensation, and other nervous system functions. Attacks generally dissipate, and the individual may go for months or years with only very mild symptoms or no discernible symptoms at all. While the exact cause of these flare-ups is not known, some individuals report having recurrences after taking a hot bath, being out in the sun, or experiencing a stressful situation.

The cause of MS is unknown, but family history of the condition is a definite risk factor. Although more women get the disease than men, men tend to have more debilitating symptoms. Most people who develop the disease have their first attack between the ages of 20 and 40. In most cases, MS does not greatly reduce the victim's life expectancy, though many sufferers become progressively more debilitated, until they cannot function on their own.

Conventional Medical Treatment

Early symptoms of multiple sclerosis are similar to those of Lyme disease, Parkinson's disease, and amyotrophic lateral sclerosis, so it is important to see your physician for an exact diagnosis. Your doctor takes a detailed medical history and may order an electroencephalogram (a charting of your brain's electrical activity) to confirm diagnosis. Other diagnostic tests for MS include lumbar puncture (to check the concentration of immune cells in your cerebrospinal fluid), simple visual stimulus exercises, and magnetic resonance imaging (MRI).

While there is currently no standard treatment for MS, there are medications that help manage symptoms. Beta interferon is thought to slow the progression of the disease, and anti-spasmodics and corticosteroids are helpful for treating myelin inflammation. Physical therapy can help patients cope with lack of motor coordination. Copaxone® (copolymer-1), a new drug under consideration

New Evidence

After studying the incidence of MS among the natural and adopted relatives of 15,000 people with multiple sclerosis, researchers believe that MS may be an inherited disease. They reasoned that if MS is caused by an environmental factor, as some experts suggest, adopted relatives—those who were exposed to the same factors as non-biological family members afflicted with MS—would be at increased risk of contracting the disease. However, these non-biological relatives were no more likely to develop MS than members of the general population. Past studies showed that an identical twin of a person with MS was 30 percent more likely than the general population to develop the disease, while close biological relatives faced a 3 to 4 percent increased risk.

by the Food and Drug Administration (FDA), was found in clinical trials to reduce the number of disease attacks in some patients.

For More Information
The Multiple Sclerosis Foundation, Inc.
6350 North Andrews Avenue
Fort Lauderdale, FL 33309
800-441-7055
www.msfacts.org

Health Notes

➤ *Studies have shown that MS sufferers who consume low-fat, vegetarian diets have fewer relapses and less severe symptoms.*

➤ *Reduce the amount of stress in your life. In some individuals, there is a link between stressful events and MS flare-ups.*

➤ *If you have MS and smoke, quit. Smoking interferes with the immune system function, possibly exacerbating MS symptoms.*

Multiple Sclerosis (MS)

National Multiple Sclerosis Society
733 Third Avenue
New York, NY 10017
800-344-4867
www.nmss.org

Complementary and Alternative Treatments

Nutrition and Supplementation

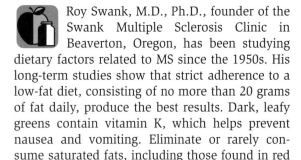

Roy Swank, M.D., Ph.D., founder of the Swank Multiple Sclerosis Clinic in Beaverton, Oregon, has been studying dietary factors related to MS since the 1950s. His long-term studies show that strict adherence to a low-fat diet, consisting of no more than 20 grams of fat daily, produce the best results. Dark, leafy greens contain vitamin K, which helps prevent nausea and vomiting. Eliminate or rarely consume saturated fats, including those found in red meat and dairy products.

Drink at least 8 8-ounce glasses of water daily to prevent toxic buildup in the muscles. "Green drinks" (those produced from chlorophyll-rich vegetables) are also beneficial for the chlorophyll they provide.

Nutritionists recommend the following daily supplements:

Most Important

- DHEA (300 mg, with food)
- flaxseed oil (2 tbsp, with food)
- vitamin B complex (50 mg)—maintains healthy nerves and aids in immune system function, supplemented with vitamin B_{12} (1000 mcg of a sublingual supplement, taken under the tongue)—prevents nerve damage, and vitamin B_6 (100 mg)—promotes red blood cell production
- phosphatidyl serine (300 mg, with food)
- complete antioxidant supplement (as directed on label)
- N-acetyl cisteine (1000 mg, on empty stomach)

- lipoic acid (200 mg, with food)
- selenium (200 mcg, with food; do not exceed 200 mcg selenium daily, taking all supplements into account)
- threonine (2 g, on empty stomach)

Also Recommended

- coenzyme Q10 (90 mg)—improves circulation and tissue oxygenation
- evening primrose oil (2000 mg)—controls symptoms
- choline (1000 mg) plus inositol (1000 mg)—stimulates the nervous system and protects the myelin sheaths
- vitamin C (1000 mg 5 times daily)—protects the immune system
- vitamin E (600 IU)—protects the nervous system, enhances circulation; take in emulsion form
- calcium (1000 to 2000 mg)—deficiency may increase your risk for developing MS; use chelate form
- magnesium (up to 600 mg daily, in divided doses)—important for myelin structure and stability

Ayurvedic Medicine

Ayurvedic practitioners may recommend the herb *ashwagandha* for strengthening the body, fighting fatigue, and reducing other symptoms of multiple sclerosis. Ayurvedic products are available at many health food stores and Indian pharmacies.

Remember to consult your doctor before embarking on any new regimen; proper care is extremely important for preventing relapses.

Traditional Chinese Medicine

Acupuncture Acupuncture can relieve muscle stiffness and promote overall relaxation, balance, and well-being, which may slow the disease's progression.

Mumps

Acupressure Acupressure can reduce stress and improve muscle tone, as well as bring about a state of balance that will enhance other therapies.

Chinese Herbal Therapy Multiple sclerosis is a very complex disease that manifests itself differently in different people. A Chinese medical doctor takes into account the patient's medical history and presenting symptoms before designing or

prescribing an herbal regimen. Herbs can be quite helpful in relieving a host of symptoms, including fatigue, incontinence, tremors, vision problems, and weak or stiff muscles. Patent formulas that may be given to boost the immune system include Panas Ginseng Capsules, Eight Immortal Long Life Pills, Ginseng and Longan, and Major Four Herbs.

MUMPS

Signs and Symptoms

- Swollen, tender salivary glands that make the cheeks appear puffy
- Fever
- Weakness and fatigue
- Lower abdominal pain (caused by swelling of the pancreas, or of the ovaries in women)
- Swollen testicles in men

Description

Although mumps is most commonly a childhood disease, affecting children between the ages of 3 and 10, adults are also susceptible. A case of the mumps is easily recognized by the telltale swelling of the cheeks just above the jaw. This swelling gradually subsides over the course of the illness.

Also known as *epidemic parotitis*, mumps is a contagious illness caused by a mild viral infection that is transmitted via droplets of saliva that are exhaled, sneezed, or coughed by an infected person. An infected person becomes contagious one day before the appearance of symptoms, and remains so for up to two weeks. Once someone has the mumps, he or she develops a natural immunity to the virus and cannot become infected again.

Conventional Medical Treatment

While there is no specific treatment for mumps, you should visit your doctor if you suspect that you or your child have the illness. Complications can sometimes arise, including *orchitis* (swelling of the testes) or neurological problems, such as encephalitis (inflamation of the brain). Recommended treatments for mumps include bed rest until fever subsides, and isolation to prevent spreading the disease. Your physician also may suggest an analgesic, such as acetaminophen.

Health Notes

➤ Getting the MMR (measles, mumps, rubella) vaccine is one of the easiest ways to prevent the mumps. All children should be vaccinated between 12 and 15 months of age and between 4 and 6 years or between 11 and 12 years.

➤ If swelling or pain is so severe that you cannot swallow, intravenous fluids and dextrose (a food replacement) may be administered.

There is a mumps vaccine available for children age one and older, and most states require that children be immunized before they begin school.

Complementary and Alternative Treatments

Nutrition and Supplementation

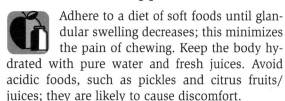 Adhere to a diet of soft foods until glandular swelling decreases; this minimizes the pain of chewing. Keep the body hydrated with pure water and fresh juices. Avoid acidic foods, such as pickles and citrus fruits/juices; they are likely to cause discomfort.

The following daily supplements are recommended. These are adult dosages. For children between 12 and 17, reduce the dose to three-quarters of the recommended amount. For children ages 6 to 12, use one-half of the recommended amount. For a child under 6, use one-quarter of the recommended amount.

- vitamin C (500 mg every 2 hours until improvement is noticed, up to 3000 to 10,000 mg daily)—destroys the virus; use sodium ascorbate form for children

- a prodophilus formula (as directed on label)—replaces friendly bacteria

- zinc (1 15-mg lozenge every 4 to 6 hours; do not exceed a total of 100 mg daily)—aids healing; do not chew, but allow to dissolve

- free-form amino acid complex (as directed on label)—repairs and heals tissue

- vitamin B complex (as directed on label)—necessary for healing

- potassium (99 mg)—restores electrolytes

(Consult your healthcare practitioner regarding duration of treatment.)

Ayurvedic Medicine

 Ayurvedic practitioners may recommend raisin water for speeding recovery, or they may suggest a sandalwood or mustard pack to reduce glandular swelling.

Traditional Chinese Medicine

 Acupuncture Acupuncture can be used to help reduce the inflamation of swollen glands. It also can alleviate earache (the practitioner will typically focus on Triple Warmer 17).

Chinese Herbal Therapy TCM practitioners may recommend that dandelion be taken internally or mixed with a little aloe vera and applied topically to swollen glands to lessen inflammation. For children, a child's dose of Ilex and Evodia Formula may be prescribed.

NASAL CONGESTION

Nasal congestion—also known as a stuffy nose—is a common symptom of many illnesses and chronic medical conditions that affect the respiratory tract. Conditions that cause nasal congestion include allergies, flu, a cold, pneumonia, sinusitis, bronchitis. This type of congestion typically occurs when the mucous membranes become inflamed and secrete excess mucus. Before self-medicating, call your physician and describe your symptoms. If an allergy is to blame, your doctor may prescribe antihistamines or recommend an over-the-counter product. For nasal congestion that accompanies a cold, flu, pneumonia, or bronchitis, your physician may recommend an over-the-counter decongestant containing ephedrine, pseudoephedrine, phenylephrine, or phenylpropanolamine, which shrinks swollen nasal tissues by causing blood vessels to constrict, reducing mucus production. Note: avoid using decongestant sprays or drops more than three days in a row because the body quickly becomes dependent on them, making congestion even worse when the medication is discontinued.

Nasal congestion also can be caused by an obstruction of normally clear breathing passages—the result be caused by more serious conditions, including nasal polyps, nasal tumors, birth-related nasal deformities, a deviated septum (the septum is the cartilage that separates the two nostrils), and nasal fractures. Many of these conditions can be diagnosed by a physical examination performed by a physician; if necessary, surgery may be required to clear the obstruction. The type of surgery depends on what is causing the obstruction.

Non-medical remedies include avoiding known allergens (for allergy-induced congestion only), drinking 10 8-ounce glasses of water a day to keep mucus liquefied, and using a humidifier if necessary to keep nasal membranes from becoming dry and irritated. Temporarily eliminating dairy foods, which can increase mucus production, can be helpful.

Herbal treatments include drinking licorice root tea, considered a natural mucus thinner; drink 2 to 3 cups per day. Licorice is one of the most commonly used medicinal herbs because of its sweet taste; herbalists also use licorice as a cough suppressant and it seems to soothe the mouth and throat as well. Osha root and pleurisy root are two other natural mucus thinners, but they have a very earthy taste and may not be palatable to some people.

Other complementary treatments include chiropractic. Although nasal congestion can be caused by many factors, such as flu, allergies, or colds, the actual symptoms and pain of nasal congestion may be chiropractically managed. It is important for the patient to first complete a standard medical workup to determine the cause of the problem. The chiropractor will most likely adjust the cervical vertebrae and may use moist heat and apply electrostimulation.

Acupressure may be helpful in relieving sinus pressure, concentrating on the points around the eyes, nose, and forehead. Practitioners also may promote sinus drainage with facial massage. In addition, they may prescribe moist heat and steam inhalation therapies to be performed at home.

n

NASAL POLYPS

Signs and Symptoms

- Constantly blocked nasal passages
- Difficulty smelling odors (in some cases)
- Frequent headaches (in some cases)

Description

The nasal lining is a mucous membrane that normally lies flat against the inside of the nose. In some instances, the lining swells and protrudes into the nasal passage, causing an overproduction of fluid in the mucous membrane—this swollen mass is known as a polyp. Polyps can appear singly or in a cluster. Polyps may be caused by hay fever or some other nasal allergy, and in some cases the cause is unexplainable. About 10 percent of asthmatics have a peculiar triad of bronchospasm, nasal polyps, and sensitivity to aspirin. Ingesting aspirin in these patients can cause a severe asthma attack and even an anaphylactic, or severe allergic, reaction.

Conventional Medical Treatment

To determine whether you have polyps, your physician examines the inside of your nose using a tong-like tool called a nasal speculum. In some cases, polyps can make it difficult for the sinuses to drain properly, contributing to sinus infection and difficulty breathing. For these reasons, many physicians recommend removing the masses surgically. Unfortunately, polyps can reappear at some point during your lifetime, so you may have to undergo more than one operation.

Health Notes

➤ Talk to your doctor about nasal sprays. Many experts believe these sprays, when overused, can increase one's risk of developing nasal polyps.

➤ If you smoke, quit. Smoking irritates the nasal membrane, aggravating symptoms of nasal polyps.

➤ If you live in an arid environment, consider getting a humidifier. Dry air can irritate the nasal membrane, aggravating symptoms of nasal polyps.

For More Information
American Academy of Otolaryngology
One Prince Street
Alexandria, VA 22314-3357
703-836-4444
www.entnet.org

Complementary and Alternative Treatments

Nutrition and Supplementation

 Diet doesn't play much of a role in the treatment of nasal polyps, although it might be helpful to eliminate dairy foods from your diet. Avoid overuse of nasal sprays and drops, and follow the recommended daily supplement program outlined below:

- vitamin C (5000 to 10,000 mg in divided doses)—can reduce the number of polyps;

studies show they have been eliminated in some cases

- multivitamin and mineral complex (as directed on label)—provides a balance of necessary nutrients

- garlic (as directed on label)—a natural antibiotic that enhances immune functions

(Consult your healthcare practitioner regarding the duration of treatment.)

SYMPTOM:

NAUSEA

Almost everyone has experienced nausea at some point in their lifetime. Nausea is characterized by a feeling of impending vomiting and is a common symptom of flu, pregnancy, motion sickness, gastrointestinal conditions such as peptic ulcer, severe pain, emotional upset, prescription or over-the-counter medication, food poisoning, substance abuse, migraine headache, a hangover, diabetes, heart attack, and other ailments. Nausea is often joined by other signs, such as pallor, headache, hypersalivation, dizziness, cold sweats, and/or vertigo.

If nausea is severe and accompanied by vomiting, extreme dizziness, vertigo, sweating, shortness of breath, or pain in any part of your body, call your doctor. Also call a physician if your nau-

sea persists on and off for more than a day or is unexplainable. You may have an underlying medical condition—such as gallstones, a migraine, or mononucleosis—that needs to be addressed.

Homecare remedies to quell nausea include chamomile or peppermint tea. Three drops of peppermint oil mixed with one tablespoon of a carrier oil and rubbed onto pulse points also can be used to alleviate nausea. Ginger—either in tea form or in capsules—has been used for centuries by practitioners of Traditional Chinese Medicine and herbalists to ease nausea related to food poisoning, morning sickness, gastrointestinal conditions, and hangover. Fresh outdoor air also can help ease mild nausea.

n

NEARSIGHTEDNESS

Signs and Symptoms

- Blurred vision when looking at distant objects

Description

Also known as *myopia*, nearsightedness lets you focus on nearby images, while you will have trouble seeing things farther away. Nearsightedness is caused by eyes that have a "stretched out," or more elongated, shape, which forces the light that enters into and is refracted by the cornea and lens to meet in front of the retina instead of at the retina, resulting in blurring of distant images. Nearsightedness tends to run in families, though it can occur naturally during the aging process. As we age, the eye tends to change shape, going from the roundness of youth to a more oval shape.

Conventional Medical Treatment

An ophthalmologist or optometrist can diagnose nearsightedness by using a series of vision exams, including the classic letter chart test. Glasses or contact lenses can correct the problem and help you see normally—or almost normally. For those desiring a more permanent solution, current laser surgeries include *radial keratotomy* (RK) and *photorefractive keratotomy*, two procedures that use lasers to change the way the eyes bend incoming light rays. Some experts believe that such operations may weaken the eye, making it more vul-

Fetal Alcohol Syndrome and Eyesight

Fetal alcohol syndrome (FAS), caused by excessive drinking during pregnancy, now surpasses Down syndrome and spina bifida as the leading cause of mental retardation in the United States. The most obvious physical defects characteristic of fetal alcohol syndrome involve the face and eyes: small head; small eyes and/or short palpebral fissures (the space between the margins of the eyelids); thin upper lip; poorly developed philtrum (the vertical groove above the upper lip); and short nose and low nasal bridge.

Visual defects are also common in children with fetal alcohol syndrome, affecting an average of 94 percent of these children. The most common of these sight problems is myopia, or nearsightedness, due to the abnormal physical shape of the eyes. While the condition cannot be corrected, eyeglasses can be prescribed. Vision experts recommend that children with fetal alcohol syndrome receive their first eye test before the age of two.

Health Notes

➤ *Don't sit too close to a television screen or computer monitor for more than an hour without resting your eyes. Some experts disagree that these activities lead to nearsightedness, while others believe that they contribute to the condition.*

➤ *Although the beneficial effects of nutrients on myopia have not been studied, many experts believe that a diet high in antioxidants (vitamins A, C, and E, and the minerals zinc and selenium) can help lessen the progression of the disease.*

nerable to injury, and the long-term results are still not known. The most likely candidates for these operations are those with mild to moderate, stable myopia.

For More Information

American Academy of Ophthalmology
P.O. Box 7424
San Francisco, CA 94120-7424
415-561-8500
www.eyenet.org

National Eye Institute
2020 Vision Place
Bethesda, MD 20892-3655
301-496-5248
www.nei.nih.gov

NECK TENSION AND PAIN

The most common source of neck pain is strain of the neck muscles. When neck muscles are strained or held unnaturally for a length of time—as in cradling a phone in the crook of the neck, sleeping in a strange position, or holding a heavy shoulder bag for a long period of time—they can become pulled. This limits the neck's comfortable range of motion. A neck nerve that has been pinched by a protruding vertebra, for example, is another cause of neck tension and pain. Other causes of neck pain and stiffness include whiplash, a cervical spine fracture, a herniated disk, muscle spasms, meningitis, neck sprain, osteoporosis, and rheumatoid arthritis.

If you can trace your neck pain to strain, then analgesics, massage, hot compresses or hot water bottles, gentle stretching, and improved pos-

ture can help ease symptoms for the three to seven days muscles need to heal. If you don't know the cause of your pain, get a doctor's diagnosis to check for an underlying cause of pain. Your physician may order X-rays, an MRI, or a CT scan. Treatment of an underlying condition can diminish or eliminate neck pain and stiffness.

For a complementary treatment, you might try chiropractic. Neck tension and pain readily respond to chiropractic treatment. After determining the cause of the discomfort, the chiropractor typically uses soft tissue massage to reduce muscle tightness. Additionally, he or she may use moist heat applications and specific chiropractic adjustment (SCA) to the cervical vertebral segments.

n

NEURALGIA, FACIAL (TRIGEMINAL)

Signs and Symptoms

- Recurring brief stabs of searing pain on one side of the lips, gums, chin, or forehead; may be accompanied by tenderness, burning, itching, or aching of affected areas
- Sweating (in some cases)
- Watery eyes (in some cases)

Description

The trigeminal nerves are tri-branched nerves located one on each side of the head; they begin just in front of each ear and branch out toward the eye, the nose, and the jaw. Trigeminal neuralgia attacks happen randomly, but can cause such

intense pain in these nerves that some people's facial muscles visibly contract—this is why the condition is sometimes called *tic douloureux*. The condition is not common—almost all sufferers are older than 50 and most are women older than 70. And although those who do suffer from the condition can find it excruciating, it is not life-threatening. The cause of trigeminal neuralgia is not known, though in some cases it occurs as a result of multiple sclerosis.

Conventional Medical Treatment

Your physician can diagnose trigeminal neuralgia by a description of symptoms, and by first ruling

Health Notes

➤ *Reduce stress. In some people with trigeminal neuralgia, stress can bring about more frequent symptoms.*

➤ *Exercise moderately (3 to 7 days a week, for 20 to 30 minutes a day). Perhaps because it helps reduce stress or because it encourages blood circulation, moderate exercise is associated with milder symptoms in people with trigeminal neuralgia.*

out any orthodontic condition that causes similar pain. Treatment includes controlling the pain with medication—often carbamazepine, phenytoin, or capsaicin. Should painkillers fail, your physician may suggest a surgical procedure to reduce the sensitivity of the trigeminal nerve.

For More Information
National Organization for Rare Diseases
P.O. Box 8923
New Fairfield, CT 06812-8923
800-999-NORD
www.rarediseases.org

Complementary and Alternative Treatments

Chiropractic

There are many forms of facial neuralgia and many causative factors. While rarely able to provide a cure, the chiropractor may be able to provide palliative (symptomatic) relief. Although the treatment can be uncomfortable, direct facial massage can be extremely effective in decreasing the pain and spasms associated with this condition.

NOSEBLEEDS

Signs and Symptoms

● Sudden stream of blood from one nostril

Description

A nosebleed is characterized by blood flowing from one nostril. This trickle of blood may be so light you may not even realize you have a nosebleed until someone points it out to you.

Small, fragile blood vessels are located in the *septum*, the cartilage that separates the two nostrils. Nosebleeds can occur when one or more of these easily damaged vessels is burst, such as from some type of trauma (for example, a blow to the nose), dry air (which makes the mucous membranes crusty and cracked), constant or forceful nose-blowing, or a scab being scraped off.

Conventional Medical Treatment

Rarely does a one-time nosebleed require medical intervention. To stop the blood flow, simply sit or stand up, pinch the end of your nose, and breathe through your mouth. In 5 to 15 minutes, the blood should stop. If the blood continues after this, see a doctor, who may suction away excess blood, then pack your nose with cotton. In severe cases, your physician may cauterize the broken blood vessel.

For More Information
National Safety Council
1121 Spring Lake Drive
Itasca, IL 60143-3201
630-285-1121
www.nsc.org

One Factor Behind Mysterious Nosebleeds

Von Willebrand's disease is a clotting disorder that is characterized by nosebleeds. The disease, which affects more people than hemophilia, also causes bleeding gums, bruising, and excessive menstrual flow in women. Von Willebrand's disease is a hereditary condition, estimated to affect as many as 1 in every 100 people. It can be transmitted to both sons and daughters by either parent (who may or may not exhibit symptoms). Many individuals do not even realize they have this health condition, which puts them at risk for excessive blood loss during medical procedures such as surgery or tooth extraction. A blood test can identify the presence of von Willebrand's disease.

Health Notes

➤ If the air in your home is dry, consider getting a humidifier. An arid environment can dry out mucous membranes in the nose, which can lead to a nosebleed.

➤ Blow your nose gently. Forceful nose-blowing can rupture a nasal capillary, causing a bloody nose.

➤ Hydrated nasal membranes are less likely to bleed. Keep the inside of your nose moisturized during dry weather or constant nose-blowing by applying a very thin layer of petroleum jelly to the inside of nostrils.

➤ When playing sports, such as football or hockey, wear a faceguard to protect your nose from injury.

Complementary and Alternative Treatments

Nutrition and Supplementation

Nosebleeds can be a symptom of vitamin deficiencies. Enhance your vitamin C intake by eating citrus fruits, tomatoes, potatoes, cabbage, and green peppers. Get your vitamin K through yogurt, alfalfa, soybean oil, and kelp. Oranges, lemons, and limes supply you with necessary bioflavonoids.

In addition, take a daily vitamin C supplement (1000 mg) with 500 mg bioflavonoids.

Ayurvedic Medicine

To stop the bleeding, Ayurvedic practitioners may recommend squeezing your nostrils together and breathing through your mouth. They also may advise holding a cool compress against your forehead while you squeeze your nose.

To prevent future nosebleeds, Ayurvedic practitioners may advise humidifying your home. If the air in your home is too dry, the mucous membranes in your nose can become very dry, and crack and bleed.

Traditional Chinese Medicine

Acupuncture Acupuncture may be useful in rechanneling the flow of blood and *chi*, which can help stop a nosebleed. Also, by strengthening the lung and spleen functions, acupuncture may help minimize or prevent chronic nosebleeds.

Acupressure The practitioner typically presses firmly on Large Intestine 4 and 20, Bladder 10, Gallbladder 20, Pericardium 6, and Governing Vessel 14 to stop a nosebleed.

Chinese Herbal Therapy For recurrent (chronic) nosebleeds, see an herb-trained acupuncturist. Herbs in combination with bioflavonoids may be helpful.

n

SYMPTOM:

NUMBNESS

Numbness—known medically as paresthesias *— is not a painful sensation, per se, but merely a strange one. Characterized by a tingling, or a "dead" feeling (that is, no feeling at all), numbness can affect any part of the body. It can appear suddenly or develop gradually.*

The most common cause of numbness is a body part that has "fallen asleep." This occurs when blood flow to an area is temporarily decreased. Unusual postures (such as tucking your legs under you while sitting for an extended period of time, or reclining with an arm or leg kept above the heart level for an extended period of time) are the most common cause of this "sleeping" state.

Simply lowering the affected part of the body below heart level and gently moving it will encourage blood flow to the area.

If feelings of numbness are not temporary, see your physician. To uncover the cause behind your paresthesias, your physician may ask when you first experienced the sensation, how long it lasted, and other pertinent questions. You also may receive a thorough physical exam.

A wide range of conditions, some very serious, may be associated with numbness, including multiple sclerosis, brain tumors, carpal tunnel syndrome, trauma, diabetes, shingles, poisoning, rabies, and migraines. When the underlying condition is treated, the numbness should disappear. See your doctor immediately if numbness occurs in one or more limbs; this could indicate a stroke.

n

OBESITY

Signs and Symptoms

- Having a body mass index (BMI) of 30 or higher in addition to one or more of the following:
- Increased blood pressure
- Low exercise tolerance
- Increased respiratory rate

Description

America is obsessed with weight control. Yet, while much of the country actively diets, fitness magazines fly off of the newsstand shelves, and low- and no-fat foods crowd supermarket shelves, many studies estimate that approximately half of this country's citizens are overweight, and this includes children.

Federal health agencies, such as the National Institutes of Health, the National Center for Health Statistics, and the Food and Drug Administration (FDA), have recently created and issued new, more stringent guidelines as to what constitutes being overweight and what constitutes obesity. Instead of centering around the classic and widely used height-and-weight-tables made popular by the Metropolitan Life Health Insurance company, the new guidelines measure something called body mass index, or BMI. Your BMI equals 704.5 multiplied by your weight in pounds divided by your height in inches squared. For example, if you are 150 pounds and 5 feet, 8 inches tall (68 inches), your BMI can be calculated this way: 704.5×150 (pounds) $\div 4624$ (that's 68^2) = BMI of 22.8. If your BMI lies between 25 to 29.9 you are considered—by these federal guidelines—to be overweight. Obesity begins at a BMI of 30.

For the general public, the word *obese* conjures images of very large individuals, perhaps weighing 300 pounds or more. In the medical community, however, the word *obese* is used to describe a weight that directly compromises health and makes an individual susceptible to various medical conditions, including hypertension, diabetes, heart disease, stroke, and certain cancers.

Obesity is caused when there is no balance between the calories one consumes and the calories one uses. Simple overeating and under-exercising is the most common reason for this excessive weight gain, though a small number of individuals have a physical reason—such as hypothyroidism or an overly slow metabolism—that makes the body store calories as fat instead of burning them.

Conventional Medical Treatment

If you choose to see your physician, he or she may run a series of tests to eliminate any medical reason for your excess weight, such as a thyroid condition. If there is no identifiable medical reason for your weight, however, your doctor will suggest a weight loss plan. How you do this depends on how overweight you are and the lifestyle you lead at the moment. With severe obesity, for example, the heart can be phenomenally taxed, prompting your physician to put you on a liquid or other quick-loss diet *only until* a specified amount of weight comes off, and you can begin to add moderate exercise to a low-fat, reduced-calorie diet. In a small number of cases, medication is prescribed to help suppress appetite or to reduce metabolism of dietary fats. *Note*: FDA guidelines state that these medications should only be prescribed to individuals with a BMI of 30 or more.

The typical weight loss plan includes a medically supervised regime of low-fat foods and low-impact aerobic exercise until you reach a goal weight. *Be warned*: Once you reach this goal, you must continue eating nutritiously and exercising—otherwise, the number on the scale will begin to creep back up to where it used to be.

O

BMI Chart

Body mass index, measured by height and weight:

BMI	21	22	23	24	25	26	27	28	29	30	31	32	33	34	35	36
Ht	Wt															
60	107	112	118	123	128	133	138	143	148	153	158	163	168	174	179	184
61	111	116	122	127	132	137	143	148	153	158	164	169	174	180	185	190
62	115	120	126	131	136	142	147	153	158	164	169	175	180	186	191	196
63	118	124	130	135	141	146	152	158	163	169	175	180	186	191	197	203
64	122	128	134	140	146	151	157	163	169	174	180	186	192	197	204	209
65	126	132	138	144	150	156	162	168	174	180	186	192	198	204	210	216
66	130	136	142	148	155	161	167	173	179	186	192	198	204	210	216	223
67	134	140	146	153	159	166	172	178	185	191	198	204	211	217	223	230
68	138	144	151	158	164	171	177	184	190	197	203	210	216	223	230	236
69	142	149	155	162	169	176	182	189	196	203	209	216	223	230	236	243
70	146	153	160	167	174	181	188	195	202	209	216	222	229	236	243	250
71	150	157	165	172	179	186	193	200	208	215	222	229	236	243	250	257
72	154	162	169	177	184	191	199	206	213	221	228	235	242	250	258	265
73	159	166	174	182	189	197	204	212	219	227	235	242	250	257	265	272
74	163	171	179	186	194	202	210	218	225	233	241	249	256	264	272	280
75	168	176	184	192	200	208	216	224	232	240	248	256	264	272	279	287

To use the Body Mass Index (BMI) table, find your height in inches in the left-hand column. Move across to find your weight. The number at the top of the column is your BMI. Pounds have been rounded off.

The National Institutes of Health established these guidelines: "overweight" is now defined as a BMI of 25 to 29.9 and "obesity" as a BMI of 30 or above.

Chart courtesy of the National Heart, Lung, and Blood Institute of the National Institutes of Health

For More Information
American Dietetic Association
216 West Jackson Boulevard
Chicago, IL 60606-6995
312-899-0040
www.eatright.org

National Health Information Center
P.O. Box 1133
Washington, DC 20013-1133
800-336-4797
http://nhic-nt.health.org

Complementary and Alternative Treatments

Nutrition and Supplementation

Sound nutrition is the key to preventing obesity, shedding excess pounds, and helping maintain a healthy weight. Balancing your calories is important. There are three components in food that provide calories: carbohydrates, protein, and fat. Let's take a look at each.

Childhood Fat, Adult Health Problems

Experts are no longer looking at baby fat as something children will outgrow. Study after study has concluded that overweight children are likely to turn into heavy adults. According to national long-term studies, about a third (26 to 41 percent) of obese preschool children were obese as adults, and about half (42 to 63 percent) of obese school-aged children were obese as adults. The risk of adult obesity was greater for children who were more obese and for children who were obese at older ages. Furthermore, research has found that heart disease may begin in children with elevated cholesterol and blood pressure, which commonly accompany obesity.

Parents are believed to play a large role in their children's obesity, for a variety of reasons. Genetics may be one factor. Scientists believe childhood obesity may be genetic, since the chance of a child's being obese is 70 percent if both parents are obese and 50 percent if only one parent is obese. Yet, there may be more at work than DNA. One controlled study found that obese parents prepare their children's food with more fat than that used by normal-weight parents. The children of obese parents had significantly less exercise and activity than children of non-obese parents. Weight maintenance (allowing a child to maintain her current weight until she grows into it) is preferred by many pediatricians to automatically placing an obese child on a diet. Recent studies have shown that children can be taught to prefer low-fat foods and to enjoy physical exercise.

Carbohydrates are plant foods that furnish your body with energy. They regulate bowel function and protect against heart disease and certain types of cancer. Low-calorie, nutrient-rich whole grains, fruits, and vegetables fall into this category and have the added advantage of being high in fiber. Healthy foods high in complex carbohydrates include whole grains, beans, lentils, and plain baked potatoes. Tofu, dried legumes, nuts, and seeds are good sources of complex carbohydrates as well as being good sources of protein.

If you're battling a weight problem, beware of refined carbohydrates, including sugar and white flour products. Such foods should be severely restricted if not totally avoided. About 30 percent of your calories should come from carbohydrates.

Protein is essential in building, repairing, and maintaining bodily tissues—your muscles and organs. Protein is a key component of enzymes, hormones, and many body fluids. It is found in all animal foods (meat, fish, poultry, dairy) as well as in vegetable sources, such as dried legumes, especially soy, nuts, and seeds. Get 40 percent of your daily calories from protein.

Fat is not necessarily evil. Healthy fats, such as those found in avocados, olives, raw nuts, seeds, and fish contain essential fatty acids. Avoid the saturated animal fats found in butter, cream, gravies, ice cream, whole milk, and rich dressings, and the hydrogenated fats found in cookies, cakes, pies, chips and crackers, fast foods, junk foods, and many prepared foods. However, if you're trying to lose weight, do not automatically cut all fats from your diet, as some fat is necessary to help your body absorb certain essential vitamins. Fats also are building blocks for hormones, cushion the organs, and provide energy. Adjust your diet so only 20 to 30 percent of your daily calories come from fats, and only 8 to 10 percent of that from saturated fats.

Balance is the key to weight loss and weight management. You need to eat a wide variety of nutrient-rich whole foods. Include more fruits, vegetables, whole grains, and plant-based proteins. Most fruits and vegetables are low in calories but high in essential nutrients. Vegetables, such as broccoli, carrots, cauliflower, collards, green beans, onions, spinach, and all whole grains, are high in fiber. Fiber is essential in maintaining a healthy weight because it keeps the colon clean and allows for easier digestion. Eat two to three servings of nutrient-rich fruits—such as cantaloupe, grapefruit, strawberries, and watermelon—each day, plus three to seven half-cup servings of vegetables.

O

419

Obesity

Unless you're a committed vegetarian, there's no need to eliminate animal products from your diet. However, by building your meals around fruits, vegetables, and grains, you'll naturally consume smaller amounts of dairy products and animal protein. When you do eat foods from these last two groups, make healthy choices: skim or 1 percent milk; non-fat or low-fat yogurt; reduced-fat cheeses; low-fat or fat-free sour cream; lean, skinless meats prepared without additional fats.

Portion control is essential, too, especially where protein is concerned. A good rule of thumb is to limit your animal protein portion to a serving no larger than the palm of your hand.

Limiting fats is a good place to start, but take it further. Excess sodium contributes to obesity as well as to high blood pressure and the risk of heart attack and stroke. To enhance the flavor of your food, use onions, fresh garlic, and ginger root. Dijon mustard, fresh lemons and limes, flavored vinegars, and plenty of herbs and spices are good replacements for salt.

It's easy to get caught up in numbers, but caloric needs vary with each individual. Do you lead a sedentary lifestyle or are you more active? What is your age? your gender? your genetic history? All of these factor into figuring out how many calories you need, so it's important that you sit down with a nutritionist to figure out a regimen that is well matched to your specific requirements.

One statistic is indisputable: To lose one pound of fat, you must burn 3,500 calories more than you take in, or consume 3,500 fewer calories than you need. If you're aiming to lose weight, it's realistic to expect to lose one pound a week if, on a daily basis, you eat 500 fewer calories than you need or burn 500 calories through exercise. A loss of one to two pounds per week is considered healthy.

All the wholesome foods in the world won't help if you don't exercise. In addition to making you feel better physically, exercise improves your emotional and mental outlook. You don't need to spend a lot of time exercising: 30 minutes of walking a day for five to seven days a week is sufficient, and will put you on a course for maintaining a healthy weight.

Nutritional supplements can help as well. Here is a daily supplement guide:

- chromium picolinate (200 to 400 mcg)—increases lean body mass and boosts energy

- L-carnitine (500 to 1000 mg)—helps burn fatty acids

- lecithin (1 tbsp)—emulsifies fat

- evening primrose oil (500 mg)—provides essential fatty acids and controls appetite

- vitamin C with bioflavonoids (3000 to 6000 mg)—speeds up a slow metabolism

- pyruvate (as directed)—helps burn fat

- garcinia (as directed)—reduces appetite

- St. John's wort (300 mg, 3 times daily)—can reduce cravings (Do not use in conjunction with antidepressants. St. John's wort may act as a mild monoamine oxidase inhibitor [MAOI]; consult your healthcare provider regarding potential dietary and medication restrictions.)

(Consult your healthcare provider regarding the duration of treatment.)

Ayurvedic Medicine

According to Ayurveda, obesity is a kapha disorder in which the gastric fire is strong but the cellular fire is weak. To control weight, Ayurvedic practitioners may suggest eating less fat and exercising more. They also may recommend taking *guggul* or *garcinia cambozia,* urge you to consume your main meal early in the day, and recommend chewing your food slowly to savor each mouthful.

Ayurvedic products are available at many health food stores and Indian pharmacies. Remember to consult with your doctor before starting a weight-management program.

Traditional Chinese Medicine

Acupuncture Acupuncture can be used to improve the flow of *chi* throughout the body (which may help boost metabolism) and to regulate any imbalances. It is also effective in curbing excessive or unhealthy food cravings that may contribute to obesity and weight gain. Acupuncture also can help stimulate metabolic change and reduce an overabundance of dampness in the body which, in turn, helps the person better control bingeing.

Acupressure Acupressure may be helpful in reducing cravings and restoring the flow of *chi* throughout the body. It also can improve the body's ability to burn fat and enhance digestion. Points that are typically manipulated during a weight-loss massage session include Bladder 20, 23, and 36; Spleen 10; and Stomach 34.

O

Chinese Herbal Therapy Chinese medicine views obesity as an overabundance of dampness and phlegm within the body—in other words, metabolic laziness. To help counteract this excess accumulation, black pepper may be prescribed to hasten and enhance digestion, while Japanese honeysuckle may be used for its diuretic properties. Joint fir (also known as ephedra or *Ma Huang*) is a time-honored anti-obesity herb that works by regulating appetite and stimulating sluggish metabolism, but must be used under the direction of an herb-trained acupuncturist to achieve the best results.

Depending upon what is determined to be the root cause of a patient's obesity, a Chinese medical expert may recommend the following over-the-counter combination preparations: Apricot Seed and Linum, Poria Five Herb Combination, Minor Bupleurum, Ledebouriella and Platycodon, or Stephania and Astragalus formulas.

Yoga and Meditation

 A routine of gentle yoga and meditation can help you stay focused on weight management, improve your strength, and acquire a healthy self-image. If you haven't exercised before, start with four or five poses, such as the Sun Salutation, Camel, Cobra, Spinal Twist, and Supported Shoulder Stand, and practice them daily. Deep breathing is also advised.

OSTEOPOROSIS

Signs and Symptoms

- Backaches (especially low back pain)
- Stooped posture
- Loss of height over time
- Fractures of the vertebrae, wrists, ankles, or hips
- Fractures that seem to happen by themselves and not in response to trauma (such as a fall or accident)

Description

You've probably seen those little old ladies—and, in some cases, men—stooped toward the ground and supported by canes. Osteoporosis is to blame for their deformed postures. Many of these individuals have a "dowager's hump" on their upper back. Osteoporosis is a bone disease that occurs when calcium stores in the bones become low. The bones then lose their density and become porous and fragile.

Osteoporosis and Osteoarthritis—What's the Difference?

Osteoporosis and osteoarthritis are easily confused: They are both bone diseases and both commonly occur in women. The difference is that osteoporosis is a painless disorder characterized by bone loss in weight-bearing sites, such as the spine or hips. Osteoporosis causes bone deterioration and weakness, leading to a forward spine curvature and frequent painful fractures. On the other hand, osteoarthritis is a painful joint disorder causing stiffness and swelling that typically affects the hands, knees, and hips of middle-aged people. The deterioration of articular cartilage causes cytokine release, leading to inflammation of the joint area. Anti-inflammatory drugs reduce the pain and swelling in osteoarthritis, while analgesics, rest, and physical therapy help manage the condition.

Health Notes

➤ If you suffer from depression, seek counseling. Studies have shown that depression seems to be a risk factor in osteoporosis, although it is not exactly known why.

➤ Ask your physician whether you are eating too much protein. Because excess protein can deplete the body's absorption of calcium, high protein consumption has been implicated in osteoporosis.

➤ Engage in regular weight-bearing exercise—such as walking, jogging, or low-impact aerobics—for 30 minutes, 3 to 7 times per week.

➤ Up your calcium intake! To prevent osteoporosis, you need at least 1000 mg each day (1500 mg each day if you are younger than 25, or postmenopausal). If you are in your 20s or older, make sure you are eating calcium-rich foods and dairy products to build up your calcium "bank." Calcium "withdrawals" begin around age 35.

➤ If you are menopausal, consider hormone replacement therapy. The estrogen this therapy contains protects against bone loss.

➤ Quit smoking. Studies have shown that smoking is a risk factor in developing osteoporosis.

➤ Lift weights. A recent study has shown that strength training can help women avoid osteoporosis. Postmenopausal women who underwent twice-weekly strength training sessions preserved bone density while improving muscle mass, strength, and balance. A good rule of thumb is to choose dumbbells at a weight that you can lift comfortably and perform 8 to 10 strength-training exercises 2 or 3 times per week. If you need guidance, ask your physician to recommend a physical therapist or physical trainer who can help you.

Because men start with a higher concentration of bone calcium, they are less likely to get the disease than women are. Those most at risk for osteoporosis are smokers, heavy drinkers, those with insufficient calcium intake, the sedentary, and postmenopausal women—all these individuals experience a loss of bone calcium. Another group at risk are individuals with small bone frames—especially Caucasians and Asians.

Conventional Medical Treatment

Bone densitometry (a bone scan) can determine whether you have osteoporosis. If you are postmenopausal or younger than 25, your healthcare provider will recommend that you get at least 1500 mg of calcium a day (1000 mg if you are premenopausal) to prevent further bone loss. You may require calcium supplements if your diet does not contain enough calcium-rich foods. Your physician also may prescribe estrogen replacement therapy, which slows the body's absorption rate of the bones' remaining calcium. The drugs alendronate and nasal calcitonin—which help preserve and restore bone mass—also may be prescribed.

Non-medical measures include weight-bearing exercise—weight lifting, walking, jogging, and low-impact aerobics—which helps bones regain a measure of calcium.

For More Information
National Arthritis and Musculoskeletal and Skin Diseases Information Clearinghouse
Building 31, Room 4C05
31 Center Drive, MSC 2350
Bethesda, MD 20892-2350
301-495-4484
www.nih.gov/niams

National Osteoporosis Foundation
1232 22nd Street, NW
Washington, DC 20037-1292
202-223-2226
www.nof.org

Complementary and Alternative Treatments

Nutrition and Supplementation

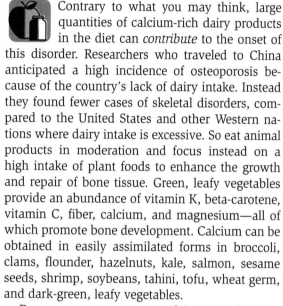

Contrary to what you may think, large quantities of calcium-rich dairy products in the diet can *contribute* to the onset of this disorder. Researchers who traveled to China anticipated a high incidence of osteoporosis because of the country's lack of dairy intake. Instead they found fewer cases of skeletal disorders, compared to the United States and other Western nations where dairy intake is excessive. So eat animal products in moderation and focus instead on a high intake of plant foods to enhance the growth and repair of bone tissue. Green, leafy vegetables provide an abundance of vitamin K, beta-carotene, vitamin C, fiber, calcium, and magnesium—all of which promote bone development. Calcium can be obtained in easily assimilated forms in broccoli, clams, flounder, hazelnuts, kale, salmon, sesame seeds, shrimp, soybeans, tahini, tofu, wheat germ, and dark-green, leafy vegetables.

Be sure to consume your calcium supplements separately from your whole grains. Whole grains contain a substance that binds with calcium, and therefore, may hinder assimilation. Calcium is absorbed best at bedtime and also promotes sleep.

Consume almonds, asparagus, cashews, rhubarb, and spinach in moderation; they contain oxalic acid, which inhibits calcium absorption. Other foods that may inhibit calcium absorption include sugar, citrus fruits, tomatoes, salt, soft drinks, and alcohol. Smoking poses the same threat. Sodas and meat products are high in phosphorus, which competes with calcium for absorption. Caffeine also has been linked to calcium loss. Nutritionists recommend the following daily supplements:

- calcium (1600 mg)—maintains strong bones; citrate form is best absorbed in older people
- boron (3 mg)—improves calcium absorption
- copper (3 mg)—aids in bone formation
- magnesium (500 to 1000 mg)—vital for calcium uptake
- vitamin A (25,000 IU; do not exceed 8000 IU if you are pregnant)—retards the aging process
- vitamin D (400 to 800 IU)—enhances calcium uptake
- zinc (30 mg; do not exceed a total of 100 mg from all supplements)—important for calcium uptake; use lozenge form
- ipraflavone (200 mg 3 times daily)—supports optimal bone density and helps prevent bone loss due to aging

(Consult your healthcare provider regarding the duration of treatment.)

Ayurvedic Medicine

To help maintain bone density, Ayurvedic practitioners advise eating a handful of sesame seeds, which are an excellent source of calcium, every day. They also may recommend drinking almond milk. In addition, the Ayurvedic herbs *shatavari* and *amla* are sometimes suggested.

Ayurvedic products are available at many health food stores and Indian pharmacies.

Traditional Chinese Medicine

Acupuncture Acupuncture may enhance the body's ability to absorb much-needed calcium by balancing the body's homeostasis. It also may be effective at lessening pain and improving energy levels.

Chinese Herbal Therapy Because TCM practitioners believe that bone health is related to kidney health, they usually recommend herbs that augment bone sinew and strengthen kidney energy, such as caltrop, eucommia, polygala, polygonatum cirrhifolium, teasel, and wild Chinese jujube. Rehmannia Eight or Rehmannia Six, two herbal combination formulas, also may be prescribed to strengthen weak bones.

Yoga and Meditation

 Do easy exercises—such as the Mountain, Tree, Warrior, and Triangle poses—daily to help strengthen your legs and back and improve posture. If you already have osteoporosis, consult your doctor to be sure the exercises are safe for you. Do not try Shoulder Stands or Head Stands without the supervision of a qualified instructor.

PARKINSON'S DISEASE

Signs and Symptoms

- Reduced ability to move face
- Mild tremors, either limited to a specific body part or involving the entire body
- Slowing of movements
- Shuffling gait
- Stiff or rigid limbs
- Slow, monotone, or low-pitched voice
- Stooped posture
- Difficulty in maintaining balance
- Difficulty talking
- Memory loss
- Fixed facial expression, with unblinking eyes, open mouth, and involuntary drooling (in late-stage cases)
- Complete inability to move arms, legs, neck and/or face (in late-stage cases)

Description

Parkinson's disease involves the progressive deterioration of nerve cells in the part of the brain that controls muscle movements. It is the job of these nerve cells to make dopamine, the brain chemical responsible for transporting signals from one brain cell to another. Once these cells lose the ability to make dopamine, a person's walking, arm movements, and facial expression become impaired. Symptoms may occur on one or both sides of the body. The disease is also called shaking palsy because of the mild, all-over shaking experienced by many sufferers.

Parkinson's disease is a progressive condition, meaning that it tends to worsen gradually over time. During the beginning of the disease symptoms are often so mild that an individual doesn't realize he or she is sick. With time, symptoms can worsen until a person is almost totally immobile and may be restricted to bed. How long this degeneration takes varies from person to person. Some people go from mild to extreme symptoms within the space of 5 years, while others experience a slower progression of symptoms over 20 or more years.

Men are slightly more likely than women to suffer from the disease. One-quarter to one-third of all Parkinson's patients have a family history of the disease, the risk being highest if a father also was affected. Most patients develop the disease at age 60 or older.

Conventional Medical Treatment

There are no standard tests to detect the presence of Parkinson's disease, yet if the condition is somewhat advanced, a physician can often recognize it by studying physical symptoms. A blood

Nicotine and Parkinson's

Cigarettes have long been implicated in a wide range of health conditions, from pneumonia to cancer to heart disease. Yet, there is one disease that cigarette smokers have a reduced risk of: Parkinson's disease. Research has confirmed that nicotine stimulates the release of dopamine, a discovery that helps explain why smokers have low incidences of Parkinson's disease. Don't expect physicians to push cigarettes as a cure for Parkinson's; however, research is currently underway to create new medications that will mimic nicotine's dopamine-stimulating abilities without the health risks traditionally associated with nicotine.

Health Notes

➤ If you are a Parkinson's patient, ask your physician about diet strategies to maximize the benefits of your medication.

➤ The Parkinson Foundation suggests that patients take Levodopa® medication an hour before meals, to allow absorption and transport of the drug to the brain before protein can interfere. Another popular approach is the protein redistribution diet, in which Levodopa® is given in the morning and virtually all the day's protein is given in the evening. Yet this can disrupt the drug's effectiveness in the evening.

➤ If chewing or swallowing become difficult, you may need to switch to a soft-food diet.

➤ To the best of your ability, engage in regular, moderate exercise. Exercise helps Parkinson's patients maintain flexibility, mobility, and even emotional stability.

➤ Depression is common in Parkinson's patients and professional psychotherapy or counseling can help patients maintain a positive attitude.

test, CT scan, and/or an MRI may be performed to rule out other diseases that may be mistaken for Parkinson's disease.

Usually a combination of drugs are used to treat Parkinson's disease. Levodopa®, a medication that helps increase the amount of dopamine in the brain, is prescribed to most Parkinson's patients. Selegiline or deprenyl (Elderpryl®) may be used early on in Parkinson's to improve symptoms. This medication works by blocking dopamine breakdown. Anticholinergic drugs, such as trihexphenidyl (Artane®) and benztropine mesylate (Cogentin®) also may be used to limit any tremors. As the disease progresses, drug therapy is continually monitored and modified as necessary; dosages are changed, certain drugs discontinued, and new drugs prescribed.

For More Information

National Foundation for Brain Research
1250 24th Street, NW - Suite 300
Washington, DC 20037-1124
202-293-5453
www.brainnet.org

Parkinson's Disease Foundation
William Black Medical Building
Columbia-Presbyterian Medical Center
710 West 168th Street
New York, NY 10032-9982
800-457-6676
www.pdf.org

Complementary and Alternative Treatments

Nutrition and Supplementation

 The healing process can be enhanced by a fresh, "live foods" diet consisting of alkaline foods and chlorophyll-rich "green" drinks. Live foods are those that are still living or growing—for example, sprouts, eaten raw—to preserve active enzymes. Consume these drinks twice daily, and use only bottled or filtered water (to minimize the ingestion of toxins).

Antioxidants are vital since they help overcome oxidative damage to the brain, and can slow the progression of this disorder. Be sure to get the amino acid phenylalanine, found in almonds, Brazil nuts, fish, pecans, pumpkin and sesame seeds, chickpeas, and lentils. Try to limit your intake of protein to 7 grams daily. This decrease in protein will help with coordination and muscle control.

If you're taking the drug Levodopa®, eat these foods in moderation, as they contain B_6, a vitamin that interferes with the drug's potency: bananas, beef, fish, liver, oatmeal, peanuts, potatoes, and whole grains.

The following recommended daily supplements should improve your condition.

Most Important

- vitamin E (3200 IU three times)—may slow progression of the disease and postpone the need for drug therapy
- selenium (200 mcg)—a powerful antioxidant
- Nicotinamide Adenine Dinucleotide (NADH; 5 mg 2 times daily)—helps activate the brain's natural production of L-dopa and dopamine
- N-acetyl cysteine (1,000 mg, on an empty stomach)
- complete antioxidant formula (as directed)
- lipoic acid (200 mg, with a meal)
- coenzyme Q10 (200 mg, with a meal)
- polyphenol supplement (120 mg)

Also Recommended

- calcium (1500 mg)—necessary for nerve impulse transmission
- magnesium (750 mg)—works with calcium
- grape seed oil (as directed on label)—contains a high level of vitamin E and linoleic acid, an essential fatty acid
- vitamin B_5 (25 mg 3 times daily)—speeds messages from one nerve cell to another
- omega-3 or flaxseed oil (as directed)—may reduce the frequency and severity of tremors

- vitamin C (3000 to 6000 mg, in divided doses)—may slow progression of the disease
- phosophatidyl serine (1500 mg)
- acetyl L-carnitine (1500 mg)
- glutathione (500 mg)

(Consult your healthcare provider regarding the duration of treatment.)

Traditional Chinese Medicine

 Acupuncture Traditional Chinese Medicine attributes Parkinson's to a liver imbalance combined with various types of weakness. Acupuncture may be helpful in controlling the tremors and muscle rigidity that characterize Parkinson's disease. It also can help alleviate the mental depression that is often associated with the disease.

Chinese Herbal Therapy Tibetan saffron and tree peony formulations may alleviate muscle tremors, while polygala can be helpful in lifting the patient's spirits. Since Chinese medicine views Parkinson's disease as an "internal wind illness," herbs also will be given to treat the underlying condition.

PELVIC INFLAMMATORY DISEASE (PID)

Signs and Symptoms

- May be asymptomatic (no symptoms)
- Mild, recurrent pain in lower abdomen
- Backache
- Irregular menstrual periods
- Heavy menstrual periods
- Vaginal discharge that may be heavy
- Pain during intercourse
- Severe pain and tenderness in the lower abdomen (in some cases)
- Fever (in some cases)
- Vomiting (in some cases)
- Severe pain in lower abdomen with nausea, vomiting, faintness, and signs of shock (emergency symptoms)

Description

Pelvic inflammatory disease (PID) is caused by one of several bacteria that are usually transmitted sexually, but also can be transmitted during an invasive medical procedure to the pelvic region (such as dilation and curettage) or childbirth. The bacteria infects one or more of the reproductive structures in the pelvis, including the fallopian tubes, ovaries, and uterus. Many women are asymptomatic or experience symptoms so mild that they do not realize that there is anything wrong. Unfortunately, the condition can become serious. If inflammation damages the fallopian tubes or ovaries, there is a higher risk for ectopic pregnancy or infertility. Should an abscess develop somewhere in the pelvic region, there's a danger that the abscess can burst and perforate one of the reproductive structures. A rarer emergency is bacteria from the pelvic infection invading the bloodstream and causing blood poisoning.

Conventional Medical Treatments

A gynecologist or physician can diagnose PID with a pelvic exam and a culture of secretions. An ultrasound may help your doctor make a diagnosis. Treatment generally entails antibiotics for the patient and her sexual partner. In severe cases, or if an abscess is present, hospitalization and intravenous antibiotics are recommended. PID returns in 10 to 25 percent of cases.

For More Information
American College of Obstetrics and Gynecology
409 12th Street SW, P.O. Box 96920
Washington, DC 20090-6920
800-673-8444
www.acog.org

Fertility Research Foundation
875 Park Avenue
New York, NY 10021
888-FRF-BABY
www.frfbaby.com

Health Notes

➤ *Get an annual pelvic exam to detect problems, such as PID, before they have a chance to grow serious.*

➤ *At the first sign of unusual pain or bleeding, visit your gynecologist for a checkup.*

➤ *Do not use douches. A recent study has found that women who douche once every three months have double the risk of PID (compared to women who never use douches), while those who douche weekly have a ten times higher risk.*

➤ *Practice safe sex (with condoms) to diminish the chance of being infected by sexually transmitted bacteria.*

➤ *Women who use an IUD (intrauterine device) as birth control have higher rates of PID than women who use other methods. The device itself is believed to make it easier for bacteria to enter the uterus.*

ⓟ

Complementary and Alternative Treatments

Nutrition and Supplementation

 Although there isn't anything in the way of diet to improve or prevent this condition, there are supplements that can be of benefit. Nutritionists recommend the following daily program:

- a prodophilus formula (as directed on label, 3 times daily)—restores friendly bacteria; especially important when taking antibiotics

- vitamin C (750 mg to 2500 mg 4 times daily)—boosts immune function and acts as an anti-viral agent

- zinc (100 mg; do not exceed this amount from all supplements)—important for the health of the reproductive organs; promotes wound healing

- colloidal silver (as directed on label)—used sublingually or topically, an antiseptic that reduces inflammation and promotes healing of lesions

- vitamin B complex (50 mg 3 times daily)—necessary in all cellular enzyme functions

- vitamin K (100 mcg)—necessary for blood clotting; destroyed by antibiotics

(Consult your healthcare provider regarding the duration of treatment.)

Traditional Chinese Medicine

Acupuncture This therapy may be used to improve circulation to the affected area, which will lessen pain and inflammation. Acupuncture also can be effective in relieving PID-related backache, abdominal pain, fever, fatigue, and vaginal discharge. The acupuncture points that practitioners focus on vary, depending upon the symptoms presented by the patient.

Acupressure The practitioner typically targets the following points to treat PID: Conception Vessel 3 and 6; Bladder 23, 31, 32, and 34; and Spleen 6 and 10—all of which will improve circulation and help manage pain.

Chinese Herbal Therapy Chinese herbs can be helpful in alleviating many of the symptoms of PID. The herbalist's recommendation may vary, depending upon the patient's specific symptoms, but may include cattail, Chinese cornbind, and ligusticum, along with herbs to fortify the kidneys and bolster the immune system.

PERIODONTITIS

p

Signs and Symptoms

- Swollen, soft and red, or recessed gums
- Gums that bleed easily
- Bad breath
- Unpleasant taste in mouth
- Pain in a specific tooth (or teeth) when eating sweet, cold, or hot foods
- Loose tooth (or teeth)

Description

If gingivitis goes untreated, periodontitis (infection around the root of the tooth) can result. Periodontitis, which can affect just a portion of the gumline or the entire gumline, is characterized by plaque-filled pockets between the teeth and gums.

As the gums become infected and inflamed, the pockets enlarge and more plaque gets trapped inside them. Pus often forms, and in severe cases, may ooze from around the affected teeth. Soon the periodontal ligament that holds the teeth (or tooth) in place becomes damaged and the alveolar bone socket that houses the teeth begins to erode. Next the affected gum detaches from the surrounding teeth, making it easy for teeth to fall out.

Conventional Dental Treatment

If you suspect periodontitis, visit your dentist, who can diagnose the condition with X-rays and a thorough exam. Treatment begins with a complete cleaning of your teeth's root surfaces. You may be

Periodontitis and Other Illnesses

Periodontitis may cause more than just missing teeth. A spate of recent studies has found that periodontal disease may significantly increase the risk for a number of health conditions. The bacteria associated with periodontitis doesn't always stay in the mouth and may travel to other parts of the body. One of the most widely-publicized links is between periodontal disease and heart disease. One study reported that people with periodontitis had a 25 percent greater risk of coronary heart disease than people with healthy gums. It is theorized that bacteria enter the bloodstream and are carried to the heart, where they weaken the cardiac muscle. Another study found that in pregnant women, bacterial toxins from infected gums can be released into the bloodstream, interfering with fetal development and retarding growth, and increasing by seven times a woman's risk of having a low-birthweight baby. Inhaling bacteria from a periodontitis-infected mouth can send germs down into the lungs and cause bacterial pneumonia. Chronic periodontal disease also has been shown to put people with diabetes at risk for poor insulin control—although it isn't exactly known how.

Health Notes

➤ If you smoke, quit. The findings of a recent study show that smoking is a risk factor in early-onset periodontitis and adult periodontitis.

➤ Consider an electric toothbrush. Researchers at the University of Buffalo, NY, found that electric toothbrushes do a better job than manual brushes in reducing levels of bacteria linked to periodontitis.

➤ If you have diabetes, your lower saliva volume puts you at an increased risk of developing periodontitis. In addition to brushing and flossing at least twice a day, talk with your healthcare provider or dentist about what you can do to lower your risk of developing gum disease.

➤ Go for regular professional teeth cleanings. Professional dental cleanings can eliminate the plaque buildup that contributes to periodontitis. Some dentists suggest twice-yearly treatments, while others recommend a professional cleaning three or four times a year.

➤ Avoid chewing tobacco. Smokeless tobacco has been implicated in the development of gum disease.

sent home with a strict regimen that includes consistent flossing and brushing. If there is no improvement with homecare—or if the periodontitis is severe—your doctor may prescribe oral antibiotics. If periodontitis is limited to one or two small areas, your dentist may instead prescribe an Actisite® patch, a tetracycline-impregnated patch that stays in place for 7 to 10 days, slowly delivering antibiotics into the site of the infection. The Food and Drug Administration (FDA) has approved the Actisite® process as another treatment for some forms of periodontal disease. In another approach now used in some European countries, a gel laced with the germ-killer metronidazole is in-

jected between teeth and gums in people with severe periodontal disease; in one study, the gel saved 94 percent of teeth. Should drug therapy not work, you may require surgery to clean the infected gum and recontour it around the teeth.

For More Information
American Dental Association
211 East Chicago Avenue
Chicago, IL 60611
312-440-2500
www.ada.org

Complementary and Alternative Treatments

Nutrition and Supplementation

 To give your teeth and gums the exercise they need, and to supply your body with the nutrients vital to healthy teeth, eat a varied diet of fresh fruits, green leafy vegetables, meat, and whole grains. Avoid carbohydrates and sugar, which inhibit the ability of white blood cells to fight bacteria.

Nutritionists recommend the following daily supplements:

- coenzyme Q10 (100 mg)—increases tissue oxygenation
- vitamin C with bioflavonoids (4000 to 10,000 mg in divided doses)—promotes healing; bioflavonoids retard plaque growth
- calcium (1500 mg)—prevents bone loss around the gums
- magnesium (750 mg)—balances the calcium
- vitamin A (25,000 IU for 1 month, then reduce to 10,000 IU; do not exceed 8000 IU if you are pregnant)—heals gum tissue; use emulsion form
- mixed carotenoid formula (as directed on label)—manufactures vitamin A as needed
- vitamin E (start with 400 IU and increase slowly to 1000 IU)—heals gum tissue
- zinc (50 to 80 mg; do not exceed a total of 100 mg from all supplements)—promotes healing
- oral glutathione spray (as directed)

(Consult your healthcare provider regarding the duration of treatment.)

Traditional Chinese Medicine

 Acupuncture Acupuncture can help treat inflammation and pain, and boost the immune system so that the body is better able to resist secondary infections. The practitioner may focus on ear points related to the mouth, adrenal gland, and upper and lower jawbone.

Acupressure In addition to massaging around the mouth itself, the practitioner also may apply pressure to Stomach 6 and 7, and Large Intestine 4, which is thought to help improve the health of the teeth by improving circulation to the area.

Chinese Herbal Therapy Achyranthes and pseudoginseng can prevent bleeding gums, and in combination with formulas that include wild Chinese jujube, polygonatum, caltrop, teasel, and polygala, can help reverse bone loss. If gums and bones weaken to the point that teeth become loose, the practitioner may recommend preparations containing eclipta.

The practitioner also may advise the patient to brush with a paste made from turmeric, cinnamon, and cloves. Because Chinese medicine regards teeth and bone problems as being related to kidney health, herbs also may be prescribed to improve kidney function.

PHLEBITIS

Signs and Symptoms

- Severe throbbing pain, redness, heat, and swelling of the leg or a vein in the leg
- Severe pain when flexing the foot or toes
- Any tender, cord-like mass under the skin of the leg

Description

Phlebitis is the inflammation of the wall of a vein, caused by the infection of tissues next to the vein or by trauma to the area. The condition also can follow a surgical procedure or result from prolonged bed rest (which contributes to poor blood circulation). Other contributing factors may include varicose veins, obesity, certain medications (including birth control pills), heredity, and arteriosclerosis. If the condition persists, it can cause a further irritation of the vein, or the vein can accumulate deposits from the blood, which may lead to the development of blood clots attached to the vein wall (a condition known as *thrombophlebitis*).

Phlebitis usually occurs in the superficial veins of the leg where it is generally not considered a serious problem. When it occurs in deeper blood vessels, there is a greater risk of blood clots breaking free, circulating in the bloodstream, and causing an obstruction in the brain, lungs, or heart.

Conventional Medical Treatment

When phlebitis occurs in a superficial vein, you can generally relieve the pain and swelling by taking analgesics, applying wet compresses, using elastic support hose, elevating your leg, and resting. Elevate your leg as much as possible to assist in blood circulation and sleep with your feet elevated on pillows. Wearing full-length support pantyhose or physician-prescribed support hose can also improve circulation. Avoid wearing knee-length hose, which can interfere with circulation. Once the pain is relieved, you may begin a regimen of mild exercise to improve blood circulation. Do not begin any exercise program, however, without consulting with your physician.

In the case of severe phlebitis, or thrombophlebitis, you should be under the care of a physician. Treatment may include anticoagulants to prevent the formation of blood clots or, in the most severe cases, surgical removal of the clot.

Phlebitis sufferers should avoid smoking, since it promotes blood clotting.

For More Information
National Heart, Lung, and Blood Institute
P.O. Box 30105
Bethesda, MD 20824-0105
301-592-8573
www.nhlbi.nih.gov

Complementary and Alternative Treatments

Nutrition and Supplementation

 Consume plenty of fresh fruits and vegetables, raw nuts and seeds, soybean products, and whole grains. Get regular moderate exercise to improve circulation.

The following daily supplements help keep the veins and blood in healthy condition:

- acetyl-L-carnitine (500 mg)—protects blood vessels from fat accumulation
- coenzyme Q10 (100 to 200 mg)—improves circulation
- flaxseed oil (2 tsp)—keeps veins soft

Pleurisy

- garlic (as directed on label)—improves circulation; thins the blood
- L-histidine (500 mg)—dilates the blood vessels
- grape seed extract (as directed on label)—reduces the risk of blood vessel disease
- vitamin C (4000 to 8000 mg)—aids circulation

(Consult your healthcare provider regarding the duration of treatment.)

Hydrotherapy

 Try contrast therapy (alternating hot and cold) to increase circulation. Use a moist, hot compress followed by a cold compress. Repeat 3 times.

Traditional Chinese Medicine

 Acupuncture Acupuncture helps improve the flow of blood to and away from the affected area. Practitioners typically focus on ear points related to the kidney, heart, liver, and adrenal gland.

Acupressure As with acupuncture, this modality can be used to stimulate circulation, thereby lessening the swelling and discomfort in veins associated with phlebitis. Bioflavonoids are often given with herbal medicines.

PLEURISY

Signs and Symptoms

- Pain in the chest that worsens when inhaling
- Fatigue

Description

Pleurisy is an inflammation of the pleural lining—the membrane that lines the lungs. The inflammation is generally viral in nature. Pleurisy can accompany other lung infections, such as pneumonia and tuberculosis. The condition also can follow a lung abscess or a blood clot in the lungs (*pulmonary embolism*).

Individuals with systemic inflammatory diseases, such as rheumatoid arthritis, are especially susceptible to pleurisy that is not accompanied by a lung infection. Studies have shown that about 20 percent of rheumatoid arthritics develop pleurisy at least once during their lives.

Health Notes

➤ *Drink in moderation or not at all. Alcoholics have been shown to have higher rates of pleural infections and pneumonia.*

➤ *At the first sign of an upper respiratory condition, consult your doctor. Early care may prevent an illness from affecting the pleural membrane.*

➤ *Help your body's immune system fight a pleural infection by eating a diet high in nutrient-dense fruits and vegetables and low in processed sugars, sodium, and fats.*

➤ *Because pneumonia can cause pleurisy, if you are in general poor health or over 65, ask your doctor about being vaccinated against the Pneumococcal bacterium and influenza.*

Conventional Medical Treatment

If you experience a sharp pain when inhaling, go to your physician immediately. A chest X-ray will be performed but may show no abnormality. Treatment is usually aimed at making the patient comfortable, including bed rest and anti-inflammatory agents, such as aspirin, ibuprofen, and indomethacin.

For More Information

The American Lung Association
1740 Broadway
New York, NY 10019
800-LUNG-USA
www.lungusa.org

Complementary and Alternative Treatments

Traditional Chinese Medicine

Acupuncture Acupuncture can help alleviate pain and inflammation in the lining of lungs. It also can be useful in strengthening the patient's weakened immune system so that the body is in a better position to fight the viral intruder responsible for this infection.

The practitioner typically focuses on auricular acupuncture points related to the lung, thorax, internal secretion, and adrenal gland.

Acupressure To reduce lung pain, the therapist may focus on points along the bladder meridian, which runs the length of the chest as well as Gallbladder 34, Liver 3, and related ear points.

Chinese Herbal Therapy The TCM practitioner may prescribe balloon flower and asarum sieboldi to treat lung infection, while mastic tree may be recommended to reduce pain. There are many herb formulations, but it is best to see an herb-trained acupuncturist for a complete diagnosis first.

PNEUMONIA

Signs and Symptoms

- Cough that may expel bloody mucus
- Chest pain
- Malaise
- Rattled-sounding breathing
- Shortness of breath
- Overall congestion (in some cases)
- High fever (in some cases)
- Chills (in some cases)
- Mental confusion (in some cases)

Description

The word *pneumonia* actually describes one of more than 50 similar illnesses that cause inflammation of the lung tissue. Thus, pneumonia can be a merely uncomfortable sickness or it can be one that is life-threatening. One reason for this range of illnesses is the cause. Pneumonia can be caused by any number of bacteria, by a range of viruses, and even by chemical irritants. Furthermore, pneumonia may start out as something else—such as a flu, cold, or bronchitis—and later turn into pneumonia.

Pneumonia and Heart Disease

Heart disease patients are more likely than the general public to have circulating in their blood antibodies to *Chlamydia pneumoniae,* one of several types of bacteria that cause pneumonia. In a recent study, analysis of diseased heart tissue and arteries revealed the presence of the bacteria in 20 out of 36 samples. The bacteria, which is spread through coughs and sneezes, causes a flu-like respiratory illness that often progresses to pneumonia. Researchers believe that after causing the initial respiratory illness, the bacterium may live in the body's tissues for years, slowly entering various blood vessels and gradually causing the inflammation that causes heart attacks and strokes.

Health Notes

➤ If you are in general poor health, are over 60, have chronic lung disease or sickle cell anemia, or have had your spleen removed, ask your doctor about being vaccinated against the Pneumococcal bacterium. Pneumococcus is the most common cause of pneumonia.

➤ Promptly treat respiratory illnesses, such as colds, flus, and bronchitis, to prevent them from progressing into pneumonia.

➤ If you smoke, quit. Several studies have found increased pneumonia rates among smokers.

➤ Avoid secondhand smoke. A four-year study by the Environmental Protection Agency (EPA) found that secondhand smoke contributes to respiratory ailments, such as pneumonia.

➤ Drink in moderation or not at all. Alcoholics have been shown to have higher rates of pneumonia.

Conventional Medical Treatment

To determine what has caused your pneumonia, your physician may listen to your breathing though a stethoscope to detect distortions that may indicate infection. Your chest may be X-rayed to uncover the location and seriousness of your infection, and a sample of your sputum may be analyzed to identify the infectious agent.

Treatment is likely to involve medication and bed rest. First, the cause of your pneumonia must be determined. Antibiotics may be prescribed to treat bacteria-caused pneumonia, anti-viral medication may be given to oust viral-induced pneumonia, and bed rest in a clean environment may be suggested for pneumonia that was sparked by a chemical irritant.

Your overall health also determines what treatment you'll receive. Healthy, young to middle-aged adults may be sent home with medication and instructions to drink plenty of fluids and rest in a warm part of the house. Elderly or frail individuals or children may be treated more aggressively, perhaps even hospitalized.

For More Information
The American Lung Association
1740 Broadway
New York, NY 10019
800-LUNG-USA
www.lungusa.org

National Heart, Lung and Blood Institute
P.O. Box 30105
Bethesda, MD 20824-0105
301-592-8573
www.nhlbi.nih.gov

Complementary and Alternative Treatments

Nutrition and Supplementation

 Liquids help thin lung secretions, so drink plenty of fresh juices. Include chlorophyll-rich, "green" vegetable juices. To increase your energy level, take a protein supplement.

The following recommended daily supplements are in adult dosages. For a child between 12 and 17, reduce the dose to three-quarters of the recommended amount. For a child between 6 and 12, cut the dose in half, and for a child under 6, use one-quarter of the recommended amount.

- vitamin A (up to 100,000 IU; do not exceed 8000 if you are pregnant)—enhances immunity and promotes repair of lung tissue
- vitamin C with bioflavonoids (5000 to 20,000 mg in divided doses)—vital for immune response
- free-form amino acid complex (as directed on label)—supplies protein; important in tissue repair
- vitamin B complex (100 mg 3 times daily)—produces antibodies; forms red blood cells; important for healthy mucous membranes
- raw thymus (500 mg twice)—promotes healing of lung tissue
- vitamin E (1500 IU)—protects lung tissue; use emulsion form
- flaxseed oil (as directed on label)—builds new lung tissue; improves stamina and speeds recovery

(Take supplements until your symptoms subside. If symptoms persist, seek the advice of your healthcare provider.)

Aromatherapy

 To speed recovery, add 3 or 4 drops of the essential oils of camphor, eucalyptus, lavender, or tea tree to steam inhalations. This modality can be used to supplement other treatments.

If you can sit up and have no fever, ask someone to massage essential oils of eucalyptus, lavender, or tea tree into your back and chest. Blend 1 or 2 drops of one of these oils into 1 teaspoon of lotion or vegetable oil, and massage gently every half hour.

Herbal Therapy

 Garlic and goldenseal have anti-microbial properties and can help fight pneumonia. Eat 8 to 10 cloves of garlic daily, or take 3 garlic capsules 3 times a day. Purchase goldenseal tincture in a health food store and follow the package directions. You also can drink coltsfoot tea.

To prepare an expectorant, combine 2 ounces powdered licorice, 1 ounce powdered wild black cherry bark, 1 ounce dried coltsfoot leaves, 3/4 teaspoon dried lobelia leaves, and 1 ounce dried horehound. Simmer 1 tablespoon of the blend in 1 cup water for 5 minutes; steep for 10 minutes; strain. Drink every 2 hours. Use only under the supervision of a qualified medical herbalist and do not exceed the recommended amount.

Homeopathy

 Pneumonia may respond to homeopathic treatment. However, the selection of a remedy—more than one is available—depends on *your* symptoms and the stage of the condition. Don't try treating this disorder yourself. See a homeopathic professional.

Hydrotherapy

 Try steam inhalation for 10 minutes every hour throughout the day. Add a few drops of essential oil of eucalyptus if desired. Alternately, a cold-water friction rub can loosen congestion and improve circulation. For instruction on these techniques, see "Hydrotherapy" in the "Introduction to Complementary Therapies" section.

Drink large amounts of water while you're recovering from this condition.

Traditional Chinese Medicine

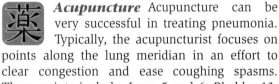 ***Acupuncture*** Acupuncture can be very successful in treating pneumonia. Typically, the acupuncturist focuses on points along the lung meridian in an effort to clear congestion and ease coughing spasms. These points include: Lung 5 and 6, Bladder 13, Pericardium 6, Governing Vessel 14, Large Intestine 11, Triple Warmer 6, and Conception Vessel 17.

Acupressure Acupressure can help lessen coughing. The practitioner may manipulate the following points: Conception Vessel 17 and 22, Lung 1, and Bladder 12 and 13, among others.

Chinese Herbal Therapy Asarum sieboldi, joint fir, anemarrhena, and burdock are often used in formulas to treat pneumonia. Dried bamboo sap and perilla seed both have expectorant properties, which can help loosen phlegm and quiet coughs. The TCM practitioner may prescribe Job's Tears if the patient's cough produces blood, and Chinese black cohosh for reducing fever and chills. There are many patent formulas available for strengthening the lungs, but the single most effective herb is cordyceps, which can be used alone or in combination.

POISON IVY, POISON OAK, POISON SUMAC

Signs and Symptoms

- Itchy rash that consists of small bumps, blisters, and general swelling
- Weals or hives (in some cases)
- Burning sensation of the eyes and mucous membranes

Description

Poison ivy, poison oak, and poison sumac all contain an oily resin called *urushiol* that causes contact dermatitis in many people. Contrary to popular perception, standing next to one of these plants isn't enough to be affected—you must touch the plant with bare skin or touch clothing or a pet that has brushed against the plant. The resin can even be carried via campfire smoke, should the plant be burned. In sensitive individuals, the rash may appear hours after contact; in

other individuals, a reaction may not appear until two days after contact.

Conventional Medical Treatment

Your general physician or a dermatologist can generally diagnose the condition after physically examining the area and asking about your exposure to outdoor plants. Treatment typically includes the use of steroid creams to lessen inflammation. In severe cases, an oral antihistamine may be used to reduce symptoms.

For More Information
American Academy of Dermatology
930 North Meacham Road
Schaumburg, IL 60173
888-462-DERM
www.aad.org

Health Notes

➤ *"Leaves of three, let them be," is a traditional rhyme used to remind people to stay away from poison ivy, poison oak, and poison sumac. However, new strains of these plants often have four, five, or six leaves. Different varieties of the plants also can grow as ground-covering or tree-climbing vines, shrubs, or small bushes. A safer bet is to ask a park ranger or plant expert to show you poisonous plants before you go hiking, so you'll know exactly what to avoid.*

➤ *If you do come in contact with a poisonous plant, wash affected skin with warm water and non-perfumed soap, then applying calamine lotion to lessen itching.*

➤ *To prevent infection of open blisters, cover with sterile gauze.*

➤ *Applying a barrier cream, such as petroleum jelly or a commercial diaper rash ointment, to your skin before going hiking to lessen your chance of developing a reaction should you touch a poisonous plant.*

➤ *Wear protective clothing with long pants and long sleeves, when you go outdoors where poisonous plants grow. Because plant resin can stick to clothes and infect skin, remove and wash clothing after hiking, touching fabrics as little as possible.*

Complementary and Alternative Treatments

Nutrition and Supplementation

Although diet cannot treat these poisons, the following daily supplements should speed up the healing process:

- vitamin C (3000 to 8000 mg)—prevents infection and spreading of the rash; reduces swelling

- vitamin A (25,000 IU; do not exceed 8000 IU if you are pregnant)—heals skin tissue; boosts immune system

- vitamin E oil or cream (as directed on label)—heals skin and prevents scarring

- zinc (50 mg; do not exceed a total of 100 mg from all supplements)—aids in skin tissue repair; use lozenge form

- topical glutathione and zinc ointments (as directed)

- pantothenic acid (B$_5$; 500 mg)

(Take supplements until your symptoms subside. If symptoms persist, seek the advice of your healthcare provider.)

Herbal Therapy

To ease intense itching, apply equal parts of tinctures of witch hazel, mugwort, white oak bark, and plantain. You also can apply a poultice of plantain. Simply mash fresh plantain leaves with a mortar and pestle, and place the mash on the skin. Hold in place with cotton or gauze strips.

To aid healing and calm the red rash, rub on aloe vera gel, available in health food stores or drug stores. Follow label directions.

Homeopathy

Homeopathic practitioners often suggest one of the following remedies, depending on your symptoms:

- *Rhus toxicodendron* (derived from poison ivy)—for itching that's accompanied by extreme restlessness; you feel better after a hot shower or bath

- *Croton tiglium*—if your skin is dry and hard, and scratching your skin feels painful

Postnasal Drip

- *Anacardium*—for extreme itching that eases after a very hot shower
- *Ledum*—for itching that lessens after a cold shower or bath

Hydrotherapy

 Add apple cider vinegar, powdered oatmeal, or powdered goldenseal to a basin of cool water. Dip a clean cloth into the water and wring out the excess. Apply cool compresses, as necessary, to control itching and diminish pain.

Traditional Chinese Medicine

 Acupuncture Acupuncture can help alleviate the itching associated with these ailments (all of which are allergic forms of contact dermatitis). The practitioner typically targets the ear points related to the lung, adrenal gland, internal secretion, back of head, and any other points corresponding to the particular affected areas of the body.

Itching is often looked at as a deficiency of *chi*. Unfortunately, the scratching associated with this condition often results in abrasion and infection. Instead of scratching, try just pressure or a quick slap, which will achieve the same relief as scratching without the abrasions.

Chinese Herbal Therapy Angelica anomala, belvedere cypress, and weeping golden bell may be used as external washes to relieve itchiness and speed healing.

SYMPTOM:

POSTNASAL DRIP

Under normal conditions, your nose and sinuses produce a cupful or more of mucus each day. This mucus has a purpose—it traps the dust and other irritating particles that we inhale. The mucus trickles in a thin stream down the back of your throat and into your stomach, where these dust specs are moved out of the body. This happens unobtrusively so that it is rarely noticed. Yet, when the air is polluted, your nose must create extra mucus to surround the larger number of irritants being inhaled. No longer traveling in a spindly stream, the increase in mucus flow doesn't go unnoticed—it's called postnasal drip. Postnasal drip also occurs when individuals with allergies happen to inhale their allergen; the

nose creates extra mucus to surround the allergens. Often, postnasal drip is accompanied by a light cough.

Treatment of postnasal drip can be as easy as removing yourself from a polluted—or allergen-filled—environment. Because the extra mucus is there to help your body, most physicians advise that you not try to suppress it. Gently blowing your nose can divert some of the mucus from the back of your throat. Steam therapy can liquefy mucus, making it easier to blow your nose: run a hot shower and shut yourself in the bathroom or hold your head over a teapot of simmering water that has just been removed from the stove.

Post-Traumatic Stress Disorder/Syndrome (PTSD)

Signs and Symptoms

In response to a specific tragedy or trauma, the appearance of one or more of the following symptoms for a minimum of three weeks:

- Feeling of detachment or estrangement from others

- Inability to have loving or friendly feelings toward others or yourself

- Persistent re-experiencing of the traumatic event in intrusive daydreams and nightmares

- Avoidance of feelings, activities, and/or locations associated with the trauma

- Negative reactions to people, sounds, smells, or other situations that remind you of the event

- Distress at the anniversary of the trauma

- Diminished interest in day-to-day activities

- Sense of shortened future or impending doom

- Depression

- Explosive anger

- Fear

- A general loss of hope

- Insomnia

- Generalized anxiety

- Difficulty concentrating

- In children, regression to infant-like behaviors, such as baby talk, thumb sucking, and loss of toilet-training habits

Description

Post-traumatic stress disorder (PTSD) (or syndrome) describes an extensive set of symptoms that occurs in response to a severe trauma. Although the syndrome has long been associated with returning soldiers, it also is very common in rape victims, victims of child abuse, persons who have survived an earthquake or bombing, individuals who have been in some type of accident, victims of a mugging or severe physical assault, and others who have suffered through some other type of physical and psychological hardship. Those who have been an eyewitness to one of these traumatic events also can develop symptoms.

Symptoms typically appear anywhere from directly after the event to six months afterward. In some cases, however, symptoms may appear one, two, or even many years after the event. How long one suffers from the syndrome varies greatly, depending on a person's psychological constitution, how horrifying the event was, what type of support the victim has, and whether the victim was physically injured. Some people suffer from PTSD for the remainder of their lives. The disorder can increase one's risk of clinical depression, generalized anxiety disorder, and suicide.

Conventional Medical Treatment

Treatment for post-traumatic stress syndrome entails both medications and psychotherapy or counseling. Tranquilizers, anti-anxiety drugs, or antidepressants may be prescribed, depending on a person's symptoms. A psychiatrist or clinical psychologist who is specifically trained to treat the condition can help a person explore and sort out the conflicting and complex feelings of guilt,

p

Health Notes

➤ If you have experienced a traumatic event, experts recommend that you seek psychiatric help immediately—even if you experience no textbook signs of post-traumatic stress syndrome. Immediate psychiatric attention has been found to greatly reduce the intensity and duration of any symptoms that may occur later.

➤ Ask your healthcare provider or psychiatrist about Eye Movement Desensitization and Reprocessing (EMDR). This treatment, which has been used for panic disorders, phobias, and anxiety disorders, involves focuses on the troubling memory while performing a series of eye exercises. It is believed that this allows the brain to convert the traumatic memories into normal, less disturbing recollections. While memories of the trauma are not entirely erased by EMDR, they no longer provoke terror.

➤ Be aware that friends or family of the traumatized individual can be strongly affected by what their loved one experienced and also may need counseling.

anxiety, detachment, depression, and fear. Not only does this process allow a patient to get much-needed validation of his or her feelings, it also eases feelings of isolation from others who have not shared the traumatic experience. A mental health professional can also give individuals guidance in dealing with the debilitating and frightening feelings of suicide, rage, and grief.

For More Information
American Academy of Child and
Adolescent Psychiatry
3615 Wisconsin Avenue NW
Washington, DC 20016-3007
202-966-7300
www.aacap.org

National Institute of Mental Health
601 Executive Boulevard
Room 8184, MSC 9663
Bethesda, MD 20892-9663
301-443-4513
www.nimh.nih.gov

Complementary and Alternative Treatments

Nutrition and Supplementation

 Nutrition is particularly important during periods of stress and recovery from trauma. Your diet should be high in fiber, full of wholesome foods. Stress reactions thicken the blood, so eat foods that thin the blood, including cantaloupe, garlic, and ginger.

Vitamin C is an important antioxidant that helps protect the body against stress. Foods high in vitamin C include strawberries, red pepper, and collard greens. Citrus fruits and juices are also good sources.

The following recommended daily supplements provide some relief of PTSD symptoms:

- vitamin B complex injections (1 cc weekly or as prescribed by a healthcare provider)—necessary for proper functioning of the nervous system, supplemented with additional oral vitamin B_5 (500 mg)—the most important of the B vitamins because it dissipates quickly during stress reactions

- zinc (50 mg; do not exceed a total of 100 mg from all supplements)—enhances immune function

- vitamin C with bioflavonoids (3000 to 10,000 mg)—depleted during stress reactions; essential to adrenal gland function

- potassium (99 mg)—excreted during stress reaction

- magnesium (1000 mg)—depleted during stress reaction; a deficiency contributes to anxiety, fear, and hallucinations

- calcium (2000 mg)—depleted during stress reactions

- melatonin (start with 1.5 mg, taken 2 hours or less before bedtime. Increase dosage up to 5 mg daily if this is not effective)—promotes sleep
- adrenal live cell support therapy (as directed)

(Consult your healthcare provider regarding the duration of treatment.)

Traditional Chinese Medicine

 Acupuncture Using acupuncture to treat the patient's stress, while he or she is receiving counseling, increases the success rate of the counseling and speeds recovery.

Yoga and Meditation

 Use a combination of breathing exercises, meditation, and yoga to clear your mind, combat stress, and relax. Choose three or four poses daily, including at least one relaxation pose, such as the Child or Corpse. Alternate nostril breathing will help you relax and compose your thoughts.

PREMENSTRUAL SYNDROME (PMS)

Signs and Symptoms

- Anxiety
- Panic attacks
- Nervous tension
- Mood swings
- Irritability
- Weight gain
- Swelling
- Breast tenderness
- Abdominal bloating
- Headaches
- Sweet cravings
- Increased appetite
- Palpitations
- Fatigue
- Dizziness
- Depression
- Difficulty concentrating
- Forgetfulness
- Crying
- Insomnia
- Sadness

Description

PMS—as premenstrual syndrome is commonly called—is not as rampant among menstruating females as many women's magazines would have their readers believe. In fact, although most women have some symptoms prior to their period, the actual number of those with clinical PMS (exhibiting eight or more of the symptoms listed above) is low. Here are a few more menstrual myths that just aren't true: Painful periods are not synonymous with PMS, nor are regular uterine cramps, irritability brought on solely by the pain of uterine cramps, or skin breakouts caused by fluctuating hormone levels during menstruation.

So what is PMS? The syndrome is a documented collection of symptoms that involve the endocrine, metabolic, reproductive, intestinal, and nervous systems of some individuals. It is unknown why some women suffer from PMS—although a hormonal imbalance is the suspected culprit and heredity is thought to play a part in deciding who gets the syndrome and who doesn't. When occurring together, the symptoms are enough to upset a woman's daily life; a small number of PMS sufferers find that they are completely incapacitated by the condition. PMS symptoms typically begin seven days before menstruation and disappear when menstruation begins.

Conventional Medical Treatment

If you suspect PMS, call your gynecologist. In order to be certain that you are not confusing it with another menstrual condition—such as painful periods or normal water gain—your doctor may ask you to keep a record for two or three menstrual cycles, detailing every symptom you experience, when you experience it, and when it disappears. After you've done this, the doctor reviews your log with you, then performs a thorough physical and pelvic examination.

Do You Crave Chocolate?

Some women who suffer from PMS crave chocolate. Yet, in the past, many doctors urged PMS sufferers to stay away from chocolate not only because it contains caffeine, a stimulant that can exacerbate PMS symptoms, but because it is high in fat and sugar. Now, a growing body of evidence points to chocolate as having a positive effect on PMS, but it's still not certain whether it's a physical or psychological effect. Researchers believe that eating chocolate may stimulate the production of endorphins, which not only give such a strong sense of pleasure, but effectively block feelings of pain. Studies also have shown that women with intense PMS may get an instant antidepressant effect from chocolate.

Health Notes

➤ *Get regular, moderate exercise. Experts recommend regular exercise for PMS sufferers, to lessen the severity of symptoms and to fight fatigue and a depressed mood.*

➤ *Change your diet. A diet low in salt, sugar, and caffeine is said by many doctors to lessen bloating, headaches, and irritability.*

➤ *Reduce stress. In many individuals, stress can exacerbate symptoms of PMS.*

➤ *Consider increasing your carbohydrate intake. Scientists have found giving in to carbohydrate cravings may actually help to reduce lethargy and other PMS symptoms in sufferers with mild to moderate symptoms.*

➤ *Keep a journal tracking daily moods and mood swings before and during PMS treatment. This can help your doctor diagnose PMS as well as alter treatment if needed.*

➤ *Avoid alcohol, which can exacerbate symptoms of PMS.*

➤ *Ask your doctor about bright-light therapy, the same therapy that is used to treat seasonal affective disorder (SAD). Some studies have shown that the therapy also lessens some women's PMS symptoms.*

PMS is a difficult condition to treat; thus, your gynecologist may treat individual symptoms separately. Oral contraceptives are often prescribed to balance the body's hormone levels which, in turn, help diminish symptoms. Some doctors may prescribe antidepressants such as fluoxetine

(Prozac®), sertraline (Zoloft®), or paroxetine (Paxil®), which increase levels of the brain neurotransmitter serotonin. Serotonin levels normally rise in women before their menstrual periods, but do not seem to rise in many PMS sufferers. Diuretics can be useful in relieving swelling and bloating.

For More Information

American College of
Obstetricians and Gynecologists
409 12th Street SW, P.O. Box 96920
Washington, DC 20090-6920
800-673-8444
www.acog.org

Women's Health America
429 Gammon Place, P.O. Box 259690
Madison, WI 53725
800-558-7046
www.womenshealth.com

Complementary and Alternative Treatment

Nutrition and Supplementation

Diet is an essential part of preventing and counteracting PMS. Eat plenty of fresh fruits and vegetables, whole grain cereals and breads, beans, peas, lentils, nuts, seeds, broiled chicken and turkey, and fish. Snack on high-protein foods, such as almonds, between meals so that your blood sugar levels remain stable.

Sodium, especially salt and the foods that contain it, should be consumed in moderation, even eliminated if possible for about one week prior to the expected onset of symptoms. Sodium increases water retention and bloating. Caffeine should also be avoided, as it's linked to breast tenderness, and is a diuretic that depletes the body of important nutrients. Alcohol and sugar also cause vital electrolytes to be lost through the urine; stay away from them at least for one week prior to the onset of symptoms.

Dairy products should be consumed in moderation, if not eliminated. They block the absorption of magnesium and cause what does get absorbed to be excreted through the urine. Refined sugars also increase magnesium excretion.

Consult your healthcare provider for individualized guidelines. However, the following daily supplement recommendations are a general guide to treating and preventing PMS:

- flaxseed oil (2 tbsp)—relieves symptoms
- calcium (1500 mg, in citrate or lactate form)—relieves cramping, backache, and nervousness
- magnesium (1000 mg, in glycinate form)—deficiency is associated with PMS
- vitamin B_5 (100 to 200 mg)—reduces stress
- vitamin B_6 (25 mg 3 times daily)—reduces water retention; aids in restoring estrogen levels to normal
- vitamin E (start with 400 IU and increase slowly to 800 IU)—relieves breast discomfort; limits free radical damage; helps relieve nervous tension, irritability, and depression
- vitamin A (10,000 IU; do not exceed 8000 if you are pregnant)—deficiency has been linked to PMS
- vitamin C with bioflavonoids (3000 to 6000 mg, in divided doses)—relieves breast discomfort

Aromatherapy

For relieving the tension that often accompanies PMS, try a relaxing aromatherapy bath. Add a few drops of lavender, geranium, clary sage, or German chamomile essential oils as the tub fills with warm water.

Ayurvedic Medicine

PMS in Ayurveda is classified and treated by three types: vata, pitta, and kapha. To correct vata PMS—which is characterized by moodiness, sleeplessness, and anxiety—Ayurvedic practitioners may suggest getting more rest, meditating, and eating comfort

p

445

foods, such as stews. For pitta PMS—which is noted for irritability, rashes, and diarrhea—they may encourage meditating and avoiding caffeine and spicy, greasy foods. If you're bothered by kapha PMS—which is distinguished by swollen breasts, weight gain, and lack of energy—practitioners might recommend exercising and eating more spicy foods and legumes. For all the doshas, they might advise a laxative to remove *ama* (wastes and impurities).

In addition, some Ayurvedic practitioners encourage the use of Ayurvedic herbs, such as *dashamoola* or *kaishore guggulu.*

Ayurvedic products are available at many health food stores and Indian pharmacies.

Herbal Therapy

 Herbalists recommend a variety of herbal remedies, including teas and a daily regimen of oils for controlling PMS symptoms.

Drink skullcap tea to reduce irritability and anxiety symptoms. Consult with a medical herbalist for instructions.

If you're bothered by water retention, try dandelion tea. For an infusion, steep 1 tablespoon dried dandelion leaves or 2 tablespoons fresh in 1 cup boiling water for 10 minutes; strain. Drink no more than 4 cups daily.

For cramping, try cramp bark tea. Simmer 2 teaspoons dried bark pieces in 1 cup boiling water for 15 minutes; strain. Drink 3 times a day when needed.

Evening primrose oil or black currant seed oil can help relieve breast tenderness and other PMS symptoms. Follow package directions, and take daily, even when you're not experiencing problems.

Herbal products are available in health food stores and in some pharmacies and supermarkets. Follow package for specific directions.

Homeopathy

 The symptoms of premenstrual syndrome may respond to homeopathic treatment. However, the selection of a remedy—more than one is available—depends on *your* symptoms and the stage of the condition. Don't try treating this disorder yourself. See a homeopathic professional.

Hydrotherapy

 For a headache accompanying PMS, place cool compresses on your forehead while soaking your feet in basin of hot water for 30 minutes.

If you're bothered by mood swings, try soaking in a neutral (slightly lower than body temperature) or lukewarm bath for 30 minutes. Replenish the water to maintain the temperature, as needed.

Traditional Chinese Medicine

 Acupuncture Irritability, depression, water retention, mood swings, sugar cravings, and breast tenderness may all be lessened or relieved altogether with acupuncture.

Acupressure To relieve the bloating, food cravings, and mood swings associated with PMS, an acupressurist may work the following points: Pericardium 6, Spleen 6, Kidney 3 and 6, and Liver 3 and 13. Additional points may be added, as symptoms dictate.

Chinese Herbal Therapy If the practitioner determines PMS is being caused by a liver imbalance, Bupleurum and Tang Gui Formula may be recommended. Premenstrual syndrome brought on by insufficient kidney and spleen yang may be treated with Rehmannia Eight or Ginseng and Atractylodes formulas. And if the condition is thought to be the result of excessive liver energy, then Tang Gui Four is the formula most often used.

Additional herbs that are used in formulas to treat PMS include angelica, leonurus, ligusticum, and white peony. Another commonly used herbal combination for this condition is called Free and Easy Wanderer Pills, which is a derivation of a traditional formula.

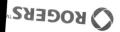

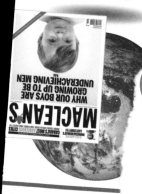
...and Meditation

Exercise is highly recommended for relieving stress and soothing PMS symptoms. Try the Reclined Cobbler, Butterfly, or Forward Bend pose. Meditate for 20 minutes daily for deep relaxation.

PROSTATE, ENLARGED

Signs and Symptoms

- Frequent need to urinate, often with an inability to sleep through the night without frequent trips to the bathroom
- Difficulty urinating
- Diminished force of urine stream
- Dribbling after the end of urination
- Recurrent urinary tract infection
- Complete inability to urinate, even though the urge is present (emergency symptom)

Description

The prostate gland is a male reproductive organ that secretes the fluid that semen needs to transport sperm. Located underneath the bladder, the prostate surrounds the urethra, which is the duct through which urine passes. The prostate does naturally enlarge somewhat as a result of aging; however, problems occur when it grows to the extent that it chokes off this passageway, making urination difficult to impossible. That said, an enlarged prostate—known medically as *benign prostatic hypertrophy* (BPH)—is an extremely common male malady, affecting 50 percent of men over 50, and 80 percent of men over 70.

Conventional Medical Treatment

To diagnose an enlarged prostate, your physician examines your prostate by inserting a gloved finger into the rectum and feeling the gland. You also may undergo a urine test, an ultrasound of the prostate gland, and/or a bladder cystoscope test. A cytoscope is passed through the urethra into the bladder and allows your doctor to visualize the inside of the bladder.

Treatment depends on how enlarged the prostate is. New federal guidelines for treating benign enlarged prostates say that men with mild to moderate symptoms may want to consider periods of doctor-monitored observation instead of choosing drug or surgical therapy right away. The guidelines were prompted by the belief that some doctors may be urging surgery or drug therapy without considering how much the condition is actually interfering with the patient's quality of life.

If symptoms are affecting your quality of life, medication is generally the first-tried option. Finasteride (Proscar®) is a new drug that shrinks the prostate by decreasing the production of dihydrotestosterone, a hormone that promotes prostatic growth. While the benefits may not be noticeable for six months, up to 75 percent taking the drug report an average 30 percent improvement in symptoms. Terazosin (Hytrin®) relaxes the muscle in the prostate and allows urine to pass more freely. In most patients, symptoms improve by about 50 percent in about a month. Drugs must be continued for life.

In severe cases, a transurethral prostate resection surgery—using a cutting device or laser to decrease the size of the gland, or a balloon procedure—in which a small balloon is moved up through the penis and is inflated in the prostate—is used to enlarge the opening through

p

Prostate, Enlarged

which the urethra travels. Complications of this surgery include impotence (erectile dysfunction) in about 5 percent of cases.

For More Information
American Medical Association
515 North State Street
Chicago, IL 60610
312-464-5000
www.ama-assn.org

Complementary and Alternative Treatments

Nutrition and Supplementation

Eat 1 to 4 ounces of raw pumpkin seeds daily. Rich in zinc, these seeds are beneficial for almost all prostate troubles. Increase your fluid intake; drink 2 to 3 quarts of spring or distilled water daily. This helps prevent cystitis and kidney infection as well as dehydration. Avoid chlorinated and fluoridated water, tobacco, alcohol, caffeine, and junk foods.

Nutritionists recommend the following daily supplements:

Most Important

- vitamin B complex (50 mg 3 times daily)—contains the anti-stress vitamins, supplemented with vitamin B_6 (50 mg twice daily)—especially helpful for its anticancer properties
- zinc (20 mg; do not exceed a total of 100 mg from all supplements)—deficiency has been linked to prostatitis; use lozenge form
- fish oil (as directed on label, 3 times daily)—important in prostate function
- L-alanine, L-glutamic acid, and L-glycine (as directed on label)—helps maintain normal prostate function
- raw prostate glandular (as directed on label)—normalizes prostate function
- vitamin E (600 IU)—enhances the immune system; a potent antioxidant
- magnesium and calcium (as directed on label)—improves prostate function

Also Recommended

- Pygeum africanum (as directed)
- saw palmetto (as directed)
- selenium (400 mcg)

(Consult your healthcare provider regarding the duration of treatment.)

Ayurvedic Medicine

Ayurvedic practitioners may recommend taking *alma* or an Ayurvedic mixture of *punarnava*, *shilajuit*, and *gokshura* to temper the symptoms of an enlarged prostate. They also may suggest drinking ginseng, hibiscus, or horsetail tea several times daily.

Ayurvedic products are available at many health food stores and Indian pharmacies.

Consult your healthcare provider before embarking on any new health regimen; early detection of serious prostate problems is critical.

Traditional Chinese Medicine

 Acupuncture To lessen pain and inflammation, acupuncturists may concentrate on working points related to the bladder, kidney, spleen, and large intestine meridians. In addition, they also may focus on Gallbladder 34, and Conception Vessel 3 and 4, along with the ear points related to the prostate gland.

Acupressure To help lessen inflammation and discomfort, the practitioner will focus on these acupressure points: Bladder 23, Conception Vessel 2 and 3, Spleen 6, Kidney 3, and Liver 3.

If urinary retention is a problem, the acupressurist also may include: Spleen 9, Bladder 28, and related ear points.

Chinese Herbal Therapy Herbs that may be given in formulas to correct the damp-heat imbalance that is believed to cause this ailment are malva, coptis, and talcum.

Plantain is often used to help relieve the swelling and pain caused by prostatitis. Other herbs may be prescribed to remedy fever or back or abdominal pain, if necessary. Most herb-trained acupuncturists will also use saw palmetto/Pygeum extracts, along with treating the constitution to speed recovery.

Yoga and Meditation

 Four yoga poses—the Wind Removal, Seated Sun, English Rooster, and Elevated Lotus—can boost circulation to the prostate area and calm prostate symptoms. In addition, a yoga exercise—the Stomach Lock—can help prevent flare-ups. Perform each daily. Consult your doctor before starting this program if you have heart problems or a hiatal hernia.

PROSTATITIS

p

Signs and Symptoms

- Difficulty urinating, even though the need to do so is frequent and urgent
- Pain in the genital area and pelvis
- Pain when ejaculating (in some cases)
- Fever and chills (emergency symptoms)
- Blood in urine (emergency symptom)
- Pain in the lower back and between the rectum and testicles (emergency symptoms)
- Pain or burning while urinating (emergency symptom)

Description

Prostatitis is an inflammation of the prostate gland in men. Prostatitis can strike at any age and accounts for one in four male visits to urologists. There are four different types of prostatitis. Acute bacterial prostatitis is caused by bacteria, and symptoms usually disappear in three to five days. Chronic bacterial prostatitis (CBP) is also caused by bacteria, but this infection persists for weeks or even months and is characterized by frequent relapses after treatment. Non-bacterial prostatitis (NBP) is the most common form of prostatitis; inflammation is present, but infection is not the cause. Prostatodynia (PD) is the form most common in young to middle-aged men. PD is a chronic condition that is often accompanied by depression, anxiety, or sexual dysfunction. Doctors do not yet understand what causes PD. The prostate appears normal and no bacteria or white blood cells are found in urine or prostate secretions.

In some men, prostatitis can be mild and recur

Health Notes

➤ *Drink 8 to 10 8-ounce glasses of water each day. Dehydration has been implicated in contributing to non-bacterial prostatitis and exacerbates existing symptoms of both non-bacterial and bacterial prostatitis.*

➤ *Drink moderately if at all. Some studies have shown that alcoholics have higher incidences of non-bacterial prostatitis.*

➤ *Limit caffeine to two cups of coffee or less a day. Caffeine aggravates symptoms in bacterial and non-bacterial prostatitis.*

➤ *Reduce stress. Stressful situations exacerbate symptoms of bacterial and non-bacterial prostatitis.*

➤ *Talk to your healthcare provider about avoiding spicy foods. Many prostatitis patients report that spicy foods contribute to painful, burning urination.*

regularly over a lifetime; other individuals may experience a severe, acute bout of the illness.

Conventional Medical Treatment

To diagnose prostatitis, your general physician or a urologist may take a urine sample, perform a digital rectal exam, in which a gloved finger is inserted into the rectum to feel the prostate, and ask for a history of symptoms.

Treatment depends on what is causing your prostatitis. If bacteria is to blame, you will be put on a course of antibiotics. If the cause is not bacterial, aspirin and anti-inflammatory medications, such as corticosteroids, will be used to reduce inflammation. In severe cases, you may need to be hospitalized.

For More Information
American Medical Association
515 North State Street
Chicago, IL 60610
312-464-5000
www.ama-assn.org

Complementary and Alternative Treatments

Nutrition and Supplementation

See "Prostate, Enlarged" entry.

Hydrotherapy

To reduce inflammation in an acute attack, try soaking in a comfortably hot sitz bath (to which you've added $1/2$ cup of dried chamomile flowers) for 30 to 45 minutes. Alternately, apply an ice pack to the area at 20-minute intervals.

Traditional Chinese Medicine

See "Prostate, Enlarged" entry.

Yoga and Meditation

Three yoga poses—Knee Squeeze, Seated Sun, and Elevated Lotus—can boost circulation to the prostate area and calm prostate symptoms. In addition, a yoga exercise—the Stomach Lock—can help prevent flare-ups. Perform the poses and exercise daily. Consult your doctor before starting these poses and exercises if you have high blood pressure, heart problems, or a hiatal hernia.

PSORIASIS

Signs and Symptoms

- Dry, red or purple patches of skin in a localized area
- Silvery scales that cover affected patches of skin
- Cracked skin (in some cases)
- Minor bleeding of affected skin (in some cases)
- Small pustules (in some cases)
- Itching of affected area (in some cases)

Description

Normal skin cells take about 30 days to make their way from the bottom skin layer up to the skin's top surface. Skin cells affected by psoriasis, however, can make the trip in four days, causing thick scales of dead skin and other glitches, such as the formation of pustules, cracking, bleeding, and itching.

Unfortunately, psoriasis is incurable. If you have it, periods of remission will occasionally be broken by flare-ups. Though it can strike at any age, most people who have the condition experience their first bout between the ages of 10 and 35. The condition, which is believed to be a genetic one, can occur anywhere on the body—from the toes to the scalp. However, an individual's outbreaks usually recur in the same spot.

Flare-ups can be prompted by a number of factors: a night of binge drinking; a bug bite, cut, or burn in the "designated" zone; a reaction to a medication; friction of clothing or shoes against the affected spot; a viral or bacterial illness somewhere else in the body (such as strep throat or a cold); or becoming overweight.

Warnings about UVA Therapy

Ultraviolet light (UVA) therapy has been shown in many studies to produce remissions in 80 to 90 percent of patients with severe psoriasis. Yet the therapy isn't without its risks. New research suggests that use of ultraviolet light for psoriasis can lead to skin cancer. For 13 years scientists studied 1,380 psoriasis patients who had undergone UVA therapy at 16 different university centers. Within this group, squamous cell carcinoma developed in more than one quarter of the patients. The cancer spread to internal organs in seven of these individuals. The study concluded that because long-term UVA therapy significantly increases the risk of squamous cell carcinoma in psoriasis patients, patients should discuss this risk with their healthcare provider before beginning this therapy.

Conventional Medical Treatment

If you've experienced a recurring rash, visit your dermatologist, who can examine the area and take a skin sample for analysis. Treatment varies, but mild cases are typically treated with over-the-counter cortisone ointments and/or coal-tar shampoos and soaps. More severe cases may be treated with Calcipotriene ointment, a vitamin D-3 derivative. In studies of 301 patients who had used the ointment twice daily for eight weeks, 10 percent had complete clearing and 70 percent had a significant improvement in symptoms. Etretinate®, a synthetic retinoid, has produced a good response in 60 to 70 percent of patients with few side effects. In extreme cases, the anti-cancer drug methotrexate may be prescribed to slow the accelerated production of skin cells. Because it causes liver and kidney damage with long-term use, this oral medication is prescribed only for the most severe cases of psoriasis.

Health Notes

➤ *Reduce stress. While stress isn't thought to cause psoriasis, it does prompt flare-ups of symptoms in psoriasis sufferers.*

➤ *In cases of stress-related flare-ups, many dermatologists now refer patients to psychotherapists or counselors.*

➤ *Talk to your doctor about any prescription or over-the-counter drugs you are currently taking. Medications that can worsen psoriasis include lithium, beta-blockers, nonsteroidal anti-inflammatory drugs, and anti-malarials.*

➤ *Drink moderately, if at all. In many people alcohol aggravates psoriasis symptoms.*

➤ *Maintain a healthy weight. Obesity has been implicated as a psoriasis risk factor; it also can worsen existing psoriasis symptoms.*

For More Information
American Academy of Dermatology
930 North Meacham Road
Schaumburg, IL 60173
888-462-DERM
www.aad.org

National Psoriasis Foundation
6600 SW 92 Street, Suite 300
Portland, OR 97223
503-244-7404
www.psoriasis.org

Complementary and Alternative Treatments

Nutrition and Supplementation

Although the underlying cause of this disorder is not known, it is likely that food sensitivities play a major role. Pso-riasis is rare in countries where the diet is low in saturated fat. The immune system also seems to play a role in this condition, as does the colon. In order to keep your colon clean and healthy, eat a diet high in fiber. Include foods such as brown rice, whole grain cereals, bran, fresh fruit, nuts, seeds, beans, fish, and fresh raw vegetables. Ideally, your diet will consist of 50 percent raw foods.

Avoid citrus fruits, fried foods, processed foods, saturated fats, and sugar. Red meat and dairy products contain arachidonic acid, a natural substance that promotes the inflammatory response and makes the lesions of psoriasis turn red and swell. Consume these foods in moderation or eliminate them from your menu. Wheat also is often a culprit in this disorder.

Glutathione creams and shampoos can be very beneficial. Use them according to package directions.

The following recommended daily supplements help improve the discomfort of psoriasis:

Most Important

• multivitamin containing vitamin A, B complex, C, and E

• flaxseed oil (1-2 tbsp daily)—supplies essential fatty acids

• mixed carotenoid formula (25,000 IU)—protects the skin tissue

• zinc (50 to 100 mg; do not exceed this amount)—essential to protein metabolism; protein is vital to healing

• a prodophilus formula

• L-glutamine (1000 mg)—protects skin

• glutathione (250 mg)

Also Recommended

• proteolytic enzymes (as directed on label)—stimulates protein synthesis and repair

• selenium (200 mcg)—has potent antioxidant properties

• shark cartilage (1 gm per 15 lbs of body weight, divided into 3 doses)—inhibits the growth of blood vessels to stop the spread of psoriasis; allow 2 to 3 months to see results

(For an *acute* condition, take supplements until your symptoms subside. If symptoms persist, seek the advice of your healthcare provider. For a *chronic* condition, consult your healthcare provider regarding the duration of treatment.)

Aromatherapy

Gentle essential oils—such as German chamomile, bergamot, and lavender—are ideal for soothing inflamed skin and controlling scaliness. Add up to 15 drops of any one of the oils to warm bath water. Following the bath, combine 1 or 2 drops of any one of the oils with 1 teaspoon of lotion or vegetable oil and gently smooth over the affected skin.

Herbal Therapy

Burdock tea and ointment can bring noticeable improvement to skin affected by psoriasis. To reduce scales and red patches, try the tea. Simmer 1 teaspoon chopped or grated dried or fresh root in 1 cup water for 10 to 15 minutes; strain. Drink 2 or 3 times a day. For itchiness and soreness, make an ointment by simmering 2 tablespoons chopped dried root in 220 grams petroleum jelly for 10 minutes; strain. Allow to cool before using. Apply as often as needed to the affected areas.

Homeopathy

Psoriasis may respond to homeopathic treatment. However, the selection of a remedy—more than one is available—depends on *your* symptoms and the stage of the condition. Don't try treating this disorder yourself. See a homeopathic professional.

Hydrotherapy

Warm salt water may help control scaliness. Add about 1 pound sea salt or table salt to the bath water and swish to distribute. Soak daily for 10 to 30 minutes. Do not use soap. Rinse with a short, cold shower and gently pat dry. Once a week try an apple cider vinegar bath. You also can try contrast therapy: apply a hot compress to the area, followed by a cold compress.

Traditional Chinese Medicine

Acupuncture To relieve the pain and dry skin associated with this condition, the acupuncturist may focus on auricular points relating to the lungs, large intestine, internal secretion, and heart meridians.

Chinese Herbal Therapy The TCM practitioner may prescribe *Gotu Kola* for its ability to heal tissue and enhance the cells' ability to repair themselves, while aloe vera can provide relief from dryness and any itching. In addition, formulas with burdock, dandelion, and Job's Tears also may be prescribed, as well as the patent formula called Dang Gui and Arctium Combination. There are different forms of psoriasis, and herb formulas vary greatly. See an herb-trained acupuncturist.

Yoga and Meditation

Psoriasis can worsen when you feel uptight and stressed. Use deep breathing, meditation, and yoga poses to calm your spirit and relax your body. Breath of Fire, a breathing exercise, can help cleanse the body of toxins. Choose three or four poses to perform daily and vary them to maintain your enthusiasm. Be sure to include one of the following relaxation poses: Baby, Corpse, or Wind Removal.

RASHES

Most people are familiar with the all-over or localized eruption of pinkish spots, small flesh-colored bumps, unusual scaling, or other out-of-the-ordinary skin symptoms that are generally known as a rash. Rashes can take on various guises: chicken pox—bodywide sprinkling of sores; hives—red reaction to an allergen; dermatitis—raw, itchy inflammation; mumps—blotchy redness; and multiple sclerosis—fine pink bumps.

Rashes can be a direct reaction to something that has touched the skin (poison ivy, diaper rash, dermatitis, and others) or can be caused by an inhaled or ingested allergen (hives). Rashes can also be a symptom of a medical condition (Lyme disease, some types of cancer, or rubella).

There is no one treatment for all rashes; how you treat a rash depends on what type of rash it is and what caused it. General guidelines include keeping skin clean and dry and refraining from scratching, which can irritate the skin and possibly cause inflammation and infection. In some cases, over-the-counter or prescription topical corticosteroid creams are used.

A complementary treatment you may wish to consider is Ayurvedic medicine. To quiet the itch and lessen the inflammation associated with skin rashes, Ayurvedic practitioners recommend applying neem oil or cilantro pulp to the affected area. They also may suggest drinking coriander tea.

r

RAYNAUD'S DISEASE

Signs and Symptoms

- Hands, fingers, feet and/or toes turn white upon exposure to cold, accompanied by stinging and pain
- Skin may turn blue or red before it recovers

Description

When exposed to cold, the blood vessels in the fingers, hands, toes, and feet constrict to prevent heat loss. The blood vessels quickly dilate once they are in a warmer temperature. In Raynaud's disease, however, the blood vessels stay constricted for up to an hour, cutting off blood to the area and causing abnormally cold hands and/or feet.

One in 20 Americans have Raynaud's disease, with women being five times more likely than men to be affected. The condition usually appears during one's 20s or early 30s. Medical professionals do not consider Raynaud's to be a disease, per se, but merely a nuisance for the sufferer. Due to the reduced flow of nutrient-rich blood, Raynaud's does weaken the skin in affected areas, leaving it prone to cuts, chafes, and bruises, and slowing the healing process. In some individuals, Raynaud's is associated with an underlying condition, such as systemic lupus or rheumatoid arthritis.

Conventional Medical Treatment

To diagnose your condition, your physician may place your hands and/or feet into a basin of cold water and observe the response. Treatment usually consists of insulating the affected extremities against cold temperatures using socks and/or gloves. In severe cases, calcium channel antagonists (or blockers) may be used to dilate blood vessels and encourage circulation to the extremities.

For More Information
National Heart, Lung, and Blood Institute
P.O. Box 30105
Bethesda, MD 20824-0105
301-592-8573
www.nhlbi.nih.gov

Health Notes

➤ *Get 30 minutes of moderate aerobic exercise every day to increase blood circulation.*

➤ *Bundle hands and feet in mittens and warm socks during cold weather.*

➤ *Reduce stress. In some people, stress worsens the symptoms of Raynaud's disease.*

➤ *Quit smoking. Smoking hampers blood circulation, exacerbating symptoms of Raynaud's disease.*

➤ *Use mittens or gloves when reaching into the refrigerator or freezer.*

➤ *Drink out of insulated glasses.*

➤ *Limit caffeine to one cup of coffee or tea per day or avoid it entirely. Caffeine can disrupt normal blood circulation, exacerbating symptoms of Raynaud's disease.*

Acrocyanosis

Raynaud's disease isn't the only cause of cold hands and feet. Acrocyanosis is a rare condition that is related to Raynaud's disease. Like Raynaud's, it involves coldness of the hands, fingers, feet and/or toes due to constricted blood vessels. Treatment for acrocyanosis is similar to treatment for Raynaud's: bundling up, exercising to boost circulation and possible calcium channel blockers.

Complementary and Alternative Treatments

Nutrition and Supplementation

 Eat a balanced diet composed of 50 percent raw foods. Avoid fatty and fried foods when possible. Caffeine and nicotine constricts the blood vessels and should be avoided, if not eliminated.

Nutritionists recommend the following daily supplements:

Most Important

- coenzyme Q10 (100 to 200 mg)—improves tissue oxygenation
- vitamin E (start with 200 IU and slowly increase to 1000 IU)—improves circulation; acts as an anticoagulant

Also Recommended

- calcium (1500 mg at bedtime)—protects arteries from stress caused by sudden blood pressure changes
- magnesium (750 mg)—works with calcium
- lecithin (1200 mg 3 times daily, with meals)—lowers blood lipid levels
- chlorophyll (as directed on label)—enhances blood flow
- dimethylglycine (1 tablet 3 times daily)—improves tissue oxygenation

- vitamin B complex (100 mg)—necessary for metabolism of fat and cholesterol
- flaxseed oil (1000 mg)—helps prevent hardening of the arteries

(Consult your healthcare provider regarding the duration of treatment.)

Herbal Therapy

Ginger tea may help improve circulation. To prepare, steep 1 teaspoon grated ginger root in 1 cup boiling water for 10 minutes; strain. Drink as needed.

Homeopathy

Raynaud's syndrome may respond to homeopathic treatment. However, the selection of a remedy—more than one is available—depends on *your* symptoms and the stage of the condition. Don't try treating this disorder yourself. See a homeopathic professional.

Traditional Chinese Medicine

Acupuncture Acupuncture can be extremely effective in improving circulation, which may lessen constriction of the blood vessels affected by Raynaud's Disease. The practitioner may focus on these points: Small Intestine 7, Heart 7, Lung 7, Pericardium 7, and the points that lie between the fingers themselves. In most cases, a hot water bottle also is very helpful.

Acupressure A practitioner may be able to alleviate cold or numbness by manipulating the fingers themselves, as well as circulation-enhancing points along various upper body meridians.

Chinese Herbal Therapy Ginger, angelica pubescens (yellow), and salvia may be used in formulas to remedy this condition. Cinnamon is often prescribed as a Chinese herb for Raynaud's disease; it works by increasing circulation to invigorate numb extremities. This requires long-term treatment and a herb-trained acupuncturist to do it right.

RETINAL DETACHMENT

Signs and Symptoms

- Blurred vision in one eye
- Vision floaters in one eye
- Sensation of flashing lights in one eye
- Shadow over a portion of one eye's field of vision

Description

A layer of minuscule blood vessels lays behind the retina. These vessels supply oxygen and other nutrients to the eye so it can function. Should the retina detach from this layer of blood vessels, the result is called retinal detachment. The portion of your visual field that corresponds to the detached part of the retina becomes lost, and instead of regular sight, you see a shadow.

You are at a higher risk for retinal detachment if you are nearsighted, male, have diabetes, are Caucasian, and/or have a family member who has experienced the condition. Aging also can facilitate retinal detachment, as can an eye injury.

Conventional Medical Treatment

Retinal detachment is an emergency situation. Should you suspect it, go immediately to an oph-

Health Notes

➤ *When playing sports that involve a ball or physical contact, wear protective goggles to ward off injury.*

➤ *People with diabetes who tightly control their blood sugar levels lower their risk of developing retinal detachment.*

➤ *To catch eye conditions early, experts recommend having a regular eye examination every two to four years between ages 40 and 65 and every one to two years after that. Annual examinations may be necessary for those with a family history of eye disease, such as nearsightedness or retinal detachment.*

thalmologist. He or she will examine the eye, using a slit lamp to visualize the edges of the retina and to determine just how serious the condition is. If addressed promptly, your ophthalmologist may be able to surgically re-attach the retina and save some or all of your vision.

For More Information

National Eye Institute
2020 Vision Place
Bethesda, MD 20892-3655
301-496-5248
www.nei.nih.gov

Prevent Blindness America
500 East Remington Road
Schaumburg, IL 60173
800-331-2020
www.preventblindness.org

Complementary and Alternative Treatments

Traditional Chinese Medicine

 Acupuncture Acupuncture can be used to invigorate the flow of blood and *chi* within the body, which may allow any built-up fluid behind the eye to drain, thereby improving vision.

Auricular points that relate to the eye also may be incorporated into an acupuncture session treating retinal detachment.

Acupressure Acupressure may be helpful in dispersing fluid that has accumulated behind the eyes. Points that may be manipulated include Bladder 1 and 2, Stomach 2, and the *Tai Yang* point at the temples.

Chinese Herbal Therapy Dendrobium Moniliforme Night Sight Pills may be prescribed to remedy this condition, along with custom-blended herbal formulas containing chrysanthemum, sickle senna, cinnamon, mishmi bitter, gentian, and joint fir, to name a few.

Because Chinese medicine attributes most eye problems to liver dysfunction, herbs are typically used to strengthen that organ and the meridian channel. Consult your conventional physician if you are considering herbal therapy to treat this disorder.

r

REYE'S SYNDROME

Signs and Symptoms

- Sudden, continuous vomiting, especially following a flu-like upper respiratory infection or chicken pox
- Confusion, irrational behavior, convulsions, or loss of consciousness
- Irritability, sensitivity to touch, personality changes
- Listlessness, excessive sleepiness, and loss of energy and aggressiveness
- For infants, symptoms include diarrhea, sometimes accompanied by vomiting, respiratory problems, and seizures

Description

Reye's syndrome was first diagnosed in 1963 and came to public attention during the 1970s, when frequent outbreaks accompanied the onset of flu season. Thanks to consistent public education campaigns, however, just two cases were reported between 1994 and 1997, down from an all-time high of 555 cases in 1980.

Reye's can affect people of all ages, although it most commonly occurs in people from infancy to young adulthood. Generally appearing three to five days following the onset of a viral illness, Reye's syndrome occurs without warning and progresses rapidly once symptoms occur. Although the disease is not contagious, it can cause serious damage to the liver and slight-to-severe brain dysfunction. Since there is no cure, early diagnosis is extremely critical. A patient should be observed carefully for symptoms for at least two to three weeks after a viral illness, such as flu or chicken pox (about one-third of cases accompany chicken pox), and a physician should be called immediately if any of the described symptoms develop.

Once physicians learned that the incidence of Reye's syndrome increased when patients treated viral illnesses with aspirin, or medications containing aspirin, they have been more successful at keeping the number of cases under control. Although there is no conclusive proof linking aspirin usage to Reye's, physicians now warn against the use of aspirin for viral illnesses.

Conventional Medical Treatment

If treatment begins as soon as possible after the onset of symptoms, there is a 50 to 90 percent chance of full recovery. The risks of lifelong injury increase significantly if Reye's syndrome is misdiagnosed or if treatment does not begin immediately, since recovery is related to the degree of swelling in the brain.

Health Notes

➤ Because research shows a link between Reye's syndrome and the use of aspirin to treat flu-like symptoms, the Centers for Disease Control recommends that children under 19 avoid medications containing aspirin.

➤ Reye's syndrome may develop without taking aspirin, so parents should be aware of symptoms even if no aspirin has been administered.

➤ Anti-nausea medications also may contain aspirin (salicylates), and because they prevent vomiting, they may mask the symptoms of Reye's syndrome.

Reye's patients should be brought or transferred immediately to an intensive care unit staffed by medical personnel experienced in the treatment of the disease. To screen for Reye's syndrome, physicians usually perform two liver function tests— SGOT (which tests for the liver enzyme *serum glutamic oxaloacetic transaminase*) and SGPT (which tests for the liver enzyme *serum glutamic pyruvic transaminase*). Test results are usually available within two to three hours.

Most patients recover completely from Reye's syndrome with prompt, effective treatment, although there is the possibility of after-effects, ranging from very slight to severe motor or learning disabilities. The amount of rehabilitation needed varies widely, according to the damage. Those recovering from Reye's syndrome should be thoroughly evaluated for problems related to memory, attention span, concentration, task completion, speech and language, fine and gross motor skills, and changes in activity levels. Parents should be aware that any of these problems also might result in learning problems in school.

Children who have been hospitalized for Reye's syndrome also may experience emotional difficulties, such as over-dependency, sleep disturbances, depression, and anxiety. If parents encounter these problems, they may want to seek professional help.

For More Information
National Institute of
Neurological Disorders and Stroke
Office of Communications and Public Liaison
P.O. Box 5801
Bethesda, MD 20824
www.ninds.nih.gov

National Reye's Syndrome Foundation, Inc.
P.O. Box 829
Bryan, OH 43506
800-233-7393
www.bright.net/~reyessyn

Complementary and Alternative Treatments

Nutrition and Supplementation

 Supplements should be given only after the recovery process has begun. Consult your healthcare provider before taking these or any other supplements. The following recommended daily doses are for persons over 18. For children between 12 and 17, use three-quarters the dose; for a child between 6 and 12, use half; for a child under 6, use one-quarter the recommended dose.

- branched-chain amino acids (as directed on label)—prevents muscle depletion

- flaxseed oil (as directed on label)—maintains and restores skin suppleness and moisture

- lecithin (1200 mg 3 times daily)—supplies choline, vital in the transmission of nerve impulses and energy production

- vitamin B complex (50 to 100 mg)—supports healing

- vitamin E (400 IU)—protects against free radical damage

(Consult your healthcare provider regarding the duration of treatment.)

r

RINGWORM

Signs and Symptoms

- Slightly raised, roundish rings of skin with a well-defined red border
- Affected areas may itch and appear scaly
- The outer border of the ring may expand outward, making individual patches larger

Description

Ringworm is a partial misnomer. While the contagious skin condition's lesions are somewhat ring-shaped, they are not caused by worms, but by a fungus. Like head lice and chicken pox, ringworm seems to be a childhood rite of passage. Ringworm is most often picked up via direct contact with infected neighborhood puppies, kittens, or people. The condition is so contagious that just touching skin after first scratching at a "ring" can spread the infection.

Conventional Medical Treatment

Ringworm can be treated with home applications of a topical over-the-counter anti-fungal ointment, spray, or liquid (follow the package directions). If ringworm does not disappear after one week of using an anti-fungal preparation, contact your physician, who may prescribe an oral anti-fungal medication.

For More Information

American Academy of Dermatology
930 North Meacham Road
Schaumburg, IL 60173
888-462-DERM
www.aad.org

Health Notes

➤ Before bringing a kitten or puppy home, take it to the veterinarian to have it checked for ringworm.

➤ Tell your children to avoid petting strange animals.

➤ Avoid contact with individuals who have ringworm.

➤ If someone in your household has ringworm, wash clothing, bedding, and linens in hot water after each use to kill fungal spores.

National Health Information Center
P.O. Box 1133
Washington, DC 20013-1133
800-336-4797
http://nhic-nt.health.org

Complementary and Alternative Treatments

Nutrition and Supplementation

 Eat an abundance of fresh vegetables and moderate amounts of broiled fish and broiled skinless chicken.

Fungi thrive on sugar, so avoid foods containing sugar or refined carbohydrates. Eliminate foods that promote the secretion of mucus, especially meat and dairy products. Cola, grains, processed foods, and fried or greasy foods should be avoided whenever possible.

Nutritionists recognize these daily supplements as helpful in treating ringworm:

- a prodophilus formula (as directed on label)—supplies friendly bacteria usually deficient in people with fungal infections

- garlic (as directed on label)—neutralizes most fungi

- vitamin B complex (50 mg 3 times daily)—balances the friendly bacteria

- vitamin C with bioflavonoids (5000 to 20,000 mg in divided doses)—necessary for proper immune function

- evening primrose oil (as directed on label)—relieves pain and inflammation

- vitamin A (25,000 IU; do not exceed 8000 IU if you are pregnant)—heals skin and mucous membranes

(Take supplements until your symptoms subside. If symptoms persist, seek the advice of your healthcare provider.)

Traditional Chinese Medicine

 Acupuncture Acupuncture may be used to speed healing and alleviate the itchiness associated with ringworm.

Chinese Herbal Therapy The TCM practitioner may recommend that a wash made with *Cnidium monnieri* be applied to the affected area to combat itchiness; this herb also has astringent properties that can counteract infection. Alum, turmeric, and camphor are other Chinese herbs used topically to treat ringworm.

ROCKY MOUNTAIN SPOTTED FEVER

Signs and Symptoms

- Chills

- High fever

- Nausea

- Red spotted rash occurring between the second and the sixth day of fever

- Severe headache

- Appetite loss

- Body-wide aches and pains

- Abdominal pain

- Vomiting

- Insomnia

- Restlessness

Rocky Mountain Fever's African Cousin

The bacterium *Rickettsia rickettsii*, which causes Rocky Mountain spotted fever, has a newly-discovered relative: *Rickettsia africae*. The recently discovered bacterium is transmitted by Amblyomma ticks in Zimbabwe and South Africa and causes an illness called African tick-bite fever. The discovery was made when seven people returned from Zimbabwe and South Africa with a strange fever, followed by body aches, swollen glands, and edema. Although there was no rash present—as there is with Rocky Mountain spotted fever—blood tests uncovered the related bacteria. Because African tick-bite fever is a potentially life-threatening infection, conventional antibiotics are recommended.

r

Rocky Mountain Spotted Fever

Description

Rocky Mountain spotted fever is caused by a bacterium called *Rickettsia ricketsii*. This microorganism is transmitted to humans by the wood tick in the western United States and the dog tick in the eastern half of the United States. Flu-like symptoms—including nausea, headache, and malaise—usually begin 3 to 10 days after being bitten by an infected tick. Between the second and sixth days of the fever, a red rash appears on your wrists and palms, as well as on your ankles and the soles of your feet. The rash slowly spreads up your arms and legs to your chest. Rocky Mountain fever can range in severity from extremely mild to near-fatal.

Health Notes

➤ When outdoors, wear long sleeves and long pants, tuck your shirt into your pants, and wear a hat. These precautions make it harder for a tick to reach bare skin.

➤ Be especially careful during late spring to late summer, when the ticks that carry Rocky Mountain spotted fever are at their most active.

➤ Wear pale-colored clothing to make it easier to find and remove ticks. You may want to avoid bright white clothing, however, since ticks are especially attracted to it.

➤ Insect repellent that contains DEET (diethyl toluamide) has been proven especially effective against ticks.

➤ After a day spent outdoors, do a thorough body and head check for ticks. If you find one, remove it immediately using tweezers. If you are concerned about Rocky Mountain spotted fever, place the tick in a glass jar and take it to your local public health department as soon as possible.

➤ Check cats and dogs regularly for ticks.

➤ While outdoors, stay as cool and dry as possible. Ticks are attracted to human sweat.

➤ To give ticks fewer places to live near your home, keep litter cleared away from your yard.

Conventional Medical Treatment

To diagnose Rocky Mountain spotted fever, your physician takes a history of symptoms and performs a blood test. If Rocky Mountain Spotted Fever is suspected, your doctor immediately begins treatment with antibiotics.

For More Information

Centers for Disease Control and Prevention
1600 Clifton Road
Atlanta, GA 30333
800-311-3435
www.cdc.gov

National Institute of Allergies and Infectious Diseases
Building 31, Room 7A50
31 Center Drive, MSC 2520
Bethesda, MD 20892-2520
301-496-5717
www.niaid.nih.gov

Complementary and Alternative Treatments

Traditional Chinese Medicine

See "Lyme Disease" entry.

ROSACEA

Signs and Symptoms

- Red areas on the face
- Facial acne
- Chronic inflammation of the cheeks, nose, forehead, and/or chin
- Pimple-like pustules in reddened areas (in some cases)
- Red, bulbous nose (more common in males)

Description

Rosacea seriously affects a sufferer's appearance, but not his or her health. The redness and inflammation that are the hallmarks of the condition are caused by enlargement of the blood vessels that lie just under the skin. Why these blood vessels enlarge in some individuals is not known, though the ailment usually strikes fair-skinned individuals of Irish descent who blush easily and is most commonly seen in those aged 30 to 50. Temporary rosacea is also common in infants after a high fever.

Conventional Medical Treatment

A dermatologist can diagnose rosacea, usually on the basis of a physical examination. About 70 to 80 percent of individuals respond successfully to long-term oral or topical antibiotic therapy—just how long-term depends on the individual. In some cases, the dose of the antibiotic is gradually reduced to control the rosacea until it can be discontinued altogether without the threat of recurrence. Why this works isn't exactly known. Sometimes, short courses of topical steroids can reduce redness. Laser therapy is another medical option currently being evaluated.

Health Notes

➤ Drink alcohol moderately or not at all. Some rosacea sufferers find that avoiding alcohol minimizes the appearance of redness.

➤ Watch your diet. Some rosacea sufferers find that avoiding hot or spicy foods and beverages alleviates symptoms.

➤ Reduce stress. In some people, stress can trigger a flare-up of rosacea.

➤ Cover your face in cold, windy outdoor weather. Some people experience flare-ups when exposed to cold, blustery air.

➤ Get enough sleep. Being well-rested can lessen the frequency and severity of flare-ups in some people.

➤ Wear sunscreen when outdoors. Ultraviolet rays can exacerbate rosacea symptoms.

➤ Avoid skin care preparations and cosmetics that contain alcohol, which can aggravate the condition.

For More Information
American Academy of Dermatology
930 North Meacham Road
Schaumburg, IL 60173
888-462-DERM
www.aad.org

National Rosacea Society
800 South Northwest Highway, Suite 200
Barrington, IL 60010
800-NO-BLUSH
www.rosacea.org

Complementary and Alternative Treatments

Nutrition and Supplementation

 Avoid saturated fats and all animal products; saturated fats promote inflammation. Also on the "no" list are alcohol, dairy products, caffeine, cheese, chocolate, cocoa, eggs, fish, salt, sugar, and spicy foods.

Improve the condition of your skin with these daily supplements:

- evening primrose oil (500 mg three times daily)—heals many skin disorders

- vitamin A (25,000 IU for 3 months, then reduce to 15,000 IU; do not exceed 8000 IU if you are pregnant)—heals and builds skin tissue

- kelp (1000 to 1500 mg)—supplies minerals needed for good skin tone

- vitamin E (start with 400 IU and increase slowly to 800 IU)—protects against free radicals

- zinc (50 mg; do not exceed a total of 100 mg from all supplements)—repairs tissue; use lozenge form

- selenium (200 mcg)—reduces inflammation

- vitamin C with bioflavonoids (3000 to 5000 mg in divided doses)—strengthens capillaries

(For an *acute* condition, take supplements until your symptoms subside. If symptoms persist, seek the advice of your healthcare provider. For a *chronic* condition, consult your healthcare provider regarding the duration of treatment.)

Traditional Chinese Medicine

 Acupuncture Acupuncture can be helpful in regulating blood flow and circulation, which may help tone down ruddiness, alleviate pustules, and repair broken blood vessels. To treat rosacea, acupuncturists typically focus on the ear points related to the lung, adrenal gland, nose, and internal secretion point. In addition, they focus on the spleen and stomach meridians to keep blood in its correct place.

Acupressure The practitioner presses firmly on Large Intestine 4 and Stomach 7 and 36, which may reduce rosacea-related breakouts.

Chinese Herbal Therapy Gentiana Combination or Dang Gui and Arctium are two patent medicines that may be used to treat rosacea.

SCABIES

Signs and Symptoms

- Itching, especially at night
- Thin, pencil-like marks on the skin

Description

Scabies are microscopic mites that can be found in bedding, but also in linens and clothing. Highly contagious, scabies can be transmitted between people through shared towels, bedding, sexual contact, hand-holding, hugging, or sitting close to someone. They are found most commonly in unhygienic, crowded environments.

Scabies burrow into the skin—and prefer the moist skin under the breasts, armpits, buttocks, back of the thighs, groin, soles of the feet, and between fingers and toes. The entry spot actually looks like a very small stab wound that could have been made with a pencil. Although scabies are not dangerous and do not carry disease, they are bothersome and annoying.

Health Notes

➤ If you have been diagnosed with scabies, avoid close contact with other people until you are treated. Use only your own bedding and linen to prevent scabies from infecting sheets, blankets, and towels that family members use.

➤ Scabies are sometimes found in ill-kept hotels and motels. If after checking into a hotel, you find the room seems unhygienic, consider informing the manager and relocating to a different establishment.

Conventional Medical Treatment

To diagnose scabies, your physician or dermatologist looks for the characteristic burrow marks. Treatment involves a topical lotion containing permethrin, such as Elmite® cream. This is typically applied from the chin down and worn overnight. One application usually kills the scabies. Your family members and anyone else you have come in close contact with must also use the product. To avoid being reinfected, all family bedding, clothing, and towels must be washed in hot water.

For More Information
The American Academy of Dermatology
930 North Meacham Road
Schaumburg, IL 60173
888-462-DERM
www.aad.org

Complementary and Alternative Treatments

Nutrition and Supplementation

 Although diet alone cannot cure scabies, you can promote the healing process by eating foods high in zinc, such as soybeans, sunflower seeds, whole grain products, and wheat bran. Do not drink soda or alcohol, and avoid sugar, chocolate, and junk foods as much as possible.

Nutritionists recommend these daily supplements:

- garlic (as directed on label)—has antiparasitic and antibiotic properties

- evening primrose oil (1000 mg 3 times daily)—helps heal most skin disorders

- vitamin A (25,000 IU for 3 months, then reduce to 15,000 IU; do not exceed 8000 IU if you are pregnant)—heals and builds skin tissue

- zinc (50 mg; do not exceed a total of 100 mg from all supplements)—repairs tissue; use lozenge form

- colloidal silver (as directed on label)—prevents secondary infection

- vitamin E (600 IU)—promotes healing

Traditional Chinese Medicine

 Acupuncture Acupuncture can be very helpful in relieving the itching and discomfort associated with this condition.

Chinese Herbal Therapy Alum, turmeric, and camphor are extremely effective in the treatment of scabies, especially when combined with sulphur, but a combination of this modality with conventional treatment will provide the fastest, most effective results.

SCOLIOSIS

Signs and Symptoms

- A sideways curvature of the spine
- Asymmetrical rib cage
- One shoulder that is higher than the other
- One hip that is higher than other
- Back pain

Description

Scoliosis is derived from a Greek word meaning "curvature." Affected individuals have an abnormal curvature of the spine. Usually the spine curves slightly to one side, causing one shoulder and hip to be higher than the other. If left untreated, the curve grows more exaggerated, causing unnatural spacing of the ribs. In extreme cases, heart and lung problems can develop.

The condition may begin in infancy, although it is more often first seen in adolescence. Mild cases of scoliosis generally cause no symptoms and are usually discovered during a routine examination by a pediatrician. Sixty to 80 percent of all cases occur in girls. The exact cause of scoliosis is not known, although it is believed that genetics play a role.

Conventional Medical Treatment

A physician can usually diagnose scoliosis with a physical exam, asking your child to bend forward so he or she can view the spine from behind. An abnormal curvature is easiest to see in this position. X-rays of the spine also may be needed to determine the extent of the curvature. Treatment depends on the severity of the disorder. Mild cases can be treated with strict adherence to a daily exercise plan to improve posture and strengthen the muscle and spine. In moderate to severe cases, the child may need to wear a custom-fitted brace to prevent further curvature. This brace extends from the lower neck to the hips and is designed to apply pressure at the apex of the curve. Usually it is worn during waking hours only, until the spine has been reasonably straightened, a process that generally takes from two to seven years. In very severe cases, surgery may be needed to realign the spine.

Health Notes

➤ *Check to see if your child's school has a scoliosis screening program. Optimally, girls should be screened between ages 11 and 14, and boys, between ages 13 and 16.*

➤ *Ask your healthcare provider about the "microstraight" device, which is currently undergoing testing. This new microchip device sounds an alarm that reminds the wearer to straighten up when he or she starts to slump. If the wearer ignores the sound, a louder alarm follows. Preliminary data have shown that the device reduces the degree of deformity by 35 to 72 percent. It was developed on the basis of evidence suggesting that traditional braces, rather than pushing and pulling the spine into the "correct" position, actually act by encouraging children to self-correct. Because the brace is uncomfortable and wearers unconsciously pull away from the pressure pads, they thereby straighten their bodies.*

For More Information
American Academy of Orthopedic Surgeons
6300 North River Road
Rosemont, IL 60018-4262
800-346-AAOS
www.aaos.org

Complementary and Alternative Treatments

Chiropractic

There are two categories of scoliosis: functional and structural. Functional scoliosis occurs as a result of muscle im-balance; the muscles on one side of the spine are tighter than those on the other side. Patients with this type of scoliosis respond extremely well to conservative chiropractic care. Structural scoliosis, on the other hand, is due to the misalignment of the vertebrae and curvature of the vertebral column. This condition often presents itself at a very early age and generally requires orthopedic intervention and, possibly, surgery.

Traditional Chinese Medicine

Acupuncture Acupuncture can be used to rechannel the flow of energy along the spine, alleviating back pain and making posture problems easier to correct. In most cases, the practitioner will work on points along the bladder, gallbladder, small intestine, and governing vessel meridians, along with auricular points related to the problematic area.

Acupressure As with acupuncture, acupressure may be used to strengthen the back muscles and correct posture to alleviate scoliosis. The practitioner typically focuses on acupressure points along the bladder, gallbladder, and governing vessel meridians.

Chinese Herbal Therapy Depending upon what the herbalist determines to be the root cause of the disorder, he or she may recommend Tu Huo and Loranthes, Rehmannia Six, or Rehmannia Eight herbal combination formulas.

Angelica Du Huo and eucommia also may be prescribed for lower back pain, while additional herbs may be given to treat scoliosis-related headaches, digestive problems, lethargy, and breathing difficulties.

S

SEASONAL AFFECTIVE DISORDER (SAD)

Signs and Symptoms

The following signs and symptoms occur annually from late fall to early spring:

- Sense of emotional numbness, despair, helplessness, hopelessness, and/or gloom
- Feelings of low self-worth
- Desire to be alone; withdrawal from others
- Worry and episodes of anxiety
- Irritability
- Belief that life is meaningless
- Decreased energy level
- Change in demeanor, either becoming more agitated or, more commonly, slowing down and dragging
- Lack of interest in once-pleasurable activities
- Abnormal sleeping patterns (nighttime insomnia, waking in the early morning, sleeping during the daytime)
- Crying for seemingly trivial reasons
- Poor appetite and weight loss or increased appetite and weight gain
- Lack of interest in appearance and grooming
- Diminished concentration and decision-making ability
- Inappropriate guilt
- Monotone speech
- Suicidal thoughts and/or behavior

Description

Seasonal affective disorder (SAD) typically sets in from late September to mid-October, grows worse in the dark months of November through January, and continues until about April. As the days grow shorter and the weather colder, you find yourself suffering from what appears to be a textbook case of clinical depression. You may feel unable to keep up at work, socialize with friends, groom and take care of yourself, maintain your household, or even venture out of the house. Once the days start growing longer and the sun comes out, you're back to your normal, even-keeled self—until next fall.

SAD is a particular type of depression that affects 2 to 10 percent of the population. Most sufferers live far north or far south of the equator. Much research has been done on the role that certain brain chemicals—called neurotransmitters—play in depression. These chemicals, which help relay electrical signals between brain cells, are believed to regulate mood. Studies have shown that a large number of depressed people exhibit reduced levels of norepinephrine, serotonin, and dopamine—three such chemicals.

While heredity is considered a primary risk factor, the exact cause of SAD is still unknown. Experts suspect that a lack of bright light may inhibit the brain's production of the mood-regulating neurotransmitter serotonin.

Conventional Medical Treatment

If you experience four or more of the preceding symptoms yearly during the period between late fall and early spring, you may have SAD. A physician may give you a physical exam to rule out any physical ailments, then refer you to a mental health expert.

Treatment consists of exposure to high levels of light. Ten to 30 minutes of outdoor time, such as a long walk, is recommended every day during the winter months—even during snowy and rainy weather. In addition, your doctor may recommend that you sit in a room in your home with a light box (available from a medical supply store), which

S

emits extremely bright light, for 15 minutes or more each day. You do not have to look at the light. In some instances, an antidepressant may be prescribed to help you get through the late fall, winter, and early spring. The most commonly prescribed antidepressants are selective serotonin reuptake inhibitors (SSRIs), such as fluoxeline (Prozac®) or sertraline (Zoloft®). These medications act by regulating the brain's neurotransmitters, thus addressing the physiological causes of depression.

For More Information
National Mental Health Association
1021 Prince Street
Alexandria, VA 22314
800-969-NMHA
TTY: 800-433-5968
www.nmha.org

Health Notes

➤ If you are house or apartment hunting, choose a home that receives lots of daylight, preferably one with a southern exposure. Sunny rooms have been shown to lessen symptoms of SAD.

➤ Increase the level of light in your current home by painting walls white, keeping drapes and blinds open, using brighter (higher watt) light bulbs and/or constructing a skylight, if possible.

➤ Get regular, moderate exercise, preferably outdoors. Regular exercise helps regulate serotonin levels which, in turn, regulate mood.

➤ Eat a low-fat, low-sugar diet high in complex carbohydrates, such as whole grains. This type of diet has been shown to lessen symptoms of SAD.

➤ Stay warm. Many SAD sufferers report that feeling chilled, either indoors or out, can exacerbate feelings of seasonal depression.

Complementary and Alternative Treatments

Nutrition and Supplementation

 See "Depression" entry.

Bodywork and Somatic Practices

 Massage, CranioSacral Therapy, Trager, Therapeutic Touch, Reiki, Oriental bodywork, polarity therapy, reflexology, Feldenkrais, and Aston-Patterning can all help this condition.

Traditional Chinese Medicine

 Acupuncture SAD may be treated with a combination of modalities, including acupuncture, which can help alleviate anxiety and improve the patient's mood. Acupuncture also may be effective at reducing lethargy and combating other SAD-related symptoms, such as overeating, loss of libido, and anti-social behavior.

Acupressure A therapist may concentrate on Large Intestine 4 and 10, Lung 9, Conception Vessel 6, Stomach 36, Kidney 3, Governing Vessel 14, and Gallbladder 20 and 21 to relieve fatigue.

If a decreased sex drive is associated with the condition, the practitioner will work additional points along the gallbladder, conception vessel, bladder, kidney and governing vessel meridians.

Chinese Herbal Therapy Depression may be treated with polygala, a decreased sex drive may be boosted with Tibetan saffron, and anxiety may be reduced with eagle wood. In addition, the herbalist may include joint fir (for overeating), licorice (for irritability), and wild Chinese jujube (for fatigue) in the herbal preparation, depending upon the symptoms.

The Chinese patent formula known as Ginseng and Dang Gui Ten Combination also may be prescribed to treat SAD. And, because Chinese medicine views sadness and anxiety as having a detrimental effect on the lungs and large intestine, herbs may be given to fortify these organs as well.

SHINGLES (HERPES ZOSTER)

Signs and Symptoms

- Tingling or painful sensation in a localized area on one side of the body or face, followed by a rash of small, red, fluid-filled blisters

Description

Shingles is caused by the *herpes zoster* virus, the very same virus that causes chickenpox. In fact, shingles usually hits only those who have already had chickenpox. After chickenpox has run its course, the herpes zoster virus retreats into the body's nerve cells, where it lies dormant. In most people, the virus remains inactive, but in some the virus reactivates, developing into shingles. Why this happens is not known.

The first symptom, a pain or tingling, occurs as the virus travels along any one of the peripheral nerves that spread out from your spine. This sensation is felt only in the area of your face or body that is served by the affected nerve. The virus causes a localized infection, and two or three days later a rash appears as the virus reaches the skin's nerve endings. For the next three to five days, the rash reaches its zenith. After that, the blisters form crusts that eventually fall off.

Though shingles can affect anyone, the condition is most common in individuals older than 60.

Conventional Medical Treatment

Your physician can diagnose shingles by physically examining the resulting rash. There is no treatment that can eradicate the virus, but antiviral drugs, such as acyclovir, may shorten the duration of symptoms. Analgesics are the mainstay of treatment to relieve pain. Fortunately, shingles is usually not a serious condition, though some individuals experience residual pain along one of their peripheral nerves for months or years after the rash disappears. Those who suffer from shingles on the face should be alert to any eye pain. If an infection develops in the eye—perhaps from rubbing the pained eye—it can result in reduced sight. Discuss this with your physician immediately.

For More Information
American Academy of Dermatology
930 North Meacham Road
Schaumburg, IL 60173
888-462-DERM
www.aad.org

Health Notes

➤ *Compresses of aluminum acetate solution, available from your doctor or pharmacy, can relieve any itching that may accompany the shingles rash.*

➤ *Talk to your healthcare provider about getting vaccinated. A chickenpox vaccine is available and can prevent shingles in some cases.*

➤ *An impaired immune system makes it more likely that you will get shingles. To boost immune system functioning, eat a low-fat diet high in antioxidants and fresh fruits and vegetables.*

Complementary and Alternative Treatments

Nutrition and Supplementation

Eat lightly and include in your diet brewer's yeast, brown rice, garlic, raw fruits and vegetables, and whole grains. Drink plenty of pure water and cleansing herbal teas. Avoid nuts, seeds, chocolate, and supplements containing the amino acid arginine.

Nutritionists recommend the following daily supplements to treat shingles:

Most Important

- L-lysine (500 mg 3 times daily, on an empty stomach)—heals and fights the virus that causes shingles

- vitamin C with bioflavonoids (2000 mg 4 times daily)—fights the virus and boosts the immune system

- vitamin B complex (100 mg 3 times daily)— necessary for nerve health

- zinc (80 mg for 1 week, then reduce to 50 mg; do not exceed a daily amount of 100 mg from all supplements)—enhances immunity and protects against infection; use lozenge form

- a prodophilus formula

- thymus live cell therapy support

Also Recommended

- calcium (1500 mg)—heals nerves and improves their function; combats stress

- magnesium (750 mg)—balances with calcium

- garlic (as directed on label)—builds up the immune system

- vitamin D (1000 IU 2 times daily for 1 week, then reduce to 400 IU)—heals tissue; necessary for calcium absorption

- vitamin E (400 to 800 IU)—prevents formation of scar tissue; can also be applied directly to affected areas of skin

- flaxseed oil (as directed on label)—promotes the healing of skin and nerve tissue

- grape seed extract (as directed on label)—pro-

tects skin cells; decreases the number of outbreaks

(Consult your healthcare provider regarding the duration of treatment.)

Aromatherapy

Mix 5 drops of one of the following essential oils into 1 teaspoon vegetable oil: bergamot, tea tree, rose, or lavender. Apply this mixture directly to the lesions to aid healing and diminish discomfort. You can also add a few drops of those oils to warm bath water for relaxation and to aid healing.

Ayurvedic Medicine

Some Ayurvedic practitioners suggest spreading a turmeric paste over the affected area to lessen pain and speed healing. Be aware that turmeric will impart a yellow stain to clothing and skin.

Bodywork and Somatic Practices

Very gentle methods, such as reflexology, CranioSacral Therapy, Therapeutic Touch, Reiki, and polarity therapy can be used.

Herbal Therapy

To numb the area, try smoothing calendula lotion or ointment over lesions several times a day. Alternatively, peppermint oil or a commercially prepared licorice gel can be applied.

You can decrease pain with an over-the-counter cream made with cayenne. The treatment works by sending the brain conflicting, or confusing, pain messages. Use only on healed lesions.

A combined tincture of oatstraw, St. John's wort, and skullcap also can bring relief. Take 1 teaspoon of the blend a day. Or mix equal parts lemon balm tincture and water; dab on lesions.

Herbal products are available in health food

stores and in some pharmacies and supermarkets. Follow package directions.

Homeopathy

A homeopathic practitioner may recommend one of the following three well-regarded remedies, depending on your symptoms:

- *Arsenicum album*—for severe burning pain that lessens if you apply warm compresses; also helpful if you feel very restless, anxious, and find it difficult to sleep

- *Mezereum*—for severe pain and itching; also helpful if scratching the lesions causes a burning sensation and the lesions have brown scabs

- *Ranunculus bulbosus*—for severe burning pain that worsens when you move or touch the lesions

Hydrotherapy

Apply ice packs, 10 minutes on and 5 minutes off, several times a day to relieve pain. Never leave the ice on for more than 20 minutes at a time; prolonged exposure to cold can damage skin. Applying ice along the spine (not on the blisters) will help. To lessen inflammation, splash apple cider vinegar on eruptions several times a day. You also can take a neutral bath (slightly cooler than body temperature) for its calming and soothing effects.

Traditional Chinese Medicine

Acupuncture Acupuncture can alleviate the pain and reduce the duration of a shingles attack. The practitioner focuses on the lung, back of head, adrenal gland, and internal secretion acupuncture points in the ear, along with points that correspond to the affected area.

Body acupuncture also may be used to treat this condition. In fact, if given at the first sign of symptoms, acupuncture has been shown to prevent post-herpetic syndrome, a chronic and very painful form of neuralgia that continues to plague the individual long after the shingles attack has abated.

Acupressure Although the rash itself should *never* be massaged directly, a practitioner may be able to relieve pain and accelerate the healing process by applying pressure to Liver 3, and to points that lie around the rash and in the ear.

As with acupuncture, acupressure—if administered in the early stages of the condition—may help prevent the development of post-herpetic syndrome, a chronic and very painful form of neuralgia.

Chinese Herbal Therapy In Chinese medicine, shingles is believed to be caused by a damp-heat imbalance, so herbs in formulas, such as gentiana (or the combination medicine, Gentiania Formula), are typically prescribed to rectify this underlying condition.

Yoga and Meditation

Use deep breathing, meditation, and yoga exercises to reduce stress and lessen the intense pain and other symptoms of shingles. Choose three or four poses that you enjoy, being sure to include at least one relaxation pose, such as the Child, Corpse, or Wind Removal. Perform daily, even after symptoms subside.

SHORTNESS OF BREATH

Sudden shortness of breath can be frightening— but it can be caused by a variety of situations, not all of them serious. If you're under 50, a non-smoker, and in good health without any other symptoms, your shortness of breath might be caused by:

- *Anxiety—If, in addition to the labored breathing, your heart is beating hard and fast and you feel panicky, you might be experiencing an anxiety attack. Practice slow, deep breathing until you can get yourself to a more calming environment.*

- *An environmental allergen—If you suspect something around you is inhibiting your breathing, remove the offending agent as soon as possible—or move to other surroundings—then relax until you can catch your breath. If your throat begins to close up at any time during an acute allergic response, get immediate medical attention.*

What if you experience shortness of breath and aren't fit or young? If you're out of shape, a smoker, or over the age of 50 and you've just exerted yourself physically, stop and rest. At your first opportunity, make an appointment with your healthcare provider for a thorough physical. You may have simply overexerted yourself. On the other hand, you don't want to overlook a possible heart or lung condition.

SICKLE CELL ANEMIA

Signs and Symptoms

- Fatigue
- Shortness of breath
- Rapid heartbeat
- Skin ulcers on lower legs
- Susceptibility to infections
- Delayed growth and development (in children)
- Vision problems (in some cases)
- Attacks of pain caused by blocked blood vessels or damaged organs (emergency symptom)
- Severe lightheadedness (emergency symptom)
- Severe shortness of breath (emergency symptom)

Description

Sickle cell anemia, also called sickle cell disease, is a blood disease that is caused by an abnormal type of hemoglobin called hemoglobin S. The condition is characterized by the transformation of normally flexible, round red blood cells to rigid, crescent-shaped cells (like sickles). These misshapen red blood cells are fragile and often break. Sickle cells also tend to clog small arteries in the bones, liver, spleen, and other organs, which can cause severe pain.

Sickle cell anemia is an inherited disease that usually appears in childhood. While not especially common among people of European descent, it is prevalent among people of African descent. Individuals of Mediterranean, Asian, and South and

S

Central American heritage also are at increased risk for the disease.

The condition is chronic with no cure. Certain situations can trigger emergencies. For instance, because a lack of oxygen at high altitudes makes red blood cells even more fragile and prone to breaking, people with sickle cell anemia often become dangerously lightheaded and breathless at high elevations. Also, people with sickle cell disease are particularly vulnerable to infectious diseases.

Conventional Medical Treatment

A blood test can detect the presence of abnormal red blood cells and hemoglobin S, confirming a diagnosis. Treatment includes daily folic acid sup-

Health Notes

➤ *You and your partner may want to undergo genetic testing before starting a family, especially if either of you has a family history of the disease. If both of you carry the sickle cell gene, there is a 25 percent chance that your children will be born with the disease.*

➤ *Sickle cell disease weakens the immune system, making the body prone to infectious illnesses. Boost your immune system with a diet high in antioxidant-rich fruits and vegetables.*

➤ *Don't smoke. Smoking weakens the immune system, making the body more prone to infectious conditions.*

➤ *Don't drink alcohol. Individuals with sickle cell anemia don't digest alcohol as efficiently as individuals without the disease. Excess alcohol can also weaken the immune system.*

➤ *Reduce stress. Stress has been shown to worsen symptoms of sickle cell anemia.*

plements, a B-family vitamin that is lacking in people with sickle cell disease. Much of the treatment for sickle cell disease is based on preventing complications. Because bacterial infections are one of the most common complications, patients are closely monitored for infection and given antibiotics, such as penicillin or erythromycin, at the first sign of bacterial illness. Blood transfusions may be given several times during a lifetime in order to strengthen a weakened blood supply.

For More Information
Sickle Cell Information Center
Grady Memorial Hospital
80 Butler Street
Atlanta, GA 30335
404-616-3572
www.emory.edu/PEDS/SICKLE

National Heart, Lung, and Blood Institute
P.O. Box 30105
Bethesda, MD 20824-0105
301-592-8573
www.nhlbi.nih.gov

Complementary and Alternative Treatments

Traditional Chinese Medicine

 Acupuncture In order to improve the flow of blood and boost the immune system (both of which are compromised in sickle cell patients), an acupuncturist may focus on Large Intestine 11, Lung 7, Bladder 18 and 19, Stomach 36, Spleen 6, Pericardium 6, Conception Vessel 12, and Governing Vessel 14.

Acupressure Acupressure may be helpful in improving circulation and reducing symptoms, including lethargy, shortness of breath, and dizziness. It also may help boost the immune system, which can stave off infections and colds.

Chinese Herbal Therapy TCM practitioners believe that sickle cell anemia (and all anemia) is caused by deficient blood, so herbs are prescribed to correct this problem. Preparations used to treat this condition may include Chinese cornbind, caltrop, ginseng, ligusticum, cordyceps, Tibetan saffron, angelica, rehmannia, and astragalus.

The Chinese combination medicines Dang Gui Four, Return Spleen Tablets, or White Phoenix Pills also may be recommended.

SINUSITIS

Signs and Symptoms

- Thick nasal discharge; runny nose
- Difficulty breathing through the nose
- Pain around eyes and/or cheeks
- Fever
- Toothache (in rare cases)

Description

Sinuses are cavities in the bone around the nose. There are four pairs of sinuses in the head, located in the forehead, between the eyes, deep in the head behind the eyes, and in the cheekbones. Each pair is connected to the nasal cavities by small openings that allow air to pass from the nasal passage through the sinuses and permit mucus to flow into the nose.

Should the tissue that lines one or more of these sinuses become inflamed and infected, the membranes of the nose itself also may swell, causing nasal stuffiness and blocking the drainage of mucus. This is called sinusitis, and it can be triggered by a bacterial, viral, or fungal infection or by severe irritation (perhaps by inhaling an irritating substance). In some cases, a person may experience sinusitis repeatedly, most often as the result of an untreated infection.

Conventional Medical Treatment

If you choose to see your physician, a physical exam, and in some cases, X-rays and/or a CAT

Health Notes

➤ Avoid pollution and cigarette smoke, which can aggravate symptoms of sinusitis. To keep your home air clean, consider getting an air purifier.

➤ Ask your healthcare provider about using a nasal saline spray to keep nasal membranes hydrated. Hydrated membranes are not irritated as easily as dehydrated nasal membranes.

➤ Don't overuse decongestants. Using these products for more than three days in a row can irritate sinuses and thicken mucus, making it more difficult to expel mucus and dry out nasal membranes.

➤ Reduce sugar intake, which some experts say impairs the immune system.

➤ Some experts say that a vegetarian diet decreases arachidonic acid concentrations. Arachidonic acid is a liquid unsaturated acid that occurs in animal fats and causes mild tissue inflammation in some people.

➤ Get regular, moderate exercise. Regular physical activity helps boost the immune system, which, in turn, wards off illness. Should you get sick, a strong immune system helps the body heal faster.

(S)

scan may be used to diagnose your condition. Treatment depends on what is causing the condition. Your physician may recommend that you try over-the-counter decongestant sprays, drops, or tablets to open the nasal passages and encourage drainage of the sinuses. In the case of a bacterial infection, antibiotics also may be prescribed.

In the case of recurring sinusitis, your physician may want to create a small opening in the bone between the nose and troublesome sinus, then clear the sinus by flushing it out with sterile water.

For More Information
Asthma and Allergy Foundation of America
1233 20th Street, NW, Suite 402
Washington, DC 20036
800-7-ASTHMA
www.aafa.org

National Institute of Allergies and
   Infectious Diseases
Building 31, Room 7A50
31 Center Drive, MSC 2520
Bethesda, MD 20892-2520
301-496-5717
www.niaid.nih.gov

Complementary and Alternative Treatments

Nutrition and Supplementation

To relieve congestion and sinus pressure, drink plenty of distilled water and fresh vegetable and fruit juices. Fresh pineapple juice is especially beneficial because it contains an enzyme called bromelain, which helps fight infection. Soups and hot herbal teas also help. Add cayenne pepper and raw onion to bring on even faster relief. Ask your healthcare provider to check for a fungal or yeast overgrowth in your sinus cavity.

Your diet should should *not* contain sugar or high amounts of salt. Dairy products increase mucus formation, so eliminate them.

The following daily supplements aid in preventing/treating sinusitis:

- vitamin C (500 mg every 2 hours)—decreases mucus and fights infection
- quercetin (as directed on label)—protects against allergies
- zinc (1 15-mg lozenge every 2 to 4 waking hours for one week; do not exceed this amount)—boosts the immune system
- coenzyme Q10 (60 mg)—stimulates the immune system
- flaxseed oil (as directed on label)—reduces pain and inflammation
- vitamin A (10,000 IU; do not exceed 8000 IU if you are pregnant)—protects against infection; maintains the health of the mucous membranes
- mixed carotenoid formula (up to 50,000 IU 3 times)—precursor of vitamin A
- N-acetyl cysteine (600 mg)

(For an *acute* condition, take supplements until your symptoms subside. If symptoms persist, seek the advice of your healthcare provider. For a *chronic* condition, consult your healthcare provider regarding the duration of treatment.)

Aromatherapy

To relieve thick congestion in your sinuses, add 3 or 4 drops essential oil of lavender, eucalyptus, red thyme, or peppermint to steam inhalations.

Ayurvedic Medicine

Ayurveda considers sinusitis to be an excess kapha problem, and practitioners say these simple remedies may help clear sinus congestion and prevent recurrences: Wash the nasal passages with a simple saline solution, which you can make at home or purchase. Place a little warm ghee or sesame oil in each nostril daily to keep passages moist.

Bodywork and Somatic Practices

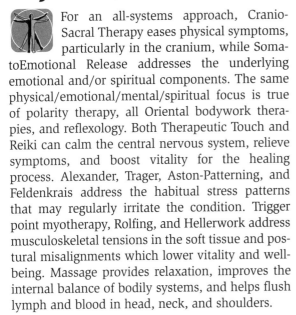

For an all-systems approach, Cranio-Sacral Therapy eases physical symptoms, particularly in the cranium, while SomatoEmotional Release addresses the underlying emotional and/or spiritual components. The same physical/emotional/mental/spiritual focus is true of polarity therapy, all Oriental bodywork therapies, and reflexology. Both Therapeutic Touch and Reiki can calm the central nervous system, relieve symptoms, and boost vitality for the healing process. Alexander, Trager, Aston-Patterning, and Feldenkrais address the habitual stress patterns that may regularly irritate the condition. Trigger point myotherapy, Rolfing, and Hellerwork address musculoskeletal tensions in the soft tissue and postural misalignments which lower vitality and well-being. Massage provides relaxation, improves the internal balance of bodily systems, and helps flush lymph and blood in head, neck, and shoulders.

Herbal Therapy

Numerous herbal remedies can combat sinusitis on several fronts: headache from stuffed sinuses, inflammation, nasal discharge, and breathing difficulties.

If you have inflammation, include 8 to 10 cloves of raw garlic in your diet daily. Alternatively, take 3 garlic capsules, 3 times a day. To further boost your immune system, try echinacea, fenugreek, or goldenseal tea. Steep 1 to 2 teaspoons dried leaves of either herb in 1 cup boiling water for 10 minutes; strain. Drink 3 times a day. To boost effectiveness, add 250 to 500 mg of bromelain (an enzyme derived from pineapple, available in health food stores) to goldenseal tea.

To fight excessive mucus, try eyebright or marshmallow tea. To make eyebright tea, steep 1 teaspoon dried leaves in 1 cup boiling water for 10 to 15 minutes; strain. For marshmallow tea, simmer 1 to 2 teaspoons finely chopped root in 1 cup boiling water for 10 to 15 minutes; strain. Drink either tea up to 3 times daily.

Homeopathy

Your homeopathic practitioner may advise one of the following treatments, depending on your symptoms:

- *Hepar sulphuricum*—for pain at the bridge of your nose; you notice an unpleasant odor, similar to pungent cheese, that seems to come from your nose; you feel better when you're warm

- *Kali bichromicum*—for pain in your cheekbones and a thick, ropy nasal discharge that's yellow or yellow-green

- *Mercurius solubilis*—for bad odors in the nose, coated tongue, and bad breath

- *Nux vomica*—if sinusitis is worse when you're outside; your nose is runny in the morning but congested at night

- *Pulsatilla*—if sinusitis is better when you're outside, and your nasal passages are more congested when you lie down or stay indoors

Hydrotherapy

Steam inhalation for 10 minutes or so every hour throughout the day is an excellent way to clear a stuffy nose. Add 1/2 cup of dried chamomile flowers to the boiling water. For directions, see "Hydrotherapy" in "Introduction to Complementary Therapies." Eucalyptus or ginger can replace the chamomile. Avoid inhalation therapy if you have asthma.

You also can use a nasal lavage (wash) to loosen secretions. Mix 1 teaspoon of salt or powdered goldenseal in 1 cup of warm (not hot) water. Use once a day.

Naturopathic doctors recommend applying warm compresses to the forehead. Others suggest applying a cold compress while soaking your feet in a basin of hot water.

Traditional Chinese Medicine

Acupuncture Sinusitis is thought to be caused by toxins in the intestines and bowels, coupled with a lack of energy to the lungs. Acupuncture may improve the flow of blood so that hazardous substances are eliminated from the body and may improve the flow of *chi* to the lungs. It also may be used to help alleviate the pain and headache caused by sinusitis.

The acupuncturist focuses on Large Intestine 4 and 20, Bladder 13 and 23, Spleen 6, and the extra point known as *Yin Tang*.

Acupressure To relieve the symptoms of sinusitis, pressure may be applied to Large Intestine 4 and 20, Spleen 6, Governing Vessel 14, Stomach 3 and 6, Bladder 2 and 6, and the *Yin Tang* point between the eyes.

Chinese Herbal Therapy Rehmannia Eight, Xanthium, and Magnolia are herbs that may be prescribed to manage sinusitis.

SLEEP APNEA/SNORING

Signs and Symptoms

- Loud snoring
- Observed episodes during sleep when breathing stops
- Morning headaches (in some cases)
- Excessive daytime sleepiness
- Intellectual impairment
- Daytime irritability

Description

Loud snoring is one of the most noticeable symptoms of sleep apnea. Sufferers have sagging throat tissue, which blocks the already-narrow airways. Snoring occurs when the breathing process pushes air past these sagging tissues, causing them to vibrate. In sleep apnea, a snore may be followed by a short stoppage of breath, which forces you awake due to lack of air. After 10 to 20 seconds or more of no breath, you let out a loud resuscitative snore or a snort accompanied by a shift in body position. You then move to a lighter level of sleep, your throat muscles regain their normal tension, and breathing becomes regular.

However, as soon as you drift back into a deeper sleep, the process repeats itself.

All this slipping back and forth between deep and light sleep leaves the sufferer feeling tired in the morning—even though it may seem that the person "slept through the night." It's not known exactly why, but sleep apnea affects mostly overweight men; the majority of sufferers are over age 40.

Conventional Medical Treatment

Most people with sleep apnea are unaware of their condition and it is usually a sufferer's bed partner who encourages him or her to seek help. For this reason, many physicians ask individuals to bring their partners with them, since it is the partners who are most familiar with the symptoms. A physician also may ask you to record yourself sleeping and bring in the cassette.

If your doctor suspects sleep apnea, he or she may ask you to spend a night in a sleep laboratory for observation and an overnight polysomnography test. Sleep centers are usually connected with a hospital or medical center. During this examination you literally spend the night in bed, hooked up to heart and brain monitors while technicians observe you. This is a very common way to confirm the diagnosis and assess the severity of your condition.

There is no one standard treatment for sleep apnea. Slimming down offers substantial improvement to most people. You also will be counseled to avoid alcohol and sleeping pills. These don't cause sleep apnea, but they do worsen the condition.

Although it isn't common, one of the most successful treatments is the use of a continuous positive airway pressure (CPAP) machine. This home apparatus features a mask connected to a small machine that blows air into nasal passages, keeping airways open during sleep. If calibrated in a sleep lab and worn properly, the machine can be very effective, though it always may be needed during nighttime sleep. If you cannot or will not wear the mask, your physician may suggest uvulopalatopharyngoplasty (UPPP), a surgical technique that removes soft tissue from the throat and

Health Notes

➤ Ask your healthcare provider about an orthodontic appliance to keep your mouth open and your tongue pulled forward. While this won't cure sleep apnea, it does lessen snoring.

➤ Avoid alcohol and other sedatives. These aggravate symptoms of sleep apnea.

➤ Maintain a normal weight. Being overweight is a risk factor for sleep apnea.

➤ Try exercises and light weight lifting to tone the upper respiratory tract. Some experts say this can reduce symptoms of sleep apnea.

➤ Sleep on a firm mattress, using a single pillow. Some people with sleep apnea claim that this lessens snoring.

Sleep Apnea and Health

A recent study found that an average of 20 percent of all patients with documented coronary artery disease (CAD) also have sleep apnea, a rate considered to be high enough to justify screening all coronary artery disease patients for the sleep disorder. Individuals with CAD and sleep apnea were also found to be at significantly greater risk for heart attack and stroke than those with CAD alone.

Another study found that people with sleep apnea had higher incidences of hypochondria, depression, and phobias than did a control population. Patients with untreated sleep apnea also have a much higher accident rate; in one study, 25 percent of patients with sleep apnea reported falling asleep at the wheel at least once a week. It is believed that deep sleep deprivation makes sleep apnea a risk factor for a wide range of health conditions.

uvula to widen airway passages. This often stops snoring and can improve apnea, but it does not eliminate it.

Complementary and Alternative Treatments

Ayurvedic Medicine

According to Ayurveda, sleep apnea may caused by excess kapha. To achieve a more restful and continuous sleep, Ayurvedic practitioners advise getting regular exercise and losing weight, if you are overweight. They also may suggest changing your sleeping position. For example, if you routinely sleep on your back or stomach, try sleeping on your side.

Remember to consult your doctor before embarking on any new health regimen; sleep apnea and snoring can be symptoms of more serious conditions.

Sprains

Traditional Chinese Medicine

 Acupuncture If the problem is caused by breathing disorders, the acupuncturist will focus on points along the lung, heart, and kidney meridians.

Chinese Herbal Therapy Herbs may be prescribed to promote relaxation, which can help you get a good night's sleep. Herbs can also be prescribed to aid in weight loss, as obesity is a contributing factor in sleep apnea and snoring. Additional herbs may be recommended to tone the kidneys, the organs responsible for sleep disorders, according to TCM experts.

SYMPTOM:

SORE THROAT

A throat may become sore for many reasons. There are mechanical causes, such as a night spent yelling for your home basketball team or too much smoking. Heavy coughing due to an irritating airborne substance also can irritate the throat and make it hurt. These types of sore throats can be prevented by speaking in a normal tone, avoiding cigarettes and secondhand cigarette smoke, keeping your home clean and well ventilated, using a humidifier if the air in your home is dry, and drinking lots of fluids to keep throat cells hydrated. To treat irritation-caused discomfort, try dissolving an aspirin and a teaspoon of sea salt in a 6- or 8-ounce glass of warm water, gargling and spitting out the water. This can be repeated every two hours.

Of course, illness is a prime cause of throat pain. Any illness that targets the throat—such as strep throat, laryngitis, or tonsillitis—will cause localized soreness. Other, more general respiratory conditions, such as colds, flus, bronchitis, and mononucleosis, also count sore throats among their characteristic symptoms.

You may want to self-treat a sore throat that accompanies a cold or flu. Yet you should see a doctor if your sore throat persists or worsens, you have a fever, your lymph nodes are swollen, swallowing is painful, you have bad breath, and/or you are coughing up mucus that is thick or greenish-yellow or is tinged with blood. After taking a culture of throat cells and/or sputum, your healthcare provider can diagnose what ails you and offer a treatment, such as antibiotics in the case of a bacterial-caused illness.

SPRAINS

Signs and Symptoms

- Rapid swelling of a joint (such as the ankle, wrist, elbow, shoulder, or knee) after the joint has been unnaturally stretched or twisted

- Pain and tenderness in affected area

- Pinkish or bluish discoloration of area (in some cases)

- Audible popping noise and inability to use affected joint (emergency symptom)

Preventing Falls in The Elderly

As we age, our bodies naturally become less flexible. In addition to putting a graceful swing in our step and allowing us to perform motions in an easy, fluid way, flexibility helps humans stay balanced and upright. When flexibility diminishes, a person's chance of trips and spills increases, which is, perhaps, why older people are especially vulnerable to falls. In fact, it is estimated that each year one-third of Americans over the age of 65 fall. Of these, 10 to 15 percent are significantly injured—breaking a bone, pulling muscles or tendons, or spraining a joint. Osteoporosis, the weakening of bones due to decreased calcium, also increases the chance of fractures when the elderly fall.

In a 1995 study published in the *New England Journal of Medicine,* researchers found that individuals who performed simple stretching exercises each morning had almost one-third fewer falls than those who did not. The three movements used in the study were the hip circle, the toe stand, and the one-leg stand. To do the hip circle, rotate your hips by making big circles, as if playing with a hula hoop. Circle five times clockwise, five times counterclockwise. Toe stands are what ballerinas call *relevés.* This simple move requires you to stand on the toes of both feet at the same time. Hold onto a table, countertop, or chair for support and stay raised on the balls of your feet for five seconds. Return your heels to the floor and repeat the move five times. To perform the one-leg stand, stand on your left leg for five seconds, with your right leg bent at the knee and raised off the ground. Return your right leg to the ground. Do ten times, then switch sides and do ten more times. To increase your flexibility further, try ballet, yoga, Pilates, and martial arts, such as tai chi, or maintain an active lifestyle with lots of stair-climbing, gardening, housecleaning, and walking. If you have movement problems, get up from seated positions slowly, wear sturdy shoes, and don't be afraid to use a cane or walker for support. Moving around with help is healthier for you—physically and mentally—than not moving at all.

It should be noted that while exercise plays an enormous role in protecting the body from falls, plain old common sense is equally important. As we age, it is essential to have regular eye and ear checkups. All the exercise in the world isn't going to keep you from tripping over a curb you didn't see or a small dog you didn't hear barking in front of you. Also, many older individuals take a variety of medications for various ailments. Once or twice a year, it's wise to bring all your medication containers to your physician for a review. Do any of the pills affect motor skills? Can any be eliminated? Are there any that are dangerous when taken together? Do any affect mental alertness? On the subject of drugs, older people are also especially sensitive to alcohol. The two glasses of wine you had with dinner when you were in your 40s may leave you staggering when you're in your 60s. For many older individuals, a half-glass of wine, or its equivalent, is all that should be consumed in one sitting.

Description

The word *sprain* means "damage to the ligaments that connect the bones." Though any joint can be sprained, the most frequently affected joints are the wrists, ankles, knees, and arches of the foot. A sprain occurs when the joint has been traumatically twisted or stretched, typically during a fall or misstep in which the weight of the body is placed on the joint in an unnatural position.

Conventional Medical Treatment

As soon as you suspect a sprain, ice the area to reduce swelling. If the sprain is a mild one, you

Health Notes

➤ *Once a joint has been sprained, it is in danger of being re-sprained during even the mildest misstep or fall. To prevent future sprains, you may want to support the area by wrapping it in an Ace® bandage when participating in sports or other physical activities.*

➤ *To prevent sprains, gently stretch muscles before physical activity. Stretching muscles after physical activity can help maintain flexibility.*

➤ *Wear sport-appropriate footwear. For instance, shoes designed for racquet sports support lateral motion and help prevent ankle sprains by preventing your feet from rolling sideways. Yet wearing these same shoes during an activity where the ankle must be kept flexible—such as aerobic dance—can actually contribute to sprains by encouraging you to land incorrectly on the side of your foot or your ankle.*

can continue with homecare: wrap the joint with a supportive wrap (such as an Ace® bandage), ice the area intermittently for a full 24 hours, and elevate the injured joint. Within 24 hours, you should be able to put weight on the joint. Use the joint as little as possible—or avoid using it altogether—and it should be completely healed within two weeks.

If the sprain seems serious, or if the pain does not improve with two or three days of homecare, see your physician for X-rays. You may have serious ligament damage or even a bone fracture—both of which require an operation, time spent in a splint, and rehabilitative physical therapy.

For More Information
American Academy of Orthopedic Surgeons
6300 North River Road
Rosemont, IL 60018-4262
800-346-AAOS
www.aaos.org

American College of Sports Medicine
P.O. Box 1440
Indianapolis, IN 46206
317-637-9200
www.acsm.org

Complementary and Alternative Treatments

Nutrition and Supplementation

 Consume plenty of juices made from fresh raw vegetables, such as garlic, beets, and radishes. These are high in valuable enzymes and vitamins.

To help ease the discomfort of sprains and promote healing, nutritionists recommend the following daily supplements:

Most Important

- hydrolysed collagen (as directed on label)
- glucosamine sulfate (1500 mg)
- proteolytic enzymes (as directed)—breaks down scar tissue

Also Recommended

- calcium (1500 to 2000 mg)—repairs connective tissue
- magnesium (750 to 1000 mg)—important for the skeletal system
- flaxseed oil (as directed on label)—promotes cellular health; speeds recovery
- grape seed extract (as directed on label)— a potent anti-inflammatory
- free-form amino acid complex (as directed on label)—repairs and strengthens connective tissue
- potassium (99 mg)—vital for tissue repair
- vitamin C (5000 to 20,000 mg in divided doses)—required for tissue growth and repair; use ascorbate form
- zinc (50 mg; do not exceed a total of 100 mg from all supplements)—important in tissue repair

(Take supplements until your symptoms subside. If symptoms persist, seek the advice of your healthcare provider.)

Aromatherapy

 Place a few drops of essential oil of camphor, chamomile, eucalyptus, lavender, or rosemary on a cold compress. Apply to the affected joint or muscle. Remove after 20 minutes; extended exposure to cold can damage skin. Reapply as necessary.

Ayurvedic Medicine

 Ayurveda considers a sprain to be a pitta condition; a strain is a vata condition. Ayurvedic practitioners may advise applying a turmeric-salt paste to the affected area. Be aware that turmeric will stain fabric and skin.

Bodywork and Somatic Practices

 Massage is not recommended. Reflexology, CranioSacral Therapy, polarity therapy, Reiki, and Therapeutic Touch are more suited to these conditions.

Chiropractic

 Sprains are usually a result of direct trauma to a joint or area of the body and generally occur during sports activities. The general chiropractic treatment for sprains includes ice applications, compression of the area by Ace® bandage, and elevation of the affected joint to facilitate drainage. Depending on the joint affected and the length of time elapsed since the injury, chiropractic therapy may facilitate healing through a combination of ice, moist heat, electromuscle stimulation, ultrasound application, gentle joint mobilizations, and specific chiropractic adjustment (SCA).

Herbal Therapy

 Herbal remedies can lessen pain and speed muscle healing. To use internally, combine equal parts of tinctures of horsetail, nettle, and willow bark. Take 1 teaspoonful of the blend 3 times a day. For an external remedy, purchase arnica tincture, cream, or ointment and apply it directly to the injured area. See package directions for specific instructions.

Herbal products are available in health food stores and in some pharmacies and supermarkets. Follow package for specific directions.

Homeopathy

 Homeopaths often recommend one of the following treatments for a sprain or strain depending on your symptoms:

- *Arnica*—for the first 24 hours after a sprain or strain to lessen the pain; at the same time, apply Arnica oil, ointment, or gel to the affected area

- *Ruta gravelones*—for sore ligaments or tendons

- *Ledum*—if the affected area is cold to the touch and the pain eases when you apply a cold compress

- *Rhus tox*—if the affected area is stiff and feels better when you move

Hydrotherapy

 Apply an ice pack to the injured area, 20 minutes on, 20 minutes off, for the first 24 to 36 hours. However, do not use longer than 20 minutes at a time, since extended exposure to cold can damage skin.

To rehabilitate the injured area without stressing it, try exercising in water.

Traditional Chinese Medicine

 Acupuncture Acupuncture can be very beneficial in the treatment of sprains, as it reduces pain and inflammation and speeds healing. The practitioner focuses on different acupuncture points, depending upon the location and severity of the sprain.

Acupressure To treat a sprained ankle, a practitioner may focus on Stomach 41, Spleen 5, and Gallbladder 40—all of which reside around the ankle. A sprained wrist is treated by applying pressure to Large Intestine 5, Small Intestine 5, Triple Warmer 4, and related ear points. Other sprains require additional acupressure points.

Chinese Herbal Therapy Pseudoginseng and Dragon Blood, *Yunnan Bai Yao,* and Tian Qi and Eucommia formulas also may be used to treat sprains. Corydalis Analgesic Tablets may be given to manage pain, and *Zheng Gu Shui* and other ointments can be used topically to relieve pain and encourage healing.

SYMPTOM:

STOMACH PAIN/STOMACHACHE

Abdominal pain, tummy ache, stomachache— no matter what you call it, pain in the gut is a common sign of a very large range of illnesses, each with a slightly different type of discomfort. Some of these conditions include:

- *Gastric upset (a cramping feeling accompanied by bloating and perhaps vomiting or diarrhea)*

- *Menstrual cramps (a constant vise-like pain sometimes accompanied by nausea)*

- *Irritable bowel syndrome (bouts of diarrhea, bloating, and/or constipation)*

- *Gallstones (intense pain that first appears at the upper right side of the abdomen, then migrates to the right shoulder blade)*

- *Appendicitis (a dull pain at the navel followed by tenderness on the lower right side of the abdomen)*

- *Ovarian cysts (dull ache in the abdomen with a sense of pressure)*

- *Food poisoning (symptoms include cramping, diarrhea, and vomiting)*

Infectious illnesses, such as the common cold and common flu, may cause mild stomachaches with fever, diarrhea, and vomiting. Peptic ulcers of the esophagus, duodenum, and stomach—as well as indigestion and gastritis—often feature a gnawing or burning pain in the upper abdomen. The pain may be lessened by eating.

In women, stomachaches may be caused by disorders of the reproductive organs. These tend to cause abdominal tenderness, often severe cramps in the mid-section of the abdomen, and may be accompanied by nausea and bloating. Menstruation is a very common cause of stomachaches. Endometriosis, pelvic inflammatory disease, ectopic pregnancy, uterine and ovarian cysts, cancer, and sexually transmitted disease also cause abdominal pains.

A stomachache also can be caused by disease or cancer in one of the abdominal organs, such as the gallbladder, pancreas, liver, or colon. Symptoms may include abdominal tenderness, pain over the diseased organ, fever, and general weakness.

With such a range of causes, it's best to let your physician diagnose what's behind your ache. You can, however, help your doctor by explaining exactly where in your abdomen the pain is located (for example, lower right), any accompanying symptoms (for example, fever or dizziness), and whether the ache is dull, constant, sharp, burning, etc. If the pain comes on suddenly and is intense and persistent, get immediate medical help—even if this means going to the emergency room. You may have appendicitis.

STRESS

Signs and Symptoms

- Stiff shoulders, neck and/or jaw
- Backache
- Intermittent headaches
- Gastric upsets
- Appetite loss or increased appetite
- Insomnia
- Acne eruptions
- Shortness of breath
- Anxiousness
- Fatigue
- Temporary memory impairment
- Increased susceptibility to infectious illnesses
- Tooth grinding
- Feelings of resentment
- Sense of hopelessness
- Irritability
- Reclusiveness
- Inability to concentrate

Description

Stress, one of the favorite buzzwords of the late twentieth century, describes our reaction to overwhelming physical, mental, or emotional stimuli. Stress can be brought on by a sudden event, such as a job loss or death of a relative, or it can be a more chronic condition brought on by daily aggravations and trying to meet the expectations of others—or ourselves. Typically, the more stressed a person feels, the greater the range of mental and physical symptoms he or she will experience.

Each of us experiences stress differently. One person may feel extreme stress working at a relatively low-pressure job, while another person may juggle a full-time job, parenthood, and night school and feel only mild stress.

Stress is actually your body's way of preparing you for an emergency. When your brain perceives danger, your pituitary gland secretes adrenocorticotropic hormone, which in turn causes your adrenal gland to release hormones called adrenaline and cortisol. These two hormones immediately cause your pulse to quicken, your muscles to tense, and your blood pressure to rise. These changes are important because during a crisis, you may need more blood in your large muscles, so your heart beats faster. To lessen the chance of bleeding to death in case of an injury, blood is directed away from your stomach and skin and your body secretes clotting chemicals into your blood. To give you quick energy, fat and sugar are released into the bloodstream. Other changes include pupil dilation for better vision, increased

Stress and the Young Child

According to several new studies, extreme stress at a young age—such as living in an emotionally, verbally, or physically abusive household—may permanently rewire the brain's circuitry. The result is an adult who is unable or less able to handle normal, everyday stress. These findings concern health officials because increasing numbers of American children are exposed to stress and violence at younger ages than ever before. Nearly half of American families with young children have at least one of the following risk factors for emotional, verbal, or physical abuse: a mother who has not finished high school, a mother who is under age 20, a mother who is unmarried at the birth of her first child, a violent male present in the household, or an estranged or distant father.

Health Notes

➤ The release of the hormone cortisol may suppress the immune system. To boost your immune system, eat a diet high in antioxidant-rich fruits and vegetables.

➤ If you suffer from stress symptoms, develop a network of close friends and family members to whom you can turn for support. A recent Swedish study shows that 50-year-old men who had recently endured high levels of emotional stress without support of family or close friends were three times more likely to die within the next seven years as those who said they had similar stresses but also had ample emotional support in their lives.

➤ Cut down or eliminate caffeine. A stressed body is already operating under the power of the natural stimulants cortisol and adrenaline. Adding another stimulant, such as caffeine, can overburden the body and suppress the immune system.

➤ Learn to set priorities and concentrate on finishing important tasks first. This can help alleviate feelings of "drowning in work."

➤ Learn to say "no"—at work and at home. If you don't have time to do your friend a favor, or if you're offered a project that seems as though it will be more trouble than it is worth, just say "no," politely yet firmly.

➤ Exercise moderately three to seven times a week. Regular exercise has been shown to be effective in lessening symptoms of stress.

➤ Keep a diary to determine what events you find particularly stressful and analyze your reactions. Many people find that writing about their troubles helps lower stress.

➤ Take time out for yourself as part of your regular routine. Do something fun, such as learning a new skill or joining a community sports team.

➤ Consider therapy to help you come to grips with the feelings of helplessness or anger that are brought on by stress.

➤ Don't use alcohol or drugs to relax. These stress an already-stressed body, and can lead to dangerous addictions.

➤ Ask yourself if you're doing something to exacerbate stress. Often it's how we react to a certain situation that creates the stress, not the situation itself.

➤ If you have trouble reducing stress on your own, consider taking a stress management class at a local college or hospital.

perspiration to keep cool, and faster breathing to increase the oxygen in the blood.

Though this "fight-or-flight" response helped cave dwellers survive, it doesn't work so well in modern times, when the stress-triggering situation can be ongoing—as in the case of financial hardship, a taxing job, or the daily pushes and pulls of work and family. When there's no letup to the stress, your body stays in this heightened "state of emergency," making you vulnerable to various health conditions, including, in extreme cases, hypertension, heart attack, and stroke.

Conventional Medical Treatment

A physical exam, a complete list of symptoms, and a detailed lifestyle history are generally all your physician needs to diagnose excess stress and rule out a mental health problem, such as anxiety disorder. Treatment depends on the person, but generally involves removing some stressors. Stress reduction techniques and lifestyle modification are usually part of a therapy plan, and in many cases, psychotherapy or counseling is recommended or required.

For More Information

American Institute of Stress
124 Park Avenue
Yonkers, NY 10703
914-963-1200
www.stress.org

National Institute of Mental Health
6001 Executive Boulevard
Room 8184, MSC 9663
Bethesda, MD 20892-9663
301-443-4513
www.nimh.nih.gov

Complementary and Alternative Treatments

Nutrition and Supplementation

Avoid foods that place stress on the system, such as processed foods, artificial sweeteners, carbonated drinks, chocolate, fried foods, junk foods, fatty meats, sugar, white flour products, chips and similar snack foods, and foods containing preservatives. Avoid caffeine, as it contributes to nervousness and can disrupt sleep patterns. Eliminate dairy products from your diet for three weeks. Reintroduce them slowly and watch for returning symptoms of your "nervous" condition. Alcohol, tobacco, and mood-altering drugs may provide temporary relief from stress, but overall, they are harmful to your health, and actually make stress worse.

Your diet should be rich in raw foods. Fresh fruits and vegetables supply valuable vitamins and minerals as well as flavonoids, which help neutralize dangerous free radicals.

Nutritionists recommend the following daily supplements:

Most Important
- vitamin B complex (50 mg)—for proper functioning of the nervous system, supplemented with vitamin B_5 (500 mg)
- vitamin C with bioflavonoids (3000 to 10,000 mg)— essential to adrenal gland function; stress depletes these hormones, which are the "anti-stress" hormones
- adrenal and thymus live cell therapy
- phosphatidyl serine (1500 mg, in divided doses, with food)

Also Recommended
- calcium (2000 mg)—lost during stress reactions
- magnesium (500 to 1000 mg)—deficiency is common in highly stressed people and can lead to anxiety, fear, even hallucinations; may cause loose bowels
- fiber (as directed on label)—improves bowel function; stress often causes bowel irritability
- potassium (99 mg)—depleted during stress reactions

(For an *acute* condition, take supplements until your symptoms subside. If symptoms persist, seek the advice of your healthcare provider. For a *chronic* condition, consult your healthcare provider regarding the duration of treatment.)

Ayurvedic Medicine

Stress can induce an imbalance in any of the doshas (vata, pitta, or kapha), depending on the person's makeup, say Ayurvedic practitioners. They often recommend meditation, relaxing baths, and massage to alleviate and control stress. They also may advise taking gota kola or the Ayurvedic formulas *Geriforte* and *Mentat*.

Ayurvedic products are available at many health food stores and Indian pharmacies.

Bodywork and Somatic Practices

Stress responds to all bodywork and somatic practices, especially when you also employ other stress reduction methods.

Chiropractic

Many patients find they are much more relaxed and less stressed following a chiropractic adjustment. The chiropractor may be able to decrease tension and pain in affected muscles, using a combination of soft tissue massage, moist heat application, and electromuscle stimulation.

In many patients, stress manifests itself in the form of headaches, neck tension and pain, or back pain (see "Headache," "Neck Tension and Pain," and "Back Pain" entries).

Traditional Chinese Medicine

Acupuncture Stress can be significantly reduced with acupuncture, which promotes feelings of calm and tranquility and releases "feel-good" endorphins that increase the patient's sense of well-being. Acupuncture also may be used to strengthen any organs that have been compromised or weakened by stress.

Acupressure Acupressure is very effective in relieving many stress-related ailments. To treat headache, the practitioner manipulates Gallblad-

der 14 and 20, Liver 3, and Large Intestine 4; for neck and shoulder stiffness, Kidney 3, Liver 3, Gallbladder 20 and 21, and Large Intestine 10; and for lethargy, Lung 9, Large Intestine 4 and 10, Stomach 36, Conception Vessel 6, and Kidney 3. Stress also can cause other symptoms—including insomnia, depression, impatience, and skin problems—and these may require the manipulation of different acupressure points.

Acupressure also can be used to enhance relaxation, and to improve the patient's outlook and ability to manage stress.

Chinese Herbal Therapy Patent formulas that may be recommended to counteract stress are Concha Marguerita and Ligustrum for anxiety and mental stress, Prunella and Scutellaria for stress-related hypertension, Minor Bupleurum for digestive upsets, Major Four Herbs to enhance immunity, and Cnidium and Tea for migraines.

Yoga and Meditation

Yoga's power to relax the body and improve circulation makes it an ideal anti-stress treatment. Use deep-breathing techniques, slow deliberate exercises, and calming meditation to achieve your stress-reduction goals. Yoga professionals recommend practicing three or four poses daily. Include at least one of the relaxation poses, such as Child, Corpse, or Wind Removal. For meditation try the Lotus, Easy, or Sun Salutation pose, and include a relaxing mantra.

S

STROKE

Signs and Symptoms

- Acute onset of one or more of the following: slurred speech, dizziness, double vision, loss of coordination, or difficulty swallowing
- Sudden weakness or loss of sensation in one leg or an arm and leg (generally on the same side of the body)
- Rapid onset of extremely severe headache
- Decline in vision, speech, or sensation over a period of minutes or hours
- Abrupt loss of consciousness (emergency symptom)
- Sudden onset of partial or complete paralysis of leg, arm, and/or face (emergency symptom)

Description

The medical term for a stroke is *cerebrovascular disease.* A stroke is caused by lack of blood flow to the brain. There are actually many different

The Monday Factor

Boston University investigators found that an average of 17 percent of strokes occur on a Monday—more than any other day of the week. Furthermore, working men were twice as likely to have a stroke on Monday as those without jobs. About 35 percent of Monday strokes occur between 8 a.m. and noon. According to research, strokes are least likely to occur on a Saturday. While popular wisdom has it that Monday strokes occur because of the mental stress of returning to work, researchers are quick to say that they don't know what mechanism may be responsible for the Monday increases. One theory is that a Monday morning stroke may be triggered by changes in physical activity from the weekend and/or a greater likelihood of smoking or drinking alcohol on the weekend.

Warning Signs of a Stroke

If you experience a sudden onset of any of the following symptoms, contact your physician or go to an emergency room immediately:

- Severe headache with no known cause
- Numbness
- Dimness of vision, especially in one eye
- Difficulty communicating or understanding speech
- Unexplained dizziness
- Weakness of the face, arm, or leg on one side of the body

types of strokes, depending on what part of the brain is cut off from blood flow. All, however, involve the loss of function related to whatever brain tissue was severed by the stoppage.

Strokes can occur suddenly and severely over the space of a few minutes, or progress gradually over several hours. An estimated 10 to 30 percent of all stroke victims first experience a mini-stroke, which has much milder symptoms than a regular stroke, usually lasts less than five minutes, and does not cause brain damage. Also known as transient strokes, these typically occur hours, days, weeks, or months before a regular stroke.

Each year, an estimated 300,000 Americans suffer a stroke. One-quarter of this number die; the rest are left with mild to severe disabilities, including brain damage, paralysis of one or both sides of the face, paralysis of one or both sides of the body, loss of speech, memory loss, impaired reasoning,

Health Notes

➤ The carotid arteries, which are in the neck, can get clogged by a cholesterol-heavy diet, just like arteries around the heart. Clogged carotid arteries can lead to a stroke. Speak to your doctor if you feel you may be at risk.

➤ Eat a diet rich in fruits and vegetables that contain vitamin C. A British study adds further support to the belief that vitamin C can help prevent disease. The study found that elderly people with low serum vitamin C levels had an increased risk of death from stroke.

➤ Quit smoking. Cigarette smoking increases the level of clot-promoting substances in the blood, decreases the beneficial high-density lipoprotein (HDL), damages blood vessels, and raises blood pressure—all of which are risk factors for stroke.

➤ If you are female and using birth control, ask your doctor or gynecologist whether oral contraceptives are safe for you. In women with other risk factors—such as obesity or smoking—oral contraceptives can increase the risk for stroke by causing blood clots.

➤ If you have high blood pressure, talk to your healthcare provider about ways to lower it. High blood pressure is thought to be the primary cause of strokes.

➤ If you've had a stroke, talk to your healthcare provider about any medication you are taking. Recent research has found that patients taking commonly prescribed drugs may be slower to recover motor function than those not receiving these drugs. The investigators found that, two to three months following a stroke, patients taking benzodiazepine tranquilizers such as diazepam (Valium®), prochlorperazine (Compazine®), haloperidol (Haldol®), antihypertensive drugs such as clonidine (Catapres®) and prazosin (Minipress®), and anticonvulsant drugs such as phenytoin (Dilantin®) and phenobarbital, were significantly less likely than the others to recover muscle strength or be able to perform simple daily tasks.

➤ Consider eliminating or cutting down on meat. In a study of older men, those who ate meat (including poultry, fish, specialty meats, and organ meats) every day were almost twice as likely to suffer a stroke compared to those who ate meat just three to six times a week.

➤ A diet high in fruits and vegetables and low on meats could greatly reduce the risk of stroke. Research has shown that individuals who consume three or more servings of fruits and vegetables daily lowered their risk of stroke by two-thirds.

➤ Practice regular, moderate exercise. A sedentary lifestyle has been identified as a risk factor for stroke.

➤ Talk to your doctor about aspirin. For some people, a daily aspirin can thin the blood, reducing one's chance of having a blood clot in the brain.

and diminished sight. Disabilities correspond to the part of the brain that was damaged. Stroke victims face a multitude of physical discomforts and challenges. Because of the loss of function, many become dependent on family members and/or private nurses, making the disease especially dreaded. The prognosis is better in younger patients because their brains are more adaptable.

The greatest risk factor for stroke is age. In fact, your chance of having a stroke doubles each decade after the age of 35. Additional risk factors include high blood pressure (70 percent of all strokes in this country occur in individuals with high blood pressure), heart conditions (in those with heart conditions, blood clots from the heart are more likely to travel up the major arteries to the brain, where they get stuck), a family history of strokes, and being of African descent. Smoking, high blood cholesterol, and diabetes also are thought to be contributing factors.

Conventional Medical Treatment

A stroke is an emergency condition. Should you or anyone you know develop any of the preceding symptoms, go straight to the nearest hospital emergency room. Diagnosis may be based upon symptoms and patient history, or may involve an MRI or CAT scan of the brain to see whether there is any leakage or any "backed-up" blood in the brain. Treatment may include immediate administration of the drug t-PA (tissue-plasminogen acti-

vator). This drug can help prevent brain damage or death by dissolving the blood clots that cause most strokes. Patients receiving t-PA within three hours of the onset of symptoms are 30 percent more likely to make a complete or near complete recovery.

Overall treatment varies widely, depending on what risk factors have contributed to the stroke and what area of the brain is affected. Typical treatment includes intensive care and a combination of life support and intravenous feeding. Also, depending on what function has been lost, a stroke victim may require some type of long-term physical therapy and/or nursing care. To prevent a second stroke, you may be given a prescription for an anti-clotting drug, such as warfarin (Coumadin®), or told to take one aspirin every day.

For More Information
Brain Research Foundation
120 South LaSalle Street, Suite 1300
Chicago, IL 60603
312-759-5150

National Stroke Association
9707 Easter Lane
Englewood, CO 80112
800-STROKES
www.stroke.org

Complementary and Alternative Treatments

Nutrition and Supplementation

As is always the case, prevention is easier than cure. Eat high-fiber foods that are low in fat and cholesterol. Meals should be planned around fruits, vegetables, and grains. Eat dark-green, leafy vegetables, legumes, nuts, seeds, soybeans, wheat germ, and whole grains to get a healthy supply of vitamin E (which improves circulation).

Foods to avoid include candies, chips, fried foods, gravies, junk food, pies, processed foods, red meat, and saturated fats. Also stay away from stimulants such as coffee, colas, tobacco, and alcohol. Drink plenty of pure water.

These are good daily supplements for you to take:

Most Important

- calcium (1500 mg)—maintains proper muscle tone in the blood vessels

- magnesium (750 mg)—balances the calcium

- vitamin D (400 mg)—aids calcium uptake

- coenzyme Q10 (100 mg)—improves tissue oxygenation

- flaxseed oil (as directed on label)—reduces blood pressure; lowers cholesterol levels; maintains proper elasticity of blood vessels

- vitamin E (start with 200 IU and increase by 200 IU each week until you reach 1000 IU daily)—helps to block the first steps leading to the disease

- selenium (200 mcg)—promotes the action of vitamin E

- vitamin B complex, containing vitamins B_6 (50 mg), B_{12} (600 mcg), and folate (200 mcg)

Also Recommended

- germanium (200 mg)—lowers cholesterol and improves cellular oxygenation

- L-methionine (500 mg, on empty stomach)—helps prevent fatty buildup in the arteries

- zinc (50 mg; do not exceed a total of 100 mg from all supplements)—aids in the healing process

- copper (3 mg)—balances with zinc

(Consult your healthcare provider regarding the duration of treatment.)

Bodywork and Somatic Practices

 Stroke patients have responded well to Feldenkrais and CranioSacral Therapy. Other methods to try would be Aston-Patterning, massage, Trager, Oriental bodywork, and polarity therapy.

Traditional Chinese Medicine

 Acupuncture Acupuncture can be used to lower cholesterol and blood pressure, as well as improve the flow of blood through the arteries in order to prevent a stroke. It also may be helpful in unblocking energy pathways following a stroke, which can hasten the patient's recovery and help prevent paralysis.

Acupressure Acupressure may prevent a stroke by rejuvenating blood flow through clogged arteries. It also helps stimulate muscles that may have been weakened by a stroke and increase energy and stamina in patients with impaired immune systems.

Chinese Herbal Therapy Chinese medicine views a stroke as an internal damp-wind condition that impairs brain and circulatory functioning, and herbs are typically prescribed to remedy this underlying disorder as well.

STY

Signs and Symptoms

- One or more painful, reddish lumps on the edge of the eyelid near the lashes
- Slightly blurred vision in the affected eye (in some cases)

Description

Sties are similar to pimples in that they are caused by bacteria—but instead of erupting around a hair follicle on the face or body, a sty erupts from a eyelash follicle. Also, like pimples, sties usually enlarge gradually as they fill with pus. Eventually, sties either burst or slowly diminish in size. If a sty grows large, it can press on the eye, causing vision to blur temporarily.

Conventional Medical Treatment

Sties generally are harmless and can be treated with homecare. The first piece of advice is to refrain from squeezing the sty in attempt to remove pus. This can spread bacteria and cause additional sties. Instead, apply a warm compress to the sore for about 10 to 15 minutes, 4 or 5 times daily. If and when the sty bursts, gently wash the area to remove pus.

Visit your physician or ophthalmologist if the sty has lasted longer than six days or is severely infected. The doctor may prescribe a topical antibiotic cream and/or lance the sty and drain the pus.

For More Information

American Academy of Dermatology
930 North Meacham Road
Schaumburg, IL 60173
888-462-DERM
www.aad.org

National Eye Institute
2020 Vision Place
Bethesda, MD 20892-3655
301-496-5248
www.nei.nih.gov

Health Notes

➤ If you suffer from recurring sties, talk to your doctor about increasing your vitamin A intake. Some health experts say there is a correlation between recurring sties and low vitamin A intake.

➤ Do not rub or touch the sty. This can aggravate the infection and spread it to unaffected areas of the eye.

Complementary and Alternative Treatments

Traditional Chinese Medicine

 Acupuncture A sty is considered a heat imbalance in Chinese medicine, so an acupuncturist may focus on Spleen 10 and Large Intestine 11; Stomach 44; or Urinary Bladder 65 in order to remedy the infection.

Chinese Herbal Therapy See an herb-trained specialist for this treatment.

S

SUBSTANCE ABUSE

Signs and Symptoms

- Using drugs every other day, daily, or several times a day

- Using drugs in non-social settings, such as work or home

- Feeling you need drugs to get through the day

- Desire to continue using drugs after others have said you've had too much

- Preoccupation with drug-taking

- Denial that you take too many drugs

- Irritation and/or arguing with friends and family who express concern about your drug use

- Underestimating or lying to friends and family about the amount of drugs you use

- Relying on drug use to help induce relaxation, relieve pain, or overcome social inhibitions

- Regret over words said or actions performed while using drugs

- Feelings of guilt about the amount of drugs you use

- Stealing or selling belongings to afford drugs

- Increased susceptibility to anxiety, depression, and/or insomnia

- Loss of memory and/or concentration

- Irregular eating habits while using drugs, either bingeing or avoiding food altogether

- Health problems and susceptibility to infectious diseases

- Blackouts (in some cases)

- The inability to remember what happened the night before, even though you didn't black out (in some cases)

- Child or spousal abuse (in some cases)

- Driving accidents or arrests while under the influence of drugs (in some cases)

- Employment problems, including tardiness, absenteeism, low productivity, and/or interpersonal problems (in some cases)

Description

Substance abuse and chemical dependency are terms that describe a condition in which a person is addicted to alcohol, prescription medication, and/or street drugs. (See "Alcoholism" entry.)

What causes substance abuse is not known exactly, but the condition affects more men than women. Some people have a genetic disposition toward chemical dependency. Many substance abusers have had a mother or father who was "a heavy drinker" or a "pill popper." That individual becomes an adult and discovers that having a couple glasses of wine with dinner helps him forget the stress of the day, or that a couple of prescription sleeping pills promotes relaxation, or that cocaine makes him lively and outgoing. Over time, the person relies more and more on chemical substances to induce a desired state. This dependency may affect relationships, short-term and long-term health, and, if the person drives, there may be accidents and/or brushes with the law. It's a vicious cycle, and to cope with the new stresses created by the substance abuse—and with the cravings that may develop—the pattern of abuse intensifies.

Conventional Medical Treatment

If you suspect that you or someone you care about is abusing alcohol or drugs, a consultation with a physician is essential. Medical treatment isn't normally used to treat substance abuse, per se, but it's important to discover whether one's health has in some way been affected—whether, for instance, the drinking has caused a vitamin deficiency or cirrhosis of the liver, or if shared needles have caused hepatitis. To address the substance abuse itself, your physician may recommend psychotherapy and/or group therapy.

One of the most well-known therapy networks is Narcotics Anonymous (NA). In return for group help, the organization asks that you eradicate all forms of drugs from your life. In weekly, twice-weekly, or even nightly NA meetings (attendance depends on how much help and support you need), you report your progress, talk about the problems and emotions you're facing, and listen to others do the same. Group members offer one another advice, wisdom, and support.

Some physicians may treat drug users with new synthetic medications known as "blockers." These can ease withdrawal symptoms and protect against relapse by acting on the same brain mechanisms that cause addiction. Another option currently under investigation is ibogaine, a quasi-psychedelic plant-derived substance that eliminates drug cravings and alters drug-seeking behavior. One dose of ibogaine can eliminate heroin, cocaine, and alcohol cravings for two or three weeks. Buprenorphine, a prescription painkiller, is also being tested for addiction-fighting potential. For heroin addicts, a new chemical called l-alpha-acetyl-methadol

Children of Drug Users

Child psychologists and criminologists have long believed that a parent's drug use plays a role in a child's mental health, and research supports this. Several new studies have documented how being raised by substance-abusing parents results in a variety of emotional characteristics and deviant behaviors, including low self-esteem, depression, anger, delinquency, and violence. It is estimated that there may be at least 22 million children who have been or are currently being raised in homes with one or two substance-abusing parents.

Health Notes

➤ Talk to your children about the health dangers of alcohol and drug use, and ask your child's school how it addresses this issue in the curriculum. One recent study has identified the pre-adolescent years (from age 10 to 12) as a particularly vulnerable period for the development of early alcohol and drug abuse.

➤ If a parent or another family member is or was dependent on alcohol, prescription medication, or street drugs, there's an increased chance that you will have the same problem. Be careful around these substances or avoid them altogether.

➤ If you notice that you are unable to get through a day without using drugs, and/or if you find yourself using drugs at work, immediately seek help from your local chapter of Narcotics Anonymous or from a trained psychotherapist, before your dependency grows stronger.

➤ Be aware that needle-sharing can lead to hepatitis and AIDS.

(LAAM) can ease addiction symptoms without producing a high of its own.

For More Information
Alcoholic Anonymous Headquarters
475 Riverside Drive
New York, NY 10015
212-870-3400
www.alcoholics-anonymous.org

Narcotics Anonymous
P.O. Box 9999
Van Nuys, CA 91409
818-773-9999
www.na.org

National Institute on Drug Abuse
6001 Executive Boulevard
Bethesda, MD 20892
301-443-6245
www.nida.nih.gov

Complementary and Alternative Treatments

Nutrition and Supplementation

Your well-balanced diet should emphasize fresh, raw foods. Add high-protein drinks, and avoid heavily processed foods, all forms of sugar, and junk food.

Nutritionists recommend the following daily supplements. The dosages are for adults. For children under the age of 17, use half to three-quarters the recommended amount.

- vitamin B complex injections (2 cc daily or as prescribed by a healthcare provider)—needed when under stress to rebuild the liver; injections are the most effective form
- calcium (1500 mg)—nourishes the central nervous system; helps control tremors
- magnesium (1000 mg)—balances the calcium
- free-form amino acid complex (as directed on label)—supplies protein in a readily assimilable form
- L-glutamine (500 mg 3 times daily)—promotes healthy mental functioning
- L-tyrosine (500 mg 2 times daily)—gives good results for cocaine withdrawal when taken with valerian root every four hours
- glutathione (as directed on label)—detoxifies drugs to reduce their harmful effects; reduces the desire for drugs
- L-phenylalanine (1500 mg, taken upon awakening)—relieves withdrawal symptoms; do not take if you are pregnant, nursing, or suffer from panic attacks, diabetes, high blood pressure, or PKU
- vitamin C (2000 mg every 3 hours)—detoxifies the system and lessens the craving for drugs

(Consult your healthcare provider regarding the duration of treatment.)

Bodywork and Somatic Practices

Many bodywork and somatic practice methods can be effective within a total rehabilitation program.

Traditional Chinese Medicine

Acupuncture Acupuncture is so effective at treating substance abuse problems that many rehabilitation facilities now include it as a mandatory part of their program. To date, there are more than 300 such programs in the United States.

Countless studies have shown that people who include acupuncture as part of their recovery program have a much higher success rate (and a much lower recidivism rate) than those who do not. Acupuncture works by significantly reducing withdrawal symptoms, including cravings and discomfort, and by enhancing feelings of relaxation and well-being.

When treating substance abuse, an acupuncturist focuses on points along the conception vessel, governing vessel, gallbladder, stomach, kidney, spleen, pericardium, lung, heart, large intestine, small intestine, and triple warmer meridians. Auricular, or ear, acupuncture may be utilized as well.

In general, acupuncture treatments for substance abuse last from 20 to 50 minutes and are given every day during the initial withdrawal phase (twice a day, if necessary), then reduced to two or three times a week as symptoms—night sweats, palpitations, chills, irritability, vomiting—abate. Once the patient's condition shows an obvious improvement, treatments may be reduced to just once a week, in order to prevent a relapse. It is always combined with counseling.

Chinese Herbal Therapy Depending upon what is determined to be the root cause of the addiction, the practitioner may recommend the following formulas to ease withdrawal: Bupleurum and Dragon Bone, Concha Marguerita and Ligustrum, Ginseng and Longan, Gentiana Formula, and Bupleurum and Tang Gui. Herbs also will be given to strengthen impaired immunity and to improve the health of any organs that have been compromised by the addiction.

SUDDEN INFANT DEATH SYNDROME (SIDS)

Signs and Symptoms

- Unexplainable death of an infant during sleep

Description

Sudden infant death syndrome, also known as SIDS or crib death, has no symptoms, other than the sudden, unexplainable death of a seemingly healthy infant. An autopsy on the baby usually shows no specific cause of death.

Babies aged two to four months are especially vulnerable to SIDS. Premature babies have been found to die of SIDS more often that babies born at term. Also, babies born weighing 6 pounds or less have higher rates of SIDS than heavier babies.

The American Association of Pediatrics recommends that babies be placed on their backs to sleep, and very young infants may need to be propped with a rolled up baby blanket. Exposure

A Possible Cause of SIDS

A new study has uncovered a clue that may help solve the puzzle of sudden infant death syndrome. Researchers believe that a cell defect involving a chemical receptor in a very small section of a baby's brain stem may keep such an infant from detecting dangerously high levels of carbon dioxide. These babies—particularly if they are sleeping on their stomachs—may breathe in higher levels of carbon dioxide in stale air trapped between their heads and the mattresses. The defect is not fully understood and researchers point out that while it might be a factor, it is not necessarily the sole cause of the syndrome. This means parents should continue to use preventative measures.

Health Notes

➤ Avoid all secondhand cigarette smoke while pregnant. Don't smoke and don't allow anyone else to smoke in your home or around your baby. Secondhand cigarette smoke before birth and after birth has been found by numerous studies to be a primary risk factor for SIDS.

➤ Put your baby on his or her back to sleep. Sleeping on the stomach or side has been associated with higher rates of SIDS.

➤ Ask your doctor or pediatrician about the use of baby blankets. A significant number of infants who died of SIDS were found with covers loosely around or over their head. Autopsies, however, report that these babies did not die of suffocation, but of unknown causes.

➤ Consider placing your baby's crib in your bedroom for the first year. That's the suggestion of a recent New Zealand study that found higher rates of SIDS among infants who did not share a room with their parents.

➤ For unexplained reasons, SIDS is more likely to occur in winter than any other season, perhaps because parents may be more inclined to overdress or overswaddle their infants in cold weather.

➤ Ask your doctor whether or not your baby should be given a pacifier. A British study has found lower rates of SIDS among infants who sleep with pacifiers.

S

to secondhand smoke either before or after birth, and being overly wrapped or extremely over-dressed are also primary risk factors for SIDS.

Conventional Medical Treatment

None—prevention and parent education are the only courses to take.

For More Information
National SIDS Resource Center
2070 Chain Bridge Road, Suite 450
Vienna, VA 22182
703-821-8955
www.circsol.com/SIDS/index.htm

Sudden Infant Death Syndrome Alliance
1314 Bedford Avenue, Suite 210
Baltimore, MD 21208
800-221-7437
www.sidsalliance.org

SYMPTOM:

SUNBURN

Just as the name implies, sunburn is a skin burn caused by the ultraviolet (UV) rays of the sun or by artificial light sources. Symptoms can range from a mild redness (a first-degree burn), to swelling and blistering (second-degree burn), to deep open sores (third-degree burn). Extreme sunburn also can lead to dizziness, nausea, and shock. A lifetime of heavy tanning also dries the skin and leads to premature wrinkles and an older appearance.

Even more important, sunburns can be life-threatening. We now know that the sun's UV rays not only burn the skin, but can also alter or mutate the DNA in skin cells. Years of such skin damage can leave the skin prone to skin cancer. Half of all new cancers are skin cancers, with about 1 million cases diagnosed in the United States each year.

Sunburn can begin within 15 minutes of exposure to UV rays. With continuous exposure, the skin produces more of the natural pigment melanin, which creates the protective skin coloring commonly called a tan. But the sun also can burn areas that do not tan, such as the eyes and lips, so these areas are even more vulnerable to sunburn.

Despite the problems associated with sunburn, many people still like the look of a summer tan and continue a pattern of overexposure. Although fair-skinned, fair-haired people burn more readily (and, therefore, are more vulnera-

ble to developing skin cancer), African Americans and other dark-skinned people also are at risk. The soft, tender skin of babies and small children is particularly vulnerable to burning.

The best way to combat the painful effects of sunburn is prevention. The American Cancer Society, the National Cancer Institute, and the American Academy of Dermatology unanimously recommend the regular use of a sunscreen with an SPF (skin protection factor) of 15 or higher. Apply the lotion at least 20 minutes before going into the sun to allow the active ingredients time to soak into the skin. Even water-resistant sunscreen should be reapplied every two hours or immediately after swimming.

A sunscreen with an SPF of 30 does not give twice the protection, as you might think. An SPF 15 sunscreen absorbs 93 percent of the sun's rays, while an SPF 30 sunscreen absorbs 97 percent; an SPF 2 absorbs 50 percent. If a fair-skinned person normally burns within 10 minutes of unprotected sun exposure, applying an SPF 2 lotion would double the time before burning to 20 minutes, and an SPF 15 lotion would increase the time to 150 minutes. Certain medications, such as some antibiotics and birth control pills, make your skin more sensitive to the sun, so read package inserts carefully.

As a general preventative guideline, it's a good idea to stay out of direct sunlight between the hours of 10 a.m. and 4 p.m. If you must be out in the sun regularly, cover up with light-weight protective clothing. A hat with a brim at least four inches wide can help prevent painful burns on the scalp and the nausea and dizziness often associated with sun exposure. Protect vulnerable areas under the eyes or chin with zinc oxide (a white, opaque ointment). Protective sunglasses are also recommended.

Treatment for sunburn varies according to its intensity. If you do get a sunburn:

- Run the reddened area under cool (not icy) water to halt the burning process.

- Apply a cool washcloth to the affected area.

- Take aspirin or ibuprofen within the first hour of being burned.

- Use skin moisturizer, especially products with aloe vera.

- Drink lots of fluids, especially drinks with electrolytes, to prevent dehydration.

- Eat foods rich in beta-carotene, vitamin E, zinc, selenium, and vitamin C to promote skin healing.

- To prevent scarring after overexposure to the sun, apply vitamin E oil from vitamin capsules or water-soluble creams. Apply vitamin C creams and lotions before sun exposure to help prevent burning. Both, however, must be used along with sunscreens.

- In more severe cases, gently clean the burned area with soap and water, and protect small burns from infection with anti-bacterial ointment and adhesive bandages.

- In general, leave blisters intact to prevent infection. If you have widespread blistering, or the burned area exudes pus or has open sores, seek medical help.

Nutrition therapies include eating raw fruits and vegetables, which supply necessary vitamins and minerals, and high-protein foods, which repair skin tissue. Sunburn dehydrates your body, so drink ample amounts of fluids.

The following daily supplements enhance recovery from sunburn:

Most Important

- coenzyme Q10 (60 mg)—increases the supply of oxygen to the cells

- colloidal silver (as directed on label)—promotes healing and subdues inflammation

- free-form amino acid complex (as directed on label)—repairs tissue

- l-cysteine (500 mg)—promotes healing of burns

- potassium (99 mg)—replaces potassium lost through burning

- vitamin C with bioflavonoids (10,000 mg)—repairs and heals tissue; reduces scarring

- vitamin A (100,000 IU for 2 weeks, then reduce to 50,000 IU until healed; do not exceed 8000 IU daily if you are pregnant)—destroys free radicals; repairs and heals tissue

- vitamin E (400 IU, increase to 1600 IU until healed)

Also Recommended

- calcium (2000 mg)—balances pH; aids in potassium utilization

- magnesium (500 to 1000 mg)—reduces stress on tissues

- vitamin B complex (100 mg)—heals tissue

- zinc (80 mg for one month; then reduce to 50 mg; do not exceed 100 mg from all supplements)—heals tissue

- vitamin E cream (apply 3-4 times)

Other complementary treatments include Chinese herbal therapy. The practitioner may recommend aloe vera as an external ointment to soothe a sunburn. An over-the-counter preparation called Beijing Absolute Red may also be helpful in relieving sunburn pain.

S

SYMPTOM:

SWEATING, EXCESSIVE

Excessive sweating, or hyperhydrosis, is a common complaint. The condition is usually a normal, temporary physiological response to stress, anxiety, heat, fever, or even eating spicy foods. But excessive sweating can be a sign of a medical problem such as hyperthyroidism. Menopause is the most common cause of generalized sweats, which occurs mostly at night. Certain medications can also cause excessive sweating. To prevent excessive sweating, use a topical agent for the hands or underarms. Preparations containing aluminum are the most effective.

Diaphoresis, the sudden onset of profuse perspiration, is usually associated with dizziness, a cold clammy feeling, and sometimes nausea. Diaphoresis is often an emergency symptom of hypoglycemia, chemical poisoning (especially by an agricultural pesticide), or a serious heart condition.

SWIMMERS' EAR

Signs and Symptoms

- Malodorous, yellowish, or yellowish-green pus draining from the ear
- Pain in the ear, particularly when the head moves
- Flaking skin in the ear canal
- Itching in the ear canal
- Hearing loss (in some cases)

Description

Medically known as external otitis, swimmer's ear is a condition marked by persistent irritation and inflammation of the outer ear canal. Swimmer's ear occurs most commonly during the summer swimming season. Water may be trapped in the ear canal after swimming, especially in individuals who repeatedly attempt to clean the ear canal with cotton swabs. Swabbing the canal disrupts the ear's own mechanism for ridding itself of debris and strips the protective coat of wax in the ear canal, leaving the area more susceptible to infection. The ailment also can develop if the canal has been physically irritated or torn by using inappropriate objects (such as toothpicks or hairpins) to clean the ear canal. Chemicals from hair products (such as sprays, mousses, and hair-coloring agents) can also cause external otitis.

Conventional Medical Treatment

If treated promptly, swimmer's ear poses no threat to general health—but if allowed to worsen, the infection can spread to underlying cartilage. Therefore, if you notice any itching or pain in your ear, visit your physician. A physical exam using a otoscope is usually enough to diagnose the condition, though a pus sample may be taken for lab analysis.

To treat the condition, your physician may clean the ear canal with a suction device. Eardrops containing a corticosteroid (to relieve itching and inflammation) may be prescribed, along with an

Health Notes

➤ *When using hair styling products, take special care to keep the product away from the outer ear canal.*

➤ *Place something warm over the affected ear to help ease the pain. Try a warm electric heating pad, hot water bottle, or a warm, wet wash cloth.*

➤ *Prevent swimmer's ear by using commercial ear drops containing aluminum acetate. According to many doctors, homemade drops are equally effective. Mix equal parts white vinegar, 70 percent isopropyl alcohol, and water, and apply one or two drops to the outer ear canal before and after swimming.*

antibiotic to fight infection. In serious cases, an oral antibiotic may be prescribed. If the pain is severe, you may be given painkillers.

For More Information
American Medical Association
515 North State Street
Chicago, IL 60610
312-464-5000
www.ama-assn.org

Complementary and Alternative Treatments

Nutrition and Supplementation

See "Ear Infection" entry.

Aromatherapy

To ease pain, gently rub the area around the outer ear with 5 drops of lavender or chamomile oil. Mix the essential oil with 1 teaspoon of canola oil before using.

Herbal Therapy

To reduce inflammation, aid healing, and boost immunity, place 2 or 3 drops of mullein oil or garlic oil in the infected ear canal every 3 hours.

Homeopathy

Your homeopathic practitioner may recommend *Pulsatilla* if hearing is difficult and you feel as if something were being forced out of the ear.

Hydrotherapy

To lessen intense pain, hold a warm hot water bottle wrapped in a light towel against the infected ear. Rewarm the bottle as necessary.

Traditional Chinese Medicine

Acupuncture Acupuncture may alleviate the inflammation and pain of swimmer's ear. The practitioner will typically work points related to the kidney (the organ responsible for ear functioning, according to traditional Chinese medicine) and to the ear itself.

Acupressure Acupressure may help relieve the symptoms of swimmer's ear. The therapist will typically focus on the following acupressure points to relieve pain and outer ear inflammation: Small Intestine 19, Gallbladder 2, Triple Warmer 17 and 21, along with additional points in and around the ear.

Chinese Herbal Therapy Mint may also be used to soothe the earache. Chinese herbal formulas such as Gentiana or Anemarrhena, Phellodendron, and Rehmannia may also be prescribed.

SWOLLEN GLANDS

Lymph glands, also known as lymph nodes, range in size from a caper to a large olive and are located throughout your body. Their function is to create lymphocytes, the disease-fighting white blood cells that help protect the body from invasion by harmful microorganisms. Should any type of harmful microbe—whether it be the latest flu bug or a type of cancer like lymphoma—attack the body, the glands enlarge to churn out lymphocytes. These busy, swollen glands may even be tender to the touch when working overtime.

The lymph glands that are most easily moni-tored are located at the side of the upper neck and under the armpits. Swelling in these nodes is a good indication that your body is fighting off infection. Sometimes, feelings of illness may appear a day or two after the glands swell. If your glands have been noticeably swollen for a week or more, or are accompanied by other symptoms (such as fever, nausea, body aches, vomiting, and so on), visit your physician.

Glands generally return to their normal size once the underlying illness is treated and they are no longer creating microbe-fighting lymphocytes.

SYPHILIS

Signs and Symptoms

- Painless sores or ulcers on genitalia and/or rectum
- Enlarged lymph nodes in the groin

In later stages, the following signs and symptoms may be present:

- Rash on palms of hands and soles of feet
- Rash on limbs or torso
- Mouth sores
- Fever
- Headache
- Soreness and aching in the bones and joints
- Patchy hair loss

Description

Syphilis is a sexually transmitted disease (STD). It is caused by a type of bacterium called *Treponema pallidum* that lives in the penile or vaginal secretions of an infected person and infects others through small cuts or abrasions in the genital area, or through the mucous membranes of the vagina. It can also be transmitted by infected blood.

Anywhere from 10 days to six weeks after exposure to the bacterium, you develop mild symptoms—usually a single painless sore on the genitals or rectum and enlarged lymph nodes in the groin. This is called the first stage. The sore usually heals in three to twelve weeks. As the bacteria enters the bloodstream and spreads through the body, the second stage appears. This is characterized by a rash on the palms of the hands and the soles of the feet and perhaps on the torso and limbs, mouth sores, and fever. Less common symptoms include intermittent headaches, aching bones and joints, and/or eye inflammation. If an infected individual is not treated, the disease can progress to a third or latent stage. During this stage the heart and nervous system may become damaged.

Syphilis had become relatively uncommon until recently, when it has begun to make a comeback. Rates among drug users are especially high.

Conventional Medical Treatment

If caught early, syphilis can be completely cured, so if you notice symptoms, it is important to see your physician, gynecologist, or urologist. To diagnose the condition, your doctor will perform a physical exam and a blood test to detect the presence of the causative bacteria. Treatment involves antibiotic therapy, usually penicillin. Follow-up blood tests are required at regular intervals for at least one year, to ensure that all bacteria have been killed.

Health Notes

➤ *Abstinence and protected sex with condoms are the best ways to prevent syphilis. Always practice safe sex with a new partner or with a partner who is not monogamous.*

➤ *Talk to your teenagers about the importance of abstinence and safe sex in preventing STDs like syphilis.*

➤ *If you are diagnosed with syphilis, alert all recent partners.*

➤ *To prevent infecting others, avoid sexual contact until your antibiotic therapy is over.*

For More Information

American College of Obstetrics and Gynecology
409 12th Street SW, PO Box 96920
Washington, DC 20090-6920
800-673-8444
www.acog.org

Centers for Disease Control and Prevention
1600 Clifton Road
Atlanta, GA 30333
800-311-3435
www.cdc.gov

Complementary and Alternative Treatments

Nutrition and Supplementation

 A whole-foods diet rich in plant foods and free of sugar, caffeine, and alcohol can assist healing. In addition, nutritionists recommend the following daily supplements:

Most Important

- a prodophilus formula (as directed on label)—restores friendly bacteria; important when taking antibiotics
- garlic (as directed on label)—stimulates the immune system and acts as a natural antibiotic
- free-form amino acid complex (as directed on label)—repairs tissue
- vitamin C (750 to 2500 mg 4 times daily)—boosts immune function
- zinc (100 mg; do not exceed this amount)—promotes healing; important for the health of the reproductive organs
- thymus and liver live cell therapy support (as directed on label)

Also Important

- colloidal silver (as directed on label)—rapidly reduces inflammation and promotes healing of lesions
- kelp (1000 to 1500 mg)—supplies balanced vitamins and minerals

S

Syphilis

- vitamin B complex (50 mg 3 times daily)—necessary in cellular enzyme system functions

- coenzyme Q10 (30 to 60 mg)— a potent free radical scavenger

- vitamin K (100 mcg)—gets destroyed by antibiotics; necessary for blood clotting

(Consult your healthcare provider regarding the duration of treatment.)

Traditional Chinese Medicine

 Acupuncture After a diagnosis has been made by your healthcare provider, acupuncture may be helpful in improving immune function and reducing stress, both of which can hasten healing and prevent recurrences.

Acupressure As with acupuncture, this modality may be effective in enhancing the patient's well-being and boosting the immune system, which can be effective in the treatment and prevention of STDs.

Chinese Herbal Therapy Chinese herbs can be quite helpful in treating a variety of sexually transmitted diseases, but you should *always* be diagnosed and treated by a conventional practitioner before using any alternative therapies. (Some STDs only can be cured with conventional antibiotics, and serious complications can arise if they are not treated properly.)

That said, there are a variety of herbs that may be beneficial in conjunction with conventional treatment, depending upon the STD and the patient's specific symptoms. Formulas with Astragalus, Japanese wax privet, and ginseng, for instance, are often used as supplemental therapy in cases of AIDS (as is Ginseng and Atractylodes Formula).

Dianthus Formula may be suggested for the treatment of gonorrhea. Sandalwood has been used to treat several types of venereal disease. Bupleurum, angelica, and cordyceps may be used to bolster the immune system.

TEMPOROMANDIBULAR JOINT SYNDROME (TMJ)

Signs and Symptoms

- Headaches (in some cases)
- Jaw pain and tenderness
- Clicking sound or grating sensation when eating or opening the mouth
- Dull pain in front of the ear
- Difficulty opening or closing the mouth due to locking of the joint
- Pain in the neck, back, shoulders, face, ear, and/or throat (in some cases)

Description

Your temporomandibular joints—located in front of each ear—connect your mandible (lower jaw) to each side of your skull. When working correctly, the two joints move at the same time. Temporomandibular joint syndrome (TMJ)—also known as temporomandibular disorder (TMD)—occurs when these joints are out of sync. As a result, the discs that sit between these joints and the skull slip out of position, resulting in irritation and inflammation of the joints and malfunction of the jaw.

Though stress does not cause TMJ, it contributes to the problem. Generally there is an underlying physical reason for the syndrome. In fact, it is commonly triggered by some kind of trauma to the head, neck, or jaw—including whiplash, a physical blow to the head, jaw, or face, regular and extreme clenching of the teeth, and regular grinding of the teeth while sleeping.

Conventional Medical Treatment

To diagnose TMJ, your physician or dentist examines your bite (the way your teeth close) for alignment abnormalities, and may perform X-rays.

Treatment may include anti-inflammatory medications. In more serious cases, a corticosteroid is injected into the jaw. You may be given a plastic bite plate to wear over your teeth to encourage proper alignment of the mandible and simultaneous functioning of the joints. Also called a splint, the device may relieve jaw-locking, pain, and noise. Such conservative therapy should be continued for at least six months before resorting to other measures. At this point, your physician or dentist may order a CAT scan or MRI to understand why you are not responding to treatments. Additional measures may include *arthrocentesis*, in which a fluid is injected into the joint, often releasing a locked jaw with no or few complications. Additional measures can include physical therapy,

An Operation Gone Wrong

In the mid-1970s many dentists began treating TMJ with Proplast® implants designed to connect the lower jaw to the skull. Yet these implants—which were made from a Teflon® compound—were insufficiently tested. Many of them shattered shortly after being inserted, releasing materials into the body which ultimately could lead to pain, disfigurement, and immune system supression. There even have been a small number of suicides that have been traced to Proplast® implants. In 1991, eight years after the implant was approved, the Food and Drug Administration (FDA) recalled it. A subsequent TMJ implant made of Silastic®—the same silicone material that's been linked to autoimmune diseases in breast-implant patients—was withdrawn from the market in January 1993. Many doctors and oral surgeons believe all TMJ implants should be removed immediately, as the risk of the implants breaking down in the body is too great.

Temporomandibular Joint Syndrome (TMJ)

ultrasound (a method of delivering deep heat), biofeedback, or transcutaneous electrical nerve stimulation. With another, more expensive procedure, *arthroscopy*, the doctor uses optics to look into the jaw and remove any tissue or debris that may keep the jaw from working properly. Your doctor may prescribe anti-inflammatory relaxants to ease muscle tightness and pain.

For More Information
American Dental Association
211 East Chicago Avenue
Chicago, IL 60611
312-440-2500
www.ada.org

Complementary and Alternative Treatments

Nutrition and Supplementation

Your diet should consist of lightly steamed vegetables, fresh fruits, whole grains, white fish, skinless chicken and turkey, brown rice, and homemade soups and breads. Foods that increase stress include all forms of sugar, white flour products, junk foods, candy, colas, potato chips, and fast foods. Caffeine also increases tension, which aggravates the problem. Avoid alcohol, as it is a contributing factor in tooth-grinding, which can cause or aggravate TMJ.

To rest your body and jaws, do not chew gum, and cut back on foods that require heavy chewing, such as red meat and bagels.

These daily supplements should help treat TMJ:

* calcium (2000 mg)—has a calming effect

* magnesium (1500 mg in divided doses)—relieves stress

* vitamin B complex (100 mg 3 times daily)—the anti-stress vitamins

* coenzyme Q10 (60 mg)—improves oxygenation of tissues

* vitamin C (4000 to 8000 mg in divided doses)—combats stress; heals and repairs connective tissue

* glucosamine sulfate (1500 mg)

(For an *acute* condition, take supplements until your symptoms subside. If symptoms persist, seek the advice of your healthcare provider. For a *chronic* condition, consult your healthcare provider regarding the duration of treatment.)

Bodywork and Somatic Practices

CranioSacral Therapy is a leading therapy in this area.

Chiropractic

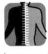

TMJ syndrome may be caused by a variety of factors, including stress, improper alignment of the teeth, and direct trauma to the jaw as a result of a car accident or blow to the chin. After a complete dental workup, the patient may find that chiropractic care, including massage and muscle stimulation to the affected muscles, provides significant relief.

Traditional Chinese Medicine

Acupuncture By using what's known as "oral acupuncture" and focusing on points behind the last molar, an acupuncturist can mitigate the neck, face, and jaw pain caused by TMJ, along with related headaches or ringing in the ears. Distal points are also used.

Acupuncture also may be helpful in reducing stress, which can prevent recurrent episodes.

Acupressure The practitioner may focus on Large Intestine 4, Gallbladder 2, Stomach 7, Small Intestine 8 and 19, Stomach 44, and related auricular points to treat this condition.

Chinese Herbal Therapy Herbs may be prescribed to treat stress, headache, tinnitus, and other TMJ symptoms (see these individual entries for more information).

TENDINITIS

Signs and Symptoms

- Pain and tenderness just outside a joint
- Swelling just outside the affected joint (in some cases)

Description

Tendinitis means "inflammation of the tendon," the tissue that connects muscles to bones, and it can occur in any joint. This inflammation is due to a small tear or tears in the tendon. The condition can be caused by an injury or by everyday overuse of the joint, such as carrying a briefcase. It most commonly affects the shoulder or the elbow.

In tennis elbow, a type of tendinitis, the pain is felt just below the crease of the elbow on the outside of the upper forearm and may extend down to the wrist. Tennis elbow is caused by repeated rotary motion of the forearm.

Conventional Medical Treatment

To diagnose tendinitis, your physician may physically examine the area and perform an X-ray. Treatment involves homecare: for the first 72 hours, rest the joint (use an Ace® bandage, sling, or brace if you need to immobilize the area); intermittently ice the area to reduce swelling; and use aspirin to reduce pain and swelling. In more serious cases, a corticosteroid may be injected into the joint to decrease inflammation, or an operation may be necessary to reconstruct the tendon.

After the area has healed, your physician may prescribe a regimen of gentle range-of-motion exer-

Tendinitis

De Quervain's Tenosynovitis

In some cases, tendon pain is not caused by tendinitis—inflammation of the tendon—but by *tenosynovitis,* an inflammation of the protective sheath that surrounds the tendon.

One of the most common forms of tenosynovitis is de Quervain's tenosynovitis, an inflammation that occurs when one of the tendon sheaths in the thumb muscles becomes too narrow for the tendon to move comfortably within it. The condition is characterized by pain in the hand, and is distinguishable from tendinitis by a catching or "triggering" sensation that occurs when the thumb is moved toward the pinky finger. Most sufferers develop the condition by performing jobs or activities requiring repetitive wrist and hand use. Women often experience the condition in the last three months of pregnancy or following delivery.

Treatment for tenosynovitis is similar to treatment for tendinitis. Generally, physicians begin therapy with immobilization of the joint. If necessary, steroid injections, or even surgery may be necessary to open up the sheath and to eliminate symptoms.

cises to keep the healed joint from becoming stiff and immobile.

For More Information

National Arthritis and Musculoskeletal and
  Skin Diseases Information Clearinghouse
Building 31, Room 4C05
31 Center Drive, MSC 2350
Bethesda, MD 20892-2350
301-495-4484
www.nih.gov/niams

Complementary and Alternative Treatments

Nutrition and Supplementation

Although there really is no change that can be generated through diet, supplements play an important role in treating tendinitis. Nutritionists recommend the following daily regimen:

Most Important

- calcium (1500 mg)—repairs connective tissue
- magnesium (750 mg)—necessary for proper muscle function
- free-form amino acid complex (as directed on label)—promotes healing
- proteolytic enzymes (as directed on label)—fights inflammation
- vitamin A (15,000 IU; do not exceed 8000 IU if you are pregnant)—repairs tissue
- mixed carotenoid formula (25,000 IU)—an antioxidant and precursor of vitamin A
- vitamin C with bioflavonoids (3000 to 8000 mg in divided doses)—reduces inflammation; forms connective tissue
- zinc (30 mg; do not exceed a total of 100 mg from all supplements)—important in all enzyme systems and tissue repair

Also Recommended

- hydrolyzed collagen (as directed on label)
- bromelain (as directed on label)
- sea cucumber (as directed on label)—reduces inflammation

(For an *acute* condition, take supplements until your symptoms subside. If symptoms persist, seek the advice of your healthcare provider. For a *chronic* condition, consult your healthcare provider regarding the duration of treatment.)

Ayurvedic Medicine

Ayurvedic practitioners may advise using a turmeric-salt paste or an Indian *bdellium* paste to reduce swelling and inflammation caused by tendinitis. (Be aware that turmeric will stain fabric and skin.) They also may recommend cool compresses and gentle stretching to improve circulation.

Bodywork and Somatic Practices

Any manual therapy that can open the restricted connective tissue is most effective in reducing pain, inflammation, and immobility. Look into sports massage, trigger point myotherapy, Trager, Hellerwork, Rolfing, CranioSacral Therapy, and Oriental bodywork. Therapeutic Touch can help reduce inflammation. Further on in the healing, use Feldenkrais, Alexander Technique, Trager, and Aston-Patterning for postural alignment and enhanced structural efficiency.

Traditional Chinese Medicine

Acupuncture The inflammation and pain caused by tendinitis may be lessened with acupuncture, which improves the flow of blood to the affected area, thereby speeding recovery. The acupuncturist focuses on different points, depending upon the location of the tendinitis. For shoulder pain, points along the stomach, bladder, and large and small intestine meridians are worked. Hip pain requires the manipulation of points along the gallbladder meridian, while thumb pain usually involves inserting needles into points on the arm, hand, and wrist that are related to the small intestine and lung lines.

Acupressure To alleviate shoulder pain, the acupressurist may concentrate on Large Intestine 11 and 14, Gallbladder 21, Stomach 38, Bladder 57, and Triple Warmer 14. An aching hip may be remedied by working Gallbladder 29, 30, and 34; Stomach 31; and painful points in the affected area. Thumb pain may be treated by firmly pressing on Large Intestine 4 and 5.

Chinese Herbal Therapy Herb formulas that may be helpful in strengthening weakened tendons include polygala, polygonatum cirrhifolium, and caltrop. Pseudoginseng and Dragon Blood is an herbal combination remedy often prescribed to treat tendinitis. There also are many liniments for this condition.

Tetanus

Signs and Symptoms

- Stiffness of the jaw, neck, and perhaps other muscles of the torso
- Painful spasms of jaw and neck muscles
- Irritability
- Difficulty swallowing
- Body-wide convulsions (emergency symptom)

Description

Because tetanus causes extreme stiffness of the jaw, it is also known as lockjaw. The condition is caused by a soil-dwelling bacteria called *Clostridium tetani*. This bacteria-tainted soil can enter the body via a deep wound, such as a puncture wound created by stepping on a nail or garden implement. If the bacteria travel to the deepest part of the wound, where there is no oxygen, they germinate and produce a toxin that interferes with the nerves controlling your muscles. Tetanus symptoms generally appear five days to three weeks after an injury. If allowed to progress un-

treated, tetanus can cause body-wide convulsions and death. Tetanus is especially dangerous to young children and the elderly.

Conventional Medical Treatment

If you have received a deep wound that is or could be contaminated with soil, promptly clean the area thoroughly and see your physician immediately. If you've never had a tetanus shot, your doctor will give you one. If you've had a tetanus shot, but it has been more than ten years since the inoculation—or you can't remember the date of your last vaccination or the wound shows signs of infection—your physician will clean and disinfect the wound site and give you a booster shot. Your body will then begin manufacturing antibodies to protect you against the bacteria that may have contaminated the wound.

If you are already showing signs of tetanus, your physician will hospitalize you and place you on antibiotic therapy, and perhaps, administer anti-toxin antibodies. A tetanus infection does not protect you from future re-infection. Therefore, you should receive the full series of vaccinations after recovering. It may be necessary to surgically remove the damaged tissue at the site of the wound.

For More Information

Centers for Disease Control and Prevention
1600 Clifton Road
Atlanta, GA 30333
800-311-3435
www.cdc.gov

National Institute of Allergies and Infectious Diseases
Building 31, Room 7A50
31 Center Drive MSC 2520
Bethesda, MD 20892-2520
301-496-5717
www.niaid.nih.org

Tetanus and Older Adults

Individuals over 60 years old account for about 59 percent of reported cases of tetanus and 75 percent of deaths from tetanus each year in the United States. According to the Centers for Disease Control and Prevention, the majority of these infections could have been prevented with a booster tetanus vaccine given once every ten years. Although it is recommended that children be inoculated against tetanus, an individual's immunity fades with age. Yet many adults are not aware of this and do not receive the necessary booster shots.

➤ *Have your child vaccinated against tetanus. The tetanus vaccine is a five-part vaccine given in combination with the diphtheria and whooping cough vaccines. It is recommended that infants receive their first vaccination at age 2 months, with the remaining parts administered at ages 4 months, 6 months, 18 months, and 5 years.*

➤ *If it has been more than five years since your last booster shot, talk to your health-care provider. While some doctors recommend receiving a booster every ten years, other healthcare providers recommend a booster every five years.*

➤ *Always wear heavy-soled shoes when gardening or walking outdoors.*

Complementary and Alternative Treatments

Traditional Chinese Medicine

 Acupuncture To treat tetanus (commonly called lockjaw), the practitioner may focus on the following points: Gallbladder 14; Stomach 4, 6, and 7; Large Intestine 4 and 20; and Governing Vessel 26.

Acupressure The therapist typically manipulates points on the face and jaw to help relieve tetanus symptoms.

Chinese Herbal Therapy Arisaema is often prescribed for tetanus. Many of the immune-enhancing formulas are used most often with herbs for spasm, usually in combination with conventional treatment.

THRUSH, ORAL

Signs and Symptoms

- Slightly raised, whitish patches in the mouth or throat
- Patches may be tender or sore and may bleed slightly if brushed with a toothbrush

Description

The *Candida* fungus occurs naturally in the mouth in small amounts. When the level of this fungus increases, you develop a problem called thrush. The overgrowth is most likely to happen when your resistance is lowered by illness or when you've been taking corticosteroids, immunosuppressive drugs, or antibiotics—all of which can upset your mouth's natural *Candida* balance. People with immune-suppressive illnesses, such as AIDS, have especially high rates of oral thrush.

Conventional Medical Treatment

Your dentist or physician can diagnose thrush with a physical exam. Treatment involves 7 to 10 days of an oral anti-fungal medication.

Health Notes

➤ *Keep hands and fingers away from the mouth. It is possible to spread a fungal infection from one area of the body to another.*

➤ *Eat one cup of yogurt every day. Studies performed on other fungal infections have shown that the live cultures in yogurt (called* lactobacillus acidophilus*) help prevent infection and lessen the severity of current infections. Because oral thrush is a fungal infection, it is believed yogurt also can play a role preventing it.*

➤ *Garlic is a natural anti-fungal. Help prevent thrush or lessen symptoms by eating two or more cloves a day. Garlic cloves can be crushed raw into salads or used in cooking.*

For More Information

American Dental Association
211 East Chicago Avenue
Chicago, IL 60611
312-440-2500
www.ada.org

Complementary and Alternative Treatments

Nutrition and Supplementation

Since thrush is a kind of fungus, it is important to eat plain yogurt containing live cultures, which will replace friendly bacteria. Your diet should be fruit-free, sugar-free, and yeast-free. To prevent the *Candida* fungus from thriving, eat foods low in carbohydrates, which basically means no sugar. Avoid aged cheeses, alcohol, baked goods, chocolate, dried fruits, fermented foods, all grains containing gluten (wheat, oats, barley, rye), ham, honey, nut butters, pickles, potatoes, raw mushrooms, soy sauce, sprouts, and vinegar. *Candida* thrive on fruits, such as oranges, grapefruit, lemons, tomatoes, pineapples, and limes, so eliminate them from your diet at the onset of an infection and for up to one month after healing. Add them back to your diet, but only in moderation. Eat lots of vegetables, fish, and gluten-free grains, such as brown rice and millet. Drink plenty of pure water.

Nutritionists suggest the following daily supplements:

Most Important

- flaxseed oil (as directed on label)—heals and prevents the fungus from destroying cells

- a prodophilus formula (as directed on label)—fights infection

- quercetin (500 mg 2 times daily)—speeds healing

- calcium (1500 mg)—often deficient in people with thrush

- magnesium (750 mg)—balances with calcium

- vitamin C (1000 mg 3 times daily)—protects the body tissues from damage by toxins released from *Candida*

- chewable coenzyme Q10 (as directed)

- glutathione mouth spray (as directed)

Also Recommended

- biotin (50 mg 3 times daily)—maintains healthy skin

- vitamin B_{12} (2000 mcg 3 times daily)—needed for metabolism of carbohydrates, fats, and proteins

(Take supplements until your symptoms subside. If symptoms persist, seek the advice of your healthcare provider.)

Traditional Chinese Medicine

Acupuncture Chinese medical practitioners have successfully treated thrush and other candidiasis disorders by using acupuncture. Typically, the practitioner focuses on points that improve immunity to reduce recurrences, along with points related to the mouth, throat, and larynx to ease immediate symptoms.

Acupressure Although acupressure cannot cure oral thrush, it may help tone the immune system to prevent future episodes. Points that may be manipulated during this treatment are Conception Vessel 6 and 12, Stomach 36, and Spleen 6 and 9.

Chinese Herbal Therapy Herbs that may be recommended to treat yeast infections include garlic, licorice, ginger, cinnamon, ginseng, and aloe vera—all of which have anti-fungal properties. However, the best treatment is to build and strengthen the whole system.

TINNITUS

Signs and Symptoms

- Continuous or intermittent ringing, buzzing, whistling, roaring, hissing, crackling, or other noise in the ear
- Continuous or intermittent hearing loss

Description

Tinnitus is not actually an illness; it is a symptom—one that accompanies numerous medical conditions, including almost all ear ailments, anemia, cardiovascular disease, hypothyroidism, and head trauma. Tinnitus also can be caused by more than 200 prescription and over-the-counter drugs. In some instances, tinnitus can accompany noise-induced or age-induced hearing loss. Why a condition causes tinnitus is not well understood.

Conventional Medical Treatment

To determine what medical condition is triggering your tinnitus, your physician may perform a thorough physical exam and conduct a series of tests, including a hearing exam, a CAT scan, blood tests, and/or cardiovascular tests. Tinnitus itself is merely annoying—not harmful. Although most attempts to identify and treat the disorder causing tinnitus are unsuccessful, there are a number of techniques that can ease the problem. One such intervention is a tinnitis masker, a hearing-aid-like device that emits a pleasant noise into the ear, covering up the more annoying sound associated with tinnitus.

For More Information
American Speech-Language-Hearing
  Association
10801 Rockville Pike
Rockville, MD 20852
800-321-ASHA
TTY: 301-571-0457
www.asha.org

When Lightning Strikes

For your hearing's sake, the next time you're caught outdoors during a lightning storm, find cover—although not near a tree, water, or metal. Tinnitus is common in individuals who have been struck by lightning, although how the two are associated is not clear. Other health side effects of lightning electrocution include burns, depression, memory problems, and insomnia.

Tinnitus

Health Notes

➤ *Reduce your sodium intake. A low-sodium diet has been shown to lessen symptoms of tinnitus.*

➤ *If your tinnitus is a known side effect of a medication you take, talk to your health-care provider. You may be able to substitute another medication.*

➤ *Drink no more than two cups of coffee or tea (or the equivalent) daily. Caffeine can aggravate tinnitus.*

➤ *Avoid alcohol, which can worsen tinnitus.*

➤ *If you smoke, quit. The nicotine in cigarettes aggravates tinnitus.*

➤ *Avoid loud noises and carry earplugs with you for those times where loud noise is unavoidable. Loud noises increase tinnitus symptoms in some people.*

➤ *Playing soft background music or other "white noise" can be useful in masking the sounds caused by tinnitus.*

➤ *Ask your physician about the anti-anxiety drug Xanax®. A team of researchers from Oregon Health Sciences University in Portland discovered that the drug was effective in dampening tinnitus sounds.*

➤ *Choose a non-aspirin pain reliever. Aspirin can aggravate tinnitus in some people.*

➤ *Limit stress. Research has found that stress worsens tinnitus.*

➤ *Increase your zinc intake. Some studies have shown that 15 to 25 mg of zinc a day lessens the ringing of tinnitus.*

American Tinnitus Association
P.O. Box 5
Portland, OR 97207
503-248-9985
www.ata.org

Lightning Strike and Electric Shock
   Survivors International
P. O. Box 1156
Jacksonville, NC 28541-1156
910-346-4708
www.mindspring.com/~lightningstrike

Complementary and Alternative Treatments

Nutrition and Supplementation

 There is a high correlation between tinnitus and poor nutrition. A diet high in vegetable proteins and complex carbohydrates is vital to ear health. Freshly made juices are excellent sources of healing vitamins and minerals as well as valuable enzymes, and they are easily assimilated.

Some of the more important nutrients that can be supplemented daily include:

* vitamin A (25,000 IU; do not exceed 8000 IU if you are pregnant)—strengthens mucous membranes

* vitamin E (600 IU)—increases circulation

* vitamin D (400 IU)—enhances immunity

* potassium (99 mg)—important for transmission of nerve impulses

* zinc (50 mg; do not exceed a total of 100 mg from all supplements)—quickens immune response; reduces infection

- vitamin B complex injections (as prescribed by doctor)—reduces ear pressure
- gingko biloba (as directed)

Ayurvedic Medicine

 Ayurvedic practitioners consider tinnitus to be a vata problem. Ringing, buzzing, and whistling in the ears may be quieted by several Ayurvedic remedies. They may suggest sipping comfrey-cinnamon tea or taking *yogaraj guggulu* for relief.

Ayurvedic products are available at many health food stores and Indian pharmacies.

Bodywork and Somatic Practices

 Manual therapies, such as CranioSacral Therapy, trigger point myotherapy, Hellerwork, or Rolfing would be a good first line of action. Strong backup methods include Oriental bodywork, Trager, reflexology, and massage.

Traditional Chinese Medicine

 Acupuncture Acupuncture has been shown to be very successful at reducing or curing tinnitus. In addition to working on acupuncture points along the kidney meridian, the practitioner also may work on the kidney, back of head, and internal and external ear points in the ear itself.

Acupressure To alleviate tinnitus, the acupressurist may focus on Gallbladder 2 and 20, Small Intestine 3 and 19, Kidney 3, Triple Warmer 17 and 21, and Bladder 23 and 52, along with related auricular points.

Chinese Herbal Therapy Caltrop, schisandra, and curculigo are Chinese kidney-fortifying herbs often used in formulas to treat tinnitus. Patent medicines that may be given to remedy tinnitus include Anemarrhena, Phellodenedron and Rehmannia, Rehmannia Six, Rehmannia Eight, and Gentiana formulas.

TONSILLITIS

Signs and Symptoms

- Sore throat
- Headaches
- Pain when swallowing
- Fever and chills
- Soreness and/or tenderness in the glands of the jaw and throat
- Specks of white discharge on the tonsils (in some cases)

Description

The tonsils, which are located on each side at the back of the throat, are actually lymph nodes, which means their job is to filter out harmful microorganisms that could infect the body. Once in a while, however, they can become overwhelmed by bacterial or viral invaders. The result is infection and inflammation, accompanied by a host of flu-like symptoms. This is tonsillitis, which is particularly common among children.

Health Notes

➤ *If you smoke, quit. Smoking weakens the body's immune system and irritates the throat, making the tonsils more prone to infection by the bacteria and viruses that cause tonsillitis.*

➤ *Eat a diet rich in fruits and vegetables. The phytonutrients and antioxidants found in these foods strengthen the immune system and boost its ability to fight bacterial or viral infections.*

➤ *If your child needs his or her tonsils removed, ask if the two of you can tour the hospital beforehand to become familiar with the hospital. Be honest in explaining the procedure.*

➤ *If your physician prescribes antibiotics to treat tonsillitis, make an effort to add yogurt to your daily diet while you're on the medication. Yogurt contains* lactobacillus acidophilus, *a substance that occurs naturally in the digestive tract, but is diminished with antibiotic therapy.*

tomies were a fairly routine practice in the past, most experts now believe that the tonsils protect against infection, and therefore, this surgery is performed only when absolutely necessary. Having these glands removed does not guarantee a lifetime free from sore throats. The same bacteria that infect the tonsils also can infect the throat—though people who've had tonsillectomies generally have fewer throat infections.

For More Information
American Medical Association
515 North State Street
Chicago, IL 60610
312-464-5000
www.ama-assn.org

National Health Information Center
P.O. Box 1133
Washington, DC 20013-1133
800-336-4797
http://nhic-nt.health.org

Complementary and Alternative Treatments

Aromatherapy

 A gentle massage with essential oils may ease discomfort. Add 5 drops bergamot, eucalyptus, or peppermint oil to 1 teaspoon vegetable oil or lotion. Gently rub into the neck and throat.

Ayurvedic Medicine

 Ayurvedic practitioners often advise taking *Septilin*, an Ayurvedic formula, for easing the discomforts of tonsillitis. They also may recommend drinking mint tea or taking a powder or pill of Indian *bdellium*. Ayurvedic products are available at many health food stores and Indian pharmacies. Be sure to consult your doctor if symptoms persist.

Conventional Medical Treatment

To distinguish tonsillitis from similar-appearing illnesses, such as the flu and strep throat, your physician may take a throat culture. Treatment includes rest, an over-the-counter analgesic (such as aspirin or acetaminophen), and possibly a course of oral antibiotics. Even though you should start feeling better after a few days on antibiotics, continue taking the medication until all pills are gone to prevent reinfection.

When the glands become infected three or more times per year, or an infection is particularly severe, your physician may recommend a tonsillectomy—removing the tonsils. Though tonsillec-

Bodywork and Somatic Practices

 Polarity therapy, reflexology, and Oriental bodywork techniques can be helpful.

Herbal Therapy

 Infusions of cleavers, sage, and red sage can help combat inflammation and soreness. To use cleavers, steep 1 teaspoon dried leaves in 1 cup boiling water for 10 to 15 minutes; strain. Drink several times a day.

For sage and red sage infusions, steep 1 teaspoon dried or fresh leaves in 1 cup boiling water for 10 to 15 minutes; strain. Gargle with the warm tea up to 5 times a day. *Caution:* Do not swallow.

A blend of tinctures of cleavers and echinacea also can temper tonsillitis. Combine equal parts of each tincture and take 1 teaspoon, 3 times daily as needed.

Herbal products are available in health food stores and in some pharmacies and supermarkets. Follow package for specific directions.

Homeopathy

 Tonsillitis may respond to homeopathic treatment. However, the selection of a remedy—more than one is available—depends on *your* child's symptoms and the stage of the condition. Don't try treating this disorder yourself. See a homeopathic professional.

Hydrotherapy

 Two hydrotherapies are easy and effective for blunting pain and reducing inflammation. Try gargling with comfortably hot water or applying a cold compress to the throat area.

Traditional Chinese Medicine

 Acupuncture Acupuncture can be used to reduce the swelling and sore throat associated with tonsillitis. The practitioner typically focuses on Lung 1, Bladder 10 and 12, and Large Intestine 4 and 11, along with ear points related to the pharynx and tonsils.

Acupuncture also can be used in place of anesthesia during tonsillectomy surgery. In most cases, the practitioner focuses on points along the large intestine, pericardium, and triple warmer meridians.

Acupressure To reduce the swelling and throat pain associated with tonsillitis, the practitioner may focus on Large Intestine 4, Lung 11, and Stomach 9 and 36. Difficulty swallowing may be relieved by applying pressure to Conception Vessel 17 and Governing Vessel 13.

Chinese Herbal Therapy Laryngitis Pills and Superior Sore Throat Powder Spray are over-the-counter remedies that may be recommended to treat tonsillitis.

TRICHOMONIASIS

Signs and Symptoms

- May be asymptomatic
- Unusual yellowish or greenish discharge from the vagina or urethra (in some cases)
- Discharge may be frothy (in some cases)
- Pain during intercourse and/or urination (in some cases)
- Itching, irritation, and/or burning sensation (in some cases)
- Pain in the lower abdomen (in some cases)
- Vaginal or penile bleeding (in some cases)

Trichomoniasis

Description

Trichomoniasis is caused by a parasite called *trichomonas*. The parasite is usually transmitted by sexual contact. Though often trichomoniasis is asymptomatic, the vagina (in women) or urethra (in men) can become inflamed and there may be discharge, burning, itching, and lower abdominal pain. (Also see "Yeast Infection" and "Vaginitis" entries.)

Conventional Medical Treatment

Your gynecologist takes a sample of secretions from the vagina or urethra to uncover the presence of any unusual organisms. Treatment of trichomoniasis typically entails metronidazole tablets to kill the parasite.

For More Information
American College of Obstetrics and Gynecology
409 12th Street, SW
Washington, DC 20024
800-673-8444
www.acog.org

Centers for Disease Control and Prevention
1600 Clifton Road
Atlanta, GA 30333
800-311-3435
www.cdc.gov

Complementary and Alternative Treatments

Traditional Chinese Medicine

Acupuncture To treat trichomoniasis-related discharge, the acupuncturist inserts needles along the stomach, spleen, and conception vessel meridians.

Acupressure A practitioner may treat this condition (and specifically vaginal discharge) by applying pressure on points along the bladder, gallbladder, stomach, spleen, and governing vessel meridians.

Chinese Herbal Therapy Herbal formulas that may be helpful in treating discharge include Gentiana and Rehmannia Eight. An herbalist also may concoct a remedy containing *cnidium monnieri*, alum, *angelica anomala*, Chinese yam, cuscuta, psoralea, and foxnut to treat trichomoniasis in both men and women.

TUBERCULOSIS

Signs and Symptoms

- May be asymptomatic at the beginning
- Mild cough that progresses to a cough that occasionally produces bloody sputum
- Fatigue
- Slight fever
- Night sweats
- Weight loss (later symptom)

Description

Tuberculosis (TB), also called consumption, is a bacterial infection that is transmitted via infected droplets that are sprayed into the air when someone with the illness sneezes or coughs. You can be infected when you breathe these released bacteria into your lungs. Mild symptoms generally appear one to three months after infection. Symptoms grow worse as the disease spreads to your lymph nodes and is carried by the lymphatic system throughout the body. If left untreated, tuberculosis can be fatal.

In the 1940s, with the introduction of medications to treat TB, the disease became rare. However, the number of TB cases in the United States began to rise again in the 1980s, especially in large cities. The most recent outbreaks have occurred among individuals with AIDS, people who live in crowded homeless shelters, and immigrants from Asia, Latin America, and Africa, where the disease is prevalent.

Conventional Medical Treatment

A physician can diagnose tuberculosis with a chest X-ray and a sputum culture, in which sputum is tested for the presence of *mycobacterium*

Health Notes

➤ Alert individuals with whom you have come in contact that you have TB. They may need to be tested and possibly treated.

➤ Your healthcare provider may need to treat members of your household, whether or not they show signs of infection.

➤ There is a TB vaccine available. Called the Bacillus Calmette-Guerin (BCG) vaccine, it consists of a weakened form of the bacterium that causes TB. It is not widely used in the United States because medical authorities here question its value.

➤ Individuals who work in the healthcare field should have a tuberculin test yearly. If the test has changed from negative to positive and the chest X-ray examination reveals no active disease, you will need to take isoniazid (INH) for six months to prevent an active TB infection from developing.

➤ If you work with individuals who are homeless, you may want to ask your physician for a TB test. Studies of homeless populations in several American cities have found TB rates among this group to be much higher than in the general population.

tuberculosis, the bacteria responsible for TB. A tuberculin skin test also may be used. This entails injecting a small amount of tuberculin purified protein derivative (PPD) into your skin. If you have TB, the injection causes a welt within 72 hours. Treatment consists of total isolation until you are no longer contagious and antibiotics to kill the TB-causing bacteria. Patients must take at least two antibiotics every day for six months or more to kill the bacteria. The most commonly prescribed drugs are isoniazid, rifampin, and pyrazinamide. Although you will feel better in three or four weeks and will no longer be infectious, you must continue to take the medication for the full course of treatment to completely eradicate the bacteria. If treatment is interrupted, the bacteria can mutate into a drug-resistant form of TB. Only about 50 percent of patients who develop this drug-resistant strain can be cured.

For More Information

American Lung Association
1740 Broadway
New York, NY 10019
800-LUNG-USA
www.lungusa.org

Centers for Disease Control and Prevention
1600 Clifton Road
Atlanta, GA 30333
800-311-3435
www.cdc.gov

National Institute of Allergies and Infectious Diseases
Building 31, Room 7A50
31 Center Drive, MSC 2520
Bethesda, MD 20892-2520
301-496-5717
www.niaid.nih.org

Complementary and Alternative Treatments

Nutrition and Supplementation

To promote healing, eat a diet consisting of at least 50 percent raw fruits and vegetables plus adequate amounts of high-quality protein. Include alfalfa sprouts, fish, fowl, organic eggs, pomegranates, raw seeds and nuts, whole grains, and garlic. Asparagus stimulates the immune function and is anti-carcinogenic, so eat it often. Drink fresh pineapple and carrot juice and a chlorophyll-rich "green" drink daily. Fresh raw potato juice also is helpful, as it contains compounds that block carcinogens and prevent cell mutation.

Get sunlight daily to assist healing.

Nutritionists recommend these daily supplements:

Most Important

- garlic (as directed on label)—a natural antibiotic that keeps infection in check

- vitamin A (25,000 IU; do not exceed 8000 IU if you are pregnant)—vital for healing lung tissue

- vitamin E (400 to 800 IU)—heals lung tissue; protects against free radicals

- coenzyme Q10 (75 mg)—carries oxygen to tissues

- colloidal silver (as directed on label)—heals lesions

- free-from amino acid complex (as directed on label)—repairs tissue

- L-cysteine and L-methionine (500 mg 2 times daily)—protects lungs and liver by detoxifying

- selenium (200 mcg)—promotes a healthy immune system

- vitamin B complex (100 mg 3 times daily)—produces red blood cells and antibodies

- vitamin C (5000 to 20,000 mg in divided doses)—promotes healing

- vitamin E (start with 400 IU and increase slowly to 1600 IU over the course of one month)—protects lung tissue

Also Recommended

- essential fatty acids (as directed on label)—aids in the formation of lung tissue

- glutathione (500 mg)—protects the lungs and cells from oxidant damage

- zinc (50 to 80 mg; do not exceed a total of 100 mg from all supplements)—promotes healing

Traditional Chinese Medicine

 Acupuncture Acupuncture may be used to treat many of the symptoms caused by tuberculosis, including fever, night sweats, weight loss, coughing spasms, chest pain, inability to catch one's breath, and swollen glands. It also can be used to strengthen the kidneys and bladder, both of which are weakened by TB.

To invigorate lung functioning and hasten the patient's recovery, the acupuncturist typically focuses on Stomach 36 and 40, Bladder 12 and 13, and Lung 5 and 9. Additional points may be added, as symptoms warrant.

Acupressure To relieve a tuberculosis-related cough, the practitioner may apply pressure to the Conception Vessel 17 and 22, Bladder 12 and 13, and Lung 1 points.

Chinese Herbal Therapy Tiger thistle and *bletilla striata* are effective formulations for reducing the production of bloody phlegm. Dried bamboo sap, balloon flower, and sargassum may be recommended to rid the body of yellow phlegm. Ginkgo biloba can strengthen cardiovascular functioning while quieting a cough. Garlic is known for its anti-bacterial properties and its ability to strengthen the immune system, which is greatly compromised in cases of tuberculosis.

Chinese patent medicines that are used to treat TB include Rehmannia Six and Pinellia Expectorant Pills.

t

ULCER, PEPTIC OR DUODENAL

Signs and Symptoms

- Gnawing feeling, aching, and/or burning in the upper abdomen or lower chest that may subside with antacids
- Pain that awakens you at night
- Nausea and vomiting (in severe cases, vomit may be tinged with bright red blood)

Description

Because it has to withstand constant contact with digestive juices and acids, the inner lining of esophagus, duodenum, and stomach is quite resistant to injury. Sometimes, however, breaks or holes occur in this lining. This condition is known as a peptic ulcer (sometimes referred to as a duodenal ulcer when it appears in the duodenum, the upper portion of the small intestine), and is actually quite common, affecting an estimated one out of every 10 people.

New research by the Centers for Disease Control and Prevention has uncovered that an estimated 90 percent of duodenal ulcers are caused by a *Helicobacter pylori* bacterium infection. It is not known how the bacteria actually contribute to ulcer formation.

The remaining 10 percent of ulcers are believed to be caused by several different factors—including heavy aspirin use, nonsteroidal anti-inflammatory use, and cigarette smoking—that weaken the lining of the esophagus, duodenum, or stomach and prompt the development of ulcers.

Ulcers affect people of all ages, emotional makeup, and socioeconomic levels. Stress may contribute to peptic ulcers, yet many individuals who are relatively stress-free develop ulcers.

The Ulcer Bug

For decades the medical world believed that all peptic ulcers occurred when excess acid created holes in the lining of the esophagus, duodenum, or stomach. Yet in 1983, an Australian scientist discovered that a specific bacterium, *Helicobacter pylori*, is responsible for most ulcers. To support his research, the scientist drank a concoction containing the *H. pylori* bacteria—then promptly developed an ulcer. While this theory was completely opposite from the prevailing view, within 18 months of this discovery, 70 scientific papers were published on the subject and the majority supported the bacteria-ulcer connection. Even after a decade of study, scientists still don't understand how the *H. pylori* bacterium manages to thrive in the highly acidic environment of the stomach, and they know even less about how the bacterium causes disease.

Conventional Medical Treatment

If you suspect you have an ulcer, see your physician. To establish a diagnosis he or she may perform an endoscopy or order a barium X-ray. Endoscopy is now the preferred method because during this procedure, in which a narrow tube is passed through the mouth into the intestines, a biopsy can be performed and tissue cultured to greatly aid in diagnosis. A blood test is also available to detect infection with *Helicobacter pylori* bacterium.

There are three main strategies for treating peptic ulcers. The first involves acid reduction using over-the-counter antacids, H_2 blockers (cimetidine, ranitidine, famotidine) and emoprazole. Sometimes a combination of antibiotics and bismuth subsalicylate (the active ingredient in Pepto-

Health Notes

➤ *To soften the burning sensation that often accompanies ulcers, avoid chocolate, peppermint, and fatty foods, all of which can worsen symptoms.*

➤ *Food may or may not relieve pain, depending on the location of the ulcer. With a duodenal ulcer, food relieves pain. With a stomach ulcer, food can provoke pain.*

➤ *If you smoke or use smokeless tobacco products, quit. Tobacco use has been implicated in acid-caused ulcers and aggravates symptoms.*

➤ *To prevent ulcers that are caused by excess stomach acid, avoid taking aspirin and ibuprofen unless absolutely necessary.*

➤ *Avoid or limit caffeine intake to two cups of coffee a day or the equivalent. This can help prevent acid-caused ulcers.*

➤ *In Thailand, cayenne pepper is used to prevent ulcers. American research has shown that daily cayenne intake does lower your risk of developing a bacterial ulcer by possibly killing the bacterium that causes ulcers.*

➤ *Limit your alcohol intake to two drinks a day or less, or abstain altogether. Alcohol can cause irritation of the stomach lining.*

Bismol®) is prescribed to eradicate *H. pylori.* Some doctors prescribe sucralfate, which works by forming a protective coating over the ulcer, allowing it to heal.

Surgery is rarely needed because medications are so effective. Surgery is used mainly to treat complications from peptic ulcers, such as perforations, recurrent bleeding from the ulcer, or bowel obstruction.

For More Information

American Medical Association
515 North State Street
Chicago, IL 60610
312-464-5000
www.ama-assn.org

National Digestive Diseases Information
  Clearinghouse
2 Information Way
Bethesda, MD 20892-3570
301-654-3810
www.niddk.nih.gov

Complementary and Alternative Treatments

Nutrition and Supplementation

 First, let's address what you *should* eat and drink. Dark-green, leafy vegetables contain vitamin K, which is necessary for healing and is usually deficient in people with ulcers. To keep the colon clean, supplement with psyllium fiber daily. Eat frequent small meals. Drink barley, wheat, and alfalfa juice, as they are potent anti-ulcer treatments.

The list of what you *shouldn't* eat is a bit longer. Avoid caffeine and alcohol. Avoid fried foods, salt, chocolate, strong spices, animal fats, and carbonated drinks. When you drink hot beverages, let them cool a while; hot beverages may trigger gastric discomfort. Do not drink cow's milk; the calcium and protein it contains stimulate the production of more acid. And finally, do not smoke. Smoking can delay or prevent healing and it may lead to relapses.

In addition to a sound diet, these daily supplements help ease the discomfort of ulcers:

Most Important

- pectin (as directed on label)—creates a soothing protective coating in the intestines, thereby relieving the discomfort of duodenal ulcers

- L-glutamine (500 mg 3 times daily)—repairs stomach lining

- vitamin E (400 to 800 IU)—reduces stomach acid; promotes healing
- arabinogalactan (as directed)
- lactobacillus sporogenes (as directed)

Also Recommended

- curcumin (25 mg 2 to 3 times daily)—promotes healing
- evening primrose oil (as directed on label)— protects the stomach and intestinal tract from ulcers
- vitamin A (50,000 IU for one month, then 25,000 IU, then reduce to 10,000 IU; do not exceed 8000 IU daily if you are pregnant)—necessary for healing; protects mucous membranes of the stomach and intestines; use emulsion form
- vitamin B complex (50 mg 3 times daily)— needed for proper digestion
- vitamin C (3000 mg)—promotes wound healing; protects against infection
- vitamin K (100 mcg)—helps prevent bleeding
- calcium carbonate (as directed)—a natural antacid

(For an *acute* condition, take supplements until your symptoms subside. If symptoms persist, seek the advice of your healthcare provider. For a *chronic* condition, consult your healthcare provider regarding the duration of treatment.)

Ayurvedic Medicine

 According to Ayurveda, ulcers are a pitta disorder that may be remedied by reducing excess pitta. To regain internal balance, practitioners may recommend taking a little licorice powder or a combination of ground cinnamon, ground cardamom, and ground cloves several times daily.

Ayurvedic products are available at many health food stores and Indian pharmacies.

Remember to consult your doctor before embarking on any new regimen; stomach pain can be an indication of a serious condition.

Bodywork and Somatic Practices

 Try reflexology, polarity therapy, Reiki, Therapeutic Touch, or Oriental bodywork.

Herbal Therapy

 Herbalists and naturopaths often suggest licorice for treating ulcers anywhere along the gastrointestinal track. Licorice has natural compounds that can soothe and heal mucous membranes. To make a licorice decoction, simmer 1 teaspoon chopped or powdered licorice root in 1 cup water for 15 minutes; strain. Drink 3 times a day. Alternatively, you can take licorice capsules under the supervision of your healthcare provider and herbal practitioner.

Teas made from marshmallow root, chamomile, or myrrh can also be effective in tempering ulcer pain. Herbalists also recommend ginger for the treatment of ulcers.

Herbal products are available in health food stores and in some pharmacies and supermarkets. Follow package for specific directions.

Homeopathy

 Ulcers of the digestive tract may respond to homeopathic treatment. However, the selection of a remedy—more than one is available—depends on *your* symptoms and the stage of the condition. Don't try treating this disorder yourself. See a homeopathic professional.

Traditional Chinese Medicine

 Acupuncture Duodenal ulcers are found in the small intestine, so an acupuncturist may focus on strengthening this organ by concentrating on auricular points that include the duodenum, stomach, sympathy, and *she-men* (a point related to the heart).

To treat a gastric ulcer the practitioner typically focuses on Pericardium 6, Stomach 36, Bladder 21, and Conception Vessel 12. The point known as Stomach 25 may be added if there is abdominal distention, and if the patient presents blood in his stool, Liver 3 may be included in the session as well. Additional points may be added to control ulcer-induced nausea and vomiting.

Acupressure To relieve the pain of a duodenal ulcer, the acupressurist may apply pressure to the following points: Conception Vessel 6 and 12; Stomach 21, 25, and 36; and Bladder 20 and 22.

To treat abdominal pain often associated with a gastric ulcer, the practitioner may work on Triple Warmer 6, Bladder 36, Conception Vessel 12, Spleen 6 and 9, and Liver 14, and related auricular points. In cases of abdominal distention, the practitioner typically focuses on Stomach 25 and 36, Spleen 6, and several points on the back of the ear.

Chinese Herbal Therapy To treat a duodenal ulcer, a Chinese herbalist may recommend herbs that have a soothing, healing effect, such as aloe vera, ginger, Job's Tears, and Solomon's Seal. The patent medicines called Internal Formula, Bupleurum, Inula, and Cyperus Formula, and Corydalis Analgesic Tablets also may be prescribed to combat the pain of a duodenal ulcer.

For a gastric ulcer, the practitioner may recommend Japanese honeysuckle, pseudoginseng, and tiger thistle. Licorice and aloe vera may help relieve the pain while trifoliate orange can be used to alleviate stomach distention. The herbal medicine known as Cyperus and Ligusticum Formula also can help reduce acid reflux and abdominal distention, while Major Four Herbs Formula may be given to help strengthen the digestive system and improve the flow of *chi.*

VAGINITIS

Signs and Symptoms

- May be asymptomatic
- Any change in vaginal discharge (change in color, volume, odor)
- Itching, irritation, or burning sensation
- Pain on urination or during intercourse (in some cases)
- Vaginal bleeding (in some cases)
- Thick, cheesy, white to off-white discharge (yeast infection)
- White, grayish-green, or yellow, sometimes frothy discharge (trichomoniasis)
- White, gray, or yellowish discharge with fishy odor (bacterial infection)

Description

Vaginitis is the most common infection of the female reproductive tract, affecting most women at some point in their lives. There are three major types of infections that can cause vaginitis: vaginal candidiasis (fungal, or yeast infection), trichomoniasis (a form of parasitic infection), and bacterial vaginosis. (See "Trichomoniasis" and "Yeast Infection" entries.)

Sexual activity is not the only way to pick up one of these organisms. Vaginal yeast infections are caused by a fungus called *Candida. Candida* is found normally in the vagina but under certain circumstances this fungus grows out of control, causing symptoms.

Predisposing factors include use of antibiotics, oral contraceptives, diabetes, pregnancy, use of feminine hygiene products, such as douches and feminine deodorant sprays, and moist environments (spending the day in a damp bathing suit).

Trichomoniasis is caused by *Trichomonas*, a par-

Bacterial Vaginosis and Premature Birth

It is estimated that bacterial vaginosis affects up to 25 percent of all pregnant women. Yet, because the condition is often asymptomatic, many are not aware they are infected. According to new research, pregnant women with untreated vaginitis have a 40 percent higher risk of pre-term delivery. Premature babies account for about 75 percent of all infant deaths in the first month of life, and these infants also have a higher risk of retardation, blindness, and learning disabilities. Exactly how the infection triggers premature birth is unclear, although experts suspect that the bacteria interfere with the amniotic fluid or the membranes that surround the fetus. In addition, bacterial vaginosis can cause serious infection during and after pregnancy and following gynecological surgery, such as Caesarean deliveries, abortion, and hysterectomy. Bacterial vaginosis also may cause pelvic inflammatory disease (PID).

Treatment for bacterial vaginosis during pregnancy usually involves topical antibiotics. In severe cases, oral antibiotics may be prescribed.

asite that is transmitted through sexual activity, but is also more common during pregnancy and after menopause. In this condition, the vaginal discharge is usually white, grayish-green, or yellow, and often appears shortly after a menstrual period. Menstrual blood raises the vaginal pH, which creates an ideal environment for *Trichomonas* to grow. Itching is usually intense.

Bacterial vaginosis is usually caused by a bacteria called *Gardnerella vaginalis.* It differs from *Candida* and trichomoniasis in that there is usually

Health Notes

➤ *Do not use feminine hygiene products, which disrupt the pH of the vagina, making it prone to vaginitis-causing bacteria. The vagina is self-cleaning and needs only soap and water washing to stay healthy.*

➤ *Wear cotton undergarments that "breathe." These prevent moisture from being trapped in the genital area, which creates a breeding ground for vaginitis-causing microbes.*

➤ *Practice safe sex. Always use a condom with a new partner or with a partner who is not monogamous.*

➤ *Chlamydia and gonorrhea are other infections of the cervix but can cause abnormal vaginal discharge. Expect your doctor to screen for these infections if you are concerned about an abnormal vaginal discharge.*

little or no inflammation of the vagina and no accompanying symptoms. Bacterial vaginosis is more common during pregnancy, lactation, and in women using an IUD, and like the other causes of vaginitis, is associated with sexual activity.

Conventional Medical Treatment

If you suspect vaginitis, see your gynecologist, who can make a diagnosis based on the characteristics of the discharge. Your doctor performs a pelvic examination and a Pap smear (if you have not had one in the past year) and collects and examines a sample of the discharge to detect the presence of one of the organisms described.

Bacterial vaginosis is treated with metronidazole or clindamycin either orally or in the form of vaginal suppositories.

For More Information
American College of Obstetricians and Gynecologists
409 12th Street, SW
Washington, DC 20024
800-673-8444
www.acog.org

Complementary and Alternative Treatments

Nutrition and Supplementation

 Vaginitis may be caused by a number of things including bacterial or fungal infection. To be safe, eat a diet that is fruit-free, sugar-free, and yeast-free. Avoid aged cheeses, alcohol, chocolate, dried fruits, fermented foods, all grains containing gluten (wheat, oats, rye, and barley), ham, honey, nut butters, pickles, raw mushrooms, soy sauce, sprouts, and vinegar. In addition, eliminate citrus and acidic fruits (oranges, grapefruits, lemons, tomatoes, pineapple, and limes) from your diet until inflammation subsides. Then reintroduce them slowly.

Eat plain yogurt that contains live yogurt cultures. (You can even apply it directly to the vagina.) This fights infection and soothes inflammation. Eating brown rice and taking prodophilus supplements helps also.

Nutritionists recommend these daily supplements to relieve discomfort:

• a prodophilus formula (as directed on label 3 times)—restores friendly bacteria

• biotin (300 mcg 3 times daily)—inhibits yeast

• essential fatty acids (as directed on label)—aid healing

• vitamin B complex (50 to 100 mg 3 times daily)—often deficient in people with vaginitis

• colloidal silver (as directed on label)—subdues inflammation and promotes healing

Vaginitis

- vitamin A (50,000 IU; do not exceed 8000 IU if you are pregnant)—aids healing
- vitamin E (400 IU)
- vitamin C (2000 to 5000 mg)—stimulates the immune system

(For an *acute* condition, take supplements until your symptoms subside. If symptoms persist, seek the advice of your healthcare provider. For a *chronic* condition, consult your healthcare provider regarding the duration of treatment.)

Aromatherapy

 Add several drops of one of the following essential oils to a warm bath for soothing relief from itching: German chamomile, tea tree, or myrrh.

Ayurvedic Medicine

 To manage vaginitis Ayurvedic practitioners may advise avoiding fermented foods, such as cheese and yeast breads, using a douche of mugwort, and taking the combination formula *Septilin*.

Remember to consult your doctor before embarking on any new regimen; vaginitis can be a symptom of a more serious condition, such as a sexually transmitted disease.

Herbal Therapy

 To relieve itching and fight inflammation, steep 1 to 2 teaspoons fresh chickweed in 1 cup of boiling water for 5 minutes; strain. Let cool and use to bathe the perineal area.

A salve made with calendula or St. John's wort also can calm itching and irritation. Look for these preparations in health food stores, and follow the directions on the label.

Herbalists also recommend boosting your intake of garlic, which is known for its anti-bacterial, antifungal, and anti-viral properties. Incorporate at least 8 to 10 cloves a day into your diet. If you can't eat that much fresh garlic, you can take 3 garlic capsules, 3 times a day instead.

Homeopathy

 Vaginitis may respond to homeopathic treatment. However, the selection of a remedy—more than one is available—depends on *your* symptoms and the stage of the condition. Don't try treating this disorder yourself. See a homeopathic professional.

Traditional Chinese Medicine

 Acupuncture To treat the discharge associated with vaginitis, an acupuncturist may concentrate on acupoints Stomach 29, Spleen 6, and Conception Vessel 1 and 5, while treating the overall imbalance as determined by a diagnosis.

Acupressure To stop the discharge caused by vaginitis, the practitioner may apply pressure to Stomach 29 and 36, Bladder 23 and 28, Governing Vessel 1, Gallbladder 26, and Spleen 6 and 10.

Chinese Herbal Therapy If vaginitis is caused by a yeast infection, the herbs sandalwood, garlic, and *cnidium monnieri* may help.

Ginseng and Atractylodes, Rehmannia Eight, Gentiana, and Tang Gui and Ginseng Eight are Chinese combination formulas that also may be prescribed to remedy the symptoms of vaginitis.

VARICOSE VEINS

Signs and Symptoms

- Enlarged veins of the legs that are easily seen under the skin
- Brownish or grayish skin discoloration on the ankle (in some cases)
- Skin ulcers near the ankles (in some cases)
- Dull aching of the affected leg(s) (in some cases)
- Itchy and/or dry skin over the varicose veins (in some cases)

Description

Most people easily recognize a varicose vein: twisted, large, and visible, it sits just below the skin of the thighs, calves, and/or ankles. Women are about twice as likely to develop these veins as men. Obese individuals of either sex have a high incidence, as do individuals with a family history of varicose veins. The condition can develop during pregnancy, but usually gets better two to three weeks after delivery.

It is not entirely clear what causes varicose veins, but the problem probably begins with a weakness in the walls of the superficial veins. The weakness causes the veins to stretch and become wider and longer. In the veins are valves that help propel blood to the heart. As the veins change shape, these valves may separate to the point that they cannot close normally. Blood then pools in the veins, enlarging and distorting them, creating varicose veins.

Conventional Medical Treatment

If you have varicose veins, it's likely they have become worse over time. Your physician may pre-

More Than Varicose Veins

When varicose veins appear suddenly over the course of a month or less and are accompanied by a feeling of heaviness, it's important to see your doctor. You may have deep venous thrombosis (DVT). The condition occurs when blood clots form in the veins in the legs. These clots can work their way up to the lungs, causing a fatal pulmonary embolism. Because DVT is so dangerous, you must check into the hospital for observation and treatment. Treatment includes heparin, an intravenous medication that thins the blood and aids in dissolving clots. After treatment, compression stockings dramatically reduce the incidence of recurrent DVT and pulmonary embolism. You also may need to take an oral blood thinner for three to six months after your hospitalization.

scribe special stockings that compress and provide support for the varicose veins and the weakened valves.

Surgical removal of varicose veins is a more permanent measure, although new varicose veins can develop even after surgery. Your doctor may suggest laser surgery to cauterize the veins.

For More Information

American Academy of Dermatology
930 Meacham Road
Schaumburg, IL 60173
888-462-DERM
www.aad.org

National Heart, Lung, and Blood Institute
P.O. Box 30105
Bethesda, MD 20824-0105
301-592-8573
www.nhlbi.nih.gov

Varicose Veins

Complementary and Alternative Treatments

Nutrition and Supplementation

Maintaining a healthy weight and a moderate level of exercise helps prevent varicose veins. A diet high in fiber that ensures daily bowel movements is also helpful. Your diet should also be low in fat and refined carbohydrates and include plenty of fish and fresh fruits and vegetables. You should cut back on animal protein, processed and refined foods, sugar, ice cream, fried foods, cheeses, peanuts, junk foods, tobacco, alcohol, and salt.

To improve circulation and relieve the discomfort of varicose veins, nutritionists recommend these daily supplements:

- coenzyme Q10 (100 mg)—increases circulation
- dimethylglycine (50 mg 3 times daily)—improves oxygen utilization in the tissues
- omega-3 fatty acids (flaxseed or fish oil, as directed on label)—reduces pain; keeps blood vessels pliable
- vitamin C (3000 to 6000 mg)—reduces blood clotting tendencies
- bioflavonoid complex (100 mg)—promotes healing; prevents bruising
- rutin (50 mg 3 times daily)—maintains the strength of the blood vessels

- vitamin E (start with 400 IU and slowly increase to 1000 IU)—improves circulation
- antioxidant formula containing zinc or selenium (as directed on label)

(Consult your healthcare provider regarding the duration of treatment.)

Aromatherapy

The essential oils of cypress, Helichrysum, lemon, and juniper can ease pain and soothe swelling. Blend into a carrier oil and use to massage the area above the affected vein.

Bodywork and Somatic Practices

Massage is contraindicated unless the veins are light and spidery. CranioSacral Therapy, polarity therapy, Oriental bodywork, Trager, Reflexology, and Feldenkrais are excellent substitute methods.

Herbal Therapy

Lotions made with witch hazel or horse chestnut, or a combination of the two herbs, can help reduce the discomfort of inflamed veins. Witch hazel lotion can be purchased at most health food stores and drugstores. To prepare a horse chestnut mixture, combine 1/2 teaspoon of the powder with 2 cups of water. Moisten a cloth and gently apply to the affected area. For a combination lotion, blend 10 parts distilled witch hazel and 1 part tincture of horse chestnut. Use as often as necessary.

Hydrotherapy

Sponge or spray your legs with cold water to relieve the aches of minor varicose veins.

For fairly swollen veins, alternate hot and cold compresses. Place a hot compress on the affected area for 1 minute; switch to a cold compress for 30 seconds. Repeat the process 3 times. Finish with a cold compress. Apply daily, as needed.

Traditional Chinese Medicine

Acupuncture Because it can improve blood flow and unblock valvular constrictions, acupuncture may be extremely helpful in treating varicose veins.

Acupressure Acupressure may be helpful in reducing pain and inflammation, and in improving the flow of blood through the affected area.

Chinese Herbal Therapy To enhance circulation the practitioner may prescribe achryanthes, corydalis, garlic, mastic tree, and white peony. (Caution: white peony should not be used during pregnancy.) Ginseng and Astragalus Formula or Central Qi Pills also may be prescribed to treat varicose veins.

Yoga and Meditation

Deep breathing, which improves circulation and helps the body relax, can help ease the pain that is often associated with varicose veins. If you're adding yoga to your routine, inverted poses—particularly the Shoulder Stand—can be very helpful.

Vertigo

VERTIGO

Vertigo is often confused with dizziness. However, while dizziness is a nonspecific sensation of imbalance, vertigo is a sensation of actual movement—that you are revolving in space (called subjective vertigo) or that your surroundings are revolving around you (called objective vertigo). During a bout of vertigo, your coordination may be physically unaffected, but you may develop what is called a vertiginous (unstable) gait if you try to walk.

By itself, vertigo is not dangerous and is a common symptom of numerous illnesses. These include inner ear infections, herpes zoster infections, head trauma, multiple sclerosis, Ménière's disease, brain tumors, and temporal lobe seizures. Vertigo also can accompany alcohol intoxication, drug use, and hyperventilation.

The easiest and most effective way to lessen feelings of vertigo is to lie down, since moving only exacerbates vertigo. Vertigo usually subsides once the underlying cause is treated.

For a complementary treatment, you may wish to try chiropractic. After proper medical evaluation to determine the cause of vertigo, many patients experience a decrease in symptoms with chiropractic care. The areas affected are usually the upper cervical (neck) vertebrae, more specifically the first and second cervical vertebrae. The chiropractor may apply moist heat and electromuscular stimulation to the muscles at the base of the head to decrease spasms and facilitate relaxation. These therapies may be followed by specific chiropractic adjustment (SCA) to those areas.

VOMITING

Vomiting is the forceful expulsion of the stomach contents through the mouth. A symptom of many illnesses—some severe (such as gastric cancer and appendicitis), some common (such as food poisoning, viral gastroenteritis, peptic ulcer, and morning sickness)—vomiting is usually preceded by nausea.

Fortunately, vomiting is usually nothing to worry about and can be eased with homecare. While you're affected, avoid eating. Drink as much water as you can to replace lost fluid and prevent dehydration—which is vomiting's greatest danger.

When vomiting is severe with little rest between bouts, when you are vomiting blood, or when you've been vomiting for more than 24 hours, seek medical attention. Your physician may want to put you on intravenous fluid therapy to replace fluids and monitor you for the presence of a more serious condition.

WARTS, GENITAL

Signs and Symptoms

- Small red or brown bumps in the genital area
- Several warts that grow close together and may appear in a cauliflower shape

Description

Genital warts, also called venereal warts, are surprisingly common, affecting both men and women. They look like common skin warts, though they appear only in the genital region. In women, warts may show up on the vaginal lips, around the anus, or inside the vagina, even on the cervix. In men, they usually appear near the top of the penis and at times on the penis shaft and scrotum.

The human papillomavirus (HPV) causes genital warts. The virus is spread through sexual contact; therefore, venereal warts are a type of sexually transmitted disease (STD).

Conventional Medical Treatment

While venereal warts are usually not a serious condition, it is important to have a gynecologist or physician examine you if you suspect them (or any other genital abnormality). In some cases, venereal warts on a woman's cervix can lead to

Menstruation and HPV

A recent study of 208 women, ages 13 to 21, found a correlation between menstruation, initiation of sexual activity, and genital warts. Research uncovered that among individuals who had genital warts, the average interval between the beginning of menarche and initiation of sexual activity was 26.6 months. For individuals who did not have genital warts, the average time span between their first period and sexual activity was 35.7 months. Researchers concluded that losing one's virginity within 18 months of one's first period was associated with a significantly higher risk of human papillomavirus (HPV) infection, compared to adolescents who postpone their first sexual intercourse three to four years. No concrete reason was found for the discovery, although it is suggested that women with immature reproductive tracts are more vulnerable to infection with HPV.

Health Notes

➤ *Practice safe sex. Be aware, however, that a condom will not protect you against warts on a partner's scrotum or vulva.*

➤ *Women who have been diagnosed with genital warts should talk to their gynecologist about having twice-yearly vaginal and uterine Pap smears. Genital warts are associated with an increased risk of cervical cancer.*

➤ *If you have a sexually-active teenager, discuss the importance of safe sex or abstinence in the prevention of STDs such as genital warts. Several studies have shown that the younger a person is when he or she begins sexual activity, the higher the chance of getting one or more STDs.*

cervical lesions, which, in turn, increases her risk of cervical cancer.

Treatment includes disclosing your condition to any present and past sexual partners who may have been affected. There are medications that can be applied directly to the warts to make them disappear, or they can be frozen off. Large venereal warts or heavy outcroppings of warts may be removed by lasers or electrical currents while the patient is under anesthesia.

For More Information
American Academy of Dermatology
930 Meacham Road
Schaumburg, IL 60173
888-462-DERM
www.aad.org

American College of Obstetrics and
   Gynecology
409 12th Street, SW
Washington, DC 20024
800-673-6444
www.acog.org

Complementary and Alternative Treatments

Ayurvedic Medicine

 Ayurvedic practitioners may advise taking an herbal combination of *shatavari*, *guwel sattva*, *kamadudha,* and *neem* after meals. They also may suggest taking *tikta ghee* on an empty stomach twice daily or *triphala* every night. Additionally, *tikta ghee* may be applied directly to the affected area. Ayurvedic products are available at many health food stores and Indian pharmacies.

Homeopathy

 Genital warts may respond to homeopathic treatment. However, the selection of a remedy—more than one is available—depends on *your* symptoms and the stage of the condition. Don't try treating this disorder yourself. See a homeopathic professional.

Warts, Skin

Signs and Symptoms

- Small, hard lump(s) on the skin that are flesh-toned, with perhaps a pinkish or whitish cast
- Though warts can occur anywhere on the body, they most commonly appear on the hands, fingers, knees, and feet

Description

Common warts are called *verrucae vulgaris.* Though they are unsightly, warts are harmless and many disappear without treatment within a two-year period. They are much more common in school-aged children and young adults than in older people.

Warts are caused by one of the more than 60 varieties of human papillomavirus (HPV). This virus, which is transmitted by direct contact—that is, touching another person's wart—causes rapid multiplication of skin cells in the infected area.

Conventional Medical Treatment

Many warts go away by themselves in six months to two years. Before seeing a dermatologist, you can try over-the-counter topical products that

Warts and Cancer

Several studies have concluded that in some individuals, warts may develop into squamous cell carcinoma, a type of skin cancer. HPV has been reported to play a role here, especially in people with suppressed immune systems, such as AIDS patients and individuals taking immune-suppressive drugs after organ transplants. More studies are currently underway to uncover exactly how HPV is linked with squamous cell carcinoma.

contain salicylic acid, lactic acid, or glycolic acid. These medications work by sloughing off the infected skin cells and usually take about three months to fully eradicate a wart. In more severe cases, a dermatologist can remove warts by freezing, cutting out the affected tissue, or laser treatments. Regardless of the treatment, warts will return in approximately one-third of all cases.

For More Information
American Academy of Dermatology
930 Meacham Road
Schaumburg, IL 60173
888-462-DERM
www.aad.org

Health Notes

➤ *Avoid directly touching a wart.*

➤ *Consume a diet high in vitamin C and zinc, both of which have strong antiviral properties.*

➤ *Individuals who take medications to suppress the immune system—such as those who have received an organ transplant—are more prone to develop warts.*

Complementary and Alternative Treatments

Nutrition and Supplementation

 Try to eat more asparagus, citrus fruits, eggs, garlic, and onions. These foods are rich in sulfur, which prevents and treats warts.

Nutritionists recommend the following daily supplements:

- vitamin B complex (50 mg 3 times daily)— important in normal cell multiplication

- vitamin C (4000 to 10,000 mg)—has powerful antiviral properties

- L-cysteine (500 mg 2 times daily)—supplies sulfur

- vitamin A (10,000 IU for 1 month, then 50,000 IU for 1 month, then 25,000 IU for 1 month or until warts disappear; do not exceed 8000 IU daily if you are pregnant)—normalizes skin and epithelial membranes

- vitamin E (400 to 800 IU; can be applied topically)—improves circulation; promotes tissue repair and healing

- zinc (50 to 80 mg; do not exceed a total of 100 mg from all supplements)—increases immunity

(Consult your healthcare provider regarding the duration of treatment.)

Aromatherapy

 All of the following essential oils are helpful for removing warts: lemon, garlic, and tea tree. Place 1 drop of any of the oils directly in the center of the wart every day until the wart falls off.

Bodywork and Somatic Practices

 To provide good lymph and blood circulation, massage may help. (Avoid massage if there are rashes, open cuts, or sores.) CranioSacral Therapy decreases stress, strengthens the immune system, and balances fluid and energy flow throughout the body. However, best results come from addressing the body holistically, as in a variety of Oriental bodywork therapies, reflexology, or Reiki. Therapeutic Touch lowers inflammation and irritability and allows the body to heal more swiftly.

Herbal Therapy

To help remove a wart, apply the sticky juices from one of the following fresh herbs directly to the affected skin twice a day, taking care not to get the liquid on surrounding skin: garlic, dandelion, milkweed, or celandine.

Alternatively, you might try *thuja* ointment, available in health food stores. Follow the package directions.

Homeopathy

Warts may respond to homeopathic treatment. However, the selection of a remedy—more than one is available— depends on *your* symptoms and the stage of the condition. Don't try treating this disorder yourself. See a homeopathic professional.

Traditional Chinese Medicine

Acupuncture Acupuncture may be used to bolster the immune system so that the body is better able to fight the viral infection that causes warts.

Chinese Herbal Therapy Evoda and Ilex and other formulas to build the immune system are recommended.

SYMPTOM:

WHIPLASH

Whiplash affects more than one million Americans a year and accounts for 10 percent of long-term disabilities caused by motor vehicle accidents. Whiplash is caused by a sudden, sharp, whipping movement of the head and neck. It usually occurs when the vehicle the victim has been riding in is struck from the rear, the side, or head-on. The result is that muscles, ligaments and/or connective tissues in the head, neck, and sometimes shoulders, are stretched, strained, or even torn. More serious whiplash may include head injuries and damage to blood vessels, nerves, or the spine. Whiplash may result in temporary pain and stiffness in the back of the head, chest, shoulders, or upper arms—symptoms that may not occur until several days after the accident.

Most people heal from whiplash injury in one month to a year. However, those whose symptoms persist a year or longer after the accident are less likely to make a complete recovery. They

may suffer from impaired reflexes, numbness or tingling, and osteoarthritic changes.

A physician can diagnose the condition with a physical exam. Treatment options include bed rest and medications, including muscle relaxants, nonsteroidal anti-inflammatory drugs (NSAIDs), and steroids. Mild cases of whiplash improve within a few days of the accident with rest and anti-inflammatory drugs. More severe cases may require physical therapy to rehabilitate injured muscles and ligaments. Exercises designed to relax, strengthen, and improve range of motion should be encouraged, and patients should learn about anatomy, physiology, posture, and potential reinjury situations to avoid repeated or prolonged neck pain. Heat, cold, and electrical nerve stimulation may also reduce neck pain.

The cervical collar, a former standby in the treatment of whiplash, has come under question lately. Several studies have found that these collars have little effect on the range of motion of

the neck, and may actually delay recovery by promoting inactivity.

In the arena of complementary therapies, you may wish to try chiropractic. As whiplash is characterized by a severe sprain or strain of the cervical (neck) muscles, tendons, ligaments, and supporting structures of the neck, patients typically respond well to chiropractic care. After care-ful examination and evaluation, the chiropractor may use ice or electromuscular stimulation for the first three days following the injury, followed by moist heat and more electromuscular stimulation. In addition, specific chiropractic adjustment (SCA) in the cervical segments of the spine may help minimize subluxations and fixations (immobility) in this area.

WHOOPING COUGH (PERTUSSIS)

Signs and Symptoms

- May be asymptomatic
- Sneezing (in some cases)
- Nasal congestion (in some cases)
- Loss of appetite (in some cases)
- Malaise (in some cases)
- Hacking cough often followed by explosive coughs that end in a high pitched whoop (in some cases)
- Loud inhalations (in some cases)
- Thick, clear saliva (in some cases)
- Vomiting (in some cases)

Description

Whooping cough, which is also called pertussis, is caused by the *Bordetella pertussis* bacteria. The illness gets its name from the telltale "whoop" that follows a cough. The bacteria is transmitted via infected airborne droplets that are easily inhaled. Typically, early symptoms mimic those of the common cold. It is during this period that whooping cough is most contagious. Not until 10 days to two weeks after infection does the whoop-like cough begin. About four weeks later, all symptoms begin to gradually disappear. Often, however, whooping cough has no distinguishing symptoms at any point during the illness, or symptoms are so mild that they're ignored.

Although the illness is considered a childhood disease—and occurs primarily in those under two years of age—adults can and do get whooping cough. Usually, whooping cough does not constitute a health threat. Yet infants under a year old, individuals with poor general health, and the elderly may develop complications, such as pneumonia or asphyxia, from the pressure of coughing.

Conventional Medical Treatment

A physician may diagnose whooping cough with a blood test or a saliva sample to detect the presence of the *Bordetella pertussis* bacterium. Often, no medication is needed; however, an antibiotic may be prescribed.

It is recommended that infants be vaccinated at 2 months, 4 months, 6 months, 12 to 18 months, and 4 to 6 years. Three new vaccines have recently

Whooping Cough (Pertussis)

Health Notes

➤ *Vaccinate your children against whooping cough to prevent the illness.*

➤ *Talk to your healthcare provider about the need for a periodic booster shot. Childhood vaccinations become less effective over the years, so adults may be at risk.*

➤ *If you or your child develop whooping cough, keep away from others until symptoms have completely disappeared.*

➤ *Drink at least 8 to 10 8-ounce glasses of water daily to keep saliva liquefied and keep throat tissue hydrated.*

been licensed to replace the former whooping cough vaccine, which was associated with side effects (including high fever and even seizures) that caused some parents to be reluctant to immunize.

For More Information

Centers for Disease Control and
   Prevention
1600 Clifton Road
Atlanta, GA 30333
800-311-3435
www.cdc.gov

National Institute of Allergies and
   Infectious Diseases
Building 31, Room 7A50
31 Center Drive, MSC 2520
Bethesda, MD 20892-2520
301-496-5717
www.niaid.nih.org

Complementary and Alternative Treatments

Traditional Chinese Medicine

 Acupuncture To relieve whooping cough, an acupuncturist may insert needles into Lung 5 and 9, and Conception Vessel 12 body points. In addition, the ear points related to the lung, bronchi, adrenal gland, and heart also may be included in the session. When treating children, acupuncture is usually replaced with herbal therapy.

Acupressure To quiet a cough, a practitioner may manipulate Conception Vessel 17 and 22, Lung 1 and 5, and Bladder 12 and 13. Vomiting may be alleviated by firmly pressing on Pericardium 6, Large Intestine 11, Conception Vessel 12, Stomach 36, and Bladder 20 and 22.

Chinese Herbal Therapy The combination medicines Major Six Herbs, Pulmonary Tonic Pills, and Citrus and Pinellia also may be prescribed in cases of whooping cough.

YEAST INFECTION, VAGINAL

Signs and Symptoms

- Itching, irritation, and/or burning in the vaginal area
- Unusual, white to off-white, curdled-appearing discharge from the vagina (in some cases)
- Pain during intercourse (in some cases)

Description

Vaginal yeast infections are caused by a fungus called *Candida*. This yeast-like organism is found naturally in small amounts in the mouth, gastrointestinal tract, and the female genital tract. Trouble occurs when the fungi "overgrow," irritating the surrounding tissue and causing a yeasty-smelling discharge.

This excessive fungal growth usually is caused by anything that changes the pH of the body cavity where the *Candida* live. Common culprits include feminine hygiene products, such as douches and feminine deodorant sprays and powders, contact with spermicides, and moist environments (caused, for instance, by spending the day in a damp bathing suit). The pH of the vagina also can be affected by oral contraceptives, antibiotics, diabetes, and pregnancy. (See also "Trichomoniasis" and "Vaginitis, Bacterial" entries.)

Conventional Medical Treatment

Your gynecologist can diagnose a yeast infection with a pelvic exam, although a sample of the discharge material also may be collected and examined. Over-the-counter medications for yeast infections are now available, and your doctor may recommend one if the infection is not severe. If you have frequent recurrences of yeast infection, you may be given a prescription for an anti-fungal drug such as Diflucan®.

Your physician also may discuss physical measures you can take to prevent a yeast infection from recurring, including wearing breathable cotton underwear that doesn't trap moisture and giving up douches and feminine deodorant products. Note: The use of such products is unnecessary and should be avoided. The vagina is self-cleansing and needs only a daily washing with soap and water to stay healthy. Anything more aggressive can disrupt its natural chemical balance and irritate its tissue, which, in turn, can lead to infections and other disorders.

For More Information

American College of Obstetricians
and Gynecologists
409 12th Street, SW
Washington, DC 20024
800-673-8444
www.acog.org

Complementary and Alternative Treatments

Nutrition and Supplementation

 Fungus multiplies in a sugary environment, so avoid sugar in all forms (fruit, refined carbohydrates, and sweets) until the infection has healed. Stay away from alcohol, aged cheeses, fermented foods, mushrooms, and yeast products.

Yogurt, kefir, and buttermilk contain bacterial cultures such as *Lactobacilli*, which will destroy the fungus. Be sure the label on your yogurt says it contains live cultures; do not consume sweetened yogurt, since yeast thrives on sugar. Avoid all other dairy products until the infection has cleared.

Yeast Infection, Vaginal

➤ *The only time you should self-medicate a yeast infection is when you've already been diagnosed and you develop identical symptoms a couple of months later under the same circumstances.*

➤ *Until your yeast infection is healed, you and your partner should use condoms during sex.*

➤ *To boost your immunity and maintain your body's ability to fight infection, talk to your healthcare provider about taking a daily multivitamin supplement as well as extra beta-carotene and vitamins C and E.*

➤ *Reduce your stress. Some women experience yeast infections during times of stress.*

➤ *For years, yogurt has been a popular folk remedy to prevent and cure yeast infections. Several studies have found that women plagued by yeast infections experience a dramatic decrease in the number of and severity of infections when they eat a daily cup of yogurt that contains* Lactobacillus acidophilus *live cultures.*

➤ *Some healthcare providers advise wearing only cotton undergarments and avoiding tightly fitting underwear to keep the genital area dry and avoid irritation.*

➤ *Change out of a wet swimsuit or workout clothes promptly.* Candida, *the yeast that causes yeast infections, thrives in a moist environment.*

➤ *Avoid feminine hygiene products, such as douches, powders, and sprays. These cause irritation and change the skin's pH, making the area more hospitable to* Candida.

➤ *Use unscented, dye-free menstrual products and toilet paper to avoid irritation from perfumes and dyes.*

➤ *If you have recurring yeast infections, talk to your healthcare provider about foods that contain yeasts, molds, and fungi—such as aged cheeses, beer, wine, cured meats, raw mushrooms, sauerkraut, and vinegar. Although the subject is controversial, some health practitioners believe these contribute to recurring yeast infections.*

➤ *Garlic helps kill* Candida *and may help in fighting or preventing a yeast infection. Add raw, mashed garlic to salads and cook with garlic whenever possible.*

These daily supplements are helpful in treating yeast infections:

- biotin (300 mcg 3 times daily)—inhibits yeast
- essential fatty acids (as directed on label)—speeds recovery
- garlic (as directed on label)—fights the infecting organism
- vitamin C (2000 to 5000 mg in divided doses)—improves immunity

Also Recommended

- vitamin A (50,000 IU; do not exceed 8000 IU if you are pregnant)—aids vaginal healing
- a prodophilus formula (as directed on label)—replaces friendly bacteria
- vitamin B complex (100 mg)—deficient in people with yeast infections
- vitamin D (400 IU)—extra amounts are needed when the body is fighting infection
- calcium (1500 mg)—extra amounts are needed when the body is fighting infection
- magnesium (750 mg)—extra amounts are needed when the body is fighting infection

(Consult your healthcare provider regarding the duration of treatment.)

Ayurvedic Medicine

Ayurveda considers candidiasis to be caused by *ama,* poor digestion of food. To stimulate digestion, a practitioner may advise taking grapefruit seed oil, *trikatu,* ginger, cayenne, or *neem* before meals. He or she may also suggest taking acidophilus and cleansing the system with a *pancha karma* program, which should be undertaken only with the guidance of a qualified Ayurvedic practitioner.

Ayurvedic products are available at many health food stores and Indian pharmacies.

Remember to consult your doctor before embarking on any new regimen; if not cured, yeast infections can worsen.

Herbal Therapy

To relieve itching and fight inflammation, steep 1 to 2 teaspoons fresh chickweed in 1 cup boiling water for 5 minutes; strain. Let cool and use the solution to bathe the perineal area.

A salve made with calendula or St. John's wort can also calm itching and irritation. Look for these preparations in health food stores, and follow the directions on the label.

Herbalists also recommend boosting your intake of garlic, which is known for its anti-bacterial, anti-fungal, and antiviral properties. Incorporate at least 8 to 10 cloves a day into your diet. If you can't eat that much fresh garlic, you can take 3 garlic capsules, 3 times a day instead.

Herbal products are available in health food stores and in some pharmacies and supermarkets. Follow package for specific directions.

Homeopathy

Yeast infections may respond to homeopathic treatment. However, the selection of a remedy—more than one is available—depends on *your* symptoms and the stage of the condition. Don't try treating this disorder yourself. See a homeopathic professional.

Traditional Chinese Medicine

Acupuncture To treat the vaginal discharge associated with a yeast infection, an acupuncturist may focus on the Spleen 6, Conception Vessel 1 and 5, and Stomach 29 points on the body, and on the uterus, internal secretion, heart, and ovary points on the ear.

Chinese Herbal Therapy Garlic may be taken internally or used as an external wash to alleviate the discomfort and itchiness caused by a yeast infection.

Several Chinese herbal formulas are recommended for the treatment of yeast infections, including Ginseng and Atractylodes, Gentiana Formula, Tang Gui and Ginseng Eight, and Rehmannia Eight.

RESOURCE LISTINGS

HEALTH AND MEDICAL WEB SITES

Alternative Health News Online
www.altmedicine.com

Maintained by journalists, this site provides information on the latest happenings in the rapidly growing field of alternative, complementary, and preventive health news.

The Alternative Medicine HomePage
www.pitt.edu/~cbw/altm.html

A jumpstation for sources of information on alternative and complementary therapies, hosted by the Falk Library of Sciences at the University of Pittsburgh.

American Cancer Society
www.cancer.org

A nationwide, community-based, voluntary health organization dedicated to eliminating cancer as a major health problem through research, education, advocacy, and service.

American Dental Association
www.ada.org

The professional association of dentists dedicated to serving both the public and the profession of dentistry through its initiatives in education, research, advocacy, and the development of standards.

American Dietetic Association
www.eatright.org

The largest group of food and nutrition professionals in the nation, serving the public through the promotion of optimal nutrition, health, and well-being.

American Heart Association
www.americanheart.org

Hosted by the leading authority on heart and blood vessel diseases, this site is dedicated to providing education and information on fighting heart disease and stroke.

American Lung Association
www.lungusa.org

Providing in-depth, timely information on lung issues including asthma, tobacco control, and environmental health in an effort to promote lung health and prevent lung disease.

American Optometric Association
www.aoanet.org

Maintained by the professional association of optometrists, this site provides information on a wide variety of eye disorders and treatments.

America's Doctor.Com
www.americasdoctor.com

Designed to assist consumers with their health information inquiries, this site offers free, private, real-time, one-on-one conversations with board-certified, board-eligible physicians.

Ask Dr. Weil
http://cgi.pathfinder.com/drweil

Hosted by bestselling author and complementary medical advisor Dr. Andrew Weil, this site provides information about a wide range of subjects, including nutrition, supplementation, lifestyle, and exercise strategies for optimal health.

Centers for Disease Control
www.cdc.gov

An agency of the Department of Health and Human Services designed to promote health and quality of life by preventing and controlling disease, injury, and disability.

Complemed.com
www.complemed.com

A site that strives to inform, guide and consult physicians and the interested public about the rational application of alternative treatment modalities.

Health A to Z
www.healthatoz.com

A comprehensive health and medical resource developed by health care professionals to enable every individual and family to better manage their health.

Healthanswers.com
www.healthanswers.com

A comprehensive, award-winning interactive health care Web site for consumers and professionals alike, featuring practical, credible, and up-to-the-minute health care information.

Healthfinder
www.healthfinder.gov

A user-friendly site maintained by the U.S. Department of Health and Human Services, the federal government's principal agency for protecting the health of all Americans and providing essential human services, especially for those who are least able to help themselves.

Health World Online
www.healthy.net

A virtual "health village" where you can access information, services, and products to help you design a wellness-based lifestyle.

Journals of the American Medical Association (JAMA)
http://pubs.ama-assn.org

This site contains the latest on research and other developments in medicine from the publications of the American Medical Association, a membership organization of physicians dedicated to promoting the science and art of medicine and the betterment of public health.

KidsHealth.org
www.kidshealth.org

Information for parents, kids, and teens from the pediatric medical experts at the Alfred I. duPont Hospital for Children, The Nemours Children's Clinics, and other children's health facilities nationwide.

Mayo Clinic Oasis
www.mayohealth.org

Maintained by a team of Mayo physicians, scientists, and educators, this site provides relevant, up-to-date health information available on a wide variety of topics.

National Center for Complementary and Alternative Medicine
http://nccam.nih.gov

The center, affiliated with the National Institutes of Health, was established by Congress in 1992 to evaluate alternative medical treatments and determine their effectiveness, and to serve as a public information clearinghouse.

National Council for Reliable Health Information
www.ncrhi.org

This non-profit health agency—comprised of volunteer health professionals, educators, researchers, attorneys, and concerned citizens—focuses its attention on health fraud, misinformation, and quackery as public health problems.

National Institute of Mental Health (NIMH)
www.nimh.nih.gov

Affiliated with the National Institutes of Health, NIMH provides information geared to help researchers, mental health and health care practitioners, patients, and the general public gain a better understanding of mental disorders and their treatment.

National Library of Medicine
www.nlm.nih.gov

Maintained by the world's largest medical library, this site features MedLine, an index that enables users to search for articles on specific topics. It currently contains nine million references going back to the mid 1960s.

New England Journal of Medicine
www.nejm.org

This on-line version of the prestigious publication of the Massachusetts Medical Society enables users to view abstracts and request full-text articles by mail or fax.

New York Online Access to Health (NOAH)
www.noah.cuny.edu

A user-friendly, bilingual site dedicated to providing high-quality health information that is timely and authoritative.

OnHealth
www.onhealth.com

An independent service that provides consumers with valuable ideas and inspiration about wellness, health, and medicine.

Richard and Hinda Rosenthal Center
http://cpmcnet.columbia.edu/dept/rosenthal/

Based at Columbia University in New York City, the Rosenthal Center is an internationally known resource for information about complementary and alternative therapies.

WebMD
www.webmd.com

The largest health community on the Web, providing reliable health care information from qualified professionals.

COMMON MEDICINAL HERBS

Common Name	Latin Name
Alfalfa	*Medicago sativa*
Aloe	*Aloe vera*
Anise	*Pimpinella anisum*
Arnica	*Arnica montana*
Astragalus	*Astragalus membranaeus*
Balmony	*Chelone glabra*
Bay leaf	*Laurus nobilis*
Black cohosh	*Cimicifuga racemosa*
Boneset	*Eupatorium perfoliatum*
Burdock root	*Arctium lappa*
Calendula	*Calendula officinalis*
Catnip	*Nepeta cataria*
Cayenne	*Capsicum*, spp.
Celery seed	*Levisticum officinale*
Chamomile	*Matricaria recutita*
Chaste berry	*Vitex agnus-castus*
Cleavers	*Galium aparine*
Coltsfoot	*Tussilago farfara*
Cramp bark	*Viburnum opulus*
Dandelion root	*Taraxacum officinale*
Devil's claw	*Harpagophytum procumbrens*
Dong quai	*Angelica sinensis*
Echinacea	*Echinacea* spp.
Elder flower	*Sambucus nigra*
Elecampane	*Inula helenium*
Eucalyptus	*Eucalyptus globulus*

Common Name	Latin Name
Fenugreek	*Trigonella foenum-graecum*
Fringetree bark	*Chionanthus virginicus*
Garlic	*Allium sativum*
Ginger root	*Zingiber officinale*
Ginkgo	*Ginkgo biloba*
Ginseng	*Panax quinquefolius*
Goldenrod	*Solidago virgaurea*
Goldenseal	*Hydrastis canadensis*
Gotu kola	*Centella asiatica*
Horehound	*Marrubium vulgare*
Horsetail	*Equisetum arvense*
Lavender	*Lavandula officinalis*
Lemon balm	*Melissa officinalis*
Licorice	*Glycyrrhiza glabra*
Linden flower	*Tilia europea*
Lobelia	*Lobelia inflata*
Marshmallow	*Althaea officinalis*
Meadowsweet	*Filipendula ulmaria*
Milk thistle	*Silybum marianum*
Mullein	*Mullein*
Myrrh gum	*Commiphora molmol*
Nettle	*Urtica dioica*
Oats	*Avena sativa*
Parsley	*Petroselinum crispum*

Common Medicinal Herbs

Common Name	Latin Name	Common Name	Latin Name
Passion flower	*Passiflora incarnata*	Skullcap	*Scutellaria baicalensis*
Pau d'arco	*Tabeluia impetiginosa*	Slippery elm	*Ulmus fulva*
Pennyroyal	*Mentha pulegium*	St. John's wort	*Hypericum performatum*
Peppermint	*Mentha piperita*		
Prickly ash	*Zanthoxylum americanum*	Uva ursi	*Artostaphylos uva-ursi*
Red sage	*Salvia officinalis var. rubia*	Valerian	*Valeriana officinalis*
Red raspberry	*Rubus idaeus*	Wild yam	*Dioscorea villosa*
Red clover	*Trifolium pratense*	Willow bark	*Salix*
Rosemary	*Rosmarinus officinalis*	Wintergreen oil	*Gaultheria procumbens*
		Witch hazel	*Hamamelis virginiana*
Sage	*Salvia officinalis*		
Sarsaparilla	*Smilax aristolochioefolia*	Yarrow	*Achillea millefolium*
Seed thyme	*Thymus vulgaris*	Yellow dock root	*Rumex crispus*

ESSENTIAL OILS USED IN AROMATHERAPY

Common Name	Latin Name

Basil   *Ocimum basilicum*
Not for small children; avoid with sensitive skin.

Bay   *Laurus nobilis*
Nontoxic at low levels; avoid when pregnant; possible skin irritant.

Benzoin absolute   *Styrax benzoin*
Nontoxic at low levels.

Bergamot   *Citrus bergamia*
Nontoxic at low levels; phototoxic; possible skin irritant.

Black pepper   *Piper nigrum*
Nontoxic at low levels; possible skin irritant.

Camphor   *Cinnamomum camphora*
Nontoxic at low levels; potential toxic reaction; avoid when pregnant.

Caraway   *Carum carvi*
Nontoxic at low levels.

Carrot   *Daucus carotta*
Nontoxic at low levels; avoid when pregnant.

Cedarwood   *Cedrus atlantica*
Nontoxic at low levels.

Chamomile, German   *Matricaria recutita*
Nontoxic at low levels.

Chamomile, Roman   *Anthemis nobilis*
Nontoxic at low levels; avoid in early pregnancy.

Clary sage   *Salvia sclarea*
Nontoxic at low levels; avoid when pregnant, with endometriosis, and cancer; potentially sensitizing; sedative.

Common Name	Latin Name

Clove   *Eugenia caryophyllus*
Skin and mucous membrane irritant; use only highly diluted.

Coriander   *Coriandrum sativum*
Nontoxic at low levels.

Cypress   *Cupressus sempervirens*
Nontoxic at low levels; avoid when pregnant, with high blood pressure, and with cancer.

Eucalyptus   *Eucalyptus globulus*
Nontoxic at low levels; avoid with high blood pressure and epilepsy; not for small children.

Fennel   *Feoniculum vulgare*
Nontoxic at low levels; avoid when pregnant and with epilepsy.

Fir   *Abies balsamea*
Nontoxic at low levels; possible skin irritant.

Frankincense   *Boswellia carterii*
Nontoxic at low levels; avoid when pregnant.

Garlic   *Allium sativum*
Almost always used in capsule form.

Geranium   *Pelargonium graveolens*
Ginger   *Zingiber officinale*
Nontoxic at low levels; potential skin irritant; sensitizing; phototoxic.

Grapefruit   *Citrus paradisi*
Potential skin irritant; sensitizing; possibly mildly phototoxic.

Helichrysum immortelle *Helicrysum italicum*
Nontoxic at low levels; avoid with anti-coagulant medications.

Essential Oils Used in Aromatherapy

Common Name	Latin Name
Hyssop	*Hyssopus officinale*

Avoid with high blood pressure, epilepsy; avoid when pregnant; possibly neurotoxic; not for children.

Jasmine absolute — *Jasminum grandiflorum*
Nontoxic at low levels; potentially sensitizing.

Juniper berry — *Juniperus communis*
Nontoxic at low levels; avoid extensive use on delicate skin, with kidney or bladder disease; avoid when pregnant; strong diuretic.

Lavender — *Lavandula angustifolia*
Nontoxic at low levels.

Lemon — *Citrus limon*
Nontoxic at low levels; potential skin irritant; sensitizing; phototoxic.

Lime — *Citrus latifolia*
Avoid when pregnant; not for children; phototoxic; possible skin irritant.

Mandarin — *Citrus reticulata*
Very mild; nontoxic at low levels.

Marjoram — *Origanum marjorana, sweet*
Nontoxic at low levels; avoid when pregnant, with asthma, low blood pressure; depression; sedative.

Melissa — *Melissa officinalis*
Possible skin irritant; avoid when pregnant.

Myrrh — *Commiphora myrrha*
Avoid when pregnant; possibly toxic at high levels.

Neroli — *Citrus aurantium*
Nontoxic at low levels.

Niaouli — *Melaleuca viridiflora*
Avoid when pregnant; not for children.

Nutmeg — *Myristica fragrans*
Nontoxic at low levels; possible skin irritant.

Orange — *Cirtus sinensis*
Nontoxic at low levels; potentially sensitizing; phototoxic.

Common Name	Latin Name
Oregano	*Origanum vulgare*

Avoid when pregnant; not for children; possible skin, mucous membrane irritant; potentially sensitizing.

Peppermint — *Mentha x piperita*
Nontoxic at low levels; avoid when pregnant or lactating; possible skin irritant.

Pine — *Pinus sylvestris*
Nontoxic at low levels; potentially sensitizing; avoid with allergic conditions.

Ravensara aromatica — *Ravensara aromatica*
Avoid when pregnant; not for children.

Rose — *Rosa damascena*
Nontoxic at low levels.

Rosemary — *Rosmarinus officinalis*
Nontoxic at low levels.

Sage — *Salvia officinalis*
Nontoxic at low levels; possibly toxic at high levels; avoid when pregnant or lactating; not for children.

Sandalwood — *Santalum album*
Nontoxic at low levels.

Tea tree — *Melaleuca alternifolia*
Nontoxic at low levels; possible skin irritant.

Thyme — *Thymus vulgaris*
Avoid when pregnant; not for children.

Thyme, red — *Thymus vulgaris*
Nontoxic at low levels; skin and mucous membrane irritant; avoid when pregnant and with high blood pressure.

Yarrow — *Achillea millefolium*
Avoid when pregnant; not for children.

Ylang-ylang — *Cananga odorata*
Nontoxic at low levels; possible skin irritant; do not use on inflamed skin; excess may cause headache, nausea.

TRADITIONAL CHINESE MEDICINE

CHI—THE LIFE FORCE

According to Traditional Chinese
Medicine, *chi,* the life force found in all
things, flows throughout our bodies
along 14 energy pathways, or *meridians.*
These meridians connect all organs and
systems to one another and to the skin.
When *chi* is flowing freely and in
harmony, you remain healthy; when it
is blocked or out of balance, illness
results. To restore health and prevent
illness, the practitioner works to
correct imbalances and reestablish
the normal, healthy flow of energy
throughout the body.

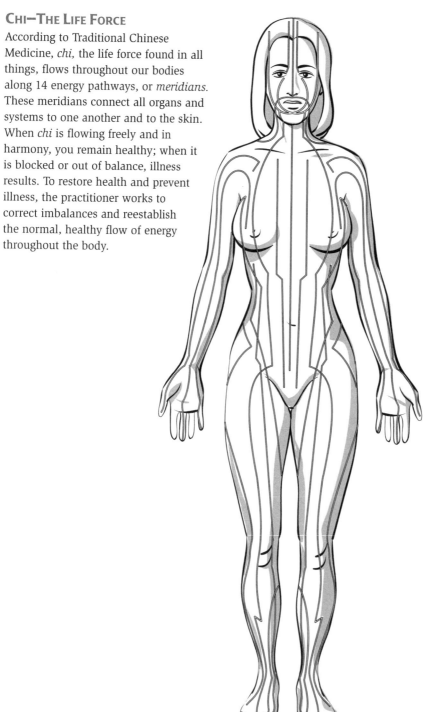

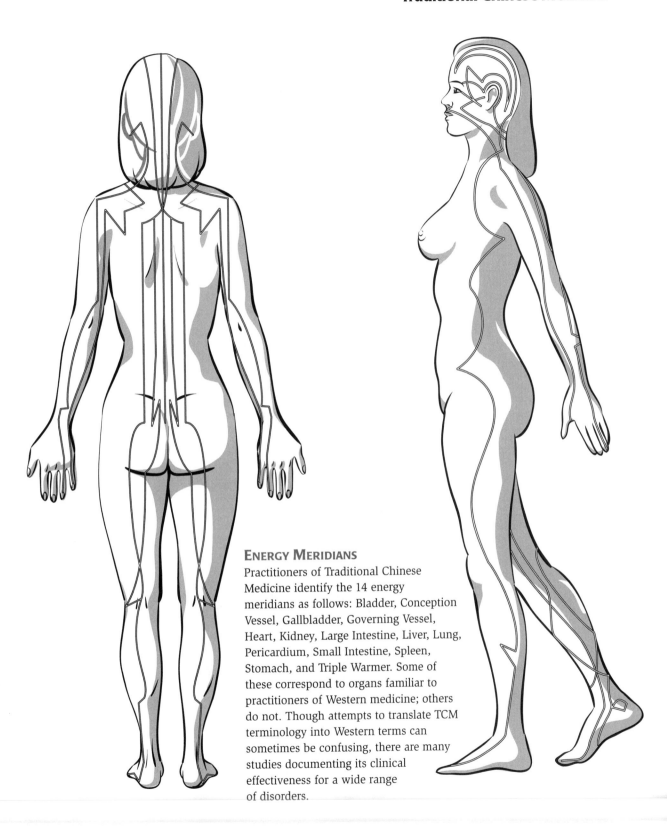

ENERGY MERIDIANS

Practitioners of Traditional Chinese Medicine identify the 14 energy meridians as follows: Bladder, Conception Vessel, Gallbladder, Governing Vessel, Heart, Kidney, Large Intestine, Liver, Lung, Pericardium, Small Intestine, Spleen, Stomach, and Triple Warmer. Some of these correspond to organs familiar to practitioners of Western medicine; others do not. Though attempts to translate TCM terminology into Western terms can sometimes be confusing, there are many studies documenting its clinical effectiveness for a wide range of disorders.

Traditional Chinese Medicine

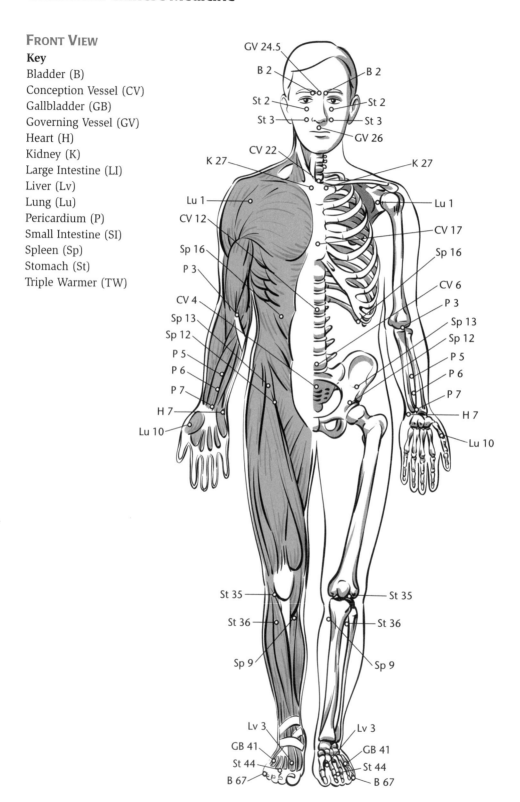

FRONT VIEW

Key
Bladder (B)
Conception Vessel (CV)
Gallbladder (GB)
Governing Vessel (GV)
Heart (H)
Kidney (K)
Large Intestine (LI)
Liver (Lv)
Lung (Lu)
Pericardium (P)
Small Intestine (SI)
Spleen (Sp)
Stomach (St)
Triple Warmer (TW)

BACK VIEW

Traditional Chinese Medicine is based on the principle that all physical functions are controlled by *chi,* the life force that flows through our bodies. By manipulating specific acupoints—either through the use of tiny, fine needles (acupuncture) or the application of finger pressure (acupressure)—TCM practitioners seek to maintain and restore health by stimulating energy flow to a particular area, system, or organ.

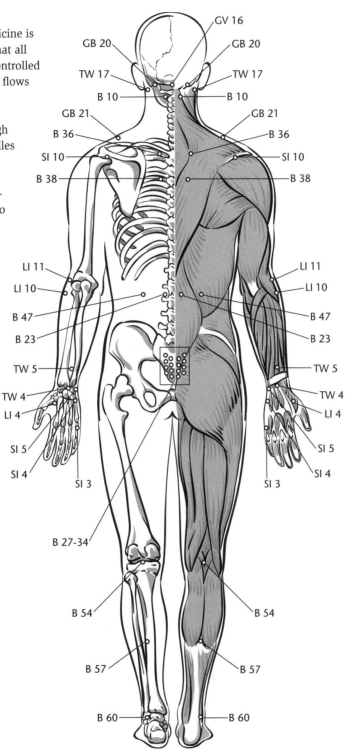

GV 16
GB 20
GB 20
TW 17
TW 17
B 10
B 10
GB 21
GB 21
B 36
B 36
SI 10
SI 10
B 38
B 38
LI 11
LI 11
LI 10
LI 10
B 47
B 47
B 23
B 23
TW 5
TW 5
TW 4
TW 4
LI 4
LI 4
SI 5
SI 5
SI 4
SI 4
SI 3
SI 3
B 27-34
B 54
B 54
B 57
B 57
B 60
B 60

Traditional Chinese Medicine

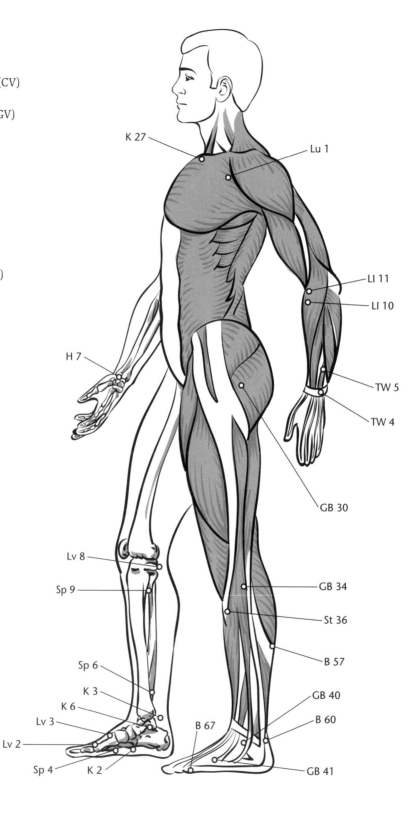

SIDE VIEW
Key
Bladder (B)
Conception Vessel (CV)
Gallbladder (GB)
Governing Vessel (GV)
Heart (H)
Kidney (K)
Large Intestine (LI)
Liver (Lv)
Lung (Lu)
Pericardium (P)
Small Intestine (SI)
Spleen (Sp)
Stomach (St)
Triple Warmer (TW)

K 27
Lu 1
LI 11
LI 10
H 7
TW 5
TW 4
GB 30
Lv 8
Sp 9
GB 34
St 36
B 57
Sp 6
K 3
K 6
GB 40
Lv 3
B 60
Lv 2
B 67
Sp 4
K 2
GB 41

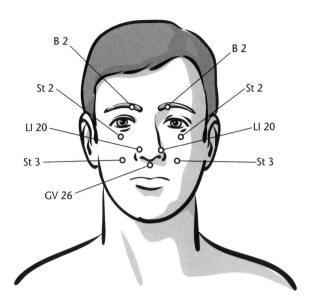

HEAD VIEWS

Over 1,000 acupoints are found on the body, 350 of which lie along the 14 energy meridians. To maintain well-being, a TCM practitioner will stimulate specific points as part of a comprehensive energy rebalancing program that may include acupuncture, acupressure, and Chinese herbal therapy.

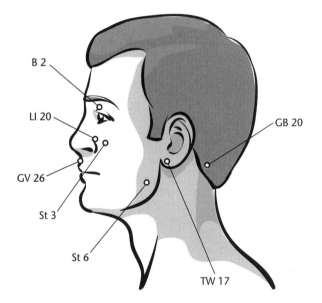

TRADITIONAL CHINESE HERBS AND HERBAL FORMULAS

Common Name	Latin Name	Traditional Chinese Name
Achyranthes	Achyranthes bidentata	Niu Xi
Acorus	Acorus gramineus	Shi Chang Pu
Agastache	Agastache rugosa	Huo Xiang
Akebia	Akebia quinata	Mu Tong
Alisma	Alisma plantago	Ze Xie
Aloe Vera	Aloe barbadensis	Lu Hui
Alum	Heuchera americana	Ming Fan
Amber	Pinites succinum	Hu Bo
Amethyst	Silica	Dze Shi Ying
Anemarrhena	Anemarrhena asphodeloides	Zhi Mu
Anemarrhena, Phellodendron, and Rehmannia Formula		Zhi Bai Di Huang Wan
Angelica	Angelica sinensis	Dang Gui
Angelica Anomala	Angelica dahurica	Bai Zhi
Angelica Du Huo (see Angelica pubescens, yellow)		
Angelica Pubescens, purple		Chiang Huo
Angelica Pubescens, yellow	Angelica grosserrata	Du Huo
Angelica and Loranthes Combination		Du Huo Ji Sheng Wan
Antelope Horn	Saiga tatarica	Ling Yang Jiao
Antelope Horn Wind Injury Remedy		Ling Yang Shang Feng Ling
Aplotaxis Carminative Pills		Mu Xiang Shun Qi Wan
Apricot Seed	Pruni armeniaca	Ku Xing Ren
Apricot Seed and Linum Formula		Ma Zi Ren Wan
Arbor Vitae	Thuja orientalis	Bai Zi Ren
Asarum Sieboldi	Asarum heterotropoides	Xi Xin
Astragalus	Astragalus membranaceus	Huang Qi
Astragalus Combination		Bu Zhong Yi Qi Tang
Balloon Flower	Platycodon grandilflorus	Jie Geng
Beijing Absolute Red		Ching Wan Hung
Belvedere Cypress	Kochia scoparia	Di Fu Zi
Biota Seeds (see Arbor vitae)		
Biota Leaves	Biota orientalis	Ce Bai Ye
Black Cardamom	Alpinia oxphylla	Yi Zhi Ren
Black Cohosh	(see Chinese Black Cohosh)	
Black Pepper	Piper nigrum	Hu Jiao
Bletilla Striata		Bai Ji
Blue Morning Glory	Pharbitis nil	Qian Niu Zi
Broomrape	Cistanche salsa	Rou Cong Rong
Buddleia Flower	Buddleia officinalis	Mi Meng Hua
Bupleurum	Bupleurum falcatum	Chai Hu
Bupleurum and Dragon Bone Forumula		Chai Hu Jia Long Gu Mu Li Tang
Bupleurum and Schizonepeta Formula		Shi Wei Bai Du Tang
Bupleurum and Tang Gui Formula		Xiao Yao Wan
Bupleurum, Inula, and Cyperus Formula		Shu Gan Wan
Bupleurum Sedative Pills		Hsiao Yao Wan
Burdock	Arctium lappa	Niu Bang Zi
Caltrop	Tribulus terrestris	Ci Ji Zi
Camphor	Cinnamomum camphora	Zhang Nao

Common Name	Latin Name	Traditional Chinese Name
Capillaris	*Artemisia capillaris*	*Yin Chen Hao*
Cardamom Seed	*Amomum villosum*	*Sha Ren*
Carmichaeli Tea Pills		*Fu Zi Li Zhong Wan*
Cattail	*Typha latifolia*	*Pu Huang*
Cerebral Tonic Pills		*Bu Bao Wan*
Chelidonium	*Chelidonium majus*	*Bai Gu Cai*
Chinaberry Bark	*Melia toosendan*	*Ku Lian Gen Pi*
Chinese Asparagus	*Asparagus conchinsinensis*	*Tian Men Dong*
Chinese Black Cohosh	*Cimicifuga foetida*	*Sheng Ma*
Chinese Cornbind	*Polygonum multiflorum*	*He Shou Wu*
Chinese Raspberry	*Rubus coreanus*	*Fu Pen Zi*
Chinese Wolfberry	*Lycium chinense*	*Gou Ji Zi*
Chinese Yam	*Dioscorea opposita*	*Shan Yao*
Chrysanthemum	*Chrysanthemum morifolium*	*Ju Hua*
Cicada	*Cryptotympana pustulata*	*Chan Tui*
Cimicifuga (*see* Chinese Black Cohosh)		
Cinnabar	*Cinnabaris*	*Zhu Sha*
Cinnabar Sedative Pills		*Ju Sha An Shen Wan*
Cinnamon	*Cinnamomum cassia*	*Rou Gui*
Cistanche (*see* Broomrape)		
Citrus Peel	*Citri reticulata*	*Chen Pi*
Clematis and Stephania Formula		*Shu Jing Huo Xue Tang*
Cnidium Monnieri	*Umbellieferae*	*She Chuang Zi*
Cnidium and Tea Formula		*Chuan Xiong Chao Tiao Wan*
Codonopsis	*Codonopsis pilosulae*	*Dang Shen*
Coix (*see* Job's Tears)		
Coix Combination		*Yi Yi Ren Tang*
Coltsfoot	*Tussilago farfara*	*Kuan Dung Hua*
Compound Cortex Eucommia Tablets		*Fu Fang Du Zhong Pian*
Concha Marguerita and Ligustrum Formula		*An Shen Bui Xin Wan*
Coptis	*Coptis sinensis*	*Huang Lien*
Cordyceps	*Cordyceps sinensis*	*Dong Chiung Xia Cao*
Cornu Cervi (*see* Deer Horn)		
Corydalis	*Corydalis ambigua*	*Yen Hu Suo*
Corydalis Analgesic Tablets		*Yan Hu Suo*
Corydalis Formula		*Shao Yao Gan Cao Tang*
Corydalis Tuber Forumula		*Yan Hu Suo Zhi Tong Pian*
Costus	*Saussurea lappa*	*Mu Xiang*
Cowherd	*Saponaria vaccaria*	*Wang Bu Liu Hsing*
Creeping Lilyturf (*see* Ophiopogon)		
Curculigo	*Curculigo orchiodes*	*Xian Mao*
Curcuma (*see* Turmeric)		
Cuscuta	*Cuscuta japonica*	*Tu Si Zi*
Cyperus and Ligusticum Formula		*Yeu Ju Wan*
Dandelion	*Taraxacum officinale*	*Pu Gung Ying*
Dang Gui and Arctium Combination		*Xiao Fen San*
Dang Gui Four		*Si Wu Tang*
Deer Horn	*Cervis nippon*	*Lu Rong*
Dendrobium Nobile	*Herba dendrobi*	*Shi Hu*
Dianthus Formula		*Ba Zheng San*
Dipsacus (*see* Teasel)		
Dodder (*see* Cuscuta)		

Traditional Chinese Herbs and Herbal Formulas

Common Name	Latin Name	Traditional Chinese Name
Dogwood Tree	Cornus officinalis	Shan Zhu Yu
Dragon Bone	Os draconis	Long Gu
Dried Bamboo Sap	Succus bambusa	Zhu Li
Duke of Chou's Centenarian Liquor		Jou Gung Bai Sui Jiou
Eagle Wood	Aquilaria agallocha	Chen Xiang
Eclipta	Eclipta prostrata	Han Lian Cao
Eight Immortal Long Life Pills		Ba Xian Chang Shou Wan
Eight Treasure Pills		Ba Zhen Wan
Eleutheros	Eleutherococcus senticosus	Wu Jia Pi
Elsholtzia Splendens	Elsholtzia cristata	Xiang Ru
Emperor's Tea		Tian Wang Bu Xin Wan
Ephedra (see Joint Fir)		
Eriocaulon Sieboldianum		Gu Jing Cao
Eucommia	Eucommia ulmoides	Du Zhong
Eupatorium	Eupatorium fortunei	Pei Lan
Fennel	Foeniculum vulgare	Hui Xiang
Fleeceflower (see also Chinese Cornbind)	Radix polygoni multiflori	He Shou Wu
Foxnut	Euryale ferox	Qian Shi
Frankincense Gum	Boswellia carterii	Ru Xiang
Free and Easy Wanderer Pills		Xiao Yao Wan
Fritillaria Extract Tablets		Chuan Bei Jing Pian
Garlic	Allium sativum	Du Suan
Gastrodia	Gastrodia elata	Tian Ma
Gentian	Gentiana scabra	Lung Dan Cao
Gentiana Formula		Long Dan Xie Gan Wan
Ginger, dried	Zingiber officinale	Gan Jiang
Ginger, fresh	Zingiber officinale	Sheng Jiang
Gingko	Ginkgo biloba	Bai Guo
Ginkgo Nut	Ginkgo biloba	Ying Xing
Ginseng	Panax ginseng	Ren Shen
Ginseng and Astragalus		Bu Zhong Yi Qi Wan
Ginseng and Atractylodes		Shen Ling Bai Zhu Pian
Ginseng and Longan Formula		Gui Pi Tang
Ginseng and Tang Gui Ten Formula		Shi Quan Da Bu Wan
Ginseng and Zizyphus Forumula		Tian Wang Bu Xin Dan
Ginseng Restorative Pills		Ren Shen Zai Zao Wan
Ginseng Stomachic Pills		Ren Shen Jian Pi Wan
Golden Book Tea		Jin Gui Shen Qi
Gotu Kola	Hydrocotyle asiatica	Di Quen Cao
Grifola (see Polyporus Fungus)		
Gynura Pinnatifida (see Pseudoginseng)		
Haliotidis	Haliotis gigantea	Shi Jue Ming
Hare's Ear (see Bupleurum)		
Hoelen and Polyporus		Zhi Zhuo Gu Ben Wan
Horny Goat Weed	Epimedium sagittatum	Yin Yang Huo
Hypertension Repressing Tablets		Jiang Ya Ping Pian
Ilex	Ilex pubescens	Mao Dong Qing
Ilex and Evodia Formula		Gan Mao Ling
Indian Madder	Rubia cordifolia	Qian Cao Gen
Internal Formula		Sai Mei An
Inula	Inula britannica	Xuan Fu Hua
Japanese Catnip	Schizonepeta tenuifolia	Jing Jie
Japanese Honeysuckle	Lonicera japonica	Jin Yin Hua

Traditional Chinese Herbs and Herbal Formulas

Common Name	Latin Name	Traditional Chinese Name
Japanese Wax Privet	*Ligustrum japonicum*	*Nu Jen Zi*
Job's Tears	*Coix lacryma-jobi*	*Yi Yi Ren*
Joint Fir	*Ephedra sinica*	*Ma Huang*
Kind Mother Decoction		*Tse Mu Tang*
Kudzu (*see* Pueraria)		
Laryngitis Pills		*Hou Yan Wan*
Ledebouriella Seselioides	*Siler divaricatum*	*Fang Feng*
Ledebouriella and Platycodon Formula		*Fang Feng Tong Sheng*
Ledebouriella and Coix Combination		*Qing Zang Fan Gen Tang Jai Yi Yi Jen*
Leonurus	*Leonurus sibiricus*	*Yi Mu Cao*
Leonurus and Achyranthes Formula		*Jiang Ya Wan*
Licorice	*Glycyrrhiza uralensis*	*Gan Tsao*
Ligusticum	*Ligusticum wallichii*	*Chuan Xiong*
Liliacea (*see* Anemarrhena)		
Little Green Dragon Formula		*Hsiao Ching Lung Tang*
Liver Strengthening Tablets		*Li Gan Plan*
Lonicera and Forsythia Formula		*Yin Chiao Chieh Tu Pien*
Lopanthus Anti-Febrile Pills		*Hou Hsiang cheng Chi Pien*
Lycium Combination		*Huan Xiao Dan*
Major Four Herbs Formula		*Si Jun Zi Tang*
Malva	*Malva verticillata*	*Dong Kui Zi*
Mastic Tree (*see* Frankincense Gum)		
Minor Bupleurum Formula		*Xiao Chai Hu Tang*
Mint	*Mentha arvensis*	*Bo He*
Mishmi Bitter (*see* Coptis)		
Morinda Root	*Morinda officinalis*	*Ba Ji Tien*
Moutan (*see* Tree Peony)		
Notoginseng (*see* Pseudoginseng)		
Nutmeg	*Myristica fragrans*	*Rou Dou Kou*
Ophiopogon	*Liriope spicata*	*Mai Men Dung*
Oyster shell	*Concha ostraea*	*Mu Li*
Panax Ginseng Capsules		*Renshen Wan*
Peony Alba	*Paeonia lactiflora*	*Bai Shao*
Peony and Licorice Formula		*Shao Yao Gan Cao Tang*
Peppermint	*Mentha arvensis*	*Bo He*
Perilla	*Perilla frutescens*	*Zi Su Zi*
Pharbitis (*see* Blue Morning Glory)		
Plantain	*Plantago asiatica*	*Che Qian Zi*
Poke	*Phytolacca acinosa*	*Shang Lu*
Polygala	*Polygala tenuifolia*	*Yuan Zhi*
Polygonatum Cirrhifolium	*Polygonatum canaliculatum*	*Huang Jing*
Polygonum Multiflorum (*see* Chinese Cornbind)		
Polyporus Fungus	*Polyporus umbrellatus*	*Zhu Ling*
Poria	*Poria cocos*	*Fu Ling*
Poria Five Herb Combination		*Wu Ling San*
Prunella	*Prunella vulgaris*	*Xia Ku Cao*
Prunella and Scutellaria Formula		*Jiang Ya Ping Pian*
Pseudoginseng	*Panax notoginseng*	*San Qi*
Pseudoginseng and Dragon Blood formula		*Chin Koo Tieh Shang Wan*
Psoralea	*Psoralea corylifolia*	*Bu Gu Zhi*
Pueraria	*Pueraria lobata*	*Ge Gen*
Rehmannia, dry	*Rehmannia glutinosa*	*Gan Di Huang*
Rehmannia, cooked	*Rehmannia glutinosa*	*Shu Di Huang*

Traditional Chinese Herbs and Herbal Formulas

Common Name	Latin Name	Traditional Chinese Name
Rehmannia and Dogwood Fruit Formula		Ming Mu Di Huang Wan
Rehmannia and Magnetitum Formula		Er Ming Zuo Ci Wan
Rehmannia Eight		Ba Wei Di Huang Wan
Rehmannia Six		Liu Wei Di Huang Wan
Return Spleen Tablets		Gui Pi Wan
Rhubarb and Scutellaria Formula		Li Dan Pian
Salvia	Salvia miltiorrhiza	Dan Shen
Sandalwood	Santalum album	Tan Xiang
Sargassum	Sargassum fusiform	Hai Zao
Saussurea and Amomum Stomach Nurturing Pills		Shiang Sha Yang Wei Wan
Schisandra	Schisandra chinensis	Wu Wei Zi
Sickle Senna	Cassia tora	Jue Ming Zi
Six Flavor Tea		Liu Wei Di Huang Wan
Six Spirit Pills		Liu Shen Wan
Solomon's Seal	Polygonatum officinale	Yu Ju
Spleen Restoration Decoction		Gui Pi Tang
Spleen Restoration Pills		Gui Pi Wan
Stephania and Astragalus Combination		Fang Ji Huang Qi Tang
Sulphur		Liu Huang
Sweet Wormwood	Artemisia annua	Huang Hua Hao
Szechuan Pepper	Zanthoxylum piperitum	Chuan Jiao
Talcum	Hydrous magnesium silicate	Hua Shi
Tang Gui and Gardenia Formula		Wen Qing Yin
Tang Gui and Ginseng Eight		Ba Zhen Tang
Tang Gui Four		Si Wu Tang
Teasel	Dipsacus asper	Xu Duan
Ten Complete Great Tonifying Pills		Shi Quan Da Bu Wan
Thistle Type	Atractylodes chinensis	Cang Zhu
Three Yellows		San Huang Xie Xin Tang
Thuja Orientalis (see Arbor vitae and Biota Leaves)		
Tian Qi and Eucommia		Tin Tzat To Chung
Tibetan Saffron	Crocus sativus	Dzang Hung Hua
Tiger Thistle	Cirsium japonicum	Da Ji Hua
Traumatic Injury Medicine		Tieh Ta Yao Gin
Tree Peony	Paeonia moutan	Mu Dan Pi
Tribulus Terrestris (see Caltrop)		
Trifoliate Orange	Poncirus trifoliata	Zhi Shi
Tuckahoe (see Poria)		
Tu Huo and Loranthus Formula		Du Huo Ji Sheng Tang
Turmeric	Curcuma longa	Jiang Huang
Uncaria	Uncaria rynchophylla	Gou Teng
Vermilion Elixir Wine		Tung Dan Jiou
Vitality Combination		Zhen Wu Tang
Weeping Golden Bell	Forsythia suspensa	Lian Qiao
Wheat	Triticum aestivum	Xiao Mai
White Peony	Paeonia lactiflora	Bai Shao
White Phoenix Pills		Wu Chi Pai Feng Wan
Wild Chinese Jujube	Ziziphus jujuba	Da Zao
Wild Chinese Violet	Viola yedoensis	Zi Hua Di Ding
Xanthium and Magnolia Formula		Bi Yan Pian
Yellow Starwort (see Inula)		
Yunnan Pai Yao Pills		

REFLEXOLOGY DIAGRAMS OF THE HANDS AND FEET

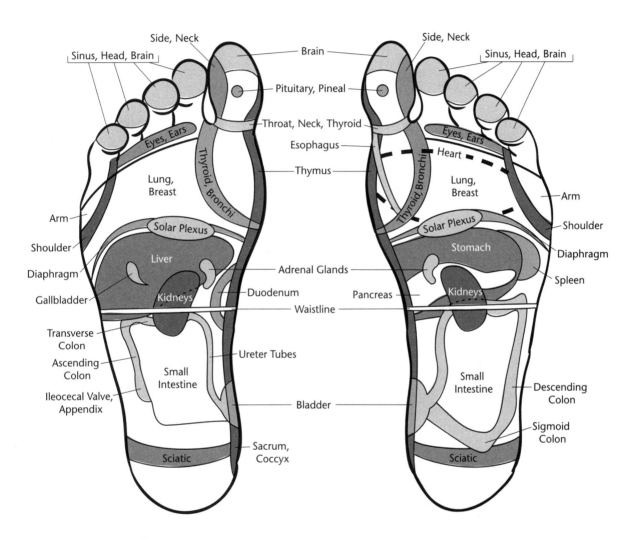

SOLES OF FEET

Reflexologists believe that the body's innate healing potential is activated by manipulating areas, or zones, located on the hands and feet. These zones correspond to each organ and organ system in the body.

Reflexology Diagrams of the Hands and Feet

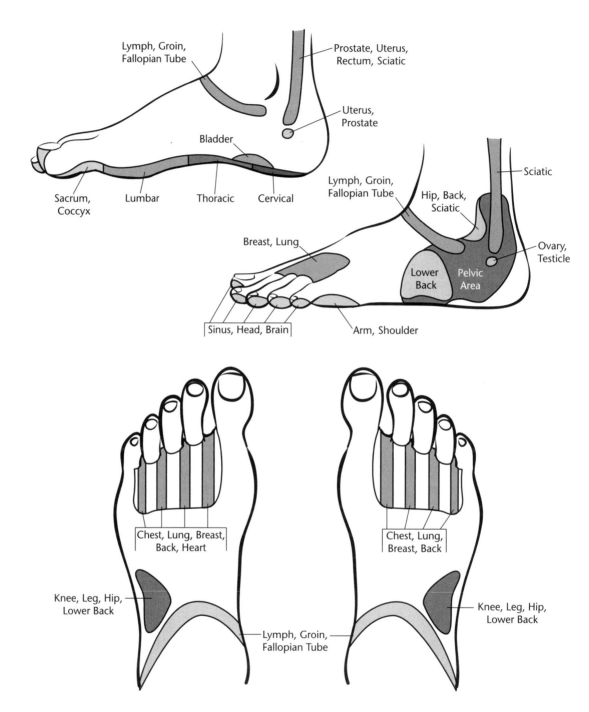

SIDES AND TOPS OF FEET

Some reflexologists believe that crystallized waste products in the hands and feet interfere with energy flow and nerve function. The pressure applied by the reflexologist breaks up these deposits and facilitates the flow of energy. Some health professionals believe that manipulating these points releases neurotransmitters called endorphins, resulting in decreased pain and increased feelings of well-being.

Reflexology Diagrams of the Hands and Feet

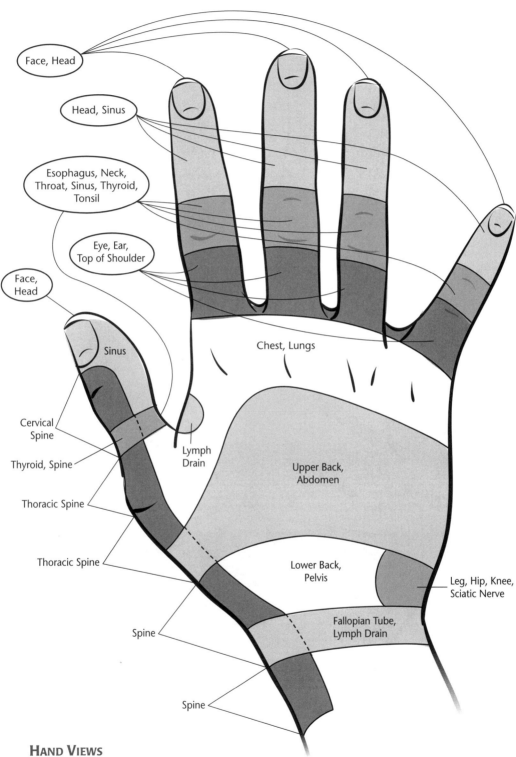

Face, Head

Head, Sinus

Esophagus, Neck, Throat, Sinus, Thyroid, Tonsil

Eye, Ear, Top of Shoulder

Face, Head

Sinus

Chest, Lungs

Cervical Spine

Thyroid, Spine

Lymph Drain

Thoracic Spine

Upper Back, Abdomen

Thoracic Spine

Lower Back, Pelvis

Leg, Hip, Knee, Sciatic Nerve

Spine

Fallopian Tube, Lymph Drain

Spine

HAND VIEWS

Reflexology is used to maintain health, to strengthen the immune system, to alleviate stress, and to provide symptom relief for a variety of conditions.

Reflexology Diagrams of the Hands and Feet

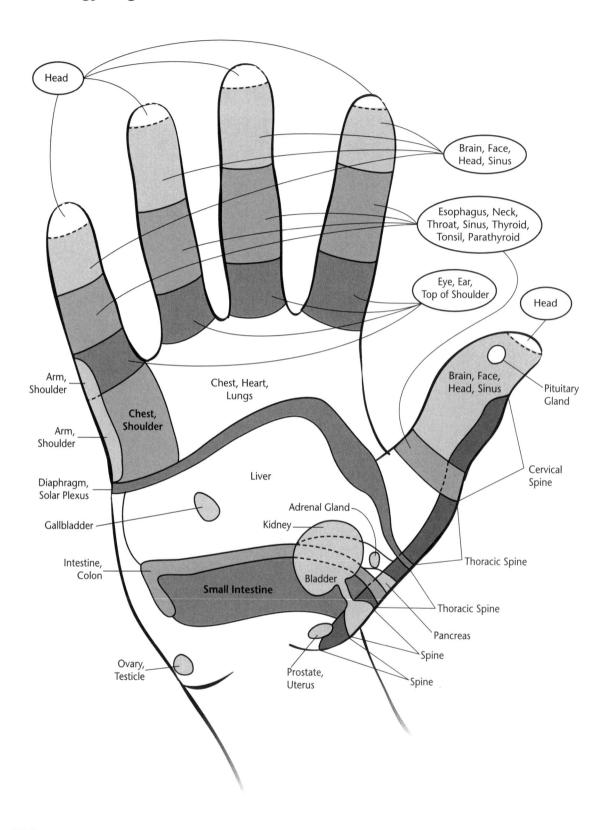

Reflexology Diagrams of the Hands and Feet

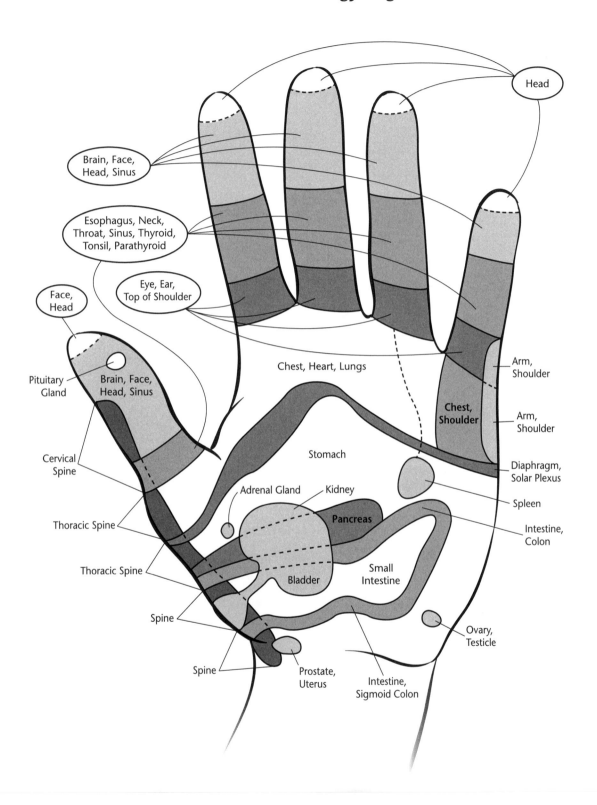

YOGA POSES

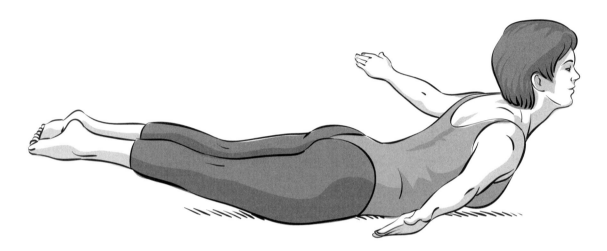

BOAT

Lie on the floor, face down, with your forehead resting against the floor and your arms at your sides with your palms down. Breathe in slowly and look up as you lift your arms, legs, and head. Hold your breath as you remain in this position for several moments. Exhale while lowering your arms, legs, and head to the resting position.

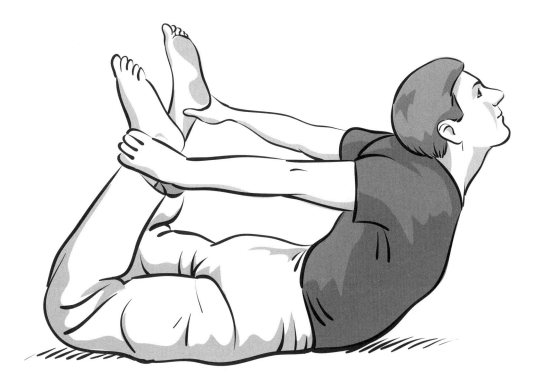

Bow

Lie on the floor, face down. Bend your knees and grasp your ankles. Breathe in as you pull up on your feet and raise your head, chest, and thighs. Hold your breath as you remain in this position for several moments. Exhale while lowering your head, chest, and thighs to the resting position.

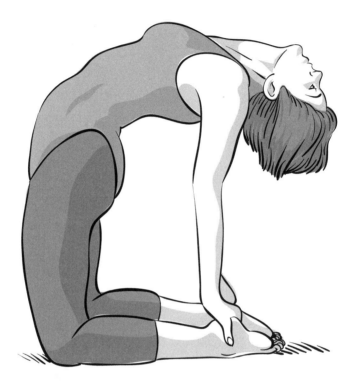

CAMEL

Kneel on the floor with your knees slightly apart. Grasp your heels, one at a time. Bend backward, exhaling as you relax your head and push your hips forward. Breathe normally; hold for several moments. Return to an upright kneeling position.

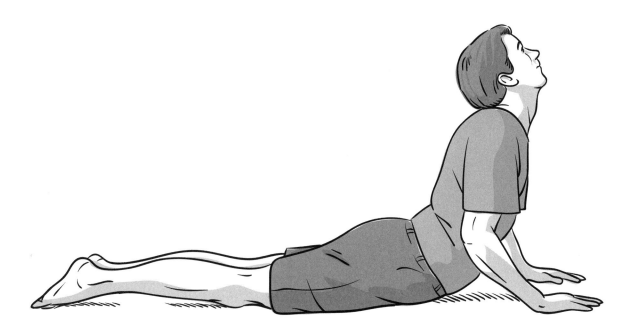

COBRA

Lie on the floor, face down, with your forehead resting on the floor and your palms on the floor next to your shoulders. Keep your feet together and breathe in as you raise your head, chest, and stomach off of the floor. Hold for several moments, then breathe out as you lower your stomach, chest, and head to the resting position.

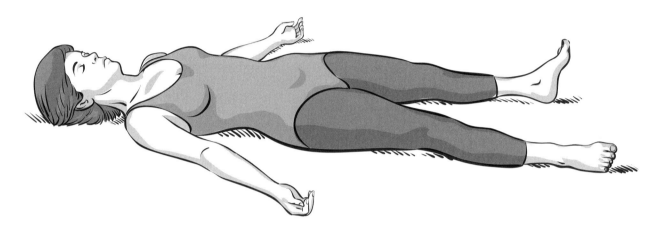

CORPSE

Lie on the floor, face up, with your feet shoulder-width apart, your feet turned outward, and your arms at your sides, palms up. Relax every part of your body, until it feels as if you are melting into the floor. Inhale and exhale deeply. Rest in this pose for a minute or so.

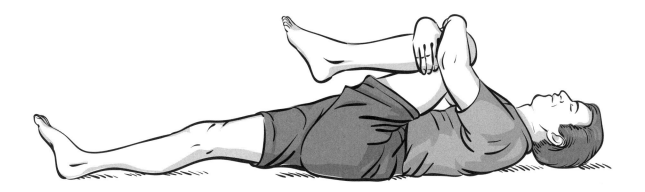

KNEE SQUEEZE

Lie on the floor, face up, with your feet together and your hands at your sides. Breathe in as you raise one knee to your chest. Hold your breath as you wrap both arms around your knee and pull it to your chest for several seconds. Breathe out as you release your knee and lower it and your head to the resting position. Repeat with the other knee.

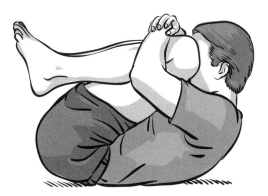

After warming up with the single Knee Squeeze, bring both knees to your chest at once, instead of one at a time, and raise your head. Breathe as above.

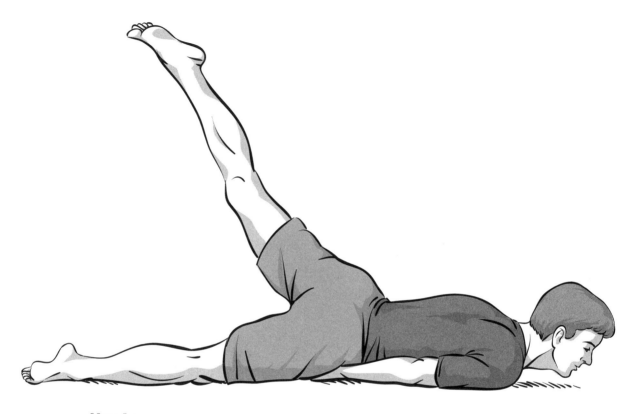

HALF LOCUST

Lie on the floor, on your stomach, with your chin resting on the floor and your hands beneath you with your thumbs facing down. Breathe in as you raise one leg, keeping your knee straight. Hold for several moments. Breathe out as you lower your leg. Repeat with the other leg.

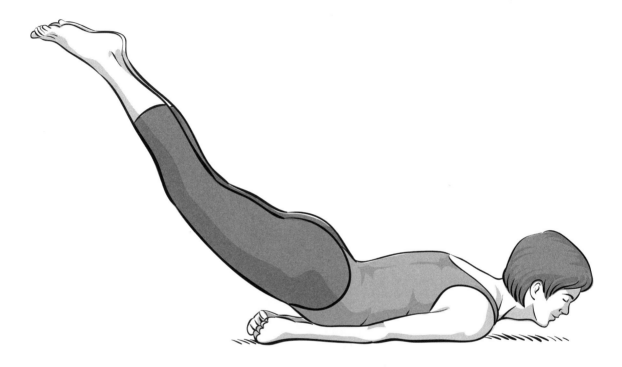

FULL LOCUST

Use the Full Locust as an advanced technique, or after warming up with the Half Locust. Lie on the floor, on your stomach, with your chin resting on the floor and your hands beneath you with your thumbs facing down. Breathe in as you raise both legs together, keeping your knees straight. Hold for several moments. Breathe out as you lower your legs.

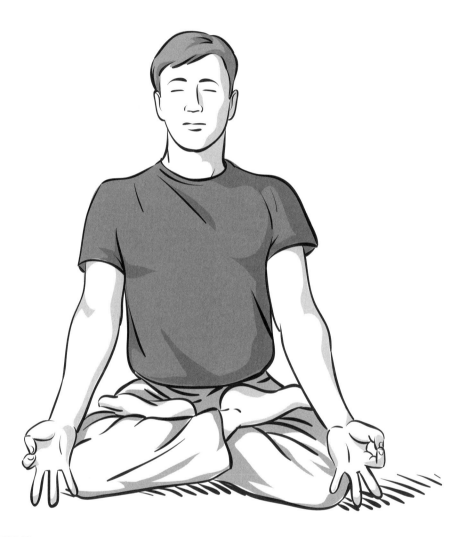

FULL LOTUS

Sit on the floor with your legs stretched in front of you. Gently bend one knee, placing your foot on top of the opposite thigh. Then bend the other knee, placing the foot on top of the opposite thigh. Breathe normally as you hold this pose for several moments.

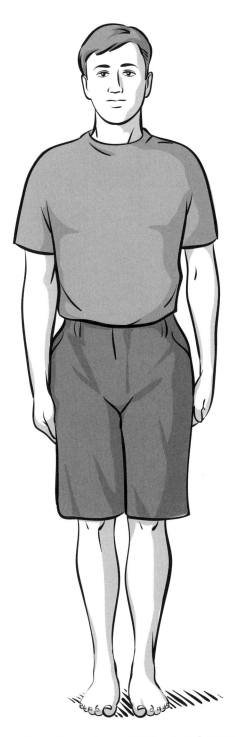

MOUNTAIN

Stand with your toes together and your heels slightly apart. Let your arms hang at your sides, with your knees relaxed, and your hips slightly forward. Stretch your spine and lift your chest and shoulders. Stretch your neck upward, keeping your chin level to the floor and your face relaxed. Breathe slowly as you hold for several seconds. Relax.

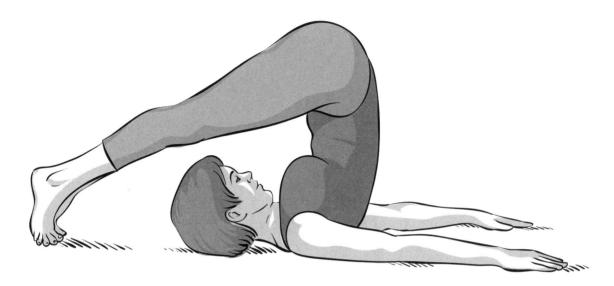

PLOW

Lie on your back with your feet together and your hands at your sides, palms against the floor. Inhale as you raise your knees to your chest. Then raise your hips from the floor, straighten your legs, and extend them over your head, touching your feet to the floor. Breathe normally as you hold this pose for several moments. Exhale as you bend your knees, bring your legs forward, and move into a sitting position.

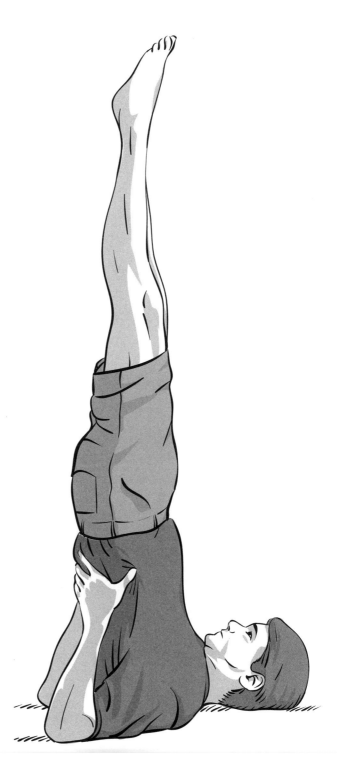

SHOULDER STAND

Lie on the floor, face up, hugging your knees to your chest. Supporting your lower back with your hands, slowly lift your hips from the floor, raising your knees until they touch your forehead. Then raise your legs until they are completely vertical. Breathe normally as you hold this position for several moments. Then bend your knees and bring them to your forehead again before rolling forward to a seated position.

INDEX

Index